Pediatric Nutrition Support

Susan S. Baker, MD, PhD
State University of New York at Buffalo
Buffalo, NY

Robert D. Baker, MD, PhD
State University of New York at Buffalo
Buffalo, NY

Anne M. Davis, PhD (ABD), RD
Executive Director of Scientific Affairs
Martek Biosciences Corporation
Columbia, MD

JONES AND BARTLETT PUBLISHERS
Sudbury, Massachusetts
BOSTON TORONTO LONDON SINGAPORE

World Headquarters
Jones and Bartlett Publishers
40 Tall Pine Drive
Sudbury, MA 01776
978-443-5000
info@jbpub.com
www.jbpub.com

Jones and Bartlett Publishers Canada
6339 Ormindale Way
Mississauga, ON L5V IJ2
CANADA

Jones and Bartlett Publishers
International
Barb House, Barb Mews
London W6 7PA
UK

Jones and Bartlett's books and products are available through most bookstores and online booksellers. To contact Jones and Bartlett Publishers directly, call 800-832-0034, fax 978-443-8000, or visit our website www.jbpub.com.

Production Credits
Publisher: Michael Brown
Production Director: Amy Rose
Associate Editor: Kylah Goodfellow McNeill
Associate Production Editor: Daniel Stone
Associate Marketing Manager: Wendy Thayer
Manufacturing Buyer: Therese Connell
Cover Design: Anne Spencer
Printing and Binding: Malloy, Inc.
Cover Printing: Malloy, Inc.

Library of Congress Cataloging-in-Publication Data
Baker, Susan, 1947-
Pediatric nutrition support handbook / Susan S. Baker, Robert D. Baker, Anne M. Davis.
p. ; cm.
Includes bibliographical references.
ISBN-13: 978-0-7637-3154-0
ISBN-10: 0-7637-3154-4
1. Artificial feeding of children--Handbooks, manuals, etc.
[DNLM: 1. Nutritional Support. 2. Child Nutrition. 3. Infant Nutrition. WS 115 B168p 2006] I. Baker, Robert Denio. II. Davis, Anne, C.N.S.D. III. Title.
RJ53.A78B35 2006
618.92'02--dc22

2006005280

6048

The authors, editor, and publisher have made every effort to provide accurate information. However, they are not responsible for errors, omissions, or for any outcomes related to the use of the contents of this book and take no responsibility for the use of the products and procedures described. Treatments and side effects described in this book may not be applicable to all people; likewise, some people may require a dose or experience a side effect that is not described herein. Drugs and medical devices are discussed that may have limited availability controlled by the Food and Drug Administration (FDA) for use only in a research study or clinical trial. Research, clinical practice, and government regulations often change the accepted standard in this field. When consideration is being given to use of any drug in the clinical setting, the health care provider or reader is responsible for determining FDA status of the drug, reading the package insert, and reviewing prescribing information for the most up-to-date recommendations on dose, precautions, and contraindications, and determining the appropriate usage for the product. This is especially important in the case of drugs that are new or seldom used.

Printed in the United States of America
10 09 08 07 06 10 9 8 7 6 5 4 3 2 1

Table of Contents

Contributors

CHAPTER 1

Cutberto Garza, MD, PhD
Academic Vice President and Dean of Faculties
Bourneuf House
Boston College
Chestnut Hill, MA

Mercedes de Onis, MD, PhD
Department of Nutrition
World Health Organization
Geneva, Switzerland

CHAPTER 2

Ronald E. Kleinman, MD
Professor of Pediatrics
Harvard Medical School
Chief, Division of Pediatric
Gastroenterology and Nutrition Unit
Massachusetts General Hospital
Boston, MA

Daniel S. Kamin, MD
Instructor in Pediatrics
Harvard Medical School
Staff Physician
Division of Gastroenterology and Nutrition
Children's Hospital Boston
Boston, MA

CHAPTER 3

Sue J. Rhee, MD
Fellow in Pediatric Gastroenterology
Harvard Medical School
Combined Program in Pediatric
Gastroenterology and Nutrition
Massachusetts General Hospital
Children's Hospital
Boston, MA

Pearay L. Ogra, MD
John Sealy Distinguished Chair Professor
(Emeritus)
Chairman (Emeritus) Department of Pediatrics
University of Texas Medical Branch, Galveston
Professor, University at Buffalo
State University of New York
Women and Children's Hospital
Buffalo, NY

W. Allan Walker, MD
Conrad Taff Professor of Nutrition and Pediatrics
Harvard Medical School
Division of Nutrition
Mucosal Immunology Laboratory
Massachusetts General Hospital for Children
Boston, MA

CHAPTER 4

Alan Lucas, MB, BChir, MA, MD, FRCP, FRCPCH, FMedSci
Director, Medical Research Council's Childhood Nutrition Research Centre
Institute of Child Health and Great Ormond Street Hospital for Children NHS Trust
University College London
London, UK

CHAPTER 5

Kristy Hendricks, ScD
Associate Professor
Nutrition/Infection
Stearns Research Building
Boston, MA

CHAPTER 6

Walter J. Chwals, MD
Professor of Surgery and Pediatrics
Case Western Reserve University School of Medicine
Rainbow Babies and Children's Hospital
Cleveland, OH

CHAPTER 7

Nancy Nevin-Folino, MEd, RD, CSP, FADA
Neonatal Nutrition Specialist
The Children's Medical Center
Dayton, OH

Robin LeBeouf-Aufdenkampe, MS, RD, LD
The University of Cincinnati Hospital
Cincinnati, OH
Dayton, OH

CHAPTER 8

Virginia A. Stallings, MD
Professor of Pediatrics
University of Pennsylvania School of Medicine
Director, Nutrition Center
Deputy Director, Stokes Research Institute
The Children's Hospital of Philadelphia
Philadelphia, PA

CHAPTER 9

Aida Miles, MMSc, RD, CSP, LD, CNSD
The Marcus Institute
Atlanta, GA

CHAPTER 10

Maria R. Mascarenhas, MBBS
Division of Gastroenterology and Nutrition
The Children's Hospital of Philadelphia
Philadelphia, PA

Lori Enriquez, RD, CSP, CNSD, LDN
Department of Clinical Nutrition
The Children's Hospital of Philadelphia
Philadelphia, PA

CHAPTER 11

Lee A. Denson, MD
Assistant Professor
Pediatric Gastroenterology, Hepatology and Nutrition
Cincinnati Children's Hospital Medical Center
Cincinnati, OH

CHAPTER 12

Joan C. Arvedson, PhD, BC-NCD
Clinical Professor
Program Coordinator, Feeding and Swallowing Services
Speech-Language Pathology and GI Division
Department of Pediatrics
Children's Hospital of Wisconsin
Medical College of Wisconsin
Milwaukee, WI

Colin D. Rudolph, MD
Professor
Chief, Pediatric Gastroenterology, Hepatology and Nutrition
Medical College of Wisconsin and Children's Hospital of Wisconsin
Milwaukee, WI

CHAPTER 13

Christina J. Valentine, MD, MS, RD
Clinical Assistant Professor of Pediatrics
The Ohio State University
Medical Advisor, Neonatal Nutrition
Children's Hospital
Columbus, OH

CHAPTER 14

Beverly W. Henry, PhD, RD, LDN
Assistant Professor
School of Family, Consumer, and Nutrition Sciences
Northern Illinois University
DeKalb, IL

CHAPTER 15

Sue Ann Anderson, PhD
Nutritionist Team Leader
Infant Formula and Medical Foods Staff
Office of Nutritional Products, Labeling, and Dietary Supplements
Center For Food Safety and Applied Nutrition
U.S. Food and Drug Administration
College Park, MD
Divison of Nutrition Science and Policy
Wahington, DC

CHAPTER 16

Mai Kamal El Mallah, MD
Pediatrics
Baylor College of Medicine
Houston, TX

Kathleen J. Motil, MD, PhD
Associate Professor of Pediatrics
Baylor College of Medicine
Section of Pediatric Gastroenterology, Hepatology and Nutrition
Houston, TX

CHAPTER 17

Beth L. Leonberg, MS, RD, CSP, FADA, CNSD, LDN
President, Nutrition Outcomes, LLC
Pipersville, PA

CHAPTER 18

Jacqueline Jones Wessel, RD, Med, CNSD, CSP, CLE, LD
Adjunct Professor
Medical Dietetics
The Ohio State University
Columbus, OH
Neonatal Nutritionist
Cincinnati Children's Hospital Medical Center
Cincinnati, OH

CHAPTER 19

Jay A. Perman, MD
Professor and Chairman, Pediatrics
University of Maryland School of Medicine
Chief of Pediatrics
University of Maryland, Hospital for Children
Baltimore, MD

Anjali Malkani MD
Clinical Assistant Professor
Pediatric Gastroenterology and Nutrition
University of Maryland
Baltimore, MD

CHAPTER 20

Valérie Marchand, MD, FRCP(C)
Gastroenterologist, Pediatrics
Division of Gastroenterology, Hepatology and Nutrition
Universite De Montreal
Hôpital Ste-Justine
Montreal
Quebec, Canada

CHAPTER 21

Anne M. Davis, MS, RD, CNSD
Senior Clinical Scientist II
Clinical Nutrition Research
Wyeth Pharmaceuticals
Collegeville, PA

CHAPTER 22

Robert J. Shulman, MD
Professor of Pediatrics
Texas Children's Hospital Foundation Chair in Gastroenterology
Baylor College of Medicine
Houston, TX

Sarah Phillips, MS, RD, CNSD
Instructor of Pediatrics
Baylor College of Medicine
Dept. Gastroenterology, Hepatology, and Nutrition
Texas Children's Hospital
Houston, TX

CHAPTER 23

Mathew P. Thomas, Pharm D
Clinical Assistant Professor of Pediatrics
Louisiana State University Health Sciences Center
Department of Pediatrics
Clinical Coordinator
Pharmacy
Children's Hospital
New Orleans, LA

John N. Udall, Jr., MD, PhD
Professor and Chairman
University of West Virginia
Health Sciences Center
Charleston Division
Department of Pediatrics
Women and Children's Hospital 830 Pennsylvania Avenue
Charleston, WV

CHAPTER 24

Susan S. Baker, MD, PhD
Professor of Pediatrics
State University of New York, Buffalo
Co-Director, Digestive Diseases and Nutrition Center
Women and Children's Hospital of Buffalo
Buffalo, NY

Robert D. Baker, MD, PhD
Professor of Pediatrics
State University of New York, Buffalo
Co-Director, Digestive Diseases and Nutrition Center
Women and Children's Hospital of Buffalo
Buffalo, NY

CHAPTER 25

Jatinder Bhatia, MBBS
Professor and Chief
Section of Neonatology
Medical College of Georgia
Augusta, GA

Amy Gates, RD, LD
Neonatal Dietitian
Medical College of Georgia
Augusta, GA

Robert D. Baker, MD, PhD
Professor of Pediatrics
State University of New York, Buffalo
Co-Director, Digestive Diseases and Nutrition Center
Women and Children's Hospital of Buffalo
Buffalo, NY

CHAPTER 26

H. Biemann Othersen, Jr., MD
Professor of Surgery and Pediatrics
Emeritus Chief, Pediatric Surgery
MUSC Children's Hospital
Medical University of South Carolina
Charleston, SC

Joshua B. Glenn, MD
Resident in Surgery
Medical University of South Carolina
Charleston, SC

Katherine Hammond Chessman, Pharm D, BCNSP, BCPS
Associate Professor of Pharmacy and Clinical Sciences
South Carolina College of Pharmacy
Medical University of South Carolina
Charleston, SC

Edward P. Tagge, MD
Professor of Surgery and Pediatrics
Chief of Pediatric Surgery
MUSC Children's Hospital
Medical University of South Carolina
Charleston, SC

CHAPTER 27

I-Fen Chang, Pharm D
Clinical Pharmacy Specialist, Solid Organ Transplant
Pharmacy Department
Texas Children's Hospital
Houston, TX

Thuy Anh Sorof, Pharm D
Clinical Pharmacist Specialist
Pharmacy Department
Texas Children's Hospital
Houston, TX

Ngoc Yen Thi Nguyen, Pharm D
Clinical Pharmacist Specialist
Pharmacy Department
Texas Children's Hospital
Houston, TX

CHAPTER 28

Shirley Ekvall, PhD, RD, LD
Professor, University of Cincinnati
Chief of Nutrition
Cincinnati Children Hospital Medical Center
Division of Developmental Disabilities
Cincinnati, OH

Valli Ekvall, PhD, RD, LD
Community Consultant
Children with Developmental Disorders and Aetna Healthcare
Indianapolis, IN
Nutrition Consultant,
Cincinnati Children's Hospital Medical Center,
Division of Developmental Disorders,
Cincinnati, OH

CHAPTER 29

Theresa Mayes, RD
Clinical Dietitian
Nutrition Services
Shriners Hospital for Children
Cincinnati, OH

Michele M. Gottschlich, PhD, RD, CNSD
Adjunct Associate Professor
Department of Dietetics and Nutrition Education
University of Cincinnati
Director of Nutrition Services
Shriners Hospital for Children
Cincinnati, OH

CHAPTER 30

Frank R. Greer, MD
Professor of Pediatrics and Nutritional Sciences
University of Wisconsin Medical School
Perinatal Center
Meriter Hospital
Madison, WI

CHAPTER 31

Robert M. Issenman, MD, FRCP
Professor, Department of Pediatrics
McMaster University
Chief, Pediatric Gastroenterology and Nutrition
McMaster Children's Hospital
Hamilton
Ontario, Canada

Tracy Hussey, MSc, RD
Clinical Dietitian, Pediatrics
McMaster Children's Hospital
Hamilton
Ontario, CA

CHAPTER 32

Nancy Spinozzi, RD, LDN
GI/Nutrition, Hunnewell Ground
Children's Hospital of Boston
Boston, MA

CHAPTER 33

Steven Yannicelli, PhD, RD
Director of Science and Education
SHS North America
Valencia, CA

Kathryn Camp, MS, RD, CSP
Assistant Professor, Pediatrics
Uniform Services University
Bethesda, MD
Pediatric Nutritionist, Pediatrics
Walter Reed Army Medical Center
Washington, DC

CHAPTER 34

Lori J. Bechard, MEd, RD, LDN
Clinical Nutrition Service
GI/Nutrition
Children's Hospital Boston
Boston, MA

Tara C. McCarthy, MS, RD, LDN
Clinical Nutrition Service
GI/Nutrition
Children's Hospital Boston
Boston, MA

CHAPTER 35

Nancy Ann Garrison, MS RD CNSD CSP
Women and Children's Hospital of Buffalo
Buffalo, NY

Chris Coburn-Miller, MS, RD, CSP
Women and Children's Hospital of Buffalo
Buffalo, NY

Robert D. Baker, MD, PhD
Professor of Pediatrics
State University of New York, Buffalo
Co-Director, Digestive Diseases and Nutrition Center
Women and Children's Hospital of Buffalo
Buffalo, NY

CHAPTER 36

Renee A. Wieman, RD, CSP, LD, CNSD
Clinical Dietitian, The Pediatric Liver and Intestinal Care Center
Nutrition Therapy/Liver Care Center
Cincinnati Children's Hospital Medical Center
Cincinnati, OH

William F. Balistreri, MD
Dorothy M.M. Kersten Professor of Pediatrics
Professor of Pediatrics
Department of Pediatrics
University of Cincinnati Medical Center
Medical Director, Liver Transplant
Division of Gastroenterology, Hepatology, and Nutrition
Cincinnati Children's Hospital Medical Center
Cincinnati, OH

CHAPTER 37

Valeria C. Cohran, MD
Assistant Professor of Pediatrics
Division of Pediatric Gastroenterology
Children's Memorial Hospital
Chicago, IL

Samuel A. Kocoshis, MD
Professor of Pediatrics
University of Cincinnati College of Medicine
Director, Nutrition and Small Intestinal Transplantation
Cincinnati Children's Hospital
Cincinnati, OH

APPENDIX A

Jodi Bettler, MA, RD, CNSD
Clinical Scientist
Clinical Nutrition
Wyeth Pharmaceuticals
Collegeville, PA

Lori Enriquez, RD, CSP, CNSD, LDN
Department of Clinical Nutrition
The Children's Hospital of Philadelphia
Philadelphia, PA

APPENDIX B

Karen Hauff, Pharm D, BCNSP
Clinical Pharmacy Specialist, Pediatrics
Department of Pharmaceutical Services
University of Minnesota Children's Hospital, Fairview
Minneapolis, MN

APPENDIX C

Steven Yannicelli, PhD, RD
Director of Science and Education
SHS North America
Valencia, CA

Kathryn Camp, MS, RD, CSP
Assistant Professor, Pediatrics
Uniform Services University
Bethesda, MD
Pediatric Nutritionist, Pediatrics
Walter Reed Army Medical Center
Washington, DC

Preface

Children are unique and present special problems for nutrition support. Growth is a distinguishing characteristic of childhood. Children's body composition, fuel reserves, nutrient needs, and growth itself change as children develop from infancy through young adulthood. Because of high and constantly changing requirements, nutrition support is complex in children and very different from that of adults. Psychological, family and social issues add further dimensions that complicate the problem of feeding children.

Nutrition support is powerful. It can reduce morbidity and offer life to children who would die otherwise. Nutrition support, however, if improperly used, causes morbidity and can increase the risk of dying. The purpose of this book is to provide health professionals the scientific rationale for nutrition support, the basic techniques needed for successful enteral and parenteral nutrition support, and ways that complications can be avoided.

This book covers a spectrum from the theoretic to the practical. For example, growth and measuring growth are discussed at the theoretic level in Chapter 1 and from a practical point of view in Chapter 5. Nutrition support for children with specific diseases such as inflammatory bowel disease, renal disease, liver disease, and cystic fibrosis is discussed. Beyond these disease entities, pediatric nutrition support, as it is practiced in different settings, the neonatal intensive care unit, pediatric intensive care unit, in the hospital, and at home is considered. This book is unique because it focuses only on infants and children and it discusses enteral and parenteral nutrition technology. In addition, the most recent advances in nutrition are incorporated, such as the DRI, a discussion of the international reference breastfeeding growth charts, and metabolic programming. The chapter authors were chosen for their expertise, their clinical experience, and their recognized stature in the medical and nutrition communities.

We believe this book will be useful to the pediatric nutrition support community, dietitians, pharmacists, nurses and doctors who perform nutrition support and to dietitians in general, physicians with an interest in nutrition, pediatric gastroenterologists, surgeons and critical care specialists, and those healthcare providers who manage home nutritional care.

We want to thank all of the infants and children who experienced nutrition support and thereby provided knowledge to the authors and ourselves to make this book possible.

Susan S. Baker
Robert D. Baker
Anne M. Davis

CHAPTER 1

An Overview of Growth Standards and Indicators and Their Interpretation

Cutberto Garza and Mercedes de Onis†*

Assessing childhood growth remains a mainstay of pediatric care in all settings, from the most advanced health care centers to those faced with severe resource constraints. It is the most widespread approach for assessing body size, weight, composition, and proportions. It can be done inexpensively and noninvasively and is of inherent interest to caretakers responsible for children's welfare. This latter feature is particularly valuable because it provides a tool for engaging parents and others in child care and provides a readily visible means of assessing the caretakers' success in their nurturing roles.

Normal growth is a necessary but not sufficient guarantee of health. It is, thus, somewhat paradoxical that this strength is also growth assessment's most salient weakness. Although the documentation of normal growth strongly suggests that all is likely well, abnormal growth signals only that something is awry and flags the need for careful diagnostic follow-up and action. This chapter focuses solely on growth and on tools for its assessment. This chapter does not discuss the differential diagnosis of abnormal growth or its treatment. Nothing is gained solely by the physical act of measuring growth. As trivial as this statement may be, it remains an issue of global importance.[1]

Growth assessment's principal utility to health care is its screening value, e.g., assessing general well being, identifying growth faltering and excessive growth, managing infant feeding, evaluating maternal lactation performance, the suitability of weaning practices, and related infant behaviors and the follow-up of children with medical conditions known to affect growth adversely, such as renal and cardiac conditions. It also is useful for population health purposes, for instance, the assessment of community levels of over- and undernutrition, the prediction and ongoing assessments of feeding emergencies, and assessments of economic resource distribution.

DEFINITION OF GROWTH

Biological growth generally refers to net gain in cell number and/or size. Such gains are reflected in multiple outcomes of an undetermined number of incompletely understood complex, metabolic processes. Outcomes of most common interest are various anthropometric characteristics that relate to body mass, size, and composition. Although the concept of physical growth traditionally has focused on fetal life and childhood, i.e., the periods preceding epiphyseal closure, it is not uncommon to apply concepts of growth to physiologic changes also characterized by hyperplastic and/or hypertrophic growth that occur during other life stages, e.g., the uterus and mammary glands during pregnancy. Concepts of growth also are used to describe pathologic processes such as the gains in mass common to neoplasms. In addition, growth may relate to developmental or functional outcomes such as maturation. Most pediatric clinical assessments of growth, however, relate to the measurement of attained weight, length or height, and head circumference. These are the emphasis of this review. Skinfold thicknesses and other measurements such as mid-arm circumference, sitting height, and bone age also are used to assess growth but are applied less commonly. These are used principally by pediatric subspecialties, endocrinologists, gastroenterologists, and nutritionists.

The complexity of biological processes that account for physical growth is daunting. This complexity is evident in the dynamics of changing growth velocities characteristic of fetal life, early infancy, childhood, preadolescence, and adolescence (Figure 1-1). Some of these phases may be unique to humans. The relatively slow rate of prepubertal growth followed by an adolescent growth spurt is described by some as a "distinct human pattern."[2] Others stress general similarities in growth patterns among humans and subhuman primates.[3] These complex growth characteristics, the large number of clinical conditions that result in growth failure, and recent studies such as those that focus on the insulin-like growth hormone system support the expectation that multiple genes are involved in growth's regulated expression.[4] Thus for growth to proceed normally, multiple genes must be present as functional alleles. The degree of genetic redundancy or degeneracy that normally regulates growth is unknown.

The normality of genetic endowments, however, is not sufficient for growth to proceed as expected. Physical growth also is sensitive to numerous environmental influences, such as constraints of socioeconomic origin as reflected by maternal education. This feature adds to the value of growth assessments as screening tools, and simultaneously makes the interpretation of abnormal growth more complex. These multiple sensitivities make measures of growth particularly useful proxies to assess metabolic well being determined by genetic endowments, disease processes that interfere with growth's normal progression, and broader aspects of health determined by environmental milieus, e.g., the nutritional adequacy and safety of the child's food supply, caretaker practices, safe water and sanitation, psychosocial support, and environmental pollutants. Until relatively recently, environmental factors of concern focused primarily on conditions that constrained growth. Growth assessments are and will be increasingly used to evaluate the food and physical activity environments created by societies for children as a means of identifying populations and individuals at risk of becoming overweight and obese.

ASSESSING GROWTH SUCCESSFULLY

The successful assessment of growth is founded on (1) the selection of an appropriate anthropometric indicator, (2) the accuracy of anthropometric measures that are obtained, and (3) the general characteristics of selected references or standards to the extent that they influence the interpretation of anthropometric measures, e.g., interpretations based on cutoffs used to assess risk or classify children according to variable degrees of under- and overnutrition.

SELECTION OF APPROPRIATE ANTHROPOMETRIC INDICATORS

In children the three most commonly used indicators to assess growth status are weight-for-age, length/height-for-age, and weight-for-length/height. Weight-for-age is the most commonly used and, for more than half of the world's countries, the sole anthropometric indicator used.[5] Although it is the easiest indicator to use where children's ages are known, weight-for-age lacks the biological specificity necessary to separate weight from length/height-related deficits or excesses in growth. Conversely, length/height-for-age and weight-for-length/height permit the distinction of stunted, wasted, and overweight children and allow the appropriate targeting of interventions.[6,7] The routine collection of length/height measurements (recumbent length up to 2 years of age and standing height for older children) is important because this enables not only the assessment of weight-for-height, but also body mass index (i.e., ratio of weight in kilo-

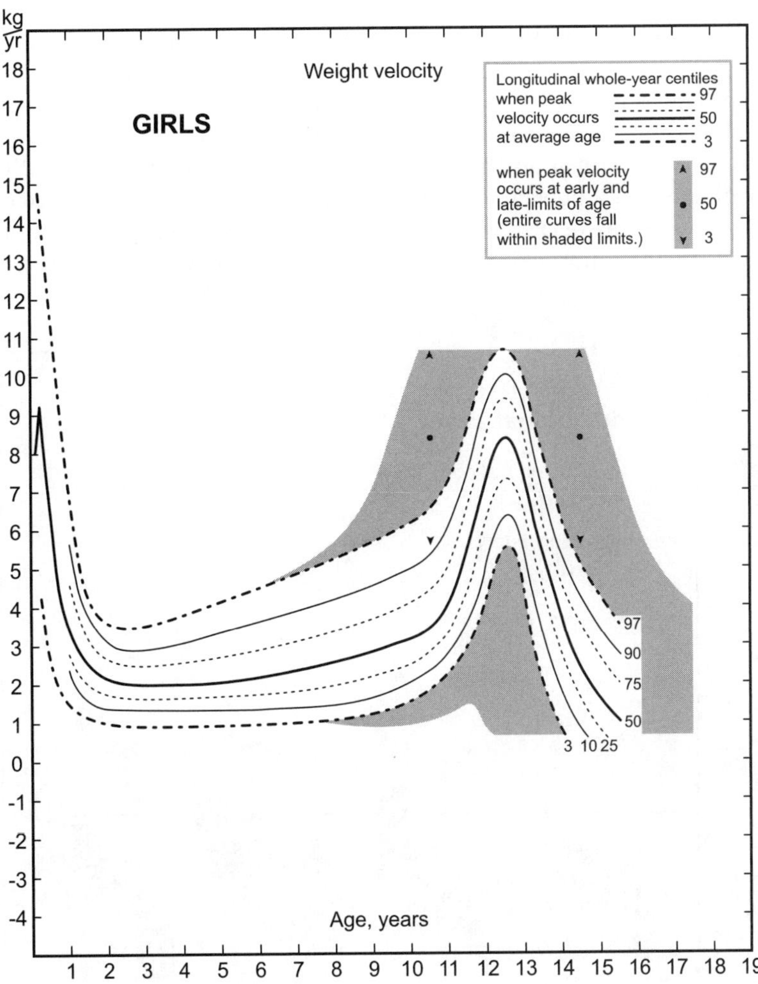

Figure 1-1 Standards for weight velocity for girls. *Source:* Tanner JM, Whitehouse RH. Clinical longitudinal standards for height, weight, height velocity, and weight velocity and the stages of puberty. *Arch Dis Child.* 1976;51:170–179. Reproduced with permission.

grams to the square of height in meters), a valuable indicator being proposed for monitoring the increasing public health problems of overweight and obesity in childhood.[8]

The interpretation of the commonly used anthropometric indicators is as follows:

Low weight-for-age: Weight-for-age reflects body mass relative to chronological age. It is influenced by both the child's height (height-for-age) and his or her weight (weight-for-height). Its composite nature makes interpretation complex. For example, weight-for-age fails to distinguish between short children of adequate body weight and tall, thin children. However, in the absence of significant wasting or stunting in a community, similar information is provided by weight-for-age and height-for-age, in that both reflect an individual's or population's long term health and nutritional experiences. Short term changes, especially reductions in weight-for-age, reveal change in weight-for-height. In general terms, the worldwide variation of low weight-for-age and its age distribution are similar to those of low height-for-age.[9]

Low height-for-age: Stunted growth reflects a process of failure to reach linear growth potential as a result of suboptimal health and/or nutritional conditions. On a population basis, high levels of stunting are associated with poor socioeconomic conditions such as low education levels (Figure 1-2) and increased risk of frequent and early exposure to adverse conditions such as illness and/or inappropriate feeding practices. Similarly, a decrease in the national stunting rate is usually indicative of improvements in overall socioeconomic conditions of a country.[10] The worldwide variation of the prevalence of low height-for-age is

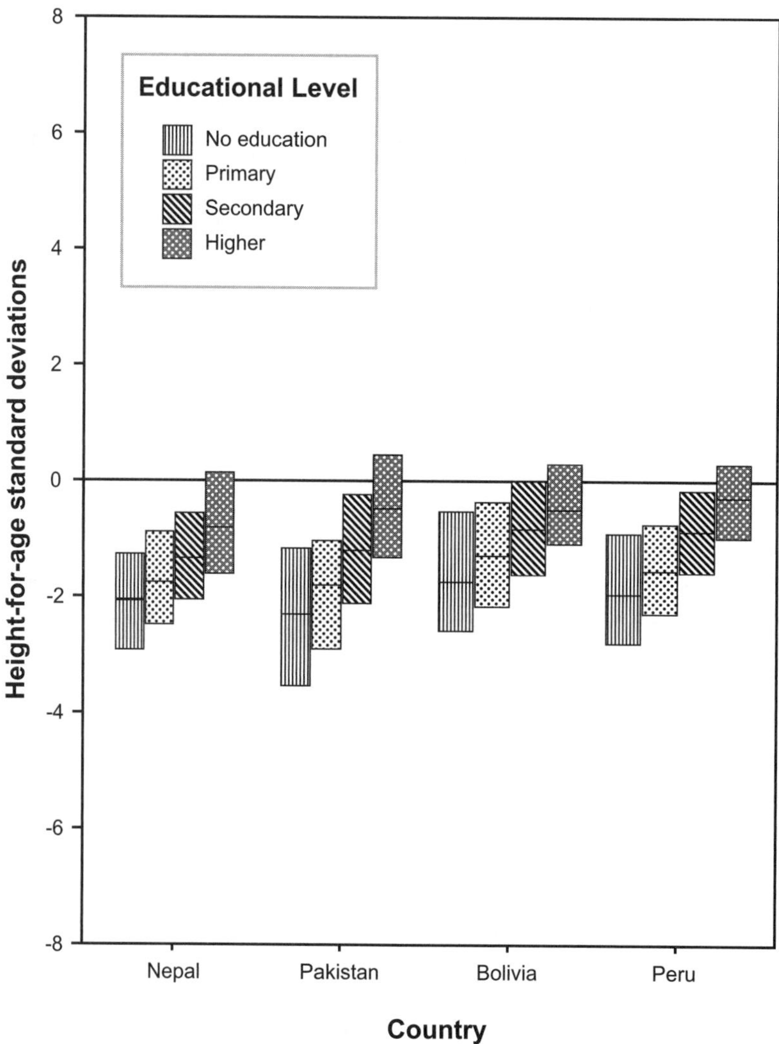

Figure 1-2 Variation of height-for-age according to maternal educational level for 4 national samples of preschool age children. *Source:* de Onis M. Socioeconomic inequalities and child growth. *Int J Epidemiol.* 2003;32:505. Reproduced with permission.

considerable, ranging from 5% to 65% among the less developed countries.[5] In many such settings, prevalence starts to rise at about 3 months of age; the process of stunting slows down at around 3 years of age, after which mean heights run parallel to the current international reference.[11] Therefore, the age modifies the interpretation of findings: for children in the age group below 2–3 years, low height-for-age probably reflects a continuing process of failing to grow or stunting; for older children, it reflects a state of having failed to grow or being stunted. From the point of view of interventions, it is important to differentiate between these two groups.

In populations without significant stunting or wasting, low height-for-age in individual children is more likely to signal deprivation due to conditions not necessarily related to poverty than in settings such as those described in the previous paragraph. Thus, for example in the United States, it is necessary to consider possibilities that include psychosocial deprivation, unmet heightened nutritional needs imposed by illness, and/or metabolic constraints imposed by the failure to transform nutrients to their active form or other mechanisms that may result in growth failure.

Low weight-for-height: Wasting or thinness indicates in most cases a recent and severe process of weight loss, which is often associated with acute starvation and/or severe disease. However, wasting also may be the result of chronic unfavorable conditions. Provided there is no severe food shortage, the prevalence of wasting is usually below 5%, even in poor countries.[12] The Indian subcontinent, where a higher prevalence of wasting is found, is an important exception. A prevalence between 10% and 14% is regarded as serious, and above or equal to 15% as critical.[9] Typically, the prevalence of low weight-for-height reaches a peak in the second year of life. Lack of evidence of wasting in a population does not imply the absence of current nutritional problems; stunting and other deficits may be present. Given these characteristics, wasting or thinness demands a careful assessment in all cases in which it is encountered.

High weight-for-height: Overweight is the preferred term for describing high weight-for-height. Even though there is a strong correlation between high weight-for-height and obesity as measured by adiposity, greater lean body mass can also contribute to high weight-for-height. On an individual basis, therefore, fatness or obesity should not be used to describe high weight-for-height. However, on a population-wide basis, high weight-for-height can be considered as an adequate indicator of obesity, because the majority of individuals with high weight-for-height are obese. Strictly speaking, the term "obesity" should be used only in the context of adiposity measurements, for example skinfold thickness.

Other available anthropometric indicators that are used to describe growth status during childhood include mid-upper arm circumference (MUAC), skinfolds, and head circumference; however, none of these has achieved such widespread use as the height- and weight-based indicators mentioned earlier due, in part, to the lack of widely acceptable pediatric reference data for their interpretation. For some of these measurements, technical difficulties result in high intra- and inter-individual variation and require skilled individuals to perform the measurements accurately and precisely. For skinfolds, the cost of equipment also has precluded their wide application in children. MUAC-for-age has been proposed as an alternative indicator for use where the collection of height and weight measurements is difficult (e.g., refugee crises); however, its proper application requires the use of age-specific reference data for its accurate interpretation. Its use also requires the ascertainment of age, an important drawback under difficult field conditions.

ACCURACY OF ANTHROPOMETRIC MEASURES

Variability in infant and child measurements can result from a number of influences: the setting in which the measurements are taken, the degree of filling of the stomach and/or bladder (in the case of weight), the behavior and cooperation of the child being measured, accuracy and precision of instruments, the anthropometrist's technical capacity (i.e., training, experience, and reliability), and the methods for recording data. Appropriate training and continual standardization, adherence to specified methods and procedures, and monitoring of data quality are essential for reducing measurement error and minimizing bias.

An important goal of standardized training is to enable trainees to measure accurately, that is, without bias. To achieve this, trainees should be taught the skills to obtain measurements that are on average equal to those measured by an expert anthropometrist who serves as a gold standard. The degree of accuracy can be assessed by a test–retest protocol in which several children are measured by both the expert and the trainee. Bias is calculated as the average deviation of the trainee's measurements from the means of the expert's corresponding values. It is equally important that the measurements taken be precise, that is, reproducible. High precision is only possible if measurement procedures are highly standardized. Precision is assessed on the basis of differences between replicate measurements taken on several subjects as prescribed by a test–retest protocol. The most commonly used parameter for assessing precision is the technical error of measurement (TEM). The TEM is calculated as the square root of the sum of squared differences between duplicate measurements, divided by 2 times the number of subjects measured.[13]

A detailed account of the measurement and standardization protocols for anthropometry used in the construction of a new international growth reference can be found elsewhere.[5] The rigorous anthropometry protocols used for the development of the international reference serve as a model for research settings. It will be difficult to be as rigorous in nonresearch settings, such as pediatric clinics. However, at the very least, the procedures should be documented carefully in training manuals, health staff collecting anthropometry data should be trained, refresher sessions should be held periodically, weighing scales and any other instruments used should be maintained in good order and calibrated before use, and health staff should be supervised.

GENERAL CHARACTERISTICS OF GROWTH REFERENCES AND STANDARDS

A clear understanding of the terms *reference* and *standard* and of the appropriate uses of those tools also is necessary. This need arises because these terms and their uses have significant implications in assessing the appropriateness of the designs of studies or approaches used to construct the tools themselves, i.e., the *reference* or *standard.* In this regard, the common interchangeable use of the terms *reference* and *standard* is inappropriate when used in conjunction with growth.

The common use of *reference* and *standard* as synonyms, however, is not surprising. The *International Dictionary for Medicine and Biology* defines *reference* as "a standard against which techniques, measurements or other observations can be compared, or upon which inferences or calculations can be based."[14] *Standard* is given two definitions of interest, "a unit, level or specification established as a *reference* for purposes of comparison or control, or for securing uniformity" and "serving as a model or magnitude against which similar entities, performances, or quantities may be compared."[14] Thus *reference* appears to be defined as a *standard,* and *standard* as a *reference.*

In the context of growth assessments, however, the distinction between a *reference* and a *standard* is important from theoretical and practical perspectives. It is much more useful to conceptualize *references* as "devices for grouping and analyzing data" and *standards* as devices that "embody the concept of a norm or target—that is a value judgment."[15] *Standards,* thus, should aid health professionals to judge current status and/or predict future outcomes. Their utility depends in large measure on their sensitivity and specificity relative to either of those objectives.[16] *References* should provide useful tools for the more limited purpose of making comparisons, i.e., measures of interest may be larger or smaller relative to the reference, but no value is assignable to observed differences.

Such theoretical considerations carry significant practical implications. There is no question that growth *references* are used in practice as *standards,* i.e., value judgments are based on them; judgments driven to a significant degree by the statistical distributions that underlie their construction. Their use thus raises basic issues that focus on the approaches used to develop commonly used national and international growth references.[17]

As background, the current international growth reference's history was reviewed in 1996.[18] Briefly longitudinal data (from 0 to 23 months) compiled by the Ohio Fels Research Institute and cross-sectional data collected by the US Health Examination Survey conducted from 1960 to 1975 in children 2 to 18 years of age were used to construct the present international growth reference for infants. Longitudinal data were obtained from various groups of infants studied before 1975. These infants were predominantly formula fed, resided in a restricted geographical area, and were of relatively high socioeconomic backgrounds. Cross-sectional data were collected by protocols designed to obtain a sample representative of older US children. On the surface, the characteristics of the US population and the compilation of data obtained from it should have resulted in the construction of tools that enabled value judgments related to attained growth and velocity for children 0 to 23 months and attained growth for children 2 to 18 years of age.

In practice, however, this expectation was not borne out by experience. This was evident from two important efforts that led to two distinct important undertakings. First, a review undertaken by WHO in the early 1990s demonstrated significant flaws in the reference it adopted for international use in 1975. The second is represented by various studies that led to the recognition of the US obesity epidemic.[19,20] Both efforts resulted in questions regarding the presumptive health status of the populations from which the current international reference drew its sample. The WHO review resulted in an international study currently under way to develop new international growth references, the WHO Multicentre Growth Reference Study (MGRS).[21] These same concerns, in part, resulted in the development of a revised US national reference.[22] Each is considered in turn in the following section.

WHO REVIEW AND THE MGRS

The WHO review assembled published and unpublished longitudinal growth data collected from infants who were exclusively or predominantly breastfed for at least 4 months and who were partially breastfed for at least the ensuing 8 months.[23] Conservative criteria were used to insure that growth was not constrained by environmental or other factors in the selected sample. Among the resulting analyses' most salient findings were that the growth of this conservatively selected sample (referred to from here as the WHO pooled breastfed group) deviated negatively from the current international reference. The deviation's magnitude was large enough to likely interfere with clinical management. These deviations were incongruent with the positive health benefits associated with breastfeeding and the group's relatively affluent living conditions and described health status. Considerations such as these led the WHO review to conclude that the current international reference did not adequately depict normal infant growth.

The same review also compared the growth of a totally distinct, more ethnically diverse group of exclusively and predominantly breastfed infants (referred to from here as the HRP group) with the current international growth reference. The second comparison group's growth also deviated negatively relative to the current international growth standard. More importantly, however, when the WHO pooled breastfed group was used as the basis for comparisons, the HRP growth pattern appeared to be sustained or improved during the 12-month follow-up period. This finding reinforced the conclusion that the present international reference was inadequate for reasons described briefly in the preceding paragraph.

The review group also observed that the variability of the WHO pooled breastfed group's growth was significantly smaller than that of the present international reference and that those differences were sustained for 12 months in both sexes. This suggested several, nonmutually exclusive possibilities, i.e., that the conservative criteria used to select the WHO pooled breastfed group resulted in an overly homogenous sample; methods used to construct the current international reference somehow artificially increased normal variability; and/or that the larger variability depicted by the current international reference was a reflection of the very broad definition of health inherent to its sampling frame, i.e., the absence of disease, with no consideration of feeding or other care practices.

Collectively, considerations such as these led to the WHO group's recommendation that a new international growth reference was needed for infants and young children. An expert group, convened to consider these and the findings of other groups assessing the uses and interpretation of anthropometry in other life stages, concurred with this recommendation and added that because of program considerations, efforts to develop new international references should be inclusive of preschool aged children.[9] More importantly, however, there was concurrence that it was time to consider the production of references that would more closely approximate standards, i.e., to describe how children *should* grow rather than to limit the effort to a description of *how* children grow in a specific setting and time.

Inherent to this recommendation are various significant implications for the construction of tools intended for assessing growth. First, effects of infant feeding practices on infant growth support the view that the definition of health for purposes of defining a sampling frame must be expanded beyond the overt absence of disease.[17] Other recommended behaviors likely to have beneficial consequences on health and influence growth also should be considered. Using the growth of breastfed infants as the *standard* is the most appropriate choice. Breastfeeding is recommended for infant feeding by all national and international health agencies for sound biological reasons.[24] Other factors likely to influence growth also were considered as inclusion (e.g., use of recommended pediatric care practices) and exclusion (e.g., use of tobacco products by the mother) criteria and were eventually adopted by the MGRS. Considerations such as these would clearly provide a sound basis for assessing normal growth and have the added value of communicating clearly to caretakers the basis on which such standards were developed, thereby also encouraging their adoption as the best means of providing optimal care to children.

Beyond such biological and practical considerations, technical aspects of the development of a *standard* also were reviewed. Among the possible explanations for the deviations between the growth of healthy infants (using the prescriptive definition introduced in the preceding paragraph) and the growth pattern depicted by the current international reference is that only relatively widely spaced measurements, i.e., 3-month intervals, were available for the current international growth reference's construction. These intervals are too long to depict dynamic patterns of human growth characteristic of infancy. It also is possible that limitations inherent to curve-fitting and smoothing techniques available at the time the current international references were constructed may account for the observed deviations. Advances in analytical capabilities and approaches should minimize such concerns in future efforts.

Revised US Growth References

The US Centers for Disease Control and Prevention (CDC) released new growth references for the United States in May 2000.[22] The new references were based principally on cross-sectional data from five surveys that employed nationally representative sampling frames. A paucity of data for infants in the National Health and Nutrition Examination Surveys II and III (NHANES II and III) led to the inclusion of data from the Pediatric Nutrition Surveillance System (PedNSS) and, to a lesser extent, from the Fels Longitudinal Study for the infant portion of the references. This effort was partially responsive to critiques of the previous National Centers for Health Statistics (NCHS) reference in that the new effort applied improved biometric techniques to smooth percentile curves, but the data available could not address issues related to a definition of health that included recommended health care practices as discussed in preceding paragraphs. Thus, for example, the new references included relatively few infants whose feeding behaviors reflect current recommendations.

The new CDC reference was reviewed recently by de Onis and Onyango.[25] Unfortunately, the new reference raises many of the same questions that were posed by the reference it replaced. In their review, de Onis and Onyango assessed the growth of the WHO pooled breastfed group, discussed earlier, relative to the new CDC reference. Breastfed infants' growth (i.e., body weight gain) is more rapid in the first 2 months than is depicted by the new reference, and less so from 3 to 12 months. Breastfed infants' linear growth also is more rapid than is depicted by the new reference until age 4 months; thereafter it declines relative to the new reference until 9 months. When these findings are compared with those reached by the WHO review group that compared the pooled breastfed group's growth to the previous NCHS reference, the new CDC reference appears to depict a heavier and shorter population (Figure 1-3).

The growth pattern depicted by the new CDC reference likely reflects the consequences of feeding practices common among US infants and the relatively infrequent growth measurements on which the new references are based. For example, Hediger et al. published a detailed description of breastfeeding patterns and duration among NCHS III infants. Approximately one half of the sample initiated breastfeeding, one fifth exclusively breastfed for 4 months, and only one sixth of those infants continued to be breastfed exclusively for 6 months.[26] Comparable breastfeeding statistics present lower estimates for both NCHS II and PedNSS samples.[27]

Another important limitation of the new CDC reference is that it is based on a sample whose average weight was higher than that of the previous 1977 NCHS reference. Growth charts updated by data from representative samples of populations undergoing increasing trends of overweight and obesity result in descriptive references that are skewed progressively to the right and, consequently, redefine previously

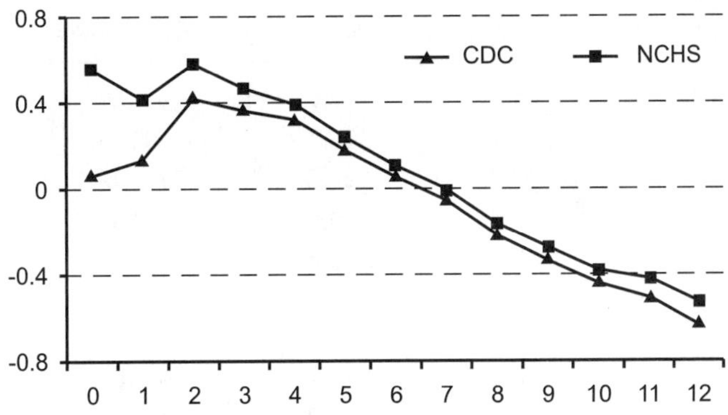

Figure 1-3 Mean weight-for-age z-scores of breast fed infants relative to the 1977 National Centers for Health Statistics (NCHS) and the 2000 Centers for Disease Control and Prevention (CDC) references. *Source:* Reproduced with permission from de Onis M, Onyango AW. The Centers for Disease Control and Prevention 2000, Growth charts and the growth of breastfed infants. *Acta Paediatrica.* 2003;92:415.

abnormal conditions as normal. This results in underestimates of true rates of overweight and obesity. The impact of such skewing by the CDC 2000 reference on evaluations of child growth has been evaluated recently using a sample of preschool-aged children.[28] In all cases, the new CDC 2000 reference substantially underestimated the weight-for-height z-scores of individual children compared to the 1977 NCHS reference. A child classified close to + 3 standard deviations (SD) using the 1977 NCHS reference was below + 2 SD when the CDC 2000 reference was applied. Similarly, a child with a z-score of + 10.7 based on the 1977 NCHS reference was below + 4 SD when using the CDC 2000 reference (Table 1-1).

Because of the implications this has for the accurate assessment and monitoring of childhood overweight and obesity, some developed countries such as the United Kingdom have recently taken the policy decision to "freeze" the British 1990 BMI reference.[29]

These considerations underscore the need to rethink the conceptual basis of future tools for assessing growth, criteria used to select groups and individuals for developing those tools, design requirements key to successfully using these tools (e.g., frequency of measurements early in infancy to depict accurately that dynamic period of growth), and updated analytical techniques that are capable of accurately depicting normal variability and other features of growth that are necessary for correctly interpreting attained and velocity measures of growth.

OTHER FACTORS AFFECTING THE INTERPRETATION OF ANTHROPOMETRIC MEASUREMENTS

Cutoffs and the bases for their designation are among the principal factors that influence the interpretation of anthropometric measurements. Their importance is similar to that of the population selected and study designs that are used to develop the assessment tools from which interpretations are derived.

Two basic approaches are used most commonly to designate cutoffs that are intended to reflect levels of adverse risks, and by inference potential benefits. Importantly, the designation

Table 1-1 Effect of increased upward skewness of CDC 2000 growth reference compared to the 1977 NCHS reference on weight-for-height z-scores.

Child	*Age (mo)*	*Weight*	*Height*	*NCHS z-score**	*CDC z-score**
Boy	48	25.3	103.0	+ 5.57	+ 3.65
Girl	48	35.1	103.7	+ 10.70	+ 3.58
Girl	74	47.8	121.2	+ 9.42	+ 3.27
Girl	78	29.4	120.1	+ 2.91	+ 1.97
Girl	52	32.3	109.4	+ 7.36	+ 2.96
Boy	22	16.8	91.3	+ 3.29	+ 2.74
Boy	43	24.3	105.4	+ 4.34	+ 2.97
Girl	62	32.9	111.4	+ 7.05	+ 2.87
Boy	58	45.2	119.0	+ 9.96	+ 2.72
Boy	42	26.4	112.5	+ 3.64	+ 2.30

* Weight-for-height standard deviations.

Source: de Onis M. The use of anthropometry in the prevention of childhood overweight. *Int J Obes Related Metab Dis.* 2004;28(suppl 3):S81–5, copyright 2004, Macmillan Publishers Ltd. Reprinted with permission.

of benefits is seldom the focus of their derivation. One approach is based exclusively on the mathematical estimation of presumed risk that depends strictly on the cutoff's distance from a given measurement's central tendency, i.e., its mean or median. The other relies on a demonstrable link between a designated outcome and a specific measurement's or indicator's observed or assumed distribution. The latter usually is intellectually and practically more satisfying because it is less abstract and relates most directly to a real life event, e.g., illness or death.

The former approach, i.e., the mathematical estimation of placement within an observed or presumed distribution, has two principal variants of interest to this discussion. One is based on a normalized measure that is expressed as multiples of a standard deviation of the targeted measure's distribution, i.e., a z-score. In this approach a z-score of 0 corresponds to the measurement's mean. Z-scores of + 1 and – 1 correspond to values 1 standard deviation above or below the mean, respectively. Z-scores of + 1.5 and – 1.5 correspond to analogous values. This approach requires that measurements of interest be either normally distributed or transformable in a manner that results in such a distribution.

The other common variant is the mathematical estimation of placement within an observed or presumed distribution. It expresses the measurement of interest as a percent of its median or mean value or as the corresponding percentile of its cumulative distribution. Neither of these variants requires a normal distribution.

The Gomez classification is an example of cutoffs intended to link mathematical estimations of placement within a presumed distribution to the risk to specified outcomes. In this classification, those with weight-for-age that fall 76–90%, 61–75%, and ≤ 60% of the theoretical average are designated as suffering from first-, second-, and third-degree malnutrition, respectively.[30] Those values are linked to presumably progressively increasing risk to serious somatic and functional—including psychological—changes and death.

WHO has recommended the z-score system because of advantages that relate to the comparability of similar z-scores across ages, sexes, and other traits that may be accounted for by this system.[9] Briefly, a z-score of + 1 always designates the same relative position within a normal distribution. This has enormous advantages whenever judgments are based on comparisons of any sort whether applied to individuals or populations.[31] The same is not necessarily true for systems that depend on percent of median or percentiles. The percent of median calculation ignores the targeted measurement's distribution, and thus, depending on a child's age, a value corresponding to 80% of the medium median may be above or below a z-score of – 2. This presents problems to the interpretation of measurements in all cases other than those that link such mathematical estimations to age-specific mortality and/or other outcomes. Because there are few examples where this is the case, this system is most often unsatisfactory.

Percentiles potentially are less likely to present similar interpretive problems if the measure of interest has been normalized. This system, however, does not require normalization, thus it can present difficulties in comparing percentile values that are not similarly distributed.

CONCLUSION

Assessments of child growth remain a mainstay of pediatric care in all settings. Their utility is determined by the measurer's ability to respond to the measurement's interpretation. The determination of normal growth should lead always to other assessments related to child health, e.g., immunization and developmental status. Similarly, the determination of abnormal growth always should lead to an evaluation of its likely determinants as suggested by the child's environment and health history, and appropriate action should be taken to treat the child and/or remedy the offending condition(s). The determination of normal and abnormal growth is dependent upon the selection of an appropriate growth indicator. The measurement's accuracy also is key. It depends on the measurer's technical skills and the appropriateness and upkeep of equipment used to obtain the desired measurements. The measurement's interpretation is dependent upon the characteristics of the reference or standard that is used and inferences that can be made may be either enhanced or limited by the reference's or standard's characteristics. New approaches for assessing young child growth promise to provide a basis for assessing the normality and abnormality of child growth more robustly than do tools that are currently available.

Since the preparation of this chapter WHO has released its growth standards. They are available at: http://www.who.int/childgrowth/en/.

REFERENCES

1. Garner P, Panpanich R, Logan S. Is routine growth monitoring effective? A systematic review of trials. *Arch Dis Child.* 2000;82:197–201.
2. Bogin B. The evolution of human growth. In: Cameron N, ed. *Human Growth and Development.* New York, NY: Academic Press; 2002:29–320.
3. Ulijasek S. Comparative growth and development in mammals. In: Ulijasek S, Johnston FE, Preece MA, eds. *Human Growth and Development.* Cambridge, UK: Cambridge University Press; 1998:96–99.
4. Rosenfield RG. Insulin-like growth factors and the basis of growth. *N Engl J Med.* 2003;349:2184–2186.
5. de Onis M, Wijnhoven TMA, Onyango AW. Worldwide practices in child growth monitoring. *J Pediatr.* 2004;144:461–465.
6. Uauy R, Kain J. The epidemiological transition: need to incorporate obesity prevention into nutrition programmes. *Public Health Nutr.* 2002;5:223–229.
7. WHO. *Management of severe malnutrition: A manual for physicians and other senior health workers.* Geneva, Switzerland: World Health Organization; 1999.
8. American Academy of Pediatrics Policy Statement. Prevention of pediatric overweight and obesity. *Pediatrics.* 2003;112:424–430.
9. WHO. *Physical status: the use and interpretation of anthropometry. Report of a WHO Expert Committee. Technical Report Series No. 854.* Geneva, Switzerland: World Health Organization; 1995.
10. Frongillo EA, de Onis M, Hanson KM. Socioeconomic and demographic factors are associated with worldwide patterns of stunting and wasting of children. *J Nutr.* 1997;127:2302–2309.
11. Shrimpton R, Victora CG, de Onis M, Costa Lima R, Blössner M, Clugston G. Worldwide timing of growth faltering: implications for nutritional interventions. *Pediatrics.* 2001;107(5):E75.
12. de Onis M, Blössner M. The World Health Organization global database on child growth and malnutrition: methodology and applications. *Int J Epidemiol.* 2003;32:518–526.
13. Malina RM, Hamill PVV, Lemeshow S. *Selected Measurements of Children 6–11 Years. United States (Vital Health and Statistics Series 11, No. 123, USDHHS).* Washington, DC: US Government Printing Office; 1973.
14. *International Dictionary of Medicine and Biology.* New York, NY: Wiley; 1986.
15. WHO. *Measuring Change in Nutritional Status: Guidelines for Assessing the Nutritional Impact of Supplementary Feeding Programmes for Vulnerable Groups.* Geneva, Switzerland: World Health Organization; 1983.
16. Garza C, Frongillo E, Dewey KG. Implications of growth patterns of breastfed infants for growth references. *Acta Paediatri Suppl.* 1994;402:4–10.
17. Garza C, de Onis M, for the WHO Multicentre Growth Reference Study Group. Rationale for developing a new international growth reference. *Food Nutr Bull.* 2004;25: S1–S4.
18. de Onis M, Yip R. The WHO growth chart: historical considerations and current scientific issues. *Bibl Nutr Dieta.* 1996;53:74–89.
19. Troiano RP, Flegal KM, Kuczmarski RJ, Campbell SM, Johnson CL. Overweight prevalence and trends for children and adolescents. The National Health and Nutrition Examination Surveys, 1963 to 1991. *Arch Pediatr Adolesc Med.* 1995;149:1085–1091.
20. Ogden CL, Troiano RP, Briefel RR, Kuczmarski RJ, Flegal KM, Johnson CL. Prevalence of overweight among preschool children in the United States, 1971 through 1994. *Pediatrics.* 1997;99(4). Available at: http://www.pediatrics.org/cgi/content/full/99/4/e1.
21. de Onis M, Onyango AW, Van den Broeck J, Chumlea C, Martorell R, for the WHO Multicentre Growth Reference Study. Measurement and standardization protocols for anthropometry used in the construction of a new international growth reference. *Food Nutr Bull.* 2004;25(suppl 1):S27–S36.
22. Kuczmarski RJ, Ogden CL, Grummer-Strawn LM, et al. *CDC Growth Charts: United States. Advance Data from Vital and Health Statistics No. 314.* Hyattsville, MD: National Center for Health Statistics; 2000.
23. WHO Working Group on Infant Growth. *An Evaluation of Infant Growth.* Geneva, Switzerland: World Health Organization; 1994.
24. WHO and UNICEF. *Global Strategy for Infant and Young Child Feeding.* Geneva, Switzerland: World Health Organization; 2003.

25. de Onis M, Onyango AW. The Centers for Disease Control and Prevention 2000 growth charts and the growth of breastfed infants. *Acta Paediatr.* 2003;92:413–419.
26. Hediger MI, Overpeck MD, Ruan WJ, Troendle JF. Early infant feeding and growth status of US-born infants and children aged 4–17 months: analyses from the third National Health and Nutrition Examination Survey 1988–1994. *Am J Clin Nutr.* 2000;72:159–167.
27. Mei Z, Yip R, Grummer-Strawn LM, Trowbridge FL. Development of a research child growth reference and its comparison with the current international growth reference. *Arch Pediatr Adolesc Med.* 1998;152:471–479.
28. de Onis M. The use of anthropometry on the prevention of childhood overweight. *Int J Obes Metab Dis.* 2004: 28(suppl 3):S83–85.
29. Wright CM, Booth IW, Buckler JM, et al. Growth reference charts for use in the United Kingdom. *Arch Dis Child.* 2002;86:11–14.
30. Gomez F, Galvan RR, Frenk S, Munoz JC, Chavez R, Vasquez J. Mortality in second and third degree malnutrition. *J Trop Pediatr.* 1956;2:77–83.
31. de Onis M, Frongillo EA, Blössner M. Is malnutrition declining? An analysis of changes in levels of child malnutrition since 1980. *Bull World Health Organ.* 2000;78:1222–1233.

CHAPTER 2

Gastrointestinal Development

Ronald E. Kleinman and Daniel S. Kamin

INTRODUCTION

Providing optimal nutrition support to infants and children requires understanding developmental changes that occur in the liver, pancreas, and gastrointestinal tract from uterine life to full maturity. Intrauterine growth, premature birth, and postnatal disease can affect the process of intestinal maturation. In this chapter we describe the functional maturation of the liver, pancreas, and intestinal tract as a nutrient assimilation organ system. We begin with a short review of gastrointestinal organogenesis and then consider the development of gastrointestinal motility and the maturation of specific liver metabolic pathways and enteric hormones, each *vis-à-vis* feeding and enteric competence. We then consider the development of nutrient absorption and digestion. The unique role of breast milk in promoting gastrointestinal maturation is discussed.

MORPHOGENESIS

Vital embryonic development begins with gastrulation—forming the three cell-layer disk that ultimately gives rise to endoderm, mesoderm, and ectoderm. This process is complete by the end of the third week of life. By 20 weeks' gestation, the fetal gut has developed sufficiently to resemble that of the mature newborn. However, most absorptive and motor functions are immature before 26 weeks, and some, particularly pancreatic exocrine functions, are not fully mature in the term newborn. Table 2-1 summarizes the timeline of gastrointestinal organogenesis and functionality.

Each aspect of development can, when perturbed, give rise to conditions that have nutritional consequences. For instance, failure of the intestine to completely recanalize (intestinal atresias), or improper rotation as the intestine reenters the abdomen at 10 weeks (midgut volvulus around a Ladd band), can result in severely compromised intestinal function. Amniotic fluid and placenta-derived growth factors present in amniotic fluid, such as epidermal growth factor, may influence growth and development of the gastrointestinal tract in utero.[1]

MOTILITY

Assimilation of nutrients is impossible without effective aboral intraluminal propagation of food and byproducts. Understanding of the motor development of the gastrointestinal tract is incomplete. However, feeding intolerance, of which dysmotility is a significant component, remains a major obstacle in providing optimal nutrition support to premature and critically ill neonates. Table 2-2 summarizes gastrointestinal motor development.

Sucking and Swallowing

Swallowing has been observed *in utero* as early as 16 weeks, and by term a fetus may swallow up to 450 ml/day of amniotic fluid.[2] Fetal swallowing of amniotic fluid is likely necessary for the proper development of intestinal anatomy,[3] motility, and absorptive function.[4] Sucking has been observed *in utero* at 6 months of gestation, but the mature coordinated suck, swallowing and breathing of the term infant generally occurs after 34–35 weeks of gestation in appropriate weight-for-gestation infants.[5,6] Thus, bypassing the mouth with nasogastric or nasoenteric feeding until approximately 34–35 weeks of gestation is standard practice in neonatal intensive care units.

Nonnutritive sucking may have psychosocial benefits for infant and parent, and it is associated with earlier hospital discharge. Nonnutritive sucking has no effect on time to full oral feeds or formula tolerance.[7]

Table 2-1 Anatomical development of gastrointestinal tract in the human fetus and gestational age of acquisition.

	Gestation (wks)
Esophagus	
• Superficial gland develop	20
• Squamous cells appear	28
Stomach	
• Gastric glands form	14
• Pylorus and fundus defined	14
Pancreas	
• Differentiation of exocrine and endocrine tissue	14
Liver	
• Lobules form	11
Small intestine	
• Crypt-villi develop	14
• Lymph nodes appear	14
Colon	
• Diameter increases	20
• Villi disappear	20

Source: Lebenthal A, Lebenthal E. The ontogeny of the small intestinal epithelium. *J Parenter Enteral Nutr.* 1999;23(5 suppl):S3-6.

Esophageal Motility

In adults, a swallow initiates relaxation of the upper esophageal sphincter, primary peristaltic wave, and coordinated relaxation of the lower sphincter. This pattern is present in term infants.[2] Preterm infants may display uncoordinated biphasic nonpropagated contractions along the esophagus.[8]

Recent work in human preterm infants[9] (gestational ages 26–33 weeks) shows that some have propagated esophageal peristalsis and lower esophageal sphincter tonic pressures similar to those of term infants. The higher frequency and longer duration of transient lower esophageal sphincter relaxation in preterm infants contributes to a higher prevalence of gastroesophageal reflux (GER). Clearance mechanisms appear intact by 31 weeks of gestation.[9]

Gastric Motility

The stomach of premature infants demonstrates immature motility.[10] Gastric emptying time increases as the density of feedings increases.[11,12] Effective contractions of the gastric antrum do not develop until approximately 30 weeks of gestation.[13] Infants with a birth weight as low as 1,400 g may demonstrate adequate gastric emptying when receiving either intermittent or continuous feeding into the stomach or small intestine.[14]

The caloric density of the feeding is the most potent trigger for gastric contractions, but fat slows gastric emptying. Full strength trophic infusions, even at infusion rates as low as 4mL/kg/hr,[11] may be more effective than dilute feed-

Table 2-2 Gastrointestinal motor development.

Organ	*Gestation age function appears (wks)*	*Mature function (wks)*
Mouth		
• Suck/swallow	16	34–35
Esophagus		
• Propagate bolus	prior to 26	31–33
Stomach		
• Mixing	20	> 8wks postpartum
• Gastric emptying	approximately 18	30
Small intestine		
• Prandial mixing	28	38
• Fasting aboral MMCs*	27	38
Large intestine		
• Defecation	Not known	Not known

*MMC—Migrating Motor Complex

ings at higher rates of delivery. Other factors influencing gastric motility in the preterm infant include serum bilirubin concentrations[15] and formula temperature.[16] Protein does not impact gastric motility in preterm infants.[17] Enterically administered insulin leads to fewer and smaller gastric residua. Both intragastric and transpyloric feedings trigger motor responses in the stomach and small intestine[11,12] and are equally effective in supporting gastrointestinal development and nutritional needs.[10]

Small Intestinal Motility

The fully mature small intestine has well defined cyclic patterns of contractile activity during fasting. The fed pattern is characterized by random mixing motor activity. Studies in animals and premature infants at 28 weeks of gestation show that fed and fasting motility patterns are similar. Progressively, the fasted and fed states become more distinct and ultimately resemble the mature motility patterns seen in the term newborn.[11]

Neuroenteric hormonal interactions are critical to maturation of small intestinal motility.[18] Small intestinal motility is enhanced maximally by full-strength trophic feeding into either the stomach or the small intestine.[12,19]

LARGE INTESTINAL MOTILITY

Little is known about the development of motility in the large intestine. Preterm infants have slow colonic motility and are more apt to have delayed meconium passage.[20]

NEUROENTERIC HORMONAL DEVELOPMENT

At no other time is the complex interplay between the central nervous system and gut more in flux than at birth. Interactions among hormones, complex neural pathways, and the relevant gastrointestinal effector cells (smooth muscle cells, enterocytes, pancreatic acinar cells, etc.) assure that nutrient assimilation is coordinated with appetite and energy expenditure.

Gut peptides are found in the early fetal intestine by the second trimester.[21] In humans and other mammals, the introduction of enteral feeding following birth provokes a massive surge in the serum concentration of regulatory peptide hormones, including enteroglucagon, gastrin, motilin, neurotensin, gastrointestinal peptide, and pancreatic polypeptide.[22] Preterm infants weighing little more than 1 kg have hormonal responses to enteral nutrition similar to term infants.[23] The type and mode of feeding have a substantial influence on enteric hormone secretion. Breast milk elicits responses of lower amplitude for some hormones, while others do not differ significantly from responses following formula feedings.[24,25] Enterally administered water,[26] intravenous dextrose, and parenteral nutrition elicit minimal enteric hormonal responses.[23,27,28] Trophic feedings stimulate enteric hormonal responses similar to full nutritive feedings.[22] The act of breastfeeding may[23,26–29] modulate hormone responses.[30] Transpyloric and intragastric feeding elicit similar hormonal responses.[29]

Hepatic Metabolism

Xenobiotic metabolism takes place primarily in the liver. The development of the relevant enzyme systems overlap with those responsible for synthesizing and recycling bile acids. The mode and type of nutrition may influence the development of enzyme systems that metabolize drugs.[31]

Drug metabolism in the liver is divided between phase 1 (oxidation and reduction via membrane-bound mixed function oxidases) and phase 2 (synthetic conjugation) reactions. Phase 1 enzymes are found in primate fetal liver at the end of the first trimester.[32] The phase 2 enzyme UDP-glucuronosyltransferase (UGT) is undetectable in human fetal liver before 20 weeks.[33] A surge in activity of phase 1 and phase 2 enzymes occurs after birth.[32] Despite the fact that drug metabolism in immature infants can be unpredictable, dietary factors influence drug metabolism. Animal models and human studies show that protein-calorie malnutrition causes decreased hepatic phase 1 activity via the P450 oxidase system.[34,35] In rats fed parenterally, demethylation and hydroxylation are decreased compared to rats fed enterally.[36] Macronutrients can affect drug metabolism. For example, in rats, enteral formulas or parenteral solutions high in protein or specific amino acids support higher P450 enzyme activity.[31]

Drug metabolism is affected by nutritional repletion after malnutrition,[37] mode of delivery of nutrients,[38] protein intake,[34] and specific amino acid composition of the diet.[39]

DIGESTION AND ABSORPTION

Carbohydrates

Carbohydrates represent approximately 40% of the energy intake of infants fed breast milk or cow's milk based formulas. Breast milk carbohydrate is approximately 80% lactose and 20% oligosaccharides.

Polysaccharides

Pancreatic amylase activity develops slowly in the newborn. Activity levels remain at approximately 0.5% of adult values for the first 6 months of life.[40] This may be due to lack of cholecystokinin (CCK) receptors on acinar cells.[41]

Salivary and breast milk amylases and mucosal glucosidases are adequate for dietary glucose polymer digestion, even in infants born as young as 26 weeks of gestation.[42] Brush border glucoamylase efficiently hydrolyzes glucose polymers 5–9 residues in length. Preterm and term infants fed glucose polymers have similar carbohydrate absorptive capacity.[41]

Breast milk amylase compensates for the attenuated activity of pancreatic amylase by hydrolyzing starch or oligosaccharides. Starch supplements are better tolerated by breastfed infants than by formula fed infants.[43] Milk produced by nonhuman mammals does not contain amylase activity.[44]

Salivary amylase cleaves internal alpha 1–4 glucose bonds of starches to maltose, maltotriose, limit dextrin, and glucose. Salivary amylases can be detected in amniotic fluid as early as 16 weeks of gestation. Salivary amylase, ineffective at pH less than 3 and undigested in the stomach, may digest starches in the small intestine.[44,45] The effect of diet, weaning, or disease on salivary amylase is unknown.

Disaccharides

All brush-border glucosidases (sucrase, isomaltase, maltase, glucoamylase) are present in intestinal epithelium by 12 weeks of gestation, and 70% of adult activity is reached between the 26th and the 34th gestational weeks. Lactase activity is detectable as early as 12 weeks, but by 34 weeks the activity is 30% that of term infants.[46]

There is controversy over the efficiency of lactose digestion in premature infants. Salvage of lactose by-products occurs in the colon where bacteria ferment lactose and the resulting short chain fatty acids (SCFA) and alcohols are absorbed. Colonocytes use SCFA and alcohol as an energy source.[47]

Monosaccharides

Galactose, 50% of the monosaccharide present in lactose, is an important energy source in milk. After digestion by lactase, glucose and galactose are readily absorbed by the same carrier-mediated mechanism.[48] Greater than 90% of absorbed simple sugars reach the portal vein; galactose is converted in the liver to glycogen or glucose.[48]

The active transport of glucose can be detected as early as 11 weeks of gestation.[41] D-xylose or stable isotope tracers[48] show monosaccharide absorption is adequate and efficient in preterm and term infants while breath hydrogen testing shows up to 71%[49,50] of infants have monosaccharide malabsorption. Monosaccharide absorption is not a limiting factor in carbohydrate absorption. Table 2-3 summarizes the functional development of carbohydrate assimilation.

PROTEIN DIGESTION

Gastric acid can be detected in the stomachs of 16-week fetuses.[42] Premature infants produce less acid than fullterm infants, but maintain gastric pH of less than 4.[51] Hydrochloric acid production doubles between birth and 1 month of age and between 2 and 12 months. Postprandial intragastric pH in infants remains above 5 for extended periods of time. The underlying mechanism involves parietal cell tissue distribution (antrum only versus body and antrum) and submaximal secretory responses to neurohumoral stimuli, both of which do not fully mature until 3–8 months of postnatal age.[42] The gastric mucosa produces pepsinogens by week 16 of gestation.[42] At 29 weeks of gestation, postprandial production of pepsin is approximately 20% that of older infants and adults. Pepsin is inactivated by the alkaline gastric environment characteristic of the neonatal postprandial state. Thus, pepsin has a limited role in neonatal protein digestion. Trace amounts of hydrolyzed proteins can be detected in the stomach between postnatal 2 and 4 weeks.[52]

Pancreatic proteases are secreted as inactive zymogens. Mucosal enterokinase activates trypsinogen to trypsin, which in turn activates other proteases. Trypsin is the most important digestive protease, and it accounts for 20% of pancreatic fluid.[44] Peptidases can be detected in the fetal pancreas as early as 3 months of gestation.[42] Protease activity in pancreatic fluid increases after birth, in term and preterm infants alike.[40] Term and preterm infants have near-adult levels of trypsin in the duodenal lumen, whereas other peptidases are 60% or less of adult activity.[41]

Mucosal enzymes digest peptides produced by pancreatic enzymes. Enterokinase can be detected in intestinal mucosa by 24 weeks of gestation, with activity highest in the duodenum. This peptidase appears late in gestation and exhibits a slow postnatal increase. The intestinal brush border contains an assortment of specific amino acid transporters to facilitate the absorption. Little is known about their ontogeny in the ma-

Table 2-3 Carbohydrate digesting enzymes in the newborn.

Enzyme	*Location of action*	*Substrate*	*First detectable (wks gestation)*	*Preterm infant, at 30 wks, % of adult activity*	*Term newborn, % of adult activity*
Polysaccharides					
• Salivary amylase	stomach, small intestine?	Amylose (glc α 1-4 glc) poly	16	Nil	20
• Pancreatic amylase	Small intestine	Amylose (glc α 1-4 glc) poly	22	Nil	Nil
• Breast milk amylase	Stomach, small intestine?	Amylose (glc α 1-4 glc) poly	NA	NA	NA
Oligosaccharides					
• Maltase-glucoamylase	Small intestine	Glc (α 1-4) glc oligos (n2-9), malt-ose	10	70	50–100
• Sucrase-isomaltase	Small intestine	Amylopectin (α 1-6) polys, sucrose	10	70	100
• Lactase	Small intestine	Lactose	10	30	>100

glc = glucose; poly = polysaccharide; oligos = oligosaccharides; n2-9 = 2-9 residues; NA = not applicable.
Source: Hamosh M. Digestion in the newborn. *Clin Perinatol.* 1996;23(2):191–209. Reprinted with permission.

turing intestine; amino acid fluxes occur across intestinal mucosa of 12–18 week fetuses.[53]

The lack of adult enzyme activity does not appear to affect efficiency of protein digestion.[41] Studies using cow's milk with varying concentrations of protein found that neonates can absorb up to 1.95 g/kg/day and 4-month-old infants can absorb 3.75 g/kg/day.[41] Immunologically significant amounts of intact protein can be absorbed by preterm infants.[44] The intestine of term infants excludes immunologically significant amounts of protein. Table 2-4 summarizes the functional development of selected enzymes involved in protein digestion.

FAT DIGESTION

Fats provide 40–50% of caloric requirements of the neonate. Gastric lipase activity is present at 25 weeks of gestation, and can be found as early as 17 weeks. It reaches significant levels of activity by 27 weeks. Preterm infants have an effective secretion mechanism. It is difficult to differentiate gastric lipase activity from swallowed salivary lipase activity.[54]

Function and expression of gastric lipases are unaffected by mode of feeding.[55] However, gastric lipolysis may be 1.5 to 2.7 times as effective when neonates are fed breast milk versus cow's

Table 2-4 Development of protein digestion.

Factor	*Location*	*First detectable (week gestation)*	*Preterm infant, 30 wks, % adult activity*	*Term infant, % of adult activity*
Acid	Stomach	Birth	< 20?	< 30
Pepsin	Stomach	16	Trace	Trace
Trypsinogen	Duodenum			Adequate
Chymotrypsinogen	Duodenum			Adequate
Enterokinase	Intestinal brush border	24	20	25
Peptidases	Intestinal brush border	12	15	Adequate
Amino acid transport	Intestinal brush border	Not known	Not known	Adequate
Macromolecular absorption	Intestinal brush border	Not known	Not known	Adequate

Source: Lebenthal E, Leung YK. The impact of development of the gut on infant nutrition. *Pediatr Ann.* 1987;16(3):211. Reprinted with permission.

milk formula (Figure 2-1).[56] Pancreatic lipase is secreted by 30 weeks of gestation. Secretagogue release and responsiveness may determine lipase activity levels in duodenal fluid, and young infants do not have as brisk a release of secretagogues in response to dietary fat as older infants.[57,58] Small-for-gestational-age and preterm infants have lower pancreatic lipase activity compared to appropriate-for-gestational-age and term infants.[59]

Adult levels of intraluminal lipolysis develop by 1–2 months' postnatal age.[60] Pancreatic lipase activity increases as a function of postnatal age after reaching an *in utero* basal level by the 28th week of gestation.[57] Initial fat absorption may be as low as 60%, but reaches 90% by 1 month of postnatal age, for both fullterm and premature infants.[61] Breast milk is absorbed more completely.[61]

Bile Acids

Bile acids are necessary for the proper digestion of most dietary fats. The relative cholestasis in neonates,[62,63] small bile acid pool size, and immature ileal bile acid transport[64,65] contribute to inadequate duodenal micellar concentrations at birth.[66] Secondary bile acids are detected by 3 months' postnatal age, likely related to a maturing colonic flora.[67,68] Preterm infants 24–34 weeks gestational age fed human milk have critical micellar concentrations by 2 weeks postpartum. Regardless of gestation age, high ratios for both duodenal cholic acid to chenodeoxycholic acid and duodenal taurine to glycine conjugates respectively approached unity by 1–2 months postpartum.[68]

SELECTED MINERALS

Absorption of calcium in premature infants occurs primarily in the upper small intestine by either passive or vitamin D related active transport. Unless calcium concentrations in the lumen are particularly low, passive absorption dominates. Vitamin D regulated transport of calcium across the intestinal mucosa is not fully opera-

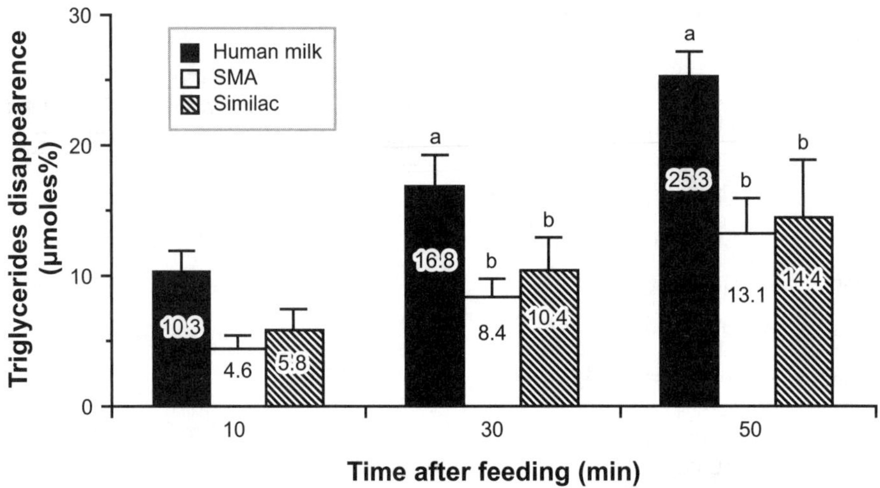

Figure 2-1 Differential lipolysis in the premature infant stomach. From Armand M, Hamosh M, Mehta NR, et al. Effect of milk or formula on gastric function and fat digestion in the premature infant. *Pediatr Res.* 1996;40(3):429–437. Reproduced with permission.

tional until near term.[69] Thus, calcium absorption in preterm infants is not significantly improved by vitamin D supplementation.

Vitamin D independent passive absorption of calcium is less effective when preterm infants are fed a lactose-free formula,[70] even though calcium absorption is enhanced by glucose-polymer containing fluids.[71] Lactose containing formulas are associated with better nitrogen absorption, magnesium and calcium retention, and fecal phosphorus excretion in both term and preterm infants.[72–74]

Magnesium absorption occurs via diffusion, solvent drag, and active transport.[75] Maximal absorption takes place in the distal small intestine.[76] Low birth weight infants are able to assimilate quantitatively similar amounts of magnesium from unsupplemented breast milk as they are from the placenta.[77]

Balance studies in human infants suggest that a developmental process underlies regulation of iron absorption and 3 cation transporters (DCT1 = Divalent Cation Transporter-1, DMT1 = Divalent Metal Transporter 1, and FPN1 = Ferroportin 1).[78,79] Expression patterns of DMT1 and FPN1 in rat duodenum suggest that negative feedback from iron stores develops later in infancy, and that early infancy may be characterized by a fixed flux of iron assimilation. These findings may be relevant to problems of ineffective or excessive iron supplementation in preterm and term infants, respectively.[79] However, interactions with other minerals, distribution along the intestine, and more specific maturational affects on regulation are not yet clear.

The mechanism by which zinc absorption takes place is not known. It is known that newborn animals absorb zinc to a higher degree than do older animals.

SELECTED VITAMINS

There is lack of detailed understanding of maturational processes that underlie vitamin assimilation. In the following sections, we highlight those for which more than minimal clinical data is available.

Vitamin B_{12}

Gastric intrinsic factor increases with postnatal age. Human milk haptocorrin, a vitamin B_{12} binding protein in human milk, can serve the same function as intrinsic factor.[80,81]

Vitamin D

At birth, relative hypocalcemia and elevated parathyroid hormone stimulate secretion of 1, 25 OH-vitamin D. Production of 25 OH-vitamin D is rate limiting in infants. There is no evidence that pharmacologic doses of vitamin D are necessary in the perinatal period.[82] The absorption pattern of isoforms of vitamin D in preterm infants are likely the same as term infants and older children.[83,84] Taurine-deficient diets in preterm infants are associated with decreased vitamin D absorption relative to term and or supplemented preterm infants.[85]

Vitamin E

Vitamin E is absorbed along the entire small intestine, but is preferentially taken up by proximal intestine. Intact micelle function is necessary for vitamin E absorption.[86] Prematurely born infants are generally considered to be vitamin E deficient, but a recent comprehensive analysis of both blood and tissue levels in 30-week-gestation neonates suggests that deficiency is not the rule.[87]

BACTERIAL FLORA

At birth, the intestine progresses from sterility to a mature and stable flora. Breast and formula fed infants develop different fecal flora. During the first days of life, the bacterial flora are heterogenous and independent of the feeding method.[88] Subsequently, lactic acid producing bifidobacteria dominate stools of breastfed infants.[89,90] Stools of formula fed infants contain bifidobacteria and *Enterbacteriaceae*. The latter exceeds the former by approximately 10 to 1,[88] but quantitative determinations of flora are controversial.[91]

Very-low-birth-weight infants and those with significant neonatal illness have profoundly altered intestinal flora because of antibiotic exposure and delay in enteral feeding. Bifidobacteria and *Lactobacillus* species are rarely identified.[92,93] Preterm infants acquire flora similar to fullterm breastfed infants by about 2 weeks.[94]

Oligosaccharides are a major component of breast milk, and they promote growth of bifidobacteria[91] to the exclusion of *Clostridia* species.[95] Studies of stools from preterm infants receiving prebiotics such as galacto- and fructo-oligosaccharides[96] and probiotics such as *bifidobacteria brev*[97] have sustained concentrations of bifidobacteria similar to stools of breastfed infants.

BREAST MILK EFFECTS ON GASTROINTESTINAL DEVELOPMENT

The composition of nutrients and other substances in breast milk support the nutritional needs of the infant during the period when some digestive and absorptive functions are not fully mature. In addition, breast milk contains a variety of bioactive substances and viable cells that may influence the maturation of neonatal digestive and immune function. These include digestive and antibacterial enzymes, growth factors, cytokines, immunoglobulins, and viable lymphocytes.

As an example, epidermal growth factor (EGF) and insulin-like growth factor (IGF-1) are secreted into breast milk in moderate quantities,[98] while colostrum may contain even higher concentrations.[99] Both factors are relatively resistant to intestinal degradation[98] and therefore are able to bind to their respective receptors on intestinal enterocytes.[100] *In vivo*[1,101–103] and *in vitro*[104–106] animal data indicate that organ growth and brush border enzyme expression is enhanced by these factors.

SUMMARY

The development of digestive function in the newborn term and preterm infant dictates how nutrition support is best accomplished in these patients. The full implications of these changes in gastrointestinal function have not been thoroughly worked out. Further work in the area of trophic enteric feeding for the promotion of intestinal growth and function will be necessary for optimal outcomes. As more is learned about the term and preterm gut, the practice of nutrition support will evolve. For instance, the robust gastric lipase activity available, even in preterm infants, may spawn new nutritional therapies in neonatal pancreatic insufficiency or alteration in enteric tube feeding strategies. Modulation of intestinal integrity, immune function, and digestive efficiency with exogenous growth factors or enteric peptide hormones is an active area of research that will continue to improve our ability to use specifically designed nutrition to optimize the health of young preterm and term infants.

REFERENCES

1. Trahair JF, Sangild PT. Fetal organ growth in response to oesophageal infusion of amniotic fluid, colostrum, milk or gastrin-releasing peptide: a study in fetal sheep. *Reprod, Fertil, & Dev.* 2000;12(1–2):87–95.
2. Bisset WM. Development of intestinal motility. *Arch Dis Child.* 1991;66(1 Spec No):3–5.
3. Trahair JF, Rodgers HF, Cool JC, Ford WD. Altered intestinal development after jejunal ligation in fetal sheep. *Virchows Arch—A Pathol Anat Histopathol.* 1993;423(1):45–50.
4. Trahair JF. Is fetal enteral nutrition important for normal gastrointestinal growth? A discussion. *JPEN.* 1993;17(1):82–85.
5. Daniels H, Devlieger H, Casaer P, Callens M, Eggermont E. Nutritive and non-nutritive sucking in preterm infants. *J Dev Physiol.* 1986;8(2):117–121.
6. Lebenthal E. Gastrointestinal maturation and motility patterns as indicators for feeding the premature infant. *Pediatrics.* 1995;95(2):207–209.
7. Premji SS, Paes B. Gastrointestinal function and growth in premature infants: is non-nutritive sucking vital? *J Perinatol.* 2000;20(1):46–53.
8. Omari TI, Barnett C, Snel A, et al. Mechanisms of gastroesophageal reflux in healthy premature infants. *J Pediatr.* 1998;133(5):650–654.
9. Omari TI, Benninga MA, Barnett CP, Haslam RR, Davidson GP, Dent J. Characterization of esophageal body and lower esophageal sphincter motor function in the very premature neonate. *J Pediatr.* 1999;135(4):517–521.
10. Liang J, Co E, Zhang M, Pineda J, Chen JD. Development of gastric slow waves in preterm infants measured by electrogastrography. *Am J Physiol.* 1998;274(3 Pt 1):G503–508.
11. Koenig WJ, Amarnath RP, Hench V, Berseth CL. Manometrics for preterm and term infants: a new tool for old questions. *Pediatrics.* 1995;95(2):203–206.
12. Baker JH, Berseth CL. Duodenal motor responses in preterm infants fed formula with varying concentrations and rates of infusion. *Pediatr Res.* 1997;42(5):618–622.
13. Hassan BB, Butler R, Davidson GP, et al. Patterns of antropyloric motility in fed healthy preterm infants. *Arch Dis Child Fetal & Neonatal Ed.* 2002;87(2):F95–99.
14. Macdonald PD, Skeoch CH, Carse H, et al. Randomized trial of continuous nasogastric, bolus nasogastric, and transpyloric feeding in infants of birth weight under 1400g. *Arch Dis Child.* 1992;67(4):429–431.
15. Costalos C, Russell G, Bistarakis L, Pangali A, Philippidou A. Effects of jaundice and phototherapy on gastric emptying in the newborn. *Biology of the Neonate.* 1984;46(2):57–60.
16. Gonzales I, Duryea EJ, Vasquez E, Geraghty N. Effect of enteral feeding temperature on feeding tolerance in preterm infants. *Neonatal Netw—J Neonatal Nurs.* 1995;14(3):39–43.
17. Riezzo G, Indrio F, Montagna O, et al. Gastric electrical activity and gastric emptying in preterm newborns fed standard and hydrolysate formulas. *J Pediatr Gastroenterol Nutr.* 2001;33(3):290–295.
18. Bueno L, Fioramonti J. Neurohormonal control of intestinal transit. *Reprod Nutr Dev.* 1994;34(6):513–525.
19. McClure RJ, Newell SJ. Randomized controlled trial of trophic feeding and gut motility. *Arch Dis Child Fetal & Neonatal Ed.* 1999;80(1):F54–58.
20. Weaver LT, Lucas A. Development of bowel habit in preterm infants. *Arch Dis Child.* 1993;68(3 Spec No):317–320.
21. Lucas A, Bloom SR, Green AA. Gastrointestinal peptides and the adaptation to extrauterine nutrition. *Can J Physiol Pharmacol.* 1985;63(5):527–537.
22. Aynsley-Green A. The endocrinology of feeding in the newborn. *Baillieres Clin Endocrinol Metab.* 1989;3(3):837–868.
23. Shulman DI, Kanarek K. Gastrin, motilin, insulin, and insulin-like growth factor-I concentrations in very-low-birth-weight infants receiving enteral or parenteral nutrition. *JPEN.* 1993;17(2):130–133.
24. Salmenpera L, Perheentupa J, Siimes MA, Adrian TE, Bloom SR, Aynsley-Green A. Effects of feeding regimen on blood glucose levels and plasma concentrations of pancreatic hormones and gut regulatory peptides at 9 months of age: comparison between infants fed with milk formula and infants exclusively breastfed from birth. *J Pediatr Gastroenterol Nutr.* 1988;7(5):651–656.
25. Aynsley-Green A, Bloom SR, Williamson DH, Turner RC. Endocrine and metabolic response in the human newborn to first feed of breast milk. *Arch Dis Child.* 1977;52(4):291–295.

26. Berseth CL, Nordyke CK, Valdes MG, Furlow BL, Go VL. Responses of gastrointestinal peptides and motor activity to milk and water feedings in preterm and term infants. *Ped Res.* 1992;31(6):587–590.

27. Lucas A, Bloom SR, Aynsley-Green A. Metabolic and endocrine consequences of depriving preterm infants of enteral nutrition. *Acta Paediatr Scand.* 1983;72(2):245–249.

28. Lucas A, Adrian TE, Christofides N, Bloom SR, Aynsley-Green A. Plasma motilin, gastrin, and enteroglucagon and feeding in the human newborn. *Arch Dis Child.* 1980;55(9):673–677.

29. Milner RD, Minoli I, Moro G, Rubecz I, Whitfield MF, Assan R. Growth and metabolic and hormonal profiles during transpyloric and nasogastric feeding in preterm infants. *Acta Paediatr Scand.* 1981;70(1):9–13.

30. Uvnas-Moberg K, Widstrom AM, Marchini G, Winberg J. Release of GI hormones in mother and infant by sensory stimulation. *Acta Paediatr Scand.* 1987;76(6):851–860.

31. Knodell RG. Effects of formula composition on hepatic and intestinal drug metabolism during enteral nutrition. *JPEN.* 1990;14(1):34–38.

32. Mannering GJ. Drug metabolism in the newborn. *Fed Proc.* 1985;44(7):2302–2308.

33. Strassburg CP, Strassburg A, Kneip S, et al. Developmental aspects of human hepatic drug glucuronidation in young children and adults. *Gut.* 2002;50(2):259–265.

34. Jorquera F, Culebras JM, Gonzalez-Gallego J. Influence of nutrition on liver oxidative metabolism. *Nutrition.* 1996;12(6):442–447.

35. Walter-Sack I, Klotz U. Influence of diet and nutritional status on drug metabolism. *Clin Pharmacokinet.* 1996;31(1):47–64.

36. Knodell RG, Steele NM, Cerra FB, Gross JB, Solomon TE. Effects of parenteral and enteral hyperalimentation on hepatic drug metabolism in the rat. *J Pharmacol & Exp Ther.* 1984;229(2):589–597.

37. Tranvouez JL, Lerebours E, Chretien P, Fouin-Fortunet H, Colin R. Hepatic antipyrine metabolism in malnourished patients: influence of the type of malnutrition and course after nutritional rehabilitation. *Am J Clin Nutr.* 1985;41(6):1257–1264.

38. Knodell RG, Wood DG, Guengerich FP. Selective alteration of constitutive hepatic cytochrome P-450 enzymes in the rat during parenteral hyperalimentation. *Biochem Pharmacol.* 1989;38(19):3341–3345.

39. Pantuck EJ, Weissman C, Pantuck CB, Lee YJ. Effects of parenteral amino acid nutritional regimens on oxidative and conjugative drug metabolism. *Anesth Analg.* 1989;69(6):727–731.

40. Lebenthal E, Lee PC. Development of functional responses in human exocrine pancreas. *Pediatrics.* 1980;66(4):556–560.

41. Lebenthal E, Leung YK. The impact of development of the gut on infant nutrition. *Pediat Ann.* 1987;16(3):211.

42. Menard D. Development of human intestinal and gastric enzymes. *Acta Paediatr Suppl.* 1994;405:1–6.

43. Hamosh M. Digestion in the premature infant: the effects of human milk. *Semin Perinatol.* 1994;18(6):485–494.

44. Hamosh M. Digestion in the newborn. *Clin Perinatol.* 1996;23(2):191–209.

45. Lebenthal E. Role of salivary amylase in gastric and intestinal digestion of starch. *Dig Dis Sci.* 1987;32(10):1155–1157.

46. Lebenthal A, Lebenthal E. The ontogeny of the small intestinal epithelium. *JPEN.* 1999;23(5 suppl):S3–6.

47. Kien CL, McClead RE, Cordero L, Jr. Effects of lactose intake on lactose digestion and colonic fermentation in preterm infants. *J Pediatr.* 1998;133(3):401–405.

48. Kien CL. Digestion, absorption, and fermentation of carbohydrates in the newborn. *Clin Perinatol.* 1996;23(2):211–228.

49. Nobigrot T, Chasalow FI, Lifshitz F. Carbohydrate absorption from one serving of fruit juice in young children: age and carbohydrate composition effects. *J Am Coll Nutr.* 1997;16(2):152–158.

50. Kneepkens CM, Vonk RJ, Fernandes J. Incomplete intestinal absorption of fructose. *Arch Dis Child.* 1984;59(8):735–738.

51. Kelly EJ, Brownlee KG, Newell SJ. Gastric secretory function in the developing human stomach. *Early Hum Dev.* 1992;31(2):163–166.

52. Mason S. Some aspects of gastric function in the newborn. *Arch Dis Child.* 1962;37:387.

53. Malo C. Multiple pathways for amino acid transport in brush border membrane vesicles isolated from the human fetal small intestine. *Gastroenterology.* 1991;100(6):1644–1652.

54. Manson WG, Weaver LT. Fat digestion in the neonate. *Arch Dis Child Fetal & Neonatal Ed.* 1997;76(3):F206–211.

55. Mehta NR, Liao TH, Hamosh M, Smith YF, Hamosh P. Effect of total parenteral nutrition on lipase activity in the stomach of very low birth weight infants. *Biol Neonate.* 1988;53(5):261–266.

56. Armand M, Hamosh M, Mehta NR, et al. Effect of human milk or formula on gastric function and fat digestion in the premature infant. *Pediatr Res.* 1996;40(3):429–437.

57. Boehm G, Bierbach U, Senger H, et al. Postnatal adaptation of lipase- and trypsin-activities in duodenal juice of premature infants appropriate for gestational age. *Biomed Biochim Acta.* 1990;49(5):369–373.

58. Githens S. Postnatal maturation of the exocrine pancreas in mammals. *J Pediatr Gastroenterol Nutr.* 1990;10(2):160–163.

59. Hernell O, Blackberg L. Molecular aspects of fat digestion in the newborn. *Acta Paediatr Suppl.* 1994;405:65–69.

60. Manson WG, Coward WA, Harding M, Weaver LT. Development of fat digestion in infancy. *Arch Dis Child Fetal & Neonatal Ed.* 1999;80(3):F183–187.

61. Jarvenpaa AL. Feeding the low-birth-weight infant. IV: fat absorption as a function of diet and duodenal bile acids. *Pediatrics.* 1983;72(5):684–689.

62. Niijima S. Studies on the conjugating activity of bile acids in children. *Pediatr Res.* 1985;19(3):302–307.

63. Heubi JE, Balistreri WF, Suchy FJ. Bile salt metabolism in the first year of life. *J Lab Clin Med.* 1982;100(1):127–136.

64. de Belle RC, Vaupshas V, Vitullo BB, et al. Intestinal absorption of bile salts: immature development in the neonate. *J Pediatr.* 1979;94(3):472–476.

65. Acra SA, Ghishan FK. Active bile salt transport in the ileum: characteristics and ontogeny. *J Pediatr Gastroenterol Nutr.* 1990;10(4):421–425.

66. Hamosh M. Lipid metabolism in premature infants. *Biol Neonate.* 1987;52(suppl 1):50–64.

67. Hammons JL, Jordan WE, Stewart RL, Taulbee JD, Berg RW. Age and diet effects on fecal bile acids in infants. *J Pediatr Gastroenterol & Nutr.* 1988;7(1):30–38.

68. Boehm G, Braun W, Moro G, Minoli I. Bile acid concentrations in serum and duodenal aspirates of healthy preterm infants: effects of gestational and postnatal age. *Biol Neonate.* 1997;71(4):207–214.

69. Bronner F, Salle BL, Putet G, Rigo J, Senterre J. Net calcium absorption in premature infants: results of 103 metabolic balance studies. *Am J Clin Nutr.* 1992;56(6):1037–1044.

70. Moya M, Cortes E, Ballester MI, Vento M, Juste M. Short term polycose substitution for lactose reduces calcium absorption in healthy term babies. *J Pediatr Gastroenterol Nutr.* 1992;14(1):57–61.

71. Stathos TH, Shulman RJ, Schanler RJ, Abrams SA. Effect of carbohydrates on calcium absorption in premature infants. *Pediatr Res.* 1996;39(4 Pt 1):666–670.

72. Moya M, Lifschitz C, Ameen V, Euler AR. A metabolic balance study in term infants fed lactose-containing or lactose-free formula. *Acta Paediatr.* 1999;88(11):1211–1215.

73. Lonnerdal B. Bioavailability of copper. *Am J Clin Nutr.* 1996;63(5):821S–829S.

74. Stack T, Aggett PJ, Aitken E, Lloyd DJ. Routine L-ascorbic acid supplementation does not alter iron, copper, and zinc balance in low-birth-weight infants fed a cows'-milk formula. *J Pediatr Gastroenterol Nutr.* 1990;10(3):351–356.

75. Kayne LH, Lee DB. Intestinal magnesium absorption. *Miner Electrolyte Metab.* 1993;19(4–5):210–217.

76. Hardwick LL, Jones MR, Brautbar N, Lee DB. Site and mechanism of intestinal magnesium absorption. *Miner Electrolyte Metabol.* 1990;16(2–3):174–180.

77. Schanler RJ, Rifka M. Calcium, phosphorus and magnesium needs for the low-birth-weight infant. *Acta Paediatr Suppl.* 1994;405:111–116.

78. Gunshin H, Mackenzie B, Berger UV, et al. Cloning and characterization of a mammalian proton-coupled metal-ion transporter. *Nature.* 1997;388(6641):482–488.

79. Leong WI, Bowlus CL, Tallkvist J, Lonnerdal B. Iron supplementation during infancy—effects on expression of iron transporters, iron absorption, and iron utilization in rat pups. *Am J Clinical Nutr.* 2003;78(6):1203–1211.

80. Adkins Y, Lonnerdal B. Mechanisms of vitamin B(12) absorption in breastfed infants. *J Pediatr Gastroenterol Nutr.* 2002;35(2):192–198.

81. Greer FR. Are breastfed infants vitamin K deficient? *Adv Exp Med Biol.* 2001;501:391–395.

82. Salle BL, Delvin EE, Lapillonne A, Bishop NJ, Glorieux FH. Perinatal metabolism of vitamin D. *Am J Clin Nutr.* 2000;71(5 Suppl):1317S–124S.

83. Kovar IZ, Mayne PD, James JJ, Barnes IC. Oral administration of active vitamin D metabolites to low birthweight infants. *Arch Dis Child.* 1986;61(8):795–797.

84. Hollis BW, Lowery JW, Pittard WB III, Guy DG, Hansen JW. Effect of age on the intestinal absorption of vitamin D3-palmitate and nonesterified vitamin D2 in the term human infant. *J Clin Endocrinol Metab.* 1996;81(4):1385–1388.

85. Zamboni G, Piemonte G, Bolner A, et al. Influence of dietary taurine on vitamin D absorption. *Acta Paediatr.* 1993;82(10):811–815.

86. Sokol RJ, Heubi JE, Iannaccone S, Bove KE, Balistreri WF. Mechanism causing vitamin E deficiency during chronic childhood cholestasis. *Gastroenterology.* 1983;85(5):1172–1182.

87. Kaempf DE, Linderkamp O. Do healthy premature infants fed breast milk need vitamin E supplementation: alpha- and gamma-tocopherol levels in blood components and buccal mucosal cells. *Pediatr Res.* 1998;44(1):54–59.

88. Yoshioka H, Iseki K, Fujita K. Development and differences of intestinal flora in the neonatal period in breastfed and bottle fed infants. *Pediatrics.* 1983;72(3):317–321.

89. Edwards CA, Parrett AM. Intestinal flora during the first months of life: new perspectives. *British J Nutr.* 2002;88(suppl 1):S11–18.

90. Iseki K. [Development of intestinal flora in neonates]. *Hokkaido Igaku Zasshi—Hokkaido J Med Sci.* 1987;62(6):895–906.

91. Mountzouris KC, McCartney AL, Gibson GR. Intestinal microflora of human infants and current trends for its nutritional modulation. *British J Nutr.* 2002;87(5):405–420.

92. Fanaro SCR, Guerrini P, Vigi V. Intestinal microflora in early infancy: composition and development. *Acta Paediatr.* 2003;91(441):48–55.

93. Dai D, Walker WA. Protective nutrients and bacterial colonization in the immature human gut. *Adv Pediatr.* 1999;46:353–382.

94. Sakata H, Yoshioka H, Fujita K. Development of the intestinal flora in very low birth weight infants compared to normal full-term newborns. *Eur J Pediatr.* 1985;144(2):186–190.

95. Butel MJ, Waligora-Dupriet AJ, Szylit O. Oligofructose and experimental model of neonatal necrotising enterocolitis. *British J Nutr.* 2002;87(suppl 2):S213–219.

96. Boehm G FS, Jelinek J, Stahl B, Marini A. Prebiotic concept for infant nutrition. *Acta Paediatr.* 2003;91(441):64–67.

97. Kitajima H, Sumida Y, Tanaka R, Yuki N, Takayama H, Fujimura M. Early administration of *Bifidobacterium breve* to preterm infants: randomised controlled trial. *Arch Dis Child Fetal & Neonatal Ed.* 1997;76(2):F101–107.

98. Lonnerdal B. Nutritional and physiologic significance of human milk proteins. *Am J Clin Nutr.* 2003;77(6):1537S–1543S.

99. Xu RJ. Development of the newborn GI tract and its relation to colostrum/milk intake: a review. *Reprod, Fertil, & Dev.* 1996;8(1):35–48.

100. Menard D, Pothier P. Radioautographic localization of epidermal growth factor receptors in human fetal gut. *Gastroenterology.* 1991;101(3):640–649.

101. Carver JD, Barness LA. Trophic factors for the gastrointestinal tract. *Clin Perinatol.* 1996;23(2):265–285.

102. Ma L, Xu RJ. Oral insulinlike growth factor-I stimulates intestinal enzyme maturation in newborn rats. *Life Sci.* 1997;61(1):51–58.

103. Young GP, Taranto TM, Jonas HA, Cox AJ, Hogg A, Werther GA. Insulin-like growth factors and the developing and mature rat small intestine: receptors and biological actions. *Digestion.* 1990;46(suppl 2):240–252.

104. Oguchi S, Shinohara K, Yamashiro Y, Walker WA, Sanderson IR. Growth factors in breast milk and their effect on gastrointestinal development. *Chung-Hua Min Kuo Hsiao Erh Ko i Hsueh Hui Tsa Chih.* 1997;38(5):332–337.

105. Hirai C, Ichiba H, Saito M, Shintaku H, Yamano T, Kusuda S. Trophic effect of multiple growth factors in amniotic fluid or human milk on cultured human fetal small intestinal cells. *J Pediatr Gastroenterol Nutr.* 2002;34(5):524–528.

106. Ichiba H, Kusuda S, Itagane Y, Fujita K, Issiki G. Measurement of growth promoting activity in human milk using a fetal small intestinal cell line. *Biol Neonate.* 1992;61(1):47–53.

Chapter 3

Mucosal Immunity

Sue J. Rhee, Pearay L. Ogra, and W. Allan Walker

INTRODUCTION

In mammals, epithelial surfaces of the respiratory tract, gastrointestinal (GI) tract, and to a smaller extent, the genitorurinary tract are the primary portals for most infectious organisms, food products, dietary antigens and a multitude of other environmental macromolecules. The immune mechanisms of defense operating at these portals represent a complex but elegant network of specialized tissues and cells collectively referred to as the "common mucosal immune system." The mucosal mechanisms of defense identified to date include *nonspecific barriers* and specific components of *innate* and *adaptive immunity*.

The *nonspecific barriers* include gastrointestinal digestive enzymes, gastric acid pH, mucin glycoproteins, trefoil factors, and defensins.[1–5]

The effector mechanisms involved in the expression of *innate immunity* include several antimicrobial peptides, phagocytic cells, neutrophils, and complement activation pathways. The host structures of innate immunity directed against recognition of pathogens are referred to as pathogen recognition receptors (PRR). These receptors belong to several structural protein families. The best characterized are the toll-like receptors (TLR). Other receptors of innate immune function include proteins with leucine-rich repeat domains, calcium dependent lectin domains, and scavenger receptor protein domains. Available evidence suggests that innate immunity plays an important role in defense against pathogenic bacterial and viral infections. Innate immunity appears to be involved in the release of inflammatory cytokines and the development of adaptive immune responses. Furthermore, innate immune mechanisms, especially TLRs, provide the host mucosa with unique abilities to distinguish different pathogen-associated molecular patterns and at the same time contribute to the development of antigen-specific T and B cell responses.

The components of *adaptive immunity* in the mucosal immune system include distinct anatomic structures such as M cells, dendritic cells, macrophages, and lymphoid elements in the epithelium, as well as the mucosa associated lymphoid follicles and the lamina propria.

This chapter will provide a broad overview of the components of mucosal defense during physiologic and pathologic states in the human gastrointestinal tract, with special emphasis on nutrition (Figure 3-1).

NONSPECIFIC MECHANISMS OF DEFENSE

Mucin Glycoproteins

Mucin glycoproteins consist of a protein skeleton coated with a complex array of oligosaccharides. They are produced by goblet cells

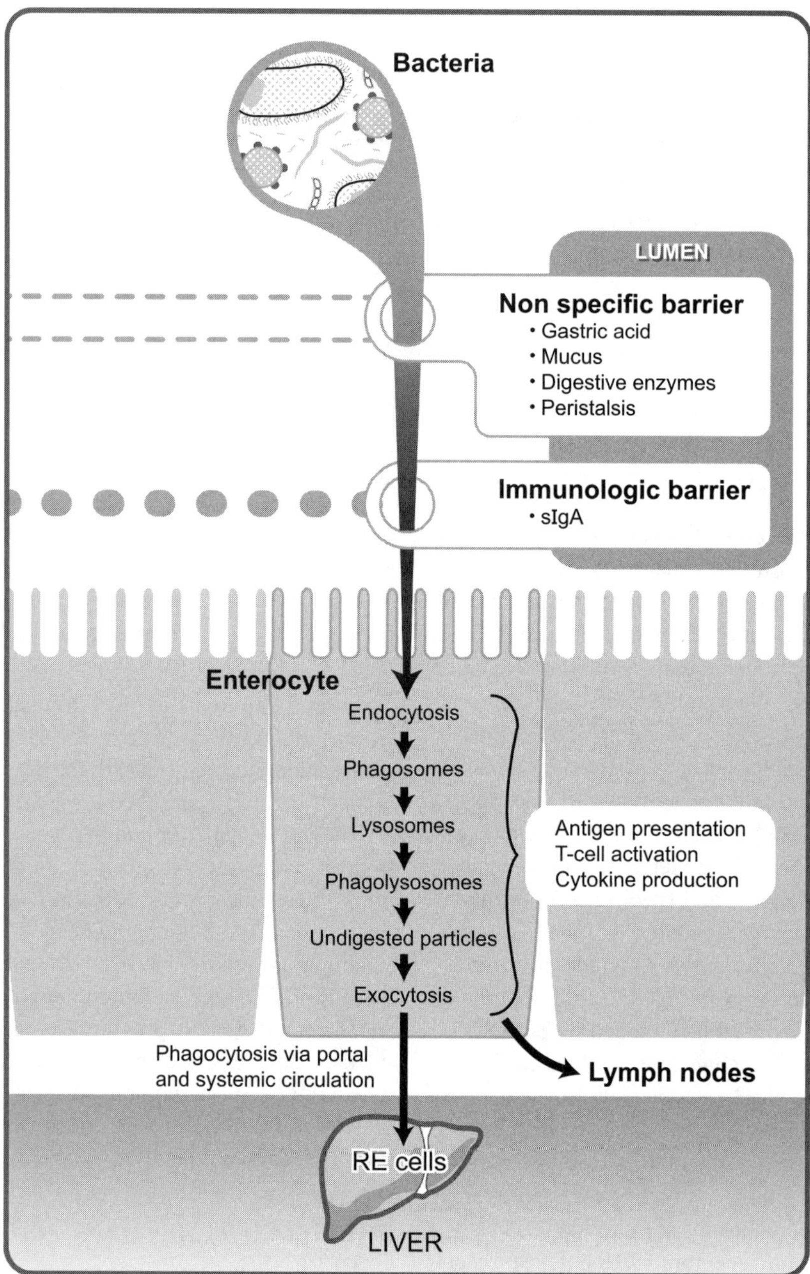

Figure 3-1 Nonimmunologic and immunologic components of the first line of gastrointestinal defense against noxious luminal stimuli. Microbes and foreign antigens can be controlled within the lumen by nonspecific gut components (e.g., mucin, etc.) or immunologic factors (e.g., sIgA). Alternatively, the enterocyte and its tight junctions provide a physical barrier for penetration of these substances or can release immune components (e.g., cytokines, etc.) that signal lymphoid cells to respond against their invasion. SIgA = Secretory IgA, RE = Reticuloendothelial

and provide a thick protective coat for the epithelium.[6,7] Particles and potential pathogens become entrapped in this sticky, viscoelastic layer and are expelled (Figure 3-2).[8]

Many mucin producing genes have been identified, and they are differentially expressed at mucosal surfaces.[9] Variation occurs in the amount of mucin produced. In the GI tract, the mucous

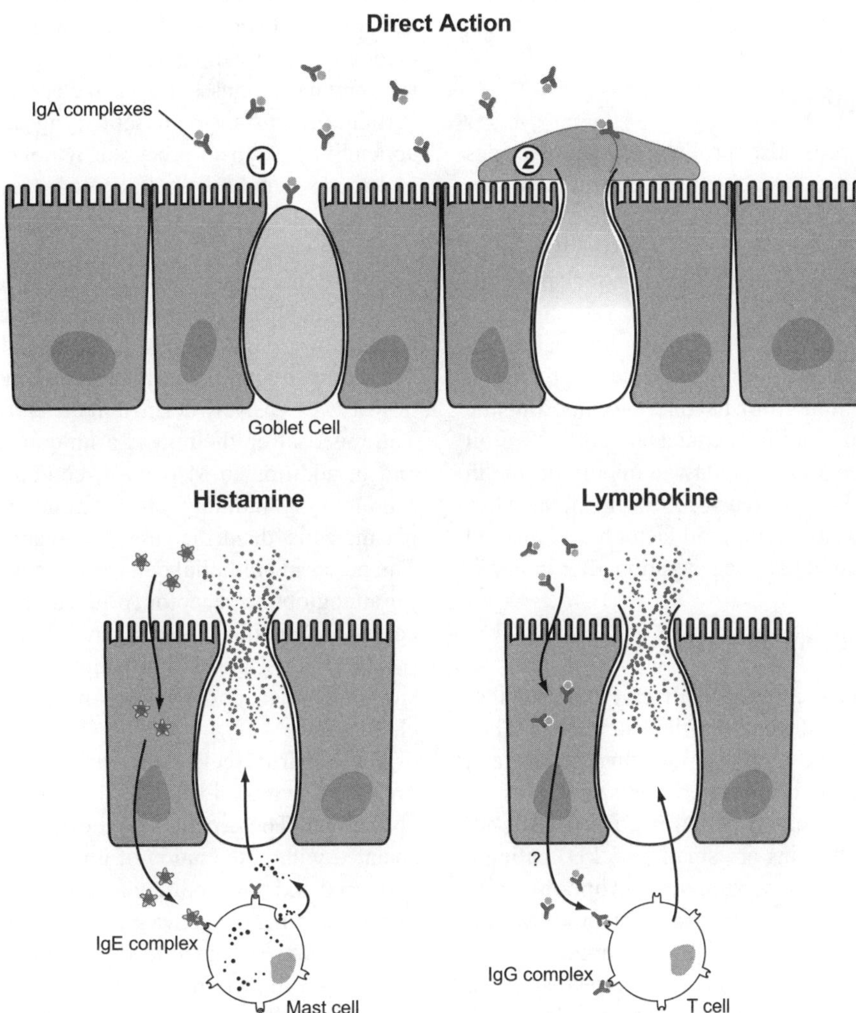

Figure 3-2 Immune complexes cause a *direct* release of mucin from goblet cells, which coat the mucosal surface and form a physical barrier to intestinal allergens. Alternatively, antigens (allergens) can be taken up by enterocytes and form either IgE-allergen complexes or absorbed IgG-allergen complexes. IgE-allergen complexes trigger mast cells to release biologically active substances, which, in turn, trigger mucin release. Absorbed IgG-allergen complexes activate T cells, releasing cytokines, which also can trigger mucus release.

blanket is thickest in the stomach and colon.[10,11] The cells least protected by mucus are the M cells, specialized epithelial cells located on the domes of Peyer's patches.[12] M cells sample luminal antigen and deliver them to underlying lymphoid tissues. Mucin gene expression can be up regulated by probiotics such as *Lactobacillus*.[13] This increase in mucin production prevents adherence of enteropathogens.[14]

Trefoil Peptides

Goblet cells also produce trefoil peptides that are found throughout the GI tract and distributed in a region-specific manner. They are highly conserved and share a distinctive motif of 6 cysteine residues that form intrachain loops held together by disulfide bonds, a structure that protects them from digestion by luminal proteases.[15] These peptides play a role in protecting the epithelium from bacterial toxins, but the mechanism is not fully characterized.[16,17] Trefoil peptides are known to play an important role in intestinal epithelial repair following injury. Mice lacking the intestinal trefoil factor have impaired mucosal healing and regeneration after injury.[18]

Paneth Cells and Defensins

Paneth cells are a specialized type of epithelial cell derived from intestinal stem cells. They are located at the base of intestinal crypts, and when stimulated by bacteria or bacterial products, produce antimicrobial peptides called defensins. Defensins are small (3-6 kD) cationic molecules with separated hydrophobic and charged regions.[19] This arrangement allows for insertion into phospholipid membranes, where they assemble to form a pore, thereby disrupting membrane function and effecting cell death.[20]

Defensins preferentially disrupt microbial membranes because they are rich in negatively charged phospholipids in contrast to human cell membranes that have a lower anionic content.[21] Defensins also exert antimicrobial effects via membrane depolarization, disruption of bacterial energy metabolism, and promotion of the adaptive immune response.[22,23] Paneth cells also secrete lysozyme and phospholipase A2, both of which have antimicrobial activity.[24]

INNATE AND ADAPTIVE MUCOSAL IMMUNE SYSTEM

The organized lymphoid follicles in the GI and bronchial subepithelial regions are considered to be the principal inductive sites of mucosal immune responses. It is also clear that under certain circumstances, nasopharyngeal tonsils, appendix, peritoneal precursor lymphoid cells, and rectal lymphoepithelial tissue (rectal tonsils) may also serve as inductive sites of local immune responses.[6,25]

The common features of all inductive mucosal sites include an epithelial surface containing M cells overlying organized lymphoid follicles. Their ultrastructural and functional characteristics were extensively defined in the early 1970s. The mucosal epithelium is a unique structure and in addition to M cells, it contains mucin producing glandular cells, lymphocytes and plasma cells, dendritic cells, and macrophages. The mucosal epithelial cells express polymeric immunoglobulin receptor (pIgR) and secretory component, major histocompatability complex (MHC) class I and II molecules, other adhesion molecules, and a variety of cytokines and chemokines.

The dendritic cells are present both in the organized lymphoid tissues and the mucosal epithelium. These cells have been strongly associated with potentiation of immune response, enhanced antigen capture via induction of TLR, and development of active immunity. Other studies have suggested that dendritic cells may also enhance the induction of mucosal tolerance in *in vivo* settings. Recent observations have suggested that dendritic cells are potent antigen presenting cells (APC) and are critical in initiating primary immune responses, graft rejection, autoimmune disease, and generation of T cell dependent B cell responses. The APC function is attributed in part to their ability to express costimulatory molecules (CD 80, CD 86), TLR, and other accessory ligands necessary for induction of immune response or induction of tolerance.[2,4,5]

The M cells are important in luminal uptake, transport, processing, and to a smaller extent, in the presentation of mucosally introduced antigens. The M cells appear to be critical in transport of luminal antigens and entry of organisms such as reovirus, poliovirus, rotavirus, and salmonella into the human host. M cell-mediated antigen uptake is characteristically associated with the development of secretary IgA responses.

The luminal appearance of SIgA in mucosal secretions results from transcytosis of polymeric IgA (pIgA) across mucosal epithelium via binding to the pIgR. The receptor is eventually cleaved, resulting in association of pIgA with a substantial part of PigR receptor. The complex of IgA and PigR is generally referred to as SIgA.

Following exposure to an antigen and its uptake via the M cells, there is a variable degree of activation of T cells, dendritic cells, and B cells, especially of the IgA isotype, (Figure 3-3). The interaction of lymphocytes with mucosal epithelium is important in differentiation of some segments of mucosal epithelium into M cells. Activation of T cells results in the release of a number of distinct cytokines or chemokines from different T cell subsets, and recognition of antigenic epitopes

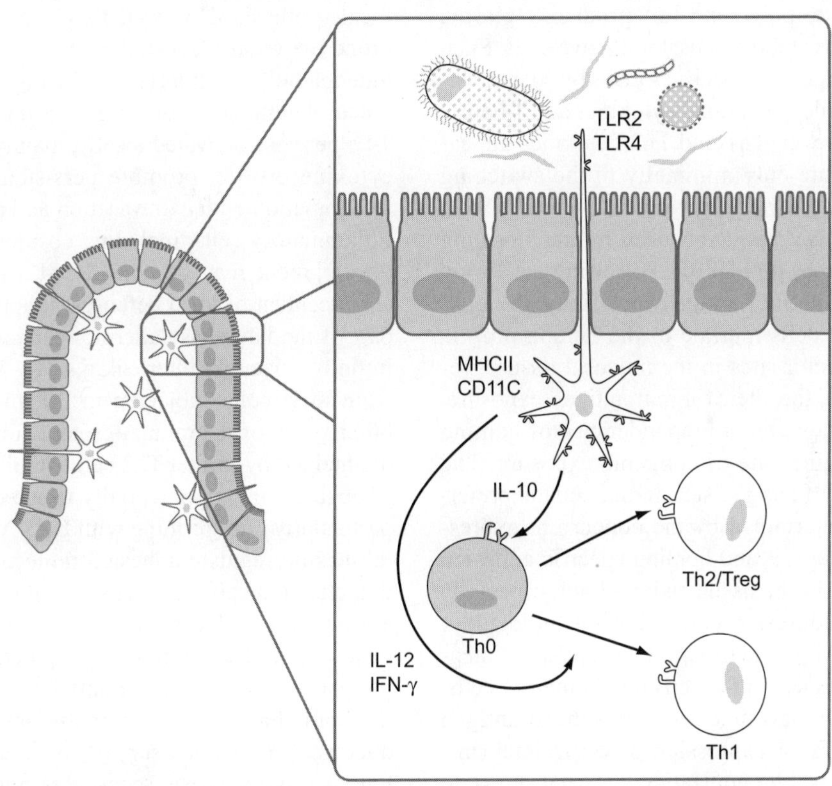

Figure 3-3 Professional antigen-presenting cells (dendritic cells) in the lamina propria can extend appendages between epithelial cells into the lumen in order to sample pathogen-associated molecular patterns (PAMPs) on microbes and food antigens via receptors such as toll-like receptors (TLR2 and TLR4). This stimulates cytokines that control T-helper cell responses (Th1 versus Th2) after antigen presentation. Treg = T regulatory cells, IFN = Interferon

involving MHC class I or II molecules. Both T cell activation and release of specific cytokines are involved in the eventual process of B cell activation, isotype switching, and specific integrin expression on antigen-sensitized B cells. Both Th1 and Th2 cells appear to benefit the development of SIgA responses. Th2 cytokines (IL-4, IL-5, IL-6, IL-9, IL-10, IL-13) are thought to be of significant help in antibody production. Secretory IgA antibody response is also enhanced by immunologic adjuvants such as cholera toxin, which results in polarized Th2 cell response.[26] Secretory IgA antibody response may also be induced through Th1 cytokines (IL-2, uterferon (IFNγ)) as shown with studies on intracellular pathogens such as salmonella.

It appears that the process of isotype switching of B cells to polymeric IgA producing plasma cells begins at the mucosal inductive sites. Such switching requires specific signals by costimulating molecules, including cytokines and T-helper cells. However, Th1 and Th2 cytokines appear to contribute only minimally to the switching of B cells to surface IgA-positive B cells. Such switching is greatly enhanced by transforming growth factor-β (TGF-β). Following activation and acquisition of antigen specificity, the IgA-producing cells migrate to the lamina propria of the effector sites in the mucosal tissues, regardless of the site of initial antigen exposure. There is, however, a preponderance of homing to the original site of antigenic exposure. The migration of antigen sensitizing cells is preferentially determined by the concurrent expression of integrins and homing specific adhesion molecules in the tissue endothelium, especially mucosal addressin cell adhesion molecule-1 (MAdCAM-1) and the specific receptors (integrins) expressed on the activated lymphoid cells. Oral (intestinal) mucosal exposure to antigen seems to favor expression of $\alpha 4\beta 7$ integrins, and intranasal immunization has been shown to induce expression of L-selectin as well as $\alpha 4\beta 7$ integrins. However, systemic immunization is generally restricted to the expression of L-selectin. The antigen-sensitized B cells undergo terminal differentiation in the mucosal lamina propria to IgA producing plasma cells. Such differentiation involves interaction with a variety of cytokines and T cell subsets.[6,25] Recently, an alternate pathway has been proposed for the switch of IgM B cells. It has been suggested that IgM B cells in the lamina propria can switch to production of IgA isotype without the need for T cell help.[4]

Locally produced IgA consists mainly of J chain-containing dimers and the larger polymeric IgA that is selectively transported through epithelial cells by the polymeric Ig receptor. The resulting secretory IgA molecules are designed to participate in immune exclusion and other immunologic functions at the mucosal surface. IgG also contributes to such surface defense. It often reaches the secretions by passive diffusion from the blood stream and, less frequently, by local synthesis. However, its proinflammatory properties render IgG antibodies of potential immunopathologic importance when IgA mediated mucosal elimination of antigens is unsuccessful. T-helper cells activated locally, mainly by a Th2 cytokine profile, promote persistent mucosal inflammation with extravasation and priming of inflammatory cells, including eosinophils. This development may be considered a pathologic enhancement of local defenses. It appears to be part of the late phase allergic reaction, perhaps initially driven by interleukin 4 (IL-4) released from mast cells subjected to IgE mediated or other types of degranulation and subsequently maintained by further Th2 cell stimulation.

Eosinophils are potentially tissue damaging, particularly after priming with IL-5. Various cytokines up regulate adhesion molecules on endothelial and epithelial cells, thereby enhancing accumulation of eosinophils and, in addition, resulting in aberrant immune regulation within the epithelium.[6,25] Soluble antigens available at the epithelial surfaces normally appear to induce various immunosuppressive mechanisms, but such homeostasis seems less potent in the airways than the induction of systemic hyporesponsiveness to dietary antigens operating in the gastrointestinal tract. Numerous cytokines and chemokines have been shown to be intimately involved in the induction and maintenance of mucosal immune responses and the level of mucosal inflammation during infections and exposure to environmental agents.

MUCOSAL IMMUNE RESPONSES AND NUTRITION

Over the past several decades, as there has been an increasing understanding of the mucosal immune system, it has become evident that nutrition plays a significant role in influencing the mucosal immune response. More specifically, factors such as malnutrition, route of admnistration, breast milk, probiotics, and specific nutritional components such as glutamine, vitamin A, zinc, and fatty acids have effects on different aspects of the mucosal immune response.

Route of Nutrition

Patients receiving total enteral nutrition (EN) compared to those receiving total parenteral nutrition (PN) after moderate to severe abdominal surgery had a lower incidence of abdominal abscesses and pneumonia[27,28]and fewer line infections.[28] A meta-analysis of 8 prospective randomized trials comparing early enteral and parenteral feeding in surgical patients demonstrated that enterally fed patients had fewer septic complications than parenterally fed patients.[28]

Patients who received enteral feeds immediately following surgery compared to patients who received enteral feeds 5 days after surgery had significantly less sepsis and lower intra-abdominal infection and fewer episodes of pneumonia.[29]

Histologic examination of intestinal tissue from both animals and humans receiving PN revealed that the lymphocyte population was decreased in the lamina propria, Peyer's patches, and in the number of intraepithelial lymphocytes.[30–32] The CD4 and CD8 ratio (2:1) remained stable within the Peyer's patches, but there was a significant decrease (to 1:1) in the laminal propria with PN.[32]

Intraluminal gastrointestinal IgA levels and respiratory tract IgA decreased with PN, reaching a nadir after 4 to 5 days.[32,33] The administration of PN solution delivered into the stomach also caused atrophy of gut-associated lymphoid tissue (GALT) and a decreased CD4:CD8 ratio when compared to a complex enteral diet.[34] The changes were entirely reversible once enteral feeding was reinstituted.[35] These observations suggest that enteral nutrition may affect mucosal immunity by altering the lymphocyte population and IgA production in the intestine.

Parenteral Nutrition: Effects on Cytokines and Endothelial Adhesion Markers

The route of nutrition has an effect on the production of cytokines and adhesion molecules.

The interaction and balance between Th1 and Th2 cytokines affects the levels of IgA produced in the small intestine. The Th1 cytokines, IFNγ and Tissue Necrosis Factor (TNF)β down-regulate IgA production, whereas the Th2 cytokines IL-4, IL-5, and IL-10 up regulate IgA production by causing SIgA- B cells in Peyer's patches to switch to SIgA+ B cells.[36,37] After 5 days of PN, IL-4 and IL-10 levels are significantly decreased. The decrease in IL-4 levels occurred with both intragastric and intravenous PN solutions, whereas the decrease in IL-10 occurred only with intravenous PN solutions. The decrease in IL-4 and IL-10 levels correlated directly with the decrease in intestinal IgA levels. There were no changes in levels of Th1 type cytokines.[38,39]

Selectins are adhesion molecules that attract polymorphonuclear leukocytes (PMNs) and cause them to adhere to endothelium. In health, the expression of P-selectin, E-selectin and intercellular adhesion molecule-1 (ICAM-1) are low. Shock, sepsis, and tissue injury increase expression of cell adhesion molecule.[40,41] Activated PMNs cause tissue injury. PN is associated with increased expression of P-selectin, E-selectin, and ICAM-1. The PN-associated decrease in IL-4 and IL-10 is associated with an increase in ICAM-1 expression.[42,43] The changes in ICAM-1 are reversible within 5 days of restarting enteral feeds.

MAdCAM-1 is a ligand found on the high endothelial venules of the Peyer's patches. It attracts naïve B and T lymphocytes that have L-selectin and α4β7 adhesion molecules on their cell surfaces.[44] Once lymphocytes are sensitized to antigen, they distribute to other extraintestinal sites such as the respiratory tract. Within hours of starting parenteral feeds, MAdCAM-1 expression in the intestine drops, reaching a nadir by 48 hours.[45] These changes caused by PN decrease lymphocytes in the intestinal mucosa and heighten the inflammatory response in the vascular endothelium.

In summary, the route of nutrition affects the GI immune system. These changes are mediated by changes in cytokine production and expression of cell adhesion molecules. PN is associated with increased risk of infection (particularly sepsis and respiratory infections), decreased lymphocyte population of the GALT, diminished IgA production and altered cytokine and adhesion molecule expression when compared to enteral feeding.

Fatty Acids

By modulating cytokine production, proliferation of lymphocytes, and antigen presentation, polyunsaturated fatty acids (PUFA) might play an important role in regulating immune function so as to prevent inappropriate inflammatory responses. In a small study, adult volunteers whose diets were supplemented with fish oil were found to have decreased production of both IL-1 and TNF.[46] Animal studies[47–49] show PUFAs are important in maintaining the intact mucosal barrier and inhibiting the proliferation of lymphocytes and other inflammatory cells.

Vitamin A, Zinc, and Glutamine

Malnutrition is often accompanied by micronutrient deficiencies. Such deficiencies may exacerbate the unfavorable effects caused by protein malnutrition. Vitamin A and zinc in particular have been shown to have effects on mucosal immunity.

Vitamin A

Vitamin A deficiency adversely affects the mucosal immune response. Animal studies have shown that low vitamin A levels are associated with a decrease in IgA producing cells, reduced IgA production and diminished ability to respond with antigen-specific IgA.[50–52] Vitamin A deficient mice have decreased Th2 cells and decreased production of IL-4 and IL-5.[53–55] Vitamin A supplementation restores the IgA concentration to normal levels.[53]

Children with vitamin A deficiency are at increased risk for developing diarrhea and respiratory infections, and even dying.[56–58] A meta-analysis of randomized clinical trials demonstrated a significant reduction (~ 30%) in infant and child mortality with vitamin A supplementation.[59] More specifically, supplementation with vitamin A was found to reduce the prevalence and severity of diarrheal disease as well as diarrhea associated mortality.[60,61]

Zinc

Zinc is a vital micronutrient in immune function.[62] Zinc deficiency leads to atrophy of lymphoid tissues, decreased antibody and cytokine production and impaired T cell proliferation.[63–66] There are conflicting data regarding the specific effects of zinc on the Th1 and Th2 responses, but it seems that zinc deficiency adversely affects both types of responses.[65,67]

Clinical studies investigating the role for zinc in intestinal immunity are limited. A randomized, controlled trial of children with acute diarrhea who were supplemented with daily elemental zinc had a less severe and shorter course of diarrhea. There was also improved growth, particularly in children who were malnourished but not necessarily zinc deficient.[68,69]

Glutamine

Glutamine is a nonessential amino acid that has significant effects on intestinal metabolism and on the mucosal immune system and is considered "conditionally essential," particularly during times of catabolic stress (see Chapter 24 for a more complete discussion of glutamine). Glutamine depletion after injury impairs immunosuppression.[70]

Glutamine is not included in standard PN solutions. Animal studies show that the addition of glutamine to PN reversed adverse effects induced by administration of standard PN. Maintenance of normal B and T cell populations, normalization of T lymphocyte population in the lamina propria, increased cytokine production (IL-4 and IL-10), and improved IgA mediated defenses were all achieved with added glutamine.[71–73] In addition, the decrease in mucus and increased intestinal permeability seen with standard PN were prevented when PN was supplemented with glutamine.[74]

There are few human studies involving glutamine supplementation. However, one randomized, double-blinded, controlled study of bone marrow patients who received glutamine supplemented PN resulted in a lower incidence of infections and lower rates of microbial colonization.[75] In a study of very-low-birth-weight infants, glutamine supplementation resulted in a blunting of the CD16 and HLADR + subsets of peripheral blood T cells, and it was speculated that the possible cause was a decreased rate of bacterial translocation.[76]

Mucosal Immunity, Probiotics, Prebiotics, and Intestinal Flora

Bacteria, normally found throughout the gastrointestinal tract,[77–81] are often regarded as pathogens. The term probiotic is defined as a "preparation of or a product containing viable, defined microorganisms in sufficient numbers, which alter the microflora (by implantation or colonization) in a compartment of the host and by that exert beneficial health effects on the host."[82] See Table 3-1. Most probiotics include the bacteria *Bifidobacterium*, *Lactobacillus casei GG* and the yeast *Saccharomyces boulardii.*[83]

Probiotics are thought to confer protective effects by enhancing the defenses of the mucosal immune system. Their mechanism of action likely involves the prevention of pathogenic bacterial colonization and translocation. More specifically, they are thought to compete for receptor sites on the intestinal surface and for intraluminal nutrients, to produce antibiotic substances, and to increase IgA production. In addition, probiotics may be capable of strengthening tight junctions, increasing mucus secretion, and enhancing production of protective nutrients such as glutamine and short chain fatty acids.[54]

A number of clinical studies have investigated the role of probiotics in the treatment of diarrhea and in the prevention of necrotizing enterocolitis (NEC). The effects of *Lactobacillus GG* in shortening both the duration of viral diarrhea and decreasing the number of watery stools have been well documented.[84–86] However, no such beneficial effect has been demonstrated with enteroinvasive diarrheal disease. A number of randomized, placebo controlled trials have demonstrated that both the incidence and duration of antibiotic associated diarrhea were decreased with the supplementation of probiotics.[87,88] In the case of *Clostridium difficile* infection, however, while there was decreased recurrence in previously infected patients, there was no effect on preventing or ameliorating an initial infection.[89,90]

In a large study of premature infants, the effects of the probiotics *Bifidobacterium infantis* and *Lactobacillus acidophillus* on the prevention

Table 3-1 Defining criteria of microorganisms that can be considered probiotics.

A probiotic should:

- Be of human origin.
- Be nonpathogenic in nature.
- Be resistant to destruction by technical processing.
- Be resistant to destruction by gastric acid and bile.
- Adhere to intestinal epithelial tissue.
- Be able to colonize the gastrointestinal tract, if even for a short time.
- Produce antimicrobial substances.
- Modulate immune responses.
- Influence human metabolic activities (i.e., cholesterol assimilation, vitamin production, etc.).

of NEC were addressed. In a randomized study, comparing infants who received probiotics and breast milk to controls receiving only breast milk without probiotics, those supplemented with probiotics had decreased incidence of and decreased severity from NEC.[91]

Prebiotics are defined as a "nondigestible food ingredient which beneficially affects the host by selectively stimulating the growth of and/or activating the metabolism of one or a limited number of health promoting bacteria in the intestinal tract, thus improving the host's intestinal balance."[92] (See Table 3-2). Examples of prebiotics are fructooligossacharides and complex oligosaccharides. Fructooligosaccharides are short and medium chains of β-D fructans, which are further classified based on their degree of polymerization. Inulin is a fructooligosaccharide that is composed of < 60 fructosyl units. Inulins are produced by a number of plant species and are found in foods such as garlic, onions, artichokes, and asparagus.[92] Inulins and oligofructoses can be prepared commercially as well. These prebiotics stimulate the growth of probiotics such as *bifidobacteria.*[93,94] As this is a relatively new concept, the health promoting effects in humans have yet to be proven.

Currently, the Food and Drug Administration (FDA) does not regulate the production of either prebiotics or probiotics. Therefore, quality assurance of these products is not established, and there could be great variability in the amount of viable bacteria.[95,96] While probiotics are generally thought to be safe and nonpathogenic, cases of septicemia have been reported in immunocompromised patients. In addition, potential side effects from prebiotics exist as well. Symptoms such as increased flatulence, borborygmi, abdominal cramping, bloating, and increased stool output have been reported.[94,97]

Table 3-2 Defining criteria to classify a food ingredient as a prebiotic.

A prebiotic should:

- Neither be hydrolyzed nor absorbed in the upper part of the gastrointestinal tract.
- Be a selective substrate for one or more potentially beneficial commensal bacteria in the large intestine.
- Stimulate bacteria to divide, become metabolically active, or both.
- Alter the colonic microenvironment toward a healthier composition.
- Induce luminal or systemic effects that are advantageous to the host.

Breastfeeding

The neonatal period is a particularly vulnerable time as newborns transition from a sterile environment *in utero* to an external world full of antigens. The mucosal immune system is not mature at birth and breastfeeding is an important means of providing passive immunity and affecting mucosal immune system development.[98]

Mammary glands are part of the mucosal immune system in that enteric antigen exposure can result in antigen-specific IgA in the breast milk.[98] The SIgA in breast milk is specific for a variety of common intestinal pathogens, to which an infant would likely be exposed.[99] Such protection may help to provide a favorable *milieu* for the development of the mucosal immune response. In addition to SIgA, oligosaccharides found in breast milk can also interfere with the adherence of pathogenic bacteria by prohibiting contact of the bacteria with the microvillous membrane.[100,101] Other factors found in breast milk are thought to enhance the development of the intestinal immune system (see Table 3-3). Lactoferrin and IL-10 and IL-1 receptor antagonists are thought to help temporize the proinflammatory response.

Studies regarding necrotizing enterocolitis (NEC) have suggested that an exaggerated inflammatory reaction may contribute to the pathogenesis of this disease. In particular, there appears to be an exaggerated production of IL-8, which stimulates neutrophil activity.[103,104] In a study examining the effects of specific factors found in breast milk on the inflammatory response,

Table 3-3 Protective factors in breast milk.

Immune related proteins:
SIgA
IL-1 receptor antagonist
IL-10

Hormones:
Cortisol
Growth hormone
Insulin-like growth factor
Erythropoietin
Thyroid hormone

Growth factors:
TGF
EGF

Antioxidant factors:
Vitamin E
Beta carotene
Ascorbic acid

Other:
Glutamine
Nucleotides
Lactoferrin

TGF-β decreased the IL-8 response, suggesting a possible mechanism for the protective effects of breast milk in NEC.[105]

Colostrum contains macrophages. A direct correlation between monocytes and IL-6 has been observed with the added finding that IL-6 seemed to have an effect on IgA production in the breast.[106] The role of this interleukin on IgA production in the neonate, however, has not yet been investigated. In addition to antimicrobial and anti-inflammatory factors, breast milk contains TGF-β, which stimulates intestinal repair.[102]

SUMMARY

There are a number of aspects of the mucosal immune response that are directly affected by nutrition. Thus far, it appears that while PN may be able to simulate the caloric, nitrogen, and micronutrient content of enteral nutrition, there are aspects of this route of nutrition that lead to dramatic alterations of mucosal immunity not seen with enteral feeds. Perhaps such changes result from an altered composition or balance of enteric flora, which may be affected by the lack of enteral stimulation.

Supplementation of PN with factors such as short chain fatty acids and glutamine may provide a means for preventing the deleterious effects on the intestinal immune system. In addition, ensuring against micronutrient deficiency is prerequisite for preserving the mucosal immune response. Ongoing research is sure to better delineate the mechanisms behind the effects of malnutrition, vitamin deficiencies, and how to best optimize formulas and PN not only to provide adequate nutrition but also to preserve the function of the mucosal immune system.

REFERENCES

1. Medzhitov R, Janeway C Jr. Innate immunity: impact on the adaptive immune response. *Curr Opin Immunol.* 1997;9:4–9.
2. Medzhitov R, Janeway C Jr. Innate immunity. *New Engl J Med.* 2000;343:338–343.
3. Akira S, Hemmi H. Recognition of pathogen-associated molecular patterns by TLR family. *Immunol Lett.* 2003;85:85–95.
4. Steinbrink K, Wolfi M, Jonuleit H, Knop J, Enk AH. Induction of tolerance by IL-10 treated dendritic cells. *J Immunol.* 1997;159:4772–4780.
5. West MA, Wallin RPA, Matthews SP, et al. Enhanced dendritic cell antigen capture via toll-like receptor-induced actin remodeling. *Science.* 2004;305:1153–1155.
6. Ogra PL. Mucosal immunity: some historical perspective on host pathogen interactions and implications for mucosal vaccines. *Immunol Cell Biol.* 2003;81:23–33.
7. McNabb PC, Tomasi TB. Host defense mechanisms at mucosal surfaces. *Ann Rev Microbiol.* 1981;35:477–496.
8. Mayer L. Mucosal immunity. *Pediatrics.* 2003;111(6 Pt 3):1595–1600.
9. Gendler SJ, Spicer AP. Epithelial mucin genes. *Ann Rev Physiol.* 1995;57:607–634.

10. Kerss S, Allen A, Garner A. A simple method for measuring thickness of the mucus gel layer adherent to rat, frog and human gastric mucosa: influence of feeding, prostaglandin, N-acetylcysteine and other agents. *Clin Sci.* 1982;63(2):187–195.
11. Sandzen B, Blom H, Dahlgren S. Gastric mucus gel layer thickness measured by direct light microscopy. An experimental study in the rat. *Scand J Gastroenterol.* 1988;23(10):1160–1164.
12. Neutra MR. Gastrointestinal mucus: synthesis, secretion, and function. In: Johnson LR, ed. *Physiology of the Gastrointestinal Tract.* New York, NY: Raven Press; 1987;975–1009.
13. Mack DR, Michail S, Wei S, McDougall L, Hollingsworth MA. Probiotics inhibit enteropathogenic *E. coli* adherence in vitro by inducing intestinal mucin gene expression. *Am J Physiol.* 1999;276(4 Pt 1):G941–950.
14. Mack DR, Ahrne S, Hyde L, Wei S, Hollingsworth MA. Extracellular MUC3 mucin secretion follows adherence of *Lactobacillus* strains to intestinal epithelial cells in vitro. *Gut.* 2003;52(6):827–833.
15. Podolsky DK. Mucosal immunity and inflammation. V. Innate mechanisms of mucosal defense and repair: the best offense is a good defense. *Am J Physiol.* 1999;277(3 Pt 1):G495–499.
16. Kindon H, Pothoulakis C, Thim L, Lynch-Devaney K, Podolsky DK. Trefoil peptide protection of intestinal epithelial barrier function: cooperative interaction with mucin glycoprotein. *Gastroenterol.* 1995;109(2):516–523.
17. Andoh A, Kinoshita K, Rosenberg I, Podolsky DK. Intestinal trefoil factor induces decay-accelerating factor expression and enhances the protective activities against complement activation in intestinal epithelial cells. *J Immunol.* 2001;167(7):3887–3893.
18. Mashimo H, Wu DC, Podolsky DK, Fishman MC, Impaired defense of intestinal mucosa in mice lacking intestinal trefoil factor. *Science.* 1996;274(5285):262–265.
19. Cunliffe RN, Mahida YR. Antimicrobial peptides in innate intestinal host defense. *Gut.* 2000;47(1):16–17.
20. White SH, Wimley SH, Selsted ME. Structure, function, and membrane integration of defensins. *Curr Opin Struct Biol.* 1995;5(4):521–527.
21. Ganz T. Defensins and host defense. *Science.* 1999;286(5439):420–421.
22. Bevins CL, Martin-Porter E, Ganz T. Defensins and innate host defence of the gastrointestinal tract. *Gut.* 1999;45(6):911–915.
23. Yang D, et al. Beta-defensins: linking innate and adaptive immunity through dendritic and T cell CCR6. *Science.* 1999;286(5439):525–528.
24. Ouellette AJ. Paneth cells and innate immunity in the crypt microenvironment. *Gastroenterology.* 1997;113(5):1779–1784.
25. Ogra PL, Faden H, Welliver RC. Vaccination strategies for mucosal immune responses. *Clin Microbiol Rev.* 2001;14:430–445.
26. Elson CO, Dertzbaugh MT. Mucosal adjuvants. In: Ogra PL, Mestecky J, Lamm ME, Strober J, Bienenstock J, McGhee JR, eds. *Mucosal Immunology.* 2nd ed. New York, NY: Academic Press; 1999:817–838.
27. Kudsk KA, Croce MA, Fabian TC, Minard G, Tolley EA, Poret HA, Kuhl MR, Brown RO. Enteral versus parenteral feeding: effects on septic morbidity after blunt and penetrating abdominal trauma. *Ann Surg.* 1992;215(5):503–511; discussion 511–513.
28. Moore FA, Feliciano DV, Andrassy RJ, McArdle AH, Booth FV, Morgenstein-Wagner TB, Kellum JM Jr, Welling RE, Moore EE. Early enteral feeding, compared with parenteral, reduces postoperative septic complications: the results of a meta-analysis. *Ann Surg.* 1992;216(2):72–83.
29. Moore EE, Jones, TN. Benefits of immediate jejunostomy feeding after major abdominal trauma—a prospective, randomized study. *J Trauma-Inj Infect Crit Care.* 1986;26(10):874–881.
30. Tanaka S, Miura S, Tashiro H, Serizawa H, Hamada Y, Yoshioka M, Tsuchiya M. Morphological alteration of gut-associated lymphoid tissue after long-term total parenteral nutrition in rats. *Cell Tissue Res.* 1991;266(1):29–36.
31. Kiristioglu I, Antony P, Fan Y, Forbush B, Mosley RL, Yang H, Teitelbaum DH. Total parenteral nutrition-associated changes in mouse intestinal intraepithelial lymphocytes. *Dig Dis Sci.* 2002;47(5):1147–1157.
32. Li J, Kudsk KA, Gocinski B, Dent D, Glezer J, Langkamp-Henken B. Effects of parenteral and enteral nutrition on gut-associated lymphoid tissue. *J Trauma-Inj Infect Crit Care.* 1995;39(1):44–51; discussion 51–52.
33. King BK, Li J, Kudsk KA. A temporal study of TPN-induced changes in gut-associated lymphoid tissue and mucosal immunity. *Arch Surg.* 1997;132(12):1303–1309.
34. King BK, Kudsk KA, Li J, Wu Y, Renegar KB. Route and type of nutrition influence mucosal immunity to bacterial pneumonia. *Ann Surg.* 1999;229(2):272–278.
35. Janu P, Li J, Renegar KB, Kudsk KA, Recovery of gut-associated lymphoid tissue and upper respiratory tract immunity after parenteral nutrition. *Ann Surg.* 1997;225(6):707–715; discussion 715–717.
36. Kramer DR, Sutherland RM, Bao S, Husband AJ. Cytokine mediated effects in mucosal immunity. *Immunol Cell Biol.* 1995;73(5):389–396.
37. Murray PD, McKenzie DT, Swain SL, Kagnoff MF. Interleukin 5 and interleukin 4 produced by Peyer's patch T cells selectively enhance immunoglobulin A expression. *J Immunol.* 1987;139(8):2669–2674.

38. Wu Y, Kudsk KA, DeWitt RC, Tolley EA, Li JI. Route and type of nutrition influence IgA-mediating intestinal cytokines. *Ann Surg.* 1999;229(5):662–667; discussion 667–668.

39. Fukatsu K, Kudsk KA, Zarzaur BL, Wu Y, Hanna MK, DeWitt RCl. TPN decreases IL-4 and IL-10 mRNA expression in lipopolysaccharide stimulated intestinal lamina propria cells but glutamine supplementation preserves the expression. *Shock.* 2001;15(4):318–322.

40. Kudsk KA. Current aspects of mucosal immunology and its influence by nutrition. *Am J Surg.* 2002;183(4):390–398.

41. Munro JM, Pober JS, Cotran RS. Recruitment of neutrophils in the local endotoxin response: association with de novo endothelial expression of endothelial leukocyte adhesion molecule-1. *Lab Invest.* 1991;64(2):295–299.

42. Fukatsu K, Lundberg AH, Hanna MK, Wu Y, Wilcox HG, Granger DN, Gaber AO, Kudsk KA. Increased expression of intestinal P-selectin and pulmonary E-selectin during intravenous total parenteral nutrition. *Arch Surg.* 2000;135(10):1177–1182.

43. Fukatsu K, Lundberg AH, Hanna MK, Wu Y, Wilcox HG, Granger DN, Gaber AO, Kudsk KA. Route of nutrition influences intercellular adhesion molecule-1 expression and neutrophil accumulation in intestine. *Arch Surg.* 1999;134(10):1055–1060.

44. Abbas AK, Lichtman AH, Pober JS. *Cellular and Molecular Immunology.* 4th ed. WB Saunders Company; Philadelphia, PA. 2000.

45. Kudsk KA. Effect of route and type of nutrition on intestine-derived inflammatory responses. *Am J Surg.* 2003;185(1):16–21.

46. Endres S, Ghorbani R, Kelley VE, Georgilis K, Lonnemann G, van der Meer JW, Cannon JG, Rogers TS, Klempner MS, Weber PC, et al. The effect of dietary supplementation with n-3 polyunsaturated fatty acids on the synthesis of interleukin-1 and tumor necrosis factor by mononuclear cells. *N Engl J Med.* 1989;320(5):265–271.

47. Kudsk KA, Croce MA, Fabian TC, Minard G, Tolley EA, Poret HA, Kuhl MR, Brown RO. Enteral versus parenteral feeding: effects on septic morbidity after blunt and penetrating abdominal trauma. *Ann Surg.* 1992;215(5):503–511; discussion 511–513.

48. Milo LA, Reardon KA, Tappenden KA. Effects of short-chain fatty acid-supplemented total parenteral nutrition on intestinal pro-inflammatory cytokine abundance. *Dig Dis Sci.* 2002;47(9):2049–2055.

49. Teitelbaum JE, Walker WA. Review: the role of omega 3 fatty acids in intestinal inflammation. *J Nutr Biochem.* 2001;12:21–32.

50. Semba RD. The role of vitamin A and related retinoids in immune function. *Nutr Rev.* 1998;56(1 Pt 2):S38–48.

51. Puengtomwatanakul S, Sirisinha S. Impaired biliary secretion of immunoglobulin A in vitamin A-deficient rats. *Proc Soc Exp Biol Med.* 1986;182(4):437–442.

52. Wiedermann U, Hanson LA, Holmgren J, Kahu H, Dahlgren UI. Impaired mucosal antibody response to cholera toxin in vitamin A-deficient rats immunized with oral cholera vaccine. *Infect Immun.* 1993;61(9):3952–3957 [erratum appears in *Infect Immun.* 1993;61(12):5431].

53. Nikawa T, Odahara K, Koizumi H, Kido Y, Teshima S, Rokutan K, Kishi K . Vitamin A prevents the decline in immunoglobulin A and Th2 cytokine levels in small intestinal mucosa of protein-malnourished mice. *J Nutr.* 1999;129(5):934–941.

54. Carman JA, Smith SM, Hayes CE. Characterization of a helper T lymphocyte defect in vitamin A-deficient mice. *J Immunol.* 1989;142(2):388–393.

55. Stephensen CB. Vitamin A, infection, and immune function. *Ann Rev Nutr.* 2001;21:167–192.

56. Duggan C, Gannon J, Walker WA. Protective nutrients and functional foods for the gastrointestinal tract. *Am J Clin Nutr.* 2002;75(5):789–808.

57. Sommer A, Katz J, Tarwotjo I. Increased risk of respiratory disease and diarrhea in children with preexisting mild vitamin A deficiency. *Am J Clin Nutr.* 1984;40(5):1090–1095.

58. Bloem MW, Wedel M, Egger RJ, Speek AJ, Schrijver J, Saowakontha S, Schreurs WH. Mild vitamin A deficiency and risk of respiratory distress and diarrhea in pre-school and school children in northeastern Thailand. *Am J Epidemiol.* 1990;131:332–339.

59. Fawzi WW, Chalmers TC, Herrera MG, Mosteller F. Vitamin A supplementation and child mortality: a meta-analysis. *JAMA.* 1993;269(7): 898–903.

60. Anonymous. Vitamin A supplementation in northern Ghana: effects on clinic attendances, hospital admissions, and child mortality. Ghana VAST Study Team. *Lancet.* 1993;342(8862):7–12 [erratum appears in *Lancet.* 1993;24;342(8865):250].

61. Barreto ML, Santos LM, Assis AM, Araujo MP, Farenzena GG, Santos PA, Fiaccone RL. Effect of vitamin A supplementation on diarrhea and acute lower-respiratory-tract infections in young children in Brazil. *Lancet.* 1994;344(8917):228–231.

62. Hansen MA, Fernandes G, Good RA. Nutrition and immunity: the influence of diet on autoimmunity and the role of zinc in the immune response. *Ann Rev Nutr.* 1982;2:151–177.

63. Keen CL, Gershwin ME. Zinc deficiency and immune function. *Ann Rev Nutr.* 1990;10:415–431.

64. Shi HN, Scott ME, Stevenson MM, Koski KG. Zinc deficiency impairs T cell function in mice with primary infection of Heligmosomoides polygyrus (Nematoda). *Parasite Immunol.* 1994;16(7):339–350.

65. Fraker P. Zinc in the immune system. *J Nutr.* 2000;130:1399S–1406S.

66. Scott ME, Koski KG. Zinc deficiency impairs immune responses against parasitic nematode infections at intestinal and systemic sites. *J Nutr.* 2000;130(5S suppl):1412S–1420S.

67. Sprietsma JE. Zinc-controlled Th1/Th2 switch significantly determines development of diseases. *Med Hypotheses.* 1997;49(1):1–14.

68. Sazawal S, Black RE, Bhan MK, Bhandari N, Sinha A, Jalla S. Zinc supplementation in young children with acute diarrhea in India. *N Engl J Med.* 1995;333(13):839–844.

69. Tomkins A, Behrens R, Roy S. The role of zinc and vitamin A deficiency in diarrhoeal syndromes in developing countries. *Proc Nutr Soc.* 1993;52(1):131–142.

70. McNurlan MA, Garlick PJ. Protein and amino acids in nutritional support. *Crit Care Clin.* 1995;11(3):635–650.

71. Alverdy JA, Aoys E, Weiss-Carrington P, Burke DA. The effect of glutamine-enriched TPN on gut immune cellularity. *J Surg Res.* 1992;52(1):34–38.

72. Li J, Kudsk KA, Janu P. Renegar KB. Effect of glutamine-enriched total parenteral nutrition on small intestinal gut-associated lymphoid tissue and upper respiratory tract immunity. *Surgery.* 1997;121(5):542–549.

73. Kudsk KA, Wu Y, Fukatsu K, Zarzaur BL, Johnson CD, Wang R, Hanna MK. Glutamine-enriched total parenteral nutrition maintains intestinal interleukin-4 and mucosal immunoglobulin A levels. *JPEN.* 2000;24(5):270–274; discussion 274–275.

74. Khan J, Iiboshi Y, Cui L, Wasa M, Sando K, Takagi Y, Okada A. Alanyl-glutamine-supplemented parenteral nutrition increases luminal mucus gel and decreases permeability in the rat small intestine. *JPEN.* 1999;23(1):24–31.

75. Ziegler TR, Young LS, Benfell K, Scheltinga M, et al. Clinical and metabolic efficacy of glutamine-supplemented parenteral nutrition after bone marrow transplantation: a randomized, double-blind, controlled study. *Ann Int Med.* 1992;116(10):821–828.

76. Neu J, Roig JC, Meetze WH, Veerman M, et al. Enteral glutamine supplementation for very low birth weight infants decreases morbidity. *J Pediatr.* 1997;131(5):691–699.

77. Hooper LV, Gordon JI. Commensal host-bacterial relationships in the gut. *Science.* 2001;292:1115–1118.

78. Nanthakumar NN, Walker WA. The role of bacteria in the development of intestinal protective functions. In: Vevey S, ed. *Allergic Diseases and the Environment. Nestle Nutrition Workshop Series Pediatric Program.* Nestec Ltd.; Karger AG, Basel, 2004;53:153–177.

79. Xavier RJ, Podolsky DK. How to get along—friendly microbes in a hostile world. *Science.* 2000;289:1483–1484.

80. Kolenbrander PE. Oral microbial communities: biofilms, interactions, and genetic systems. *Ann Rev Microbiol.* 2000;54:413–437.

81. Margulis L, Sagan D, Thomas L. *Microcosmos: four billion years of evolution from our microbial ancestors.* Berkeley, Calif: University of California Press; 1997.

82. Teitelbaum JE, Walker WA. Nutritional impact of probiotics as protective gastrointestinal organisms. *Int Semin Pediatr Gastroenterol.* 2002;11:1–7.

83. Teitelbaum JE, Walker WA. Nutritional impact of pre- and probiotics as protective gastrointestinal organisms. *Ann Rev Nutr.* 2002;22:107–138.

84. Isolauri E, Juntunen M, Rautanen T, Sillanaukee P, Koivula T. A human *Lactobacillus* strain (*Lactobacillus casei* sp strain *GG*) promotes recovery from acute diarrhea in children. *Pediatrics.* 1991;88(1):90–97.

85. Isolauri E, Kaila M, Mykkanen H, Ling WH, Salminen S. Oral bacteriotherapy for viral gastroenteritis. *Dig Dis Sci.* 1994;39(12):2595–2600.

86. Majamaa H, Isolauri E, Saxelin M, Vesikari T. Lactic acid bacteria in the treatment of acute rotavirus gastroenteritis. *J Pediatr Gastroenterol Nutr.* 1995;20(3):333–338.

87. Arvola T, Laiho K, Torkkeli S, Mykkanen H, Salminen S, Maunula L, Isolauri E. Prophylactic *Lactobacillus GG* reduces antibiotic-associated diarrhea in children with respiratory infections: a randomized study. *Pediatrics.* 1999;104(5):e64.

88. Vanderhoof JA, Whitney DB, Antonson DL, Hanner TL, Lupo JV, Young RJ. *Lactobacillus GG* in the prevention of antibiotic-associated diarrhea in children *J Pediatr.* 1999;135(5):564–568.

89. Biller JA, Katz AJ, Flores AF, Buie TM, Gorbach SL. Treatment of recurrent *Clostridium difficile* colitis with *Lactobacillus GG. J Pediatr Gastroenterol Nutr.* 1995;21(2):224–226.

90. McFarland LV, Surawicz CM, Greenberg RN, Fekety R, Elmer GW, Moyer KA, Melcher SA, Bowen KE, Cox JL, Noorani Z, et al. A randomized placebo-controlled trial of *Saccharomyces boulardii* in combination with standard antibiotics for *Clostridium difficile* disease. *JAMA.* 1994;271(24):1913–1918 [erratum appears in *JAMA.* 1994;272(7):518].

91. Lin H-C, Su B-H, Chen A-C, et al. Oral probiotics reduce the incidence and severity of necrotizing enterocolitis in very low birth weight infants. *Pediatrics.* 2005;11:1–4.

92. Gibson GR, Roberfroid MB. Dietary modulation of the human colonic microbiota: introducing the concept of prebiotics. *J Nutr.* 1995;125(6):1401–1412.

93. Simmering R, Blaut M. Pro- and prebiotics—the tasty guardian angels? *Appl Microbiol Biotechnol.* 2001;55(1):19–28.
94. Gibson GR, Beatty ER, Wang X, Cummings JH. Selective stimulation of bifidobacteria in the human colon by oligofructose and inulin. *Gastroenterology.* 1995;108(4):975–982.
95. Hamilton-Miller JM, Shah S, Smith CT. "Probiotic" remedies are not what they seem. *BMJ.* 1996;312(7022):55–56.
96. Ross S. Functional foods: the Food and Drug Administration perspective. *Am J Clin Nutr.* 2000;71(6 suppl):1735S–1738S; discussion 1739S–1742S.
97. Pederson A, Sandstrom S, VanAmelsvoort JMM. The effects of ingestion of inulin on blood lipids and gastrointestinal symptoms in healthy females. *Br J Nutr.* 1997;78:215–222.
98. Hanson LA, Ashraf R, Zaman S, Karlbert J, Lindblad BS, Jalil F. Breastfeeding is a natural contraceptive and prevents disease and death in infants, linking infant mortality and birth rates. *Acta Paediatr.* 1994;83:3–6.
99. Goldman AS. The immune system of human milk: antimicrobial, antiinflammatory and immunomodulating properties. *Pediatr Infect Dis J.* 1993;12(8):664–671.
100. Claud EC, Walker WA. Hypothesis: inappropriate colonization of the premature intestine can cause neonatal necrotizing enterocolitis. *FASEB J.* 2000;15(8):1398–1403.
101. Newburg DS. Oligosaccharides in human milk and bacterial colonization. *J Pediatr Gastroenterol Nutr.* 2000;30(suppl 2):S8–17.
102. Bernt KM, Walker WA. Human milk as a carrier of biochemical messages. *Acta Paediatr Suppl.* 1999;88(430):27–41.
103. Edelson MB, Bagwell CE, Rozycki HJ. Circulating pro- and counterinflammatory cytokine levels and severity in necrotizing enterocolitis. *Pediatrics.* 1999;103(4 Pt 1):766–771.
104. Nadler EP, Stanford A, Zhang XR, Schall LC, Alber SM, Watkins SC, Ford HR. Intestinal cytokine gene expression in infants with acute necrotizing enterocolitis: interleukin-11 mRNA expression inversely correlates with extent of disease. *J Ped Surg.* 2001;36(8):1122–1129.
105. Claud EC, Savidge T, Walker WA. Modulation of human intestinal epithelial cell IL-8 secretion by human milk factors. *Ped Res.* 2003;53(3):419–425.
106. Saito S, Maruyama M, Kato Y, Moriyama I, Ichijo M. Detection of IL-6 in human milk and its involvement in IgA production. *J Reprod Immunol.* 1991;20(3):267–276.

Chapter 4

Long Term Consequences of Early Nutrition

Alan Lucas

NUTRITION, HEALTH, AND PROGRAMMING

There has been a significant change in focus in the field of nutrition. Previously the interest was in meeting nutritional needs, preventing deficiencies, and in the practical aspects of feeding. While these remain important, the new focus is on the biological effects nutrition has on the organism, with major consequences for *health*.

Nutrition may impact on health in several ways. First, it is increasingly recognized as a factor that may profoundly alter a patient's clinical course and prognosis. Thus, the use of human milk in neonatal care substantially reduces the risk of life-threatening systemic sepsis or necrotizing enterocolitis (NEC).[1] In children with diverse conditions, such as gut disease, renal failure, neurodevelopmental disorders, allergy and surgery, nutrition may have important consequences, affecting disease severity, length of hospital stay, or need for more expensive therapies.[2] Second, nutrition is regarded as a key influence, throughout the life of the organism,[3] on health outcomes, including cardiovascular risk, obesity, and cancer. Third, diet is a vehicle for introducing a range of toxicological factors (e.g., drugs and environmental contaminants in breast milk, aluminium in parenteral nutrition solutions[4]) or pathogenic organisms including *E. Sakazaki* in formulas, and HIV in breast milk with short or long term health impact. However, this chapter considers a further, critical aspect that has important, widespread implications for both public health and clinical practice—the emerging evidence that nutrition, during critical early periods, can have lifetime consequences for health and development.

The Concept of Critical Periods

The idea that nutrition may have long term consequences is part of a broader concept concerning the importance of early life events in general. In the 1980s, Lucas proposed the term *programming* to describe the general phenomenon that a stimulus or insult, when applied at a critical or sensitive period in development, could have long term or lifetime effects on the structure or function of the organism.[5]

The first description of a critical period in development was by Spalding (1873) in relation to imprinting in birds.[6] Since then, developmentalists have demonstrated numerous examples of sensitivity during such windows, to a variety of endogenous and environmental triggers.

The sensitivity to programming stimuli may be dramatic with a brief stimulus exposure producing overt lifetime effects. For instance, during a short period in development, the rat brain, exposed to testosterone from the developing testis, is programmed for male behavior. Experimental administration of just one dose of testosterone to a female fetus at this precise, critical window in time will permanently program the brain for male behavior.[7] Environmental programming agents include light (postnatal retinal exposure to light is critical for normal programming of the visual pathway and hence squint amblyopia); temperature (in reptiles, environmental temperature before hatching of eggs determines sex); and drugs. With regard to the latter, teratogens are well recognized to operate during specific critical periods of fetal development with lifetime effects on the structure of the organism. Postnatally, Bagley showed a single dose of phenobarbital administered to a neonatal rat (a dose which at any other time would induce drowsiness) had lifetime effects on metabolism—p450 cytochrome monooxygenase activity[8] (and raised important concerns about our lack of understanding of the impact of human neonatal pharmacology). These examples are given to illustrate that when we turn to *nutrition* as an early environmental programming influence, we should not find it counterintuitive that brief periods of nutritional manipulation may also have important and enduring consequences for health.

Nutritional Programming in Animals

McCance pioneered the first formal animal experiments demonstrating lifetime effects of early nutrition.[9] By manipulating litter size in rats, he altered intake of breast milk just during the brief suckling period (21 days). Rats placed in large rather than smaller litters (and therefore relatively underfed) were smaller at 21 days. But rather than show catch-up when subsequently fed normally, they progressively diverged in size compared to those from smaller litters, so that by adulthood there was a major programmed size difference between groups. Conversely, when a similar duration of undernutrition was imposed at 9 weeks of age, complete catch-up growth occurred afterwards, showing the window of sensitivity for programming growth had already closed at that age. McCance's studies influenced 40 years of subsequent animal research showing that nutrition during early life could program in adulthood many outcomes of potential relevance to human health and development, including blood pressure, blood lipids, obesity, insulin secretion, atherosclerosis, learning, and behavior.

Much work has focused on the brain. Extensive animal data, largely on rats, show that nutrition at a vulnerable period of brain development may have permanent effects on brain size, brain cell number, behavior, learning, and memory. In Smart's review of 165 animal studies on early undernutrition and later learning, the number of studies in which undernourished animals fared worse than controls greatly outweighed those that favored the controls.[10] The extent to which these animal data had relevance to human cognitive development, however, was uncertain at that time.

Numerous animal studies have yielded results of potential relevance to adult disease in humans. Some of the first such studies were those of Hahn (1984), who manipulated litter size in neonatal rats so that rats from small litters were temporarily overfed during the brief suckling period. In these studies, Hahn found that in adulthood, these animals had permanent elevation in plasma insulin and cholesterol.[11] Weaning these animals onto a high carbohydrate diet further induced lifelong elevation in the activities of HMG-CoA reductase and fatty acid synthetase (key enzymes for cholesterol).

Perhaps the most instructive studies have been in nonhuman primates. Lewis, in a controlled experiment, overfed baboons in infancy to test long term consequences for body fatness in adulthood. Apart from a transient increase in body fatness during the early overfeeding period itself, the baboons remained normal weight until around puberty, when their weight gain accelerated and they became significantly overweight.[12] This important example of programming demonstrates the principle that programmed effects may be remembered by the organism, but the consequences not expressed until later in life. Evidence for such late emergence of programmed effects in humans is cited in the next section.

Approaches to Nutritional Programming in Humans

Animal studies are important in the programming field since they allow detailed study of *mechanism*. They also make *lifetime* studies possible. Indeed the recent work of Ozanne and Hales show that lifespan of mice may be altered by brief manipulation of early protein intake.[13] However, animal data may have uncertain applicability for humans. It is essential, therefore, to study programming directly in man. Two complementary approaches have been used: experimental intervention trials of early diet with long term prospective follow-up to detect outcome effects and retrospective observational studies.

Retrospective observations, for instance those by Barker and coworkers,[14] have shown that risk of death from ischemic heart disease increases for subjects who are small at birth. Such observations are valuable in providing rapid answers, ideal for hypothesis generation; and they allow study of major clinical endpoints. However, the shortcoming is that it is difficult to prove (nutritional) causation from an observational association and therefore the data may be an insecure basis for practice.

Experimental intervention trials of early nutrition targeted to study programming have the major disadvantage that they require investment in long term follow-up—at least to the stage that outcome findings have strong predictive value for adult health. However, their strength is the experimental design, which, by controlling (through randomization) for both known and unknown confounding factors, can be used to prove causation and hence, importantly, underpin practice. Lucas first initiated such studies, based on the pharmaceutical trial model, in the early 1980s.[15,16] As with any therapeutic trial, such studies examine not only the *efficacy* of the intervention (e.g., long term benefit for cardiovascular risk), but also its *safety*. These experimental trials were the first human studies to test nutritional programming, though because of the prospective design, long term findings of studies started in the early 1980s have only recently emerged.

An intermediate approach is to exploit past randomized trials of nutrition in mothers and infants by tracing and following up the cohorts. These trials were not originally studied with long term outcome in mind, but nevertheless have an experimental design. A large pan-European consortium will now take this approach.

Impact of Nutrition on Long Term Outcome in Humans

Now backed by extensive experimental studies in animals and both experimental and observational studies in humans for more than 2 decades, there is strong cumulative evidence of the importance of early nutrition for later outcome. Programming effects explored thus far include cardiovascular disease (CVD) and its risk factors, brain development and cognition, bone health, obesity, and immunity. Examples of these are discussed in this chapter, giving weight to outcomes established by randomized trials. Many of the first intervention trials of early nutrition were conducted in preterm infants and raise the question of whether these findings can be generalized. However, observational data and emerging evidence from newer clinical trials (again supported by animal evidence) provide a strong basis for the view that postnatal life in infants born at term is also a critical period for programming. This chapter will demonstrate that programming may occur in response to: (1) quantitative variation in overall nutrient intake (both high and low intakes), (2) qualitative aspects of the diet (e.g., breast milk versus formula), and (3) individual nutrients.

IMPACT OF EARLY NUTRITION ON THE HUMAN BRAIN

The first major studies that examined the effect of early nutrition on later cognition in humans were observational and addressed the impact of infant malnutrition and of breastfeeding.

Malnutrition

Numerous studies have shown protein-energy undernutrition is associated with later deficits in cognitive functioning.[17,18] However, malnutrition is associated with poor social circumstances, lack of stimulation, and poverty that could have confounded the results. Nevertheless, even after attempts to match controls for social background, as in a large Guatemalan study on 4 villages with similar lifestyles,[19] beneficial effects of nutritional supplementation on cognitive performance have been shown.

Breastfeeding

Studies since the 1920s have often shown superior performance of breastfed infants for cognition, verbal ability, or school performance.[20–24] These studies are subject to two possible types of confounding: (1) the intimacy of breastfeeding might affect infant development and (2) in more recent years, breastfeeding has been associated with higher socioeconomic status and education, and greater propensity to positive health-related behavior, factors which in themselves might influence infant development. In some, but not all studies, adjustment for the latter type of confounding has not removed the cognitive benefit of breastfeeding.

In preterm infants, both types of confounding can be explored. In 300 children aged 7–8 years, IQ was 8 points higher in those previously breast milk fed even after adjusting for social and educational factors. However, in this study, infants were fed human milk by nasogastric tube, also suggesting the advantage was not related to the intimacy of breastfeeding.[24]

Other studies suggesting a causal effect of breastfeeding were those conducted at a time when artificially fed children came from the most socioeconomically advantaged stratum of society. Hoeffer studied children born in the United States between 1915 and 1921 and showed that breastfed children performed better than those who were artificially fed, though children who were exclusively breastfed beyond 9 months did less well.[25] A study of elderly subjects born in the UK in the 1930s showed that despite lower socioeconomic status those who were breastfed had higher unadjusted IQ.[26]

Evidence from Randomized Trials

While the weight of the foregoing evidence is compelling, proof that nutrition is important for long term neurodevelopment has depended on *randomized trials*. Such trials of nutritional supplementation of malnourished populations in developing countries have been few, but they have provided evidence for at least medium-term effects of early nutrition on cognitive function.[27,28] Long term data are largely unavailable from these trials, and in any case more sophisticated neurocognitive testing, now possible, has not generally been applied to detect specific effects that might theoretically have been missed previously.

The strongest available evidence from clinical trials comes from a series of parallel intervention studies conducted on nearly 1,000 preterm infants, starting in 1982.[16,29] One trial compared infants fed solely on standard versus enriched preterm formula. The diets differed principally in protein and micronutrient contents. These diets were fed on average just 4 weeks. Psychomotor development indices (Bayley scales: PDI) were 15 points higher at 18 months follow-up in the group that received the enriched formula. The effect was greatest in those born small for gestational age and in males. In both cases there were significant advantages in both mental and psychomotor development indices (Bayley scales: MDI and PDI) for the preterm formula fed groups.[29]

Subsequently, at 7.5–8 years, boys previously fed standard versus enriched preterm formula had a 12-point disadvantage ($P < 0.01$) in verbal IQ. In those with highest intakes of trial diets, there were a 10-point disadvantage and a 14-point disadvantage in overall IQ ($P < 0.05$) and verbal IQ ($P < 0.01$). Consequently, more infants fed term formula had low verbal IQ (< 85): 31% versus 14% for both sexes ($P = 0.02$) and 47% versus 13% in boys ($P = 0.009$).[16] This effect of early nutrition on later verbal rather than performance skills implies that the effects of nutrition on the brain are selective, as now suggested using modern techniques to examine the effects on long term *structural* development of the brain.

Unexpectedly, the group fed the standard formula also had a significant increase in the incidence of cerebral palsy (largely spastic diplegia), raising a clinically important following hypothesis.[16] There is evidence from newborn rats and preterm monkeys that the brain may reorganize to achieve complete functional compensation if cortical damage occurs sufficiently early.[30] It is plausible that although cerebral palsy in prematurely born children might originate prenatally or at least before enteral feeding has commenced, whether the brain can subsequently achieve functional compensation at a time of rapid brain growth and development might depend on the provision of adequate nutrient substrates. Unpublished data from this cohort, followed into adulthood, shows not only persistence of the cognitive effects, notably on verbal IQ, but also effects, probably permanent, on the *structure* of the brain, using sophisticated MRI scanning techniques to compare groups of subjects. These data provide evidence on the exquisite sensitivity of the brain to suboptimal nutrition in early life and give more credibility to the numerous observational studies linking early undernutrition to later impairment of cognition.

Specific Nutrients and Brain Development

One clear instance of an irreversible nutritional influence on cognitive function is maternal iodine deficiency, which may result in frank cretinism or reduced cognitive function and school performance in the offspring.[31] Extensive literature on iron deficiency in animals and humans indicates that it has had long term and possibly permanent adverse effects on brain development.[32–34] Iron deficiency, like malnutrition, tends to occur in poor social circumstances, confounding interpretation of the consequences. More data from randomized trials are needed, but the cumulative evidence is sufficiently compelling that prevention of early iron deficiency anemia is regarded as a clinical and public health priority. Taurine has recently reemerged as a potentially critical single nutrient for neurodevelopment, notably in preterm infants emphasizing the potential importance of its incorporation in artificial feeds.[35]

Perhaps the greatest efforts have been devoted to whether dietary sources of long chain polyunsaturated fatty acids (LCPUFA), notably docosahexaenoic acid (DHA) and arachidonic acid (AA) are essential for normal neurodevelopment. These fatty acids, present in breast milk and important functional components of the nervous system, had not until recently been added to formulas. The question has been whether endogenous synthesis from precursors is inadequate, and if so, whether they can be added safely and effectively given the sources of these lipids available (fish, egg, plants, and single cell organisms). While a number of studies indicate short term benefits for cognitive or visual performance in preterm and term infants, longterm benefits have yet to be established. Current trials show neutral, positive, or even negative (Lucas, unpublished) effects on neurodevelopment according to the sources of LCPUFA used (which contain other lipids as well as LCPUFA).[36–41] These data emphasize the importance for health professionals to appraise research data carefully on any specific product used in order to choose those supported by robust efficacy and safety trials.

The evidence from animals and humans that early nutrition is critical for long term development of the brain is strong, and this must be factored into public health and clinical practice decisions (as discussed later) in order to preserve long term neurocognitive potential.

PROGRAMMING OF BONE HEALTH

Increasing evidence shows early nutrition influences long term bone health and linear growth. Metabolic bone disease (MBD) in preterm infants appears a good example of a silent programming influence. MBD, due to insufficient supply and retention of calcium and phosphorus for bone formation, may be clinically unapparent, often signalled only by late elevation in plasma alkaline phosphatase activity. Yet this condition appears to be one of the most important influences on long term linear growth that can be manipulated in practice, with reduced height detected as far as 12 years later.[42]

Of greater interest is the possibility that early nutrition could "program" adult degenerative bone disease—osteoporosis—a major and costly problem in developed countries. In trials of preterm infants, those assigned to unfortified diets (suitable for full term infants: standard formula or unfortified breast milk) as opposed to enriched diets (preterm formulas) had biochemical evidence of increased bone formation (raised plasma osteocalcin) 8–12 years later.[43] Increased bone formation and turnover is a feature of osteoporosis and raises the hypothesis, supported by other studies, that adult bone health risk can be manipulated by infant diet.

PROGRAMMING OF CARDIOVASCULAR DISEASE

For the brain and bones, meeting early nutritional needs and promoting growth appear to have favorable programming effects. For programming the risk of cardiovascular disease, the major cause of mortality in the developed world, different principles appear to apply.

Fetal Programming

Cardiovascular risk may be programmed both prenatally and postnatally. Prenatal programming by nutrition has less relevance to routine clinical care since it is more difficult to manipulate nutrition in the fetus. While animal studies show sensitivity to programming in fetal life,[44,45] in humans this has been harder to approach with few randomized trials. Most evidence is retrospective and observational and often relies on proxy measures for early nutrition such as size at birth. It is also unclear how the observed relationships between small size at birth and later cardiovascular disease risk[14] can be translated into practice recommendations. Finally, while it is undoubtedly the case that a deranged metabolic milieu *in utero*, such as a diabetic pregnancy, can have long term effects, generally the effects on cardiovascular risk for postnatal nutritional intervention are much greater (see Breast Milk and Later Cardiovascular Health) than for, say, birth weight.[15] For these reasons, this chapter is devoted to the impact of postnatal nutrition.

Postnatal Programming

In distilling the evidence for nutritional programming of later cardiovascular disease risk, there appear two potentially important influences: (1) breast milk (2) postnatal growth.

Breast Milk and Later Cardiovascular Health

Breastfed infants have been shown in observational studies to have lower risk of cardiovascular disease, hypercholesterolemia, obesity, type II diabetes, and high blood pressure.[46–49] These data could be confounded by sociobiological differences between breastfed and formula fed groups. However, a causal relationship has been testable in preterm infants. Here it has been possible to take infants whose mothers had elected not to provide breast milk and randomly assign them to human milk from a milk bank (donated by lactating mothers unrelated to the subject) versus an infant formula.[50–53]

In such trials, those fed human milk rather than formula, with as little as one month (on average) intervention period, had lower blood pressure, LDL cholesterol, leptin resistance (possible tendency to later obesity), and insulin resistance.[50–53] These effects were seen 13–16 years postintervention on prospective follow-up. The effect sizes were large (see Size of the Effect, later in this chapter), comparable to, or greater than nonpharmacological interventions to affect these risk factors in adulthood. As further evidence of causation, exploratory analyses of these trials showed clear dose-response relationships for these outcomes: the greater the breast milk intake in the neonatal period, the lower the risk factor status in adolescence. Thus, although the observational data may still be challenged as inconclusive, the combination of such evidence with that from formal intervention trials in preterm infants provides compelling overall evidence that breast milk feeding reduces risk of the metabolic syndrome.

Impact of Rapid Postnatal Growth

The trials on preterm infants, cited earlier,[50–53] compare infants fed unsupplemented human milk versus enriched (preterm) formula, and also, in parallel, a standard formula versus enriched formula. These studies provide experimental evidence that diets promoting faster neonatal growth increase later cardiovascular risk. That is, the infants who were fed on growth-promoting enriched diets had greater risk of developing features of the metabolic syndrome at follow-up.

This finding was not just a feature of prematurity: infants born full term but small for gestation, randomly assigned to a growth-promoting formula, had higher diastolic blood pressure 6–8 years later compared with those assigned to standard formula.[15] Results of further analyses of these studies on preterm and term infants suggested that it was indeed the growth acceleration that explained the adverse effects of a nutrient-enriched diet on later insulin resistance and blood pressure.[50,52]

Postnatal Growth Acceleration Hypothesis

The foregoing findings led to a proposed "postnatal growth acceleration hypothesis" as a key to the early programming of cardiovascular disease.[15] Consistent with this, later insulin resistance was found greatest in infants born preterm with accelerated growth in the first 2 weeks,[52] the period of fastest postnatal growth, and least in those who grew at a rate lower than that normally targeted (the intrauterine growth rate). Such growth was also associated with greater endothelial dysfunction in adolescence,[54] an early stage in atherosclerosis. The effect size was substantial (see Size of the Effect, later in this chapter). Therefore, early growth acceleration programmed the abnormal vascular biology associated with early atherosclerosis, whereas slower early growth was beneficial.

These findings are consistent with previous animal data showing that with a higher plane of early postnatal nutrition and a faster growth program there is a propensity to the metabolic syndrome. Adverse longterm health effects of early growth acceleration emerge as a fundamental biological phenomenon across animal species. Thus, growth acceleration during sensitive windows reduces fat deposition in Atlantic salmon, lowers resistance to starvation in speckled wood butterflies, impairs glucose tolerance and life span in rats, and reduces cardiovascular disease risk in nonhuman primates.[55,56]

Data from further studies in man strongly support this hypothesis. Childhood growth acceleration is associated with later insulin resistance, obesity, and CVD. However, growth acceleration is greatest in early infancy, suggesting that this period may be most critical. Indeed, early growth acceleration is associated with later obesity, dyslipidemia, raised concentrations of insulin in infants small for gestation, and, from as early as 4 days of age, high insulin-like growth factor-1.[57–63] Programming of the hypothalamic-pituitary axis in general probably directly affects later CVD and noninsulin-dependent diabetes mellitus (NIDDM).[64]

This hypothesis predicts that a high nutrient intake, which promotes early growth, would adversely program cardiovascular health. Several observations, in addition to the trials cited above, support this prediction. Greater nutrient intake in infancy is associated with raised blood pressure in adults.[65] The risk of later obesity increases with an earlier adiposity rebound—an indicator of faster growth—and with early introduction of weaning foods.[66] Infants of diabetic mothers fed their own mothers' milk, rather than lower-nutrient-banked donor breast milk, have a greater risk of later obesity, whereas those fed more banked milk had less risk of later impaired glucose tolerance than those fed maternal breast milk.[67] Remarkably, relative undernutrition was beneficial from as early as the first week, when growth is highly variable. An important public health inference from these findings is that the observed advantages of breastfeeding cited earlier might be due to the slower early growth of breast milk fed infants.[15]

GENERAL PROGRAMMING ISSUES

Balance of Risks

It appears from the evidence previously mentioned that early programming influences have quite different effects on different systems. Thus, in preterm neonates, while early growth promotion might favor the brain, it appears less advantageous for later cardiovascular risk. Simultaneous risks and benefits exist for many therapeutic interventions in medicine (e.g., drug therapy), and clearly in appraising the value of a public health or clinical intervention, a balancing of risks and benefits is needed.

Timing of the Programming Window

Studies on preterm and full term infants suggest that the effect size of nutrition on cardiovascular risk factors is similar in both term and preterm infants indicating that birth, at any gestation, sets the organism for subsequent, postnatal sensitivity to cardiovascular programming.[15,50] In contrast, current evidence suggests that for the brain, gestation is more critical and that those born more immature are more vulnerable to the neurocognitive programming effects of nutrition than those born beyond term.[16,68] The duration of windows of sensitivity could relate to outcome and have not yet been defined. Although it might be assumed that greatest sensitivity to programming would be in fetal or early postnatal life, it is possible that much later periods are still critical—even during adolescence when new genes are being switched on.

Emergence of the Programmed Effect

Programmed effects may be detected early. Effects of growth acceleration on increased insulin resistance may be detected within the first year (Fewtrell, unpublished). In contrast, and in keeping with studies in baboons,[12] (see Nutritional Programming in Animals, earlier in this chapter), programmed effects might not emerge until much later. For instance, the benefits of breast milk for later blood pressure were not seen in one study at 7–8 years, but large benefits were detected in adolescence.[50] Moreover, some effects may first become apparent in adulthood. The potential for late emergence of programmed effects has important implications in terms of the need for long term follow-up not only to detect efficacy but also safety of early nutritional intervention.

Critical Interactions

That there is a low prevalence of cardiovascular disease in developing countries implies the early programming environment is insufficient to affect outcome alone. There needs to be interaction with subsequent environment—notably diet. Mott and Lewis[69] provided experimental evidence for this in baboons, breast or formula fed in infancy, and then placed on a Western diet rich in saturated fats. In adulthood, the breast-fed group were more dyslipidemic and had more atherosclerosis, implying an adverse interaction between a Western diet and prior breastfeeding.

Size of the Effect

The effects of early nutrition on subsequent IQ or verbal IQ have been large in some studies reaching 12–15 quotient points, which would have a large population impact.[16,29] The effect on cardiovascular risk factor is sufficient to have a major impact on health of populations in developed countries. Thus, neonates with the greatest early weight gain had 4% lower flow-mediated endothelial dependent dilation of the brachial artery (an early marker of the atherosclerotic process), compared with those with the least early weight gain, similar to the effect of insulin-dependent diabetes mellitus (4%) and smoking (6%) in adults.[24] The impact of early nutrition in randomized trials on later blood pressure is around 3–4 mm Hg—an effect size, which, if applied to the US population as a whole, would be expected to affect cardiovascular death rate by around 150,000 cases year.[50] A 10% lowering of later LDL cholesterol with breastfeeding would, in adults, reduce cardiovascular disease by around 25% and mortality from it by around 14%.[51] Thus, early nutrition emerges as one of the most important factors that can be manipulated in clinical and public health practice.

MECHANISM

A consideration of programming mechanisms is beyond the scope of this chapter, but briefly key research issues include how storage of the "memory" of a programmed event is preserved throughout the life of the organism. This implies an epigenetic phenomenon. Those suggested include adaptive changes in gene expression, clonal selection or differential tissue proliferation in early development. Another key research issue is an understanding of "coupling mechanisms," whereby the programming stimulus (nutrition) is coupled to "receptors" in sensitive tissues.[5] Hormonal coupling mechanisms seem likely, and those proposed include insulin, gut hormones, IGF-1, and leptin.[53,64] Exploring such fundamental processes may throw light on more general mechanisms by which early endogenous and environmental factors during development may have lifetime effects. This is quintessential pediatric research—understanding the legacy of pediatrics for adult health.

FUTURE CLINICAL IMPLICATIONS

Our new understanding of the impact of early nutritional environment on later health effects will ultimately focus the practitioner on issues previously little considered. Clearly, nutrition is not simply a matter of meeting nutritional needs. It must now be regarded as a branch of therapeutics, since important health outcomes can be manipulated and clinicians will increasingly need to appraise data from efficacy and safety trials as in other areas of therapeutics.

In some areas, scientific knowledge is sufficient to underpin practice. Breastfeeding (and the use of breast milk in neonatal care) is now supported by substantial data on its effects on later health. Infant formulas, while all meet nutritional needs, are becoming differentiated by variable contents of ingredients that impact on health outcomes, such as LCPUFA. Thus balanced, scientific appraisal of efficacy and safety data of products used in practice is important. Some nutrients have specific importance for later outcome, and their adequacy in the diet must be ensured (e.g., iron). Other areas are advancing rapidly and will increasingly underpin clinical management. Such an area is growth.

Further Understanding of Growth

Clinicians are often concerned over what would be a desirable target growth rate for a patient under their care. Such considerations have had a largely theoretical basis. Normal growth is traditionally defined as the growth rate seen in others of the same age, which is the basis of growth charts. This cyclical reasoning would no longer be acceptable in other areas of therapeutics. If target body fatness, for instance, were defined in terms of US population averages, this would clearly be erroneous. Ideal body fatness is better defined as that which is not associated with excess morbidity. For infant growth, the issue is more complex.

In preterm infants we clearly have a conflict. Rapid early growth favors the brain and bones; slower early growth favors later cardiovascular risk. Thus a balance of risks is needed (as noted earlier). Although slow growth (below the intrauterine rate) has some benefit for later cardiovascular outcome, it risks undernutrition and its adverse consequences and has a profound adverse effect on later cognition. Currently, the balance of risks favors the brain, and preterm infants should be fed with specialized products to support rapid growth (at least at the intrauterine rate). In small-for-gestational-age, full term infants, however, the brain appears to be less sensitive than in preterm infants, and, in one large study, attempts to promote more rapid infant growth have not so far shown benefits for neurodevelopment follow-up to 18 months.[68] However, preliminary evidence shows that promoting growth in this population adversely elevated diastolic blood pressure 5–8 years later (as discussed previously in Impact of Rapid Postnatal Growth[15]). Thus, it may prove imprudent to aggressively promote catch-up in healthy, small-for-gestational-age infants, at least in the early postnatal period. More work is needed in this area; for instance, studies are needed to explore whether in more extreme cases of growth retardation, with head growth failure, as seen in severe disease, the balance of risks again favors growth promotion to preserve neurocognitive function. In developing countries, short term health may take precedence over long term outcome and considerable care is needed to prevent deficiencies.

CONCLUSION

Nutrition has emerged as a major environmental influence of health, with the potential for lifetime effects including cognition and risk of adult degenerative disease. It seems likely that nutritional practices will move away from the sole focus on achieving short term targets, such as normalization of immediate growth rate, but rather will be geared increasingly to their impact on long term outcomes. By analogy, the current treatment of high blood pressure is not based on the mere fact that blood pressure may be altered to keep it close to population norms, but rather because treatment reduces serious later morbidity, such as mortality from stroke. Our new understanding of the importance of nutrition clearly puts an onus on health professionals, including pediatricians, to engage in its effective practice in the interests of child health.

REFERENCES

1. Lucas A, Cole TJ. Breast milk and neonatal necrotising enterocolitis. *Lancet.* 1990;336:1519–1523.
2. Booth IW. Enteral nutrition in childhood. *Br J Hosp Med.* 1991;46:111–113.
3. Committee on Clinical Practice Issues in Health and Disease. The role and identity of physician nutrition specialists in medical school-affiliated hospitals. *Am J Clin Nutr.* 1995;61:264–268.
4. Bishop NJ, Morley R, Day JP, Lucas A. Aluminium neurotoxicity in preterm infants receiving intravenous-feeding solutions. *N Engl J Med.* 1997;336:1557–1561.
5. Lucas A. Programming by early nutrition in man: the childhood environment and adult disease. In: Bock GR, Chichester WJ, eds. *CIBA Foundation Symposium 156.* Chichester: Wiley; 1991:38–55.
6. Spalding DA. Instinct with original observations on young animals. *MacMillan's Magazine.* 1873;27:282–293. Reprinted in *Br J Anim Behav.* 1954;2:2–11.
7. Angelbeck JH, DuBrul EF. The effect of neonatal testosterone on specific male and female patterns of phosphorylated cytosolic proteins in the rat preoptic-hypothalamus, cortex and amygdala. *Brain Res.* 1983;264:277–283.
8. Bagley DM, Hayes JR. Neonatal phenobarbital administration results in increased cytochrome P450-dependent monocygencase activity in adult male and female rats. *Biochem Biophys Res Commun.* 1983;114:1132–1137.
9. McCance RA. Food growth and time. *Lancet.* 1962;2:271–272.
10. Smart J. Under nutrition, learning and memory: review of experimental studies. In: Taylor TG, Jenkins NK, eds. *Proceedings of XII International Congress of Nutrition.* London: John Libbey; 1986:74–78.
11. Hahn P. Effect of litter size on plasma cholesterol and insulin and some liver and adipose tissue enzymes in adult rodents. *J Nutr.* 1984;114:1231–1234.
12. Lewis DS, Bartrand HA, McMahan CA, McGill HC Jr, Carey KD, Masoro EJ. Preweaning food intake influences the adiposity of young adult baboons. *J Clin Invest.* 1986;78:899–905.
13. Ozanne SE, Hales CN. Catch-up growth and obesity in male mice. *Nature.* 2004;427:411–412.
14. Barker DJP. Fetal nutrition and cardiovascular disease in adult life. *Lancet.* 1993;341:938–941.
15. Singhal A, Lucas A. Early origins of cardiovascular disease. Is there a unifying hypothesis? *Lancet.* 2004;363:1642–1645.
16. Lucas A, Morley R, Cole TJ. Randomised trial of early diet in preterm babies and later intelligence quotient. *BMJ.* 1998;317:1481–1487.
17. Grantham-McGregor S. Field studies in early nutrition and later achievement. In: Dobbing J, ed. *Early Nutrition and Later Achievement.* London: Academic Press; 1987:128–174.
18. Simeon DT, Grantham-McGregor SM. Nutritional deficiencies and children's behaviour and mental development. *Nutr Res Rev.* 1990;3:1–24.
19. Freeman HE, Klein RE, Townsend JW, Lechtig A. Nutrition and cognitive development among

rural Guatemalan children. *Am J Public Health.* 1980;70:1277–1285.

20. Florey C du V, Leech AM, Blackhall A. Infant feeding and mental and motor development at 18 months of age in first born singletons. *Int J Epidemiol.* 1995;24: S21–26.
21. Rogan WJ, Gladen BC. Breast feeding and cognitive development. *Early Hum Dev.* 1993;31:181–193.
22. Fergusson DM, Beautrais AL, Silva PA. Breast feeding and cognitive development in the first seven years of life. *Soc Sci Med.* 1982;16:1705–1708.
23. Rodgers B. Feeding in infancy and later ability and attainment: a longitudinal study. *Dev Med Child Neurol.* 1978;20:421–426.
24. Lucas A, Morley R. Breast milk and subsequent intelligence quotient in children born preterm. *Lancet.* 1991;339:261–264.
25. Hoefer C, Hardy MC. Later development of breast fed and artificially fed infants. *JAMA.* 1929;92:615–619.
26. Gale CR, Martyn CN. Breast feeding, dummy use and adult intelligence. *Lancet.* 1996;347:1072–1075.
27. Super CM, Herrera MG, Mora JO. Long-term effects of food supplementation and psychosocial intervention on the physical growth of Colombian infants at risk of malnutrition. *Child Development.* 1990; 61(1):29–49.
28. Grantham-McGregor SM, Powell CA, Walker SP, Himes JH. Nutritional supplementation, psychosocial stimulation, and mental development of stunted children: the Jamaican study. *Lancet.* 1991;338:1–5.
29. Lucas A, Morley R, Cole TJ, et al. Early diet in preterm babies and developmental status at 18 months. *Lancet.* 1990;335:1477–1481.
30. Kolb B, Whishaw IQ. Development and recovery. In: Schmidt Robert, ed. *Fundamentals of Neuropsychology*. 3rd ed. New York, NY: Freeman HE; 1990;679–711.
31. Fierro-Beniter R, Casar R, Stanbury J, et al. Long-term effects of correction of iodine deficiency on psychomotor development and intellectual development. In: Dunn J, Pretell E, Dara C, Viteri F, eds. *Towards the Eradication of Endemic Goiter, Cretinism and Iodine Deficiency*. Washington, DC: Pan American Health Organisation; 1986; 140–199.
32. Lozoff B, Jimenez E, Wolf AW. Long-term developmental outcome of infants with iron deficiency. *N Engl J Med.* 1991;325:687–694.
33. Walter T. Impact of iron deficiency on cognition in infancy and childhood. *Eur J Clin Nutr.* 1993;47:307–316.
34. Lozoff B, Britenham GM, Wolf AW, et al. Iron deficiency anaemia and iron therapy effects on infant developmental test performance. *Pediatrics.* 2004;79:981–995.
35. Wharton BA, Morley R, Isaacs EB, Cole TJ, Lucas A. Low plasma taurine and later neurodevelopment. *Arch Dis Child Fetal Neonatal Ed.* 2004;89:F497–F498.
36. Fewtrell MS, Morley R, Abbott RA, et al. Double-blind randomised trial of long-chain polyunsaturated fatty acid supplementation in formula fed to preterm infants *Pediatrics.* 2002;110:73–82.
37. Fewtrell MS, Abbott RA, Kennedy K, et al. Randomized double-blind trial of LCPUFA-supplementation using fish oil and borage oil in preterm infants. *J Pediatr.* 2004;144:471–479.
38. O'Connor D, Hall R, Adamkin D, et al. Growth and development in preterm infants fed long-chain polyunsaturated fatty acids: a prospective, randomized controlled trial. *Pediatrics.* 2001;108:359–371.
39. Simmer, K. Patole, S. Longchain polyunsaturated fatty acid supplementation in preterm infants. *Cochrane Database of Systematic Reviews.* 1, 2006.
40. Simmer, K. Longchain polyunsaturated fatty acid supplementation in infants born at term. *Cochrane Database of Systematic Reviews.* 1, 2006.
41. Lauritzen L, Hansen HS, Jorgensen MH, Michaelsen KF. The essentiality of long chain n-3 fatty acids in relation to development and function of the brain and retina. *Progress in Lipid Res.* 2001;40:1.
42. Fewtrell MS, Cole TJ, Bishop NJ, Lucas A. Neonatal factors predicting childhood height in preterm infants: evidence for a persisting effect of early metabolic bone disease. *J Pediatr.* 2000;137:668–673.
43. Fewtrell MS, Prentice A, Jones SC, Lunt M, Cole TJ, Lucas A. Bone mineralization and turnover in preterm infants at 8–12 years of age: the effects of early diet. *J Bone Miner Res.* 1999;14:810–820.
44. Desai M, Crowther NJ, Ozanne SE, Lucas A, Hales CN. Adult glucose and lipid metabolism may be programmed during fetal life. *Biochem Soc Trans.* 1995;23:331–335.
45. Snoek A, Remacle C, Reusens B, Hoet JJ. Effect of a low protein diet during pregnancy on the fetal rat endocrine pancreas. *Biol Neonate.* 1990;57:107–118.
46. Fall CHD, Barker DJP, Osmond C, Winter PD, Clark PMS, Hales CN. Relation of infant feeding to adult serum cholesterol concentration and death from ischaemic heart disease. *BMJ.* 1992;304:801–805.
47. Owen CG, Whincup PH, Odoki K, Gilg JA, Cook DG. Infant feeding and blood cholesterol: a study in adolescents and a systematic review. *Pediatrics.* 2002;110:597–608.
48. Von Kries R, Koletzko B, Sauerwald T, et al. Breastfeeding and obesity: cross sectional study. *BMJ.* 1999;319:147–150.
49. Pettitt DJ, Forman MR, Hanson RL, Knowler WC, Bennett PH. Breastfeeding and incidence of non-insulin-dependent diabetes mellitus in Pima Indians. *Lancet.* 1997;350:166–168.

50. Singhal A, Cole TJ, Lucas A. Early nutrition in preterm infants and later blood pressure: two cohorts after randomised trials. *Lancet.* 2001;357:413–419.
51. Singhal A, Cole TJ, Fewtrell M, Lucas A. Breast-milk feeding and the lipoprotein profile in adolescents born preterm. *Lancet.* 2004;363:1571–1578.
52. Singhal A, Fewtrell M, Cole TJ, Lucas A. Low nutrient intake and early growth for later insulin resistance in adolescents born preterm. *Lancet.* 2003;361:1089–1097.
53. Singhal A, Sadaf Farooqi I, O'Rahilly S, Cole TJ, Fewtrell MS, Lucas A. Early nutrition and leptin concentrations in later life. *Am J Clin Nutr.* 2002;75:993–999.
54. Singhal A, Cole TJ, Fewtrell M, Deanfield J, Lucas A. Is slower early growth beneficial for long-term cardiovascular health? *Circulation.* 2004;109:1108–1113.
55. Metcalfe NB, Monaghan P. Compensation for a bad start: grow now, pay later? *Trends Ecol Evol.* 2001;16:254–260.
56. Roth GS, Ingram DK, Black A, Lane MA. Effect of reduced energy intake on the biology of ageing: the primate model. *Eur J Clin Nutr.* 2000;54:S15–20.
57. Forsen T, Eriksson J, Tuomilehto J, Reunanen A, Osmond C, Barker D. The fetal and childhood growth of persons who develop type 2 diabetes. *Ann Intern Med.* 2000;133:176–182.
58. Ong KKL, Ahmed ML, Emmett PM, Preece MA, Dunger DB. Association between postnatal catch-up growth and obesity in childhood: prospective cohort study. *BMJ.* 2000;320:967–971.
59. Eriksson JG, Forsen T, Tuomilehto J, Winter PD, Osmond C, Barker DJP. Catch-up growth in childhood and death from coronary heart disease: longitudinal study. *BMJ.* 1999;318:427–431.
60. Stettler N, Zemel BS, Kumanyika S, Stallings VA. Infant weight gain and childhood overweight status in a multicenter, cohort study. *Pediatrics.* 2002;109:194–199.
61. Finken MJJ, Keijzer-Veen MG, Van Montfoort AG, et al. Early catch-up growth in weight of very preterm low birthweight infants is associated with higher levels of LDL-cholesterol and apo-B at age 19. *Pediatr Res.* 2003;53(suppl):32A.
62. Colle E, Schiff D, Andrew G, Bauer CB, Fitzhardinge P. Insulin responses during catch-up growth of infants who were small for gestational age. *Pediatrics.* 1976;57:363–371.
63. Deiber M, Chatelain D, Naville D, Putet G, Salle B. Functional hypersomatotropism in small for gestational age (SGA) newborn infants. *J Clin Endocrinol Metab.* 1989;68:232–234.
64. Cianfarani S, Germani D, Branca F. Low birthweight and adult insulin resistance: the 'catch-up growth' hypothesis. *Arch Dis Child Fetal Neonatal Ed.* 1999;81: F71–73.
65. Martin RM, McCarthy A, Smith Davey G, Davies DP, Ben-Schlomo Y. Infant nutrition and blood pressure in early adulthood: the Barry Caerphilly growth study. *Am J Clin Nutr.* 2003;77:1489–1497.
66. Wilson AC, Forsyth JS, Greene SA, Irvine L, Hau C, Howie PW. Relation of infant diet to childhood health: seven year follow up of cohort of children in Dundee infant feeding study. *BMJ.* 1998:316:21–25.
67. Plagemann A, Franke K, Harder T, Kohlhoff R. Long-term impact of neonatal breast-feeding on body weight and glucose tolerance in children of diabetic mothers. *Diabetes Care.* 2002;25:16–22.
68. Morley R, Fewtrell MS, Abbott RA, Stephenson T, MacFadyen UM, Lucas A. Neurodevelopment in children born small for gestational age; a randomized trial of nutrient enriched versus standard formula, and comparison with a reference breast fed group. *Pediatrics.* 2004;113:515–521.
69. Mott GE, Lewis DS, McGill HC. Programming of cholesterol metabolism by breast or formula feeding: the childhood environment and adult disease. In: Bock GR, Chichester WJ, eds. *CIBA Foundation Symposium 156.* Chichester: Wiley; 1991:56–76.

CHAPTER 5

Anthropometric Evaluation

Kristy Hendricks

INTRODUCTION

Physical growth is, from conception to maturity, a complex process influenced by nutrition, environment, and genetics. Anthropometry, the study of human body measurements on a comparative basis, includes the measurement of physical dimensions at different ages and is widely used to monitor the growth and health of individuals.[1,2] Comparison with references for age and sex helps determine abnormalities in growth and development that may have resulted from nutrient deficiencies or excesses.

Accurate assessment of growth requires an appropriate growth reference, accurate measures, accurate calculation of the child's age, and appropriate interpretation of the scale used to describe the variable.[1,3] Various scales are used in the pediatric population to describe and evaluate anthropometric indicators. These measures are most frequently described as percentiles, z-scores and percent of the median.[1,3] Each scale has strengths; a comparison of their relevant issues of use and interpretation is summarized in Table 5-1. Each scale compares the individual to the reference population,

Table 5-1 Summary of the use of anthropometric scales.

	Z-scores	*Percentiles*	*Percent of median*
Uses normalized curves	Yes	Yes	No
Interpretation of extreme values consistent across age and height groups*	Yes	Yes	No
Interpretation of cut-off value consistent across indices†	Yes	Yes	No
Ability to identify children with extreme values	Good	Poor	Good
Values from a study population are distributed normally	Yes	No	Yes‡

* The physiological meaning or consequences of extreme values may differ across age and height groups.
† For example, 80% of median is about – 4 SD for height-for-age, but about – 2 SD for weight-for-age.
‡ May be skewed to upper values in weight-for-height and weight-for-age curves.

Source: Gorstein J, Sullivan K, Yip R, et al. Issues in the assessment of nutritional status using anthropometry. *Bull World Health Organ.* 1994;72:273–283. Reproduced with permission.

which presently is the revised National Center for Health Statistics (NCHS) and Centers for Disease Control (CDC) growth reference, which will be discussed in the next section.[4–6] Optimally, the nutritional risk of an individual will be classified accurately if the measure is accurate and the appropriate growth reference and scale of comparison is used.

Repeated measurements of an individual over time provide objective data on nutrition, health, and well being. While evaluating growth over time is more useful than a single measurement, single measurements can be used to screen children who may be at nutritional risk and to determine need for a more complete assessment. Accurate assessment of body composition in infants and children is fundamental to understanding normal growth and development, and growth is a marker for a variety of medical and psychosocial problems in infants and children. Errors of measurements taken at different times can be caused by poor technique and equipment[1,7] (see Chapter 1 for further discussion). Detailed descriptions of standardized techniques and equipment for anthropometry can be found in other sources.[1,7]

ANTHROPOMETRIC REFERENCE DATA FOR CHILDREN: NCHS/CDC REVISED GROWTH CHARTS FOR THE UNITED STATES

In 2000, the NCHS/CDC revised growth charts for the United States were released.[4] The new charts are based on a different reference population than the 1977 charts were, but the newer ones appear similar to the 1977 charts, which consisted of 14 charts based on age, gender, weight-for-age, length-for-age, height-for-age, weight-for-length, and weight-for-height. In addition to these, 16 new charts include charts for body mass index (BMI) for age for boys and girls aged 2 to 20 years. Data from multiple National Health Nutrition Examination Surveys (NHANES I and III) that was collected between 1963 and 1994 and other additional data sources were used to establish the growth chart data set.[4–6]

National data were lacking for infants and young children, and the revised infant growth charts reflect more racial and ethnic diversity and a better mix of bottle fed and breastfed infants. CDC promotes one set of growth charts for all racial and ethnic groups.[8] In addition, new BMI growth charts, which can be used clinically beginning at age 2 years, are available for boys and girls. It should be noted that to avoid the influence of an increase in body weight and BMI that occurred with NHANES III, experts agreed that data from subjects older than 6 years from that survey be excluded from the revised weight and BMI charts.[5]

Three sets of charts have been developed using differing percentile curves and the addition of 3rd and 97th percentiles to the graphs to better assess children at the extremes of the percentiles. The majority of clinicians will use the charts that have the 5th, 10th, 25th, 50th, 75th, 90th, and 95th percentiles. All of the revised growth charts and accompanying background information are available at http://www.cdc.gov/growthcharts.

The World Health Organization (WHO) is developing international standard growth charts for children birth to 5 years. The growth standard will be based on infants who follow WHO infant feeding recommendations of breastfeeding for 12 months and initiation of complementary feeding between 4 and 6 months. Once published, the application for use in the US population will be assessed.[6]

SCALES OF COMPARISON

Percentiles

The CDC growth charts consist of a series of curves called percentiles that graph the distribution of American children by selected body measurements. Percentiles are the common clinically used method of comparison that graphically indicate where individual children fit in context to the reference. Percentiles rank the position of a child, indicating what percent of the population would have higher or lower measurements than that individual. The growth charts are discussed in the previous section, and a summary of percentile indicators of nutritional status is shown in Table 5-2.[5] These are CDC recommended cut off criteria for screening, indicating the need for further evaluation of growth parameters as discussed in the following sections.

Z-Score

Table 5-1 summarizes scales of the various indicators of growth. Z-score denotes deviation of an individual value from the mean value of the reference population divided by the standard deviation for the reference population.[9] It may be used to express any normally distributed numerical measurement, but is most frequently used to evaluate weight, height, and weight-for-height. It is more sensitive than percentile change because it allows the clinician to numerically describe the distance of the measurement from the median; thus movement toward or away from the average is precisely expressed. This measurement is particularly useful for chronically ill children, a significant percentage of whom will fall below the fifth percentile, as children with values below (or above) the extreme percentiles can be classified accurately. Although easier to understand graphically as a percentile, the degree of deficit or improvement becomes clearer when expressed numerically, as a z-score, and patients' measurements move toward or away from the median. The following equation shows how to calculate z-score:

$$(\text{actual value} - \text{median reference value}) \div \text{standard deviation}.$$

Compared to the percentiles the following z-scores are approximate:

$$97\% = +1.88$$

$$50\% = 0$$

$$3\% = -1.88$$

Percent of the Median

The third scale commonly used to compare anthropometric measures is percent of the median. Methods vary widely in classification of malnutrition, but most use percent of the median for various measures including weight-for-height, weight-for-age, and height-for-age.[10–13] Examples of common classifications are shown in Table 5-3. The various measures can have quite different interpretations. The classification of the indices measured into discrete categories such as either wasting or stunting is important as the etiology and treatment may vary.

Weight

Body weight is a reproducible growth parameter and a good index of acute and chronic nutritional status. Accurate age and sex specific referral data for comparison is necessary for evaluation. Weight is typically evaluated in three ways: weight-for-age, weight-for-height, and

Table 5-2 Indicators of nutritional status (percentiles).

Head circumference-for-age	< 5th percentile > 95th percentile
Stunting/shortness Length- or height-for-age	< 5th percentile
Underweight Weight-for-length BMI-for-age	< 5th percentile
Overweight Weight-for-length BMI-for-age	> 95th percentile
Risk of overweight BMI-for-age	85th to > 95th percentile

Source: Adapted from Polhamus B, Thompson D, Benton-Davis SL, Reinold CM, Grummer-Strawn LM, Dietz W. Overview of the CDC growth charts: United States, 2003. Available at: http://www.medscape.com/viewprogram/2560_pnt. Accessed April 23, 2004.

BMI.[1,2,4] Weight-for-age compares the individual to reference data for weight attained at any given age whereas weight-for-height looks at the appropriateness of the individual's weight compared to his or her own height. Weight-for-age does not distinguish between short children with adequate body weight (stunting) and tall, thin children (wasting).[2,3] The use of weight-for-age for predicting or identifying "wasted" children was found to have low sensitivity and specificity in 3 US populations.[14] When a child is underweight, further assessment is necessary to determine whether this is due to wasting, stunting, or a combination. Despite limitations, as a single measure and over time, weight is a useful and primary growth indicator.[15]

Length

Measured with appropriate equipment and technique, length is a simple and reproducible growth parameter that provides, in conjunction with weight, significant information. Length-for-age growth charts assesses linear growth. Children who fall below the fifth percentile may have a severe deficit, and measurements that range between the fifth and tenth percentiles should be evaluated further.[4] Length assesses growth failure and chronic undernutrition, especially in early childhood and adolescence.[1,2] Children whose serial anthropometric data show a change in relative position on the height growth curves should be evaluated by other indices such as z-score over time or incremental growth curves (growth velocity).[3,9]

Head Circumference

Head circumference as an indicator of brain growth can be influenced by nutritional status until the age of 36 months, but deficiencies are manifest in weight and height before being seen in brain growth. Routine examination also screens for other possible influences on brain growth, such as developmental delay or neurological problems.[5]

Weight-for-Height

Weight-for-length reflects body weight independent of age, giving a better indication of appropriate body size. This ratio more accurately assesses body build and distinguishes wasting (acute malnutrition) from stunting (chronic malnutrition).[1,2] Low weight-for-height or growth faltering may be more responsive to nutrition therapy than chronic stunting, which is frequently more complex in nature.[16,17] Weight-for-height should also be interpreted in the context of weight-for-age and height-for-age. Especially in chronically ill children, weight-for-height alone may not accurately identify obesity.[18]

Table 5-3 Classification of malnutrition (percent of the median).

Anthropometric measure	*Normal*	*Mild*	*Moderate*	*Severe*
Weight-for-age	> 90 (10)	90–75	< 75–60	< 60
Weight-for-height	110–90 (11)	90–85	85–75	< 75
Weight-for-height	> 90 (13)	90–81	80–70	< 70

Sources: Developed from Gomez F, Galvan RR, Cravioto J, Frenk S. Malnutrition in infancy and childhood, with special reference to kwashiorkor. *Adv Pediatr.* 1955;7:131–169; McLean DS, Read WWC. Weight/length classification of nutrition status. *Lancet.* 1975;2:219–221; and Waterlow JC. Classification and definition of protein calorie malnutrition. *Br Med J.* 1972;3:565–567.

BMI

BMI is determined by dividing the person's weight in kilograms by their height in meters squared. The formula for BMI is:

$$\text{BMI} = \text{weight (kg)}/\text{height}^2 \text{ (meters)}$$

BMI correlates well with adiposity in adults and is recommended for use in screening for obesity. In adolescents, BMI-for-age correlates with total body fatness.[19,20] Age and sexual maturity are also highly correlated with body fatness. BMI is a major addition to the revised CDC growth charts for children older than 2 years.[4] Numerous professional organizations endorse use of BMI percentile to assess overweight, risk of overweight, and underweight in this population.[21–23] BMI-for-age is the only indicator that allows plotting a measure of weight and height with age on the same chart. BMI is gender and age specific until adulthood.[4] It is recommended that percentiles be used rather than an absolute number because this value changes throughout periods of growth. A BMI at the 95th percentile may range from 18 to 30, depending on the age and sex of the child. Currently a BMI at or above the 85th percentile for age and sex, using the NCHS growth data, indicates a need for evaluation and treatment for overweight. BMI is a screening tool, used to identify overweight or underweight (see Table 5-2). Further assessment of body composition would be warranted to determine excess fat deposition.

Growth Velocity

Growth velocity is a simple and reproducible measure that evaluates change in rate of growth over a specified time period; it generally is expressed in centimeters per year.[2] It is a sensitive way of assessing growth failure or slowed growth and is particularly helpful in the early identification of children with undernutrition. Increments in growth may occur at different times, but they follow a similar sequence in most instances. Growth velocity charts are constructed from and used for longitudinally obtained incremental data.[24–26] Either a dramatic decrease or slow deceleration in growth velocity from the norm needs further assessment as to causation.

Sex specific percentiles for increments in weight, length, head circumference, and mid-upper arm circumferences (MUAC) based on longitudinal data from the multicenter Euro-Growth Study are now available for selected intervals during the first 36 months of life.[24] The anthropometric cohort (n = 2145) came from 12 European countries with diverse socio-economic characteristics; 54% of the infants were exclusively breastfed for the first 2 months. These and previously published[25,26] incremental growth references may be useful in the evaluation of serial anthropometric measures.

Body Composition

The assessment of body composition is an important parameter in making clinical decisions about causes and treatment of growth abnormalities.[1] Lean body mass (LBM) and fat mass (FM) are the 2 compartments typically measured.[1,7] As an example, Stapelton found the deficit for z-scores of anthropometric measures of LBM (or muscularity) to be greater than the deficit in adiposity for children with cystic fibrosis.[27]

Skinfold Thickness

Nearly half of the body fat in humans is in the subcutaneous layer, and measurements of this deposit can lead to accurate estimates of total body fat. Skinfold thickness measurements are accurate, simple, and reproducible, and they can be used to monitor changes in total body fat.[1,7] Measurements for childhood through adult life were compiled by Frisancho, based on measurements of large samples of children throughout the United States.[28] Skinfold thickness measurements assess current nutritional status and body composition. They provide an index of body energy stores and can be used in conjunction with weight or height to determine chronic undernutrition or overweight and to define the athletic child who might be overweight but not "overfat." Measurement sites vary, and edema or intravenous fluids may affect accuracy. Measurements are most useful on children who can be followed over a period of time.

Tricep skinfold is the most commonly measured site; subscapular and suprailiac measurements are also frequently used, though reference data are limited.[29] Daniels and colleagues assessed the ability of different measures of body fat distribution in children and adolescents.[30] Dual-Energy X-ray Absorptiometry (DEXA), which can be used to assess body composition as well as bone mineral density, was used as the gold standard in evaluating 201 children ages 7–17 years. The strongest correlation of fat distribution was waist circumference and subscapular skinfold thickness. Age was found to be more important than pubertal maturation, and there was greater deposition of central fat with increasing age.[31] Reference data on body composition currently being obtained by NHANES, which includes DEXA, should allow assessment of the validity of various skinfold measures in children.[32]

Circumferences

Circumferences are important measurements that record the size of cross-sectional and circumferential dimensions of the body. Circumferences used alone, in combination with skinfold measurements taken at the same location, or in combination with other circumferences can provide indices of nutritional status and levels of fat patterns.[7] Circumferences of the limbs, together with skinfold measures of subcutaneous adipose tissue thickness, can provide cross-sectional areas of adipose tissue or areas of the underlying muscle plus bone.

In conjunction with triceps skinfold thickness, MUAC can be used to determine cross-sectional midarm muscle and fat areas. As with skinfold thickness, arm circumference correlates well with other more sophisticated and difficult measures of body composition.[1,7] A simple nomogram calculation requires circumference and triceps skinfold measures to determine muscle circumference and cross-sectional muscle and fat areas. A WHO expert committee recommended that MUAC for age reference values be developed and published.[33] In addition, a reference set of curves for MUAC for height have been generated and are age and sex independent.[34]

As discussed, waist circumference has been shown to correlate with most precise measures of body fat. Other anthropometric variables determined to be of use in the adult population, particularly in evaluating overweight, are currently being assessed in the pediatric population.[35] Recommendations for their use and interpretation will be particularly helpful in the adolescent age group.

BONE MINERALIZATION

Osteoporosis occurs in all populations and at all ages.[36] In children with chronic disease or nutrition related disorders, this risk is increased.[37] In these children, altered growth, delayed maturation, inflammation, or inadequate diet and activity may increase risk.[38] Assessment of bone mass, identification of causation, and risk are essential in determining treatment options.

DEXA is a precise method frequently used to assess bone mineral density (BMD) in children.[39] Interpretation of BMD in children is complicated by puberty, age, and body size, as well as racial and ethnic differences. More complete reference data with which to compare children has also helped in the evaluation process. Several investigators feel that BMD expressed as z-score more accurately defines the bone mineralization status of children.[40,41]

CONCLUSION

Tracking of a child's growth by anthropometric measures is a sensitive method of evaluating nutritional status and health. Accurate assessment of growth is essential in identifying children at nutritional risk, determining causation, and initiating potential medical nutrition therapy. The 2000 NCHS/CDC growth charts represent a significant improvement in the growth reference for assessment and are recommended for use in all children.

REFERENCES

1. Gibson RS. *Principles of Nutritional Assessment.* New York, NY: Oxford University Press; 1990.
2. Hendricks KM, Duggan C, eds. *Manual of Pediatric Nutrition.* 5th ed. Hamilton, Ontario, Canada: BC Decker; 2005.
3. Gorstein J, Sullivan K, Yip R, et al. Issues in the assessment of nutritional status using anthropometry. *Bull World Health Organ.* 1994;72(2):273–283.
4. Kuczmarski RJ, Ogden CL, Grummer-Stawn LM, et al. CDC growth charts: United States. *Vital and Health Statistics CDC/NCHS 314*; May 30, 2000.
5. Polhamus B, Thompson D, Benton-Davis SL, Reinold CM, Grummer-Strawn LM, Dietz W. Overview of the CDC growth charts: United States, 2003. Available at: http://www.medscape.com/viewprogram/2560_pnt. Accessed April 23, 2004.
6. Grummer-Strawn LM, Garza C, Johnson CL. Childhood growth charts. *Pediatrics.* 2002;109(1):141–142.
7. Lohman TG, Roche AF, Martdroll R. *Anthropometrics standardization reference manual.* Champaign, Ill: Human Kinetics Books; 1988.
8. Overpeck MD, Hediger ML, Ruan WJ, et al. Stature, weight, and body mass among young US children born at term with appropriate birth weights. *J Pediatr.* 2000;137(2):205–213.
9. Dibley MJ, Staehling N, Nieburg P, et al. Interpretation of z score anthropometric indicators derived from the international growth reference. *Am J Clin Nutr.* 1987;20:503.
10. Gomez F, Galvan RR, Cravioto J, Frenk S. Malnutrition in infancy and childhood, with special reference to kwashiorkor. *Adv Pediatr.* 1955;7:131–169.
11. McLaren DS, Read WW. Weight/length classification of nutrition status. *Lancet.* 1975;2:219–221.
12. Jelliffe D. The assessment of nutritional status of the community. In: *World Health Organization Monograph 53*. Geneva, Switzerland: World Health Organization; 1996.
13. Waterlow JC. Classification and definition of protein calorie malnutrition. *Br Med J.* 1972;3:565–567.
14. Sullivan KM, et al. Weight-for-age as a screening tool for finding children who are low weight-for-height. In: *Abstracts of the 116th Annual Meeting of the American Public Health Association, Chicago, IL, 13–17 November 1988.* Washington, DC: American Public Health Association; 1989:88.
15. Raynor P, Rudolf MCJ. Anthropometric indices of failure to thrive. *Arch Dis Child.* 2000;82(5):364–365.
16. Mascarenhas MR, Zemel B, Stallings VA. Nutritional assessment in pediatrics. *Nutrition.* 1998;14:105–115.
17. Ekvall SW. Nutritional assessment and early intervention. In: Ekvall SW, ed. *Pediatric Nutrition in Chronic Diseases and Developmental Disorders.* New York, NY: Oxford University Press;1993:53.
18. Hendricks KM, Duggan C, Gallagher L, et al. Malnutrition in hospitalized pediatric patients: Current prevalence. *Arch. Ped. Adol. Med.* 1995;149(10):1118–1112.
19. American Academy of Pediatrics Committee on Nutrition. Prevention of pediatric overweight and obesity. *Pediatrics.* 2003;112:424–430. Available at: http://pediatrics.aappublications.org/cgi/content/full/112/2/424?eaf. Accessed April 23, 2004.
20. Freedman DS, Dietz WH, Srinivasan SR, Berenson GS. The relationship of overweight to cardiovascular risk factor among children and adolescents: the Bogalusa heart study. *Pediatrics.* 1999;103:1175–1182.
21. Himes JH, Dietz WH. Guidelines for overweight in adolescent preventive services: recommendations from an expert committee—the Expert Committee on Clinical Guidelines for Overweight in Adolescent Preventive Services. *Am J Clin Nutr.* 1994;59(2):307–316.
22. Barlow SE, Dietz WH. Obesity evaluation and treatment: Expert Committee recommendations. The Maternal and Child Health Bureau, Health Resources and Services Administration and the Department of Health and Human Services. *Pediatrics.* 1998;102(3):E29.
23. Anonymous. Assessment of Childhood and Adolescent Obesity: results from an international obesity task force workshop; Dublin, June 16, 1997. *Am J Clin Nutr.* 1999;70(1):117S–175S.
24. van't Hof MA, Haschke F, Darvay S, for the Euro-Growth Study Group. Euro-growth references on increments in length, weight, and head and arm circumferences during the first 3 years of life. *J Pediatr Gastroenterol Nutr.* 2000;31(suppl):S39–S47.
25. Roche AF, Himes JH. Incremental growth charts. *Am J Clin Nutr.* 1980;33:2041–2052.
26. Tanner JM, Davis PSW. Clinical longitudinal standards for height and weight velocity for North American children. *J Pediatr.* 1985;107:317–329.
27. Stapelton D, Kerr D, Gurrin L, Sherriff J, Sly P. Height and weight fail to detect early signs of malnutrition in children with cystic fibrosis. *J Pediatr Gastro Nutr.* 2001;33(3):319–325.
28. Frisancho AR. New norms of upper limb fat and muscle areas for assessment of nutritional status. *Am J Clin Nutr.* 1981;34:2540.
29. Roche AF, Sievogel RM, Chumlea WC, Webb P. Grading body fatness from limited anthropometric data. *Am J Clin Nutr.* 1981;34(12):2831–2838.
30. Daniels SR, Khoury PR, Morrison JA. Utility of different measures of body fat distribution in children and adolescents. *Am J Epidemiol.* 2000;152(12):1179–1184.

31. Brambilla P, Roland-Cachera MF, Testolin C, et al. Lean mass of children in various nutritional states: comparison between dual-energy x-ray absorptiometry and anthropometry. *Ann N Y Acad Sci.* 2000; 904:433–436.
32. US Department of Health and Human Services, Centers for Disease Control and Prevention, National Center for Health Statistics. NHANES III reference manuals and reports [computer file]. Hyattsville, MD: National Center for Health Statistics, 1996. Available at: http://www.cdc.gov/nchs/data/nhanes/bc.pdf. Accessed December 8, 2005.
33. de Onis M, Yip R, Mei Z. The development of MUAC-for-age reference data recommended by a WHO Expert Committee. *Bull World Health Organ.* 1997;75:11–18.
34. Mei Z, Grummer-Strawn LM, de Onis M, Yip R. The development of a MUAC-for-height reference, including a comparison to other nutritional status screening indicators. *Bull World Health Organ.* 1997;75(4):333–341.
35. Gillum RF. Distribution of waist-to-hip ratio, other indices of body fat distribution and obesity and associations with HDL cholesterol in children and young adults aged 4–19 years: the third national health and nutrition examination survey. *Int J Obes Rel Metab Disorders: J Int Assoc Study Obes.* 1999;23(6):556–563.
36. Anonymous. Osteoporosis prevention, diagnosis, and therapy. [Consensus Development Conference, NIH]. *NIH Consensus Statement.* March 27–29, 2000;17(1):1–45.
37. Moreira-Andres MN, Canizo FJ, de la Cruz FJ, Gomez-de la Camara A, Hawkins FG. Evaluation of radial bone mineral content in prepubertal children with constitutional delay of growth. *J Pediatr Endocrin Metab.* 2000;13(6):591–597.
38. Leonard MB, Propert KJ, Zemel BS, Stallings VA, Feldman HI. Discrepancies in pediatric bone mineral density reference data: potential for misdiagnosis of osteopenia. *J Pediatr.* 1999;135(2 Pt 1):182–188.
39. Warner JT, Cowan FJ, Dunstan FDJ, Evans WD, Webb DKH, Gregory JW. Measured and predicted bone mineral content in healthy boys and girls aged 6–18 years: adjustment for body size and puberty. *Acta Paediatrica.* 2004;87(3):244–249.
40. Henderson RC. The correlation between dual-energy x-ray absorptiometry measures of bone density in the proximal femur and lumbar spine of children. *Skeletal Radiol.* 1997;26(9):544–547.
41. Ellis KJ, Shypailo RJ, Hardin DS, et al. Z score prediction model for assessment of bone mineral content in pediatric diseases. *J Bone Min Res.* 2001;16(9):1658–1664.

Chapter 6

Energy Metabolism and Appropriate Energy Repletion in Children

Walter J. Chwals

INTRODUCTION

Energy metabolism is based on the provision of protein and nonprotein substrates. Energy requirements in children differ from those in adults because of additional requirements for growth and physical activity. Growth velocity during early infancy is higher than at any other time during childhood and is exceeded only by intrauterine growth rates. Energy requirements are also dependent on metabolic status and nutritional reserve and can change rapidly in response to acute injury.

Energy Expenditure Measurement

Changes in energy expenditure reflect alterations in metabolism that accompany a variety of clinical states. Accurate assessment of energy expenditure allows the provision of appropriate calories, avoids excesses or deficits of nutritional substrates, and decreases morbidity and mortality.

Energy expenditure is a characteristic feature of metabolism that can be measured by the amount of heat released. This is the principle of *direct calorimetry,* in which energy release is quantified by the amount of heat required to raise the temperature of 1 mL of water by 1° C from 15.5° to 16.5° C (1 calorie). Energy required to raise the temperature of 1 liter of water by 1° C in the same fashion is 1 kilocalorie. Because direct calorimetry requires a subject to be enclosed in a calorimeter for extended periods, it is impractical for clinical use. In contrast, *indirect calorimetry* can be performed at the bedside using a metabolic cart. A metabolic cart measures the differences in O_2 and CO_2 concentrations between a known volume (liters/min) of inspired and expired gas.[1] O_2 consumption (VO_2) and CO_2 production (VCO_2) may be calculated on the basis of known and constant relationships between VO_2, VCO_2, and heat produced (energy expenditure) for a variety of metabolic processes. These include the oxidation of carbohydrates, fats, and proteins and lipogenesis. The following formula, [2,3] or variations of it, is generally employed:

$$MEE = 3.58\ VO_2 + 1.45\ VCO_2 + 1.8\ U_N$$

where MEE is measured energy expenditure (kcal/unit time) and UN is urinary nitrogen. The respiratory quotient (RQ) defined as VCO_2/VO_2 is specific and constant for each of these processes. For example, for the total oxidation of carbohydrate, RQ = 1.0, fat RQ = 0.7, and protein RQ = 0.809. For lipogenesis (the biosynthesis of fat from carbohydrate), RQ = 2.75.[4] If the macronutrient substrate (protein, carbohydrate, and fat) intake is known, indirect calorimetry can be used to calculate the amount of protein, carbohydrate, and fat oxidation and the amount of fat biosynthesis (de novo lipogenesis).[5]

Other methods have been used to calculate energy expenditure, including doubly labeled water, mass spectrometry, and the Fick equation. Doubly labeled water uses simultaneously infused tracer doses of deuterium-labeled water (^2H_2O) and ^{18}O-labeled water.[6] The initial isotope enrichment plateau is measured in the urine and the energy expenditure is calculated based on the difference in the decay rates between deuterium and ^{18}O (equivalent to net CO_2 production) as determined by subsequent decreases in urine isotope concentrations over the next 3–10 days. This method is not useful for the evaluation of acute injury states in the intensive care setting. It is better applied to stable subjects. Another isotopic method applicable to children involves the use of L-[1-^{13}C] leucine and $NaH^{13}CO_3$.[7] While this technique can be used in the intensive care setting, results depend on access to a mass spectrometer. The Fick equation can be used to calculate VO_2 and VCO_2 in critically ill children but requires cardiopulmonary vascular access to measure thermodilution.[8]

Metabolizable Energy and Energy Balance

Energy balance (EB) is the amount of energy taken in by the body over a given period of time (conventionally 24 hours), minus MEE. It is expressed in the following formula:

$$EB = E_I - MEE$$

where E_I is energy intake. A positive energy balance is generally reflective of growth in children. It is important to understand that E_I depends on the percent of energy that is actually absorbed. Furthermore, the absorption of calories from the intestinal tract requires energy. This concept is termed *diet-induced thermogenesis* and is conventionally accepted to range from 5–15% in a normally functioning bowel, depending on the percent of protein, carbohydrate, and fat in the diet.[9,10] There is no substantial energy cost for nutrient absorption for calories delivered parenterally. An increase in energy expenditure has been demonstrated with intravenous amino acid infusions and is thought to relate to hepatic amino acid degradation and urea synthesis.[11] Absorption decreases enterally with bowel malfunctions such as malabsorption or short bowel.

The amount of energy available for metabolic activity is termed *metabolizable energy,* and is approximately 88% of enteral caloric intake in breastfed infants.[12] Metabolizable energy can be calculated by subtracting fecal and urinary energy losses from energy intake. Metabolizable energy also represents the fraction of each macronutrient substrate absorbed from the intestine: 0.93 for protein, 0.98 for carbohydrate, and 0.98 for fat. These data yield the following conversion factors: 4.0 kcal/g protein, 25 kcal/g nitrogen, 9.1 kcal/g fat, 4.1 kcal/g starch (glycogen), 3.75 kcal/g glucose, and 3.4 kcal/g dextrose.[13] Metabolizable energy can be (1) expended for all of the metabolic operations that occur in the body; (2) deposited in tissue for growth, maintenance, or repair; and (3) lost to the environment through the skin and respiratory tract (insensible losses).

Energy Requirements

Energy requirements can be partitioned into energy needed for maintenance of metabolic functions such as basal metabolic rate, growth, activity, and heat loss to the environment. Energy requirements are age related, and on a weight basis, they are 3 to 4 times higher for infants than for adults (Table 6-1).

Basal metabolic rate (BMR) is defined as the energy expenditure of an individual at least 10 hours after the last meal, awake and lying supine, in a quiet, darkened room at normal body and ambient temperature, without physical or psychological stress, and following an 8-hour sleep. This is not practical for infants and young children. Instead, resting energy expenditure (REE) or resting metabolic rate (RMR) can be considered. It is assumed that REE or RMR can be measured in infants sleeping quietly without rapid eye movement and within half an hour of the next planned feeding.[14,15]

Table 6-1 Age-adjusted energy requirements.

	*Energy delivery**	
Age (yr)	*Kcal/kg/day*	*Kcal/day*
0–1	120–90	500–1000
1–7	90–75	1000–1500
7–12	75–60	1500–2000
12–18	60–30	2000
> 18	30–25	2000–1300

* The left-sided values in each column indicate requirements at the lowest age of the interval (e.g., 120 kcal/kg/day or 500 kcal/kg/day at the age of 0 years).

Source: Adapted from Wretlind A. Complete intravenous nutrition. Theoretical and experimental background. *Nutr Metab.* 1972;14(suppl):1–57.

In healthy, term babies, the BMR is about 40 to 45 kcal/kg/day, increases to about 60 kcal/kg/day by approximately the fourth to fifth month of life,[14] and then gradually declines to about 20 to 25 kcal/kg/day during adolescence, largely due to a relative decrease in the growth of parenchymal organs that have high oxygen consumption rates (brain, liver, kidney, and heart) and an increase in muscle mass (with relatively low VO_2) and fat.[16,17]

Activity: Activity related-energy expenditure is low in early infancy, approximately 5% of total energy requirement in very low-birth-weight infants, and about 15% in term infants. Energy expenditure increases gradually to approximately 40–45% of total energy requirement by the second year of life.[18] These changes coincide with increased mobility and decreased sleep time.

Environment: Energy lost to the environment includes measurable losses (predominantly stool and urine) and insensible losses (energy lost through the skin and respiratory tract). In healthy infants, fecal and urine losses comprise approximately 10–15% of energy intake.[14] Two thirds of insensible losses occur via the skin and one third via the respiratory tract. Insensible losses are higher in infants, especially preterm babies, due to decreased skin thickness (stratum cornium), decreased subcutaneous fat, and increased body surface area (relative to body weight).

Growth: In healthy, metabolically nonstressed neonates, weight gain occurs when absorbed energy (metabolizable energy) exceeds energy expenditure. Growth increases proportional to the amount of energy delivered over the BMR, 55 to 60 kcal/kg/day.[12] For every 5 kcal in excess of REE absorbed, approximately 1 g of new tissue is generated.[12,16] In term neonates, a growth rate of approximately 15 g/kg/day can be achieved with energy delivery of 110 to 120 kcal/kg/day. In low-birth-weight (< 1,500 g) infants, approximately 150 kcal/kg/day is needed to achieve adequate weight gain.[14] Normal healthy infants use about 30 to 35% of their daily calorie intake for growth during the first 6 months of life. Faster-growing preterm infants use 50% or more for growth.[12,14] At 2 years of age, only about 2–5% of energy intake is used for this purpose (Figure 6-1).

Protein Requirements

Growth can be expressed in terms of protein accretion, which is the amount of protein laid down as new tissue. Nitrogen accounts for approximately 2% of total body weight at birth and about 3% in adults. During the first year of life, infants increase body length twofold and body weight threefold. Brain mass grows to 60% of its normal adult size during the first year of life. However, energy needs take metabolic precedence, so protein is preferentially used as an energy source if nonprotein substrate delivery is inadequate to meet energy needs, even if protein delivery is low.

In the healthy infant, protein requirements are 0.93 g/kg/day and decrease progressively with age. Protein accretion is 0.5 g/kg/day during the second and third months of life, 0.26 g/kg/day during the fifth and sixth months of life, 0.18 g/kg/day from 9 to 12 months of age, and 0.08 g/kg/day between 2 and 3 years of age.[19] Protein accretion is dependent on the amount of protein actually absorbed (metabolizable protein), the

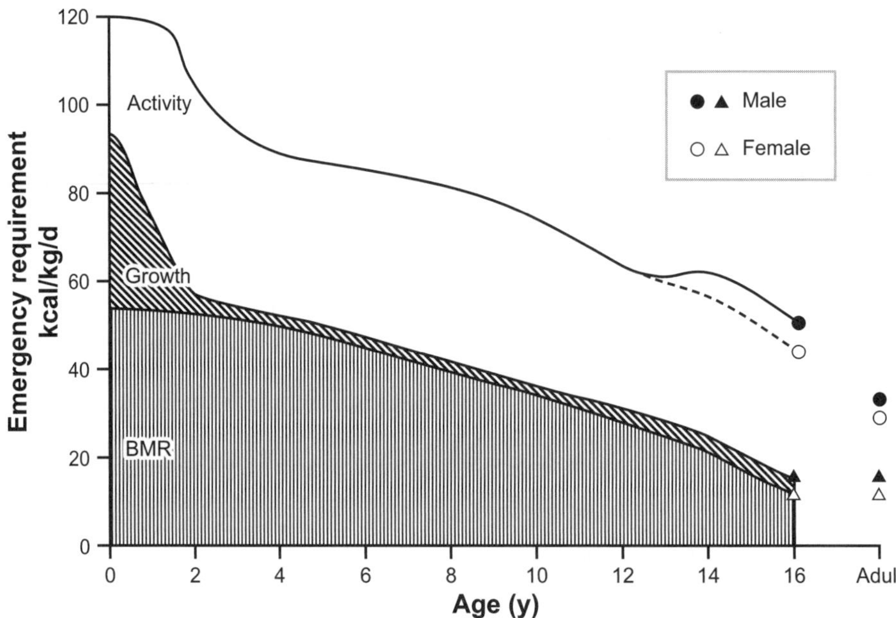

Figure 6-1 Growth. Change in energy requirements per kilogram body weight in healthy children during growth. BMR = basal metabolic rate. *Source:* Holliday MA: Body composition and energy needs during growth. In: Falkner F, Tanner JM, eds. *Human Growth: A Comprehensive Treatise.* 2nd ed. New York, NY: Plenum Publishing; 1986:2;101–115. *Postnatal Growth Neurobiology*. Reproduced with permission from Plenum Press.

efficiency of conversion of various dietary proteins into tissue protein (estimated at 90% for breast milk but only 70% for soy protein found in infant formula), and the protein lost during breakdown.

Protein lost because of incomplete enteral absorption and breakdown can be estimated by measuring stool, urine, and skin nitrogen content and is calculated to be approximately 0.95 g/kg/day during the first year of life. Taking these factors into account and allowing for interpatient variability, the estimated enteral protein requirement is approximately 2.6 g/kg/day during the neonatal period, 2.0 g/kg/day at 2 to 3 months of age, and 1.3 g/kg/day at 1 year of life. Values are less for amino acids provided parenterally.

In the premature or small-for-gestational age (SGA) infant, protein needs are higher (ranging to 3.5 g/kg/day) owing to substantially increased urinary nitrogen losses and increased catch-up growth requirements (~ 20% higher than the 3.0 g/kg/day needed to support intrauterine growth rates).[20] Because of accelerated organ growth rates, protein requirements may reach 3 to 4 g/kg/day in otherwise healthy low-birth-weight infants to achieve the desired weight gain of 15–30 g/kg/day.[21]

Nonprotein Caloric Requirements

Most infant formulas provide a relatively balanced delivery of the nonprotein calories, carbohydrates, and fats. In the postnatal period, infant metabolism is characterized by a greater dependence on lipid substrate than carbohydrate for energy needs.[21] There is evidence that premature infants, because of impaired fat absorption by the immature gut, may benefit from increased concentrations of medium chain triglycerides (MCTs) in enteral formulas.[22] Carbohydrates remain important as a source of energy for children and are optimally provided in the form of starches, such as those found in cereals.

Infant Energy Reserves

The body fat compartment is generated during the last 2 months of gestation and reaches about 10% of total body weight at term. Most body fat is contained in white adipose tissue, which serves as an insulating blanket against energy loss and for the storage of energy. A second type of fat is stored as brown adipose tissue (BAT), which can compose up to 10% of total body fat at term. Infants with intrauterine growth retardation have reduced total body fat, exhibited by decreased skinfold thickness and ponderal index. The ponderal index is defined as birth weight in grams multiplied by 100, divided by body length in centimeters.[23] Ponderal index and skinfold thickness correlate with lean body mass in premature and term infants. As gestational age increases in both SGA and appropriate-for-gestational age (AGA) infants, there is a significant decrease in percentage of lean body mass relative to total body weight, indicating increased adipose tissue stores.

Infants undergo temperature shock at birth. There are two mechanisms by which an infant can generate heat: shivering thermogenesis and nonshivering thermogenesis. In shivering thermogenesis, muscle contraction generates heat. BAT creates heat in nonshivering thermogensis. Nonshivering thermogenesis occurs immediately after birth but shivering thermogenesis cannot happen in the first few days of life.

BAT can generate large amounts of heat. BAT converts thyroxine to triiodothyronine. Biochemically, BAT is identical to white fat except for the presence of *thermogenin,* an uncoupling protein that allows BAT to generate heat.[24] In infants, BAT constitutes 1–2% of birth weight and is concentrated in the axillary and perirenal areas. BAT is strongly dependent on an adequate supply of lipids. During periods of cooling, there is a rapid redistribution of cardiac output, resulting in increased blood flow to BAT. Excess energy used to generate heat can rapidly lead to depletion of energy stores needed for homeostasis. Even routine nursing procedures performed on the premature infant in an incubator can lead to a temperature drop as great as 2 to 3°, requiring up to 2 hours for restoration of thermoneutrality.[25]

At birth, human infants are completely dependent on nonshivering thermogenesis for maintaining body temperature. The onset of nonshivering thermogenesis is delayed by a placental factor that is thought to inhibit thermogenesis. This factor disappears during the first few days of neonatal life and a gradual increase in BAT thermogenin activity occurs. As the BAT is slowly replaced by white adipose tissue, the infant becomes dependent on shivering thermogenesis. Very premature infants carry out nonshivering thermogenesis poorly because of inadequate BAT stores (which develop during the last 3 months of gestation). Fullterm infants can keep their body temperature at a level much higher than that of the environment, whereas premature infants tend to be more poikilothermic. The rate of lipid depletion in BAT and the loss of nonshivering thermogenesis are accelerated in malnourished and sick infants.

The principal goal of protein-calorie nutritional support in low-birth-weight infants is to generate postnatal growth rates that match intrauterine growth. Preterm infants are developmentally immature and energy stores in the form of hepatic glycogen content and subcutaneous adipose tissue are low. Calorie reserves in the 1,000 g infant are about 100 kcal/kg/day, in contrast to those of the term baby, which measure 1,500 to 1,800 kcal/kg/day. It is particularly important to recognize that these low energy reserves exist in the fat mass, and not as glycogen, especially in early preterm or SGA infants. Glycogen reserves are low in the preterm neonatal liver. Furthermore, brain tissue is exclusively dependent on glucose as a fuel source, and the neonatal brain represents 10% of total body weight, in contrast to the adult brain, which represents 2% of total body weight. Premature and SGA infants are at risk for the development of hypoglycemia if adequate exogenous glucose is not provided because they have a small amount of endogenous reserves to mobilize. In addition, functional immaturity of fatty acid oxidative enzymes may impede mobilization of the small fat reserves they do have.[26] For this reason, it is critically important to provide approximately 6 mg/kg/min of dextrose (8.64 g/kg/day) to meet the metabolic needs of the brain.[27]

Factors Modifying Energy Metabolism and Energy Requirements

Factors known to influence metabolic demand include age, gender, and the type, amount, and route of macronutrient substrate administration, ambient temperature, body temperature, activity level, and metabolic stress. Gender becomes a factor at about the third year of life when the metabolic rate of males exceeds that of females.[28] This difference increases rapidly at puberty due to increased muscle mass in boys and increased adipose mass in girls. The metabolic rate is dependent on body temperature and has been shown to increase 10–13% for each degree centigrade (or 7.2% for each degree Fahrenheit) of body temperature elevation (due to the Q_{10} effect, which describes the increase in the rate constant for chemical reactions associated with increased body temperature).[29] Tissue injury elicits an acute metabolic stress response, which can have complex and profound effects on energy requirements in infants and children.

Acute Metabolic Stress Response

In response to local or systemic injury, such as trauma, sepsis, or acute inflammatory conditions, a series of metabolic changes that characterize the acute injury response state occurs (Figure 6-2 and Chapter 29). Among the early features of the response is the release of cytokines, followed rapidly by alterations in the hormonal environment. As a result of this response, a sequence of metabolic events is initiated; the sequence includes the catabolism of endogenous stores of protein, carbohydrate, and fat to provide essential substrate intermediates and energy necessary to fuel the ongoing response process. Amino acids from catabolized proteins flow to the liver, where they provide substrate for the synthesis of acute phase proteins and glucose (gluconeogenesis). Acute metabolic stress is a hypermetabolic, hypercatabolic state that results

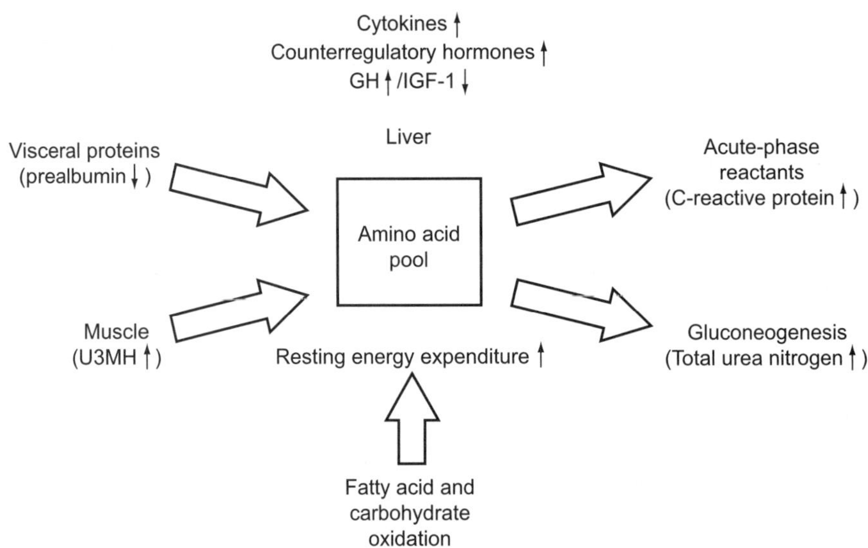

Figure 6-2 Metabolic response to acute injury. Acute metabolic stress response to acute injury. GH = growth hormone; IGF-I = insulin-like growth factor I; U3MH = urinary 3-methyl histidine.

in the loss of endogenous tissue. Growth, which is an anabolic process, is inhibited during periods of acute metabolic stress. As the acute metabolic stress response resolves, anabolic metabolism ensues to restore catabolic losses. In children, this phase is characterized by the resumption of somatic growth.

Insulin is a potent anabolic hormone responsible for glycogen synthesis, the storage form of carbohydrate, lipogenesis, and new protein synthesis. Insulin and insulin-like growth factor-1 (IGF-1) are essential hormones for somatic growth in infants and children. Acute metabolic stress is characterized by increases in the serum concentrations of catecholamines, glucagon, and cortisol, referred to as counterregulatory hormones because they oppose the anabolic effects of insulin. Serum concentrations of these metabolic stress-related hormones increase as a result of cytokine release.[30]

Glucagon induces glycolysis and gluconeogenesis, which counteract the anabolic effects of insulin. Increased glycolysis results in increased serum lactate and alanine concentrations, and they provide substrate necessary for the endogenous regeneration of glucose (Cori and alanine cycles).

Cortisol induces muscle proteolysis and promotes gluconeogenesis. Glucocorticoids cause the muscle proteolysis associated with cytokine release, and they are a predictor of protein breakdown and hypermetabolism in acutely stressed adults. The major amino acid sources for gluconeogenesis are alanine and glutamine derived from skeletal muscle and gut, respectively. Hepatic uptake of these amino acids is accelerated during acute metabolic stress.[31]

Catecholamines cause hyperglycemia by promoting hepatic glycogenolysis, by causing conversions of skeletal muscle glycogen to lactate (which is then transported to the liver for conversion to glucose through the Cori cycle), and by suppressing the pancreatic secretion of insulin. Catecholamines also induce lypolysis, which results in the mobilization of free fatty acids. Finally, catecholamines, in addition to glucagon and cortisol, induce hypermetabolism, which is associated with an increase in the basal metabolic rate.

In health, the major actions of growth hormone are to decrease protein catabolism and promote protein synthesis, to promote fat mobilization and the conversion of free fatty acids to acetyl coenzyme A, and to decrease glucose oxidation while increasing glycogen deposition. The anabolic effects of growth hormone are mediated principally by IGF-1. During acute metabolic stress, IGF-1 concentrations decrease and IGF-1 inhibitory binding concentrations increase. In this state, the substrate-mobilizing effects of growth hormone prevail and result in increased lipolysis and free fatty acid oxidation.

Both term and premature infants can generate a counterregulatory response to surgically induced injury.[32,33] The response is short lived—about 24 hours—can be dampened by fentanyl anesthesia, and may differ according to the age and physiologic maturity of the infant. For instance, children from 2 to 20 years of age do not have significant differences in cortisol production immediately after surgery despite considerable age differences and variable durations of surgically induced stress.[34] In contrast, after open-heart surgery, neonatal infants can generate only about 50% of the average 2-year-old child's surgically induced cortisol response.[33] Furthermore, neonatal infants can generate a graded response based on the degree of severity of surgical stress.[35] Studies in preterm baboons showed a graded counterregulatory hormone response based on injury severity.[33] The onset of the response is delayed and of longer duration than the hormonal response reported in more mature, stressed infants. This suggests that functional immaturity associated with earlier gestational development plays a role in this process.

Stable infants undergoing elective surgical procedures do not have an appreciable energy response to operative trauma.[36] If surgical procedures are classified on the basis of the magnitude of the procedures, a small but significant increase in energy response is observed in association with major operative trauma, compared to minor operative trauma.[37] In general, the predominant stimulus for the energy response to injury in infants is the underlying disease process that necessitated the surgery, rather than the operative procedure itself.[38]

Anabolic Hormone Resistance During Acute Metabolic Stress

Throughout human existence, the metabolic response to acute injury and disease has been characterized by an associated decrease or absence of exogenous nutrient intake (anorexia). A predominant clinical feature of serious illness in neonates is feeding intolerance, or a decreased willingness to feed. This phenomenon causes the sick infant to rely on the mobilization of endogenous fuel stores for the provision of substrates and energy required during the period of acute metabolic stress. Normal anabolic metabolism, which results in the removal of substrates from the circulation and their deposition in tissue stores, would appear to be counterproductive in the face of increased demands for substrate mobilization. Because of this, and because the advent of exogenous nutritional support occurred recently in the time frame of human development, the attenuation of anabolic hormone effects in response to acute injury states teleologically represents an important evolutionary compensatory mechanism. The suppression of, or resistance to, the anabolic effects of at least 2 key hormones, insulin and growth hormone, characterizes this mechanism.

Because the anabolic effects of these hormones are variable and depend on a multitude of associated conditions, it is important to define which of these effects and associated conditions are altered in "resistance," for example:

- Nature of the injury insult (e.g., sepsis versus burn)
- Substrate pool affected (e.g., glucose versus protein)
- Region of the body sampled (e.g., splanchnic, hepatic peripheral muscle, or systemic circulatory beds)
- Timing of samples taken relative to the injury event
- Use of exogenous hormonal supplementation

Lack of attention to these details has led to considerable controversy, especially in relation to the nature of insulin resistance.[39–43]

Insulin resistance is defined as increased glucose production, lipolysis, fatty acid oxidation, proteolysis, and decreased glucose uptake and storage associated with high serum glucose, amino acid, and insulin levels. Septic and acute injury states in adults are characterized by an inability to use glucose despite increased serum glucose, amino acid, and lipid concentrations. Thus sepsis and acute injury are associated with insulin resistance.

Early studies showed hyperglycemia occurred in association with elevated serum insulin concentrations,[40,41] which could not be reversed by the administration of exogenous insulin. Subsequent studies in septic adults and severely burned children reported failure of exogenous insulin to suppress hepatic glucose production despite concomitant provision of exogenous glucose.[43,44] Comparing septic patients with healthy adults using a euglycemic hyperinsulinemic clamp with increasing insulin doses demonstrated suppressed insulin effect in the septic group, suggesting a possible insulin receptor defect.[45] A study of severely septic adults showed glucose production and clearance increased in association with a decreased glucose-stimulated insulin secretion. This suggests that glucose uptake may be insulin independent in sepsis.[46]

Pyruvate dehydrogenase activity is dependent on the nature of the injury and its activity may partially explain whether glucose oxidation is appropriate to circulating insulin levels. For instance, the activity of this enzyme is depressed in septic adults (thus reducing aerobic metabolism and glucose oxidation),[47] whereas there is a fortyfold increase in activity in burned patients.[44]

Because insulin is known to promote protein anabolism, primarily by decreasing proteolysis, the protein breakdown observed in acute metabolic stress has been ascribed to insulin resistance.[48] However, the anabolic effect of insulin on protein is reported to be intact.[49] Furthermore, decreased leucine oxidation and improved nitrogen retention have been observed in hyperinsulinemic burned patients.[50]

Sakurai and colleagues showed that the exogenous provision of extremely large insulin doses during a 7-day period in severely burned adults increases muscle protein synthesis (approximately 350% relative to that of control subjects), and is associated with a sixfold increase in amino acid transport from the circulation to the muscle pool.[51] This report suggests that exogenous insulin may be useful in promoting protein synthesis in severely catabolic patients. To achieve this effect, insulin was infused at rates that resulted in serum concentrations of 900 μU/mL, which are more that 10 times higher than the range generally observed (55 to 70 μU/mL) in injured patients. In addition, although all study groups were fed enterally (protein intake of approximately 2.1 g/kg/day protein and 60 kcal/kg/day), the insulin group received an additional 80 kcal/kg/day as intravenous dextrose to prevent insulin-induced hypoglycemia. Although muscle protein synthesis was increased, there was no improvement in the rate of burn or wound healing compared to that of the control group.

In one study the use of exogenous insulin at much lower infusion rates improved nitrogen secretion in moderately stressed adult patients after abdominal surgery.[52] When protein intake was increased from 1.5 to 3.0 g/kg/day, however, there was no significant difference in nitrogen retention between the insulin group and the control group. A randomized prospective evaluation of the use of insulin to reduce injury-induced hyperglycemia demonstrated decreased morbidity and mortality in critically ill adults in the absence of excess caloric delivery, likely due to decreased hyperglycemia-induced immunosuppression.[53]

In health, the major actions of growth hormone are to decrease protein catabolism and promote protein synthesis, mobilize fat, and convert free fatty acids to acetylcoenzyme A, decrease glucose oxidation and increase glycogen deposition. The anabolic effects of growth hormone, particularly as they relate to protein metabolism, are mediated principally by IGF-1. During acute metabolic stress, IGF-1 levels fall, and IGF-1 inhibitory binding protein concentrations rise.[54] In this state, the substrate-mobilizing effects of growth hormone prevail and result in increased lipolysis and fatty acid oxidation. These findings describe anabolic growth hormone resistance during acute metabolic stress states.

OVERFEEDING

Overfeeding occurs when the administration of calories or other substrate exceeds requirements for metabolic homeostasis. These requirements vary according to the patient's age, state of health, and underlying nutritional status and are altered during periods of injury-induced stress. Excess nutrition delivery increases metabolic demands that occur with acute injury and places an additional burden on the lungs and liver. The result is an increase in the mortality risk. This increased risk is avoidable by ensuring that calorie intake does not exceed demand during periods of acute metabolic stress in critically ill infants and children.

Effect on Respiration

Carbohydrate overfeeding, either with or without excessive calorie delivery, can have a negative effect on respiration. Lipogenesis, an energy requiring process, is characterized by an increase in VCO_2 relative to VO_2. The RQ for pure lipogenesis is 2.75.[4] Lipogenesis is the only metabolic process where the RQ is greater than 1. Because other metabolic processes that are associated with RQ values of 1 or less occur simultaneously in vivo (e.g., in lipid oxidation, RQ = 0.707; in carbohydrate oxidation, RQ = 1.00; and in protein oxidation, RQ = 0.809), and because measured RQ represents the net effect of these processes, RQ values in excess of 1 represent high lipogenic activity and are usually associated with overfeeding. In infants, increased CO_2 production from excess carbohydrate administration causes an increase in respiratory rate necessary to remove excess CO_2.[55] Excess protein delivery exacerbates this effect in adults by increasing respiratory sensitivity to CO_2.[56] Substituting lipid for some of the carbohydrate, usually 25 to 35%, is effective in reducing CO_2 production and lipogenesis and decreasing RQ.[55,57–60]

When excessive calories are provided, hypermetabolism (increased MEE) accompanies the increases in VCO_2. Overfeeding results in increased respiratory requirements caused by increased CO_2 production,[61–63] even though it might not be completely reflected in total RQ.[64] Glucose administered in excess of maximum oxidation rates undergoes lipogenesis and causes an increase in CO_2 production.[62] The importance of overfeeding is confirmed by studies that show overfeeding causes ventilatory dependence in patients with decreased pulmonary reserve.[56,65,66] This ventilatory dependency is caused by the inability of patients with limited pulmonary function to eliminate increased CO_2 produced when excessive total calories, particularly carbohydrate, are metabolized.[66,67] Preterm infants are especially vulnerable to the respiratory effects of overfeeding because of their immature pulmonary function and limited respiratory reserve.

Effect of Hepatic Morphology and Function

In healthy subjects and clinically stable patients, excessive glucose intake causes insulin levels to increase, resulting in decreased fatty acid oxidation, reduced ketogenesis, increased glucose oxidation, and increased lipogenesis. The insulin-glucagon ratio increases in the portal vein in association with increased hepatic fat deposition. Serum transaminase levels increase, indicating hepatocellular injury.[68]

In one study of stable adult patients overfed with glucose-based parenteral nutrition (PN), (average 177% of predicted energy expenditure) liver biopsies showed fatty infiltration and incipient intrahepatic cholestasis within 5 days of the initiation of intravenous nutrition.[69] After 21 days, liver biopsies showed bile duct proliferation, canalicular bile plugs, centrilobular cholestasis with bile pigment in hepatocytes, and periportal inflammation. Liver function test results were elevated in 83% of the subjects by a mean of 14 days, and the number of liver function test abnormalities increased in proportion to histological changes. These findings are typical of a number of similar studies involving overfed subjects.[62,68,70,71]

Similar results are documented in studies of clinically stable infants receiving glucose-based PN. In infants the onset of change is more rapid.[72] Acute metabolic stress increases lipolysis and free fatty acid oxidation relative to glucose oxidation owing to counterregulatory hormone-induced insulin resistance. These endocrine effects reduce the efficiency with which exogenous carbohydrate is metabolized. With excessive carbohydrate delivery, serum insulin, glucose, glucose oxidation, and fatty acid oxidation increase, and lipogenesis remains high.[73] These events predispose the liver to hepatic cellular injury. Glucose oxidation is dependent on pyruvate dehydrogenase for entry of pyruvate into the tricarboxylic acid cycle. During sepsis, increased serum concentrations of lactate and alanine suggest that pyruvate dehydrogenase activity may be inhibited.[47] Excess glucose administration increases the hepatic work.[73]

Lipid overfeeding with long chain triglyceride (LCT) can inhibit bacterial clearing by the reticuloendothelial system.[74] Decreased hepatic clearance is associated with increased bacterial sequestration in the lung, resulting in increased pulmonary neutrophil activation and the release of inflammatory mediators. LCT contains high concentrations of linoleic acid, an arachidonic acid precursor that increases substrate availability for prostaglandin synthesis. Replacing LCT with MCT, which is absorbed directly into the blood from the gut, preserves liver reticuloendothelial system function and reduces lung bacterial sequestration.

Overfeeding during critical illness cannot reverse metabolic changes caused by stress. Instead, overfeeding further increases the negative impact of metabolic stress by increasing the demands associated with it and by augmenting the hepatic workload.[63] In addition, hepatic compromise due to overfeeding during nonstress periods may decrease hepatic metabolic function in response to subsequent acute injury, especially sepsis. Cecal ligation and puncture in rats previously overfed enterally for 6 days resulted in marked decreases in hepatic (and whole body) protein synthesis relative to the normal intake group.[75] Hepatomegaly was 67% greater in the overfed group, but liver protein per gram of tissue was significantly less relative to normally fed animals. It is noteworthy that hepatic dysfunction and pathomorphologic changes due to carbohydrate-based PN solutions are observed in infants and evolve most rapidly in preterm infants, especially those who are septic.[70]

Effect on Immunocompetence

Excess caloric delivery causes immunocompromise, likely caused by hyperglycemia. *In vitro*, a direct association exists between hyperglycemia and deficiencies in white blood cell activation and function, including impaired granulocyte adhesion, chemotaxis and phagocytosis, decreased respiratory burst, and impaired intracellular killing, as well as decreased immunoglobulin function and complement fixation. These functions improve with glucose control.[76,79] Hyperglycemia is associated with increased mortality and morbidity in critically ill adult and pediatric patients.[53,67,77,78,79]

The response to acute injury can itself cause hyperglycemia. Tissue injury results in the increased secretion of cytokines followed by counterregulatory hormones and growth hormone. Cytokine-induced elaboration of counterregulatory hormones increases hepatic glucose production (due primarily to epinephrine and glucagon) and decreases peripheral glucose uptake (primarily due to insulin resistance). Growth hormone increases peripheral lipolysis and fatty acid oxidation, which amplifies hyperglycemia by decreasing the need for serum glucose to serve as an energy source. Thus, the degree of stress-related hyperglycemia is directly related to the magnitude of the acute injury and the availability of mobilizable substrate.

Hyperglycemia is also caused by excess parenteral or enteral calorie delivery. PN is associated with overfeeding-related hyperglycemia[80] caused, in part, by the absence of natural gastrointestinal mediated functions that protect against excessive caloric nutrition. Overfeeding can be particularly harmful in critically ill patients in catabolic states where excess calories cannot be deposited in storage compartments such as adipose tissue. Excess caloric delivery further increases injury-related hyperglycemia. Indirect calorimetric assessment in the adult intensive care setting has shown that in the absence of serious burns, multiple trauma, or severe head injury, most adult patients have a resting energy expenditure of approximately 25 kcal/kg/day.[81] If caloric delivery does not exceed this amount, overfeeding-associated hyperglycemia can be avoided.[82] When energy delivery in adult patients substantially exceeds 25 kcal/kg/day, the rate of hyperglycemia and infectious complications increases.[80,83,85]

Effect on Survival

Despite the logical assumption that the damaging aspects of overfeeding during acute metabolic stress would have a negative impact on survival, proof is elusive in human studies. Further studies are needed to conclusively show an effect of overfeeding on survival in acutely ill humans. In the meantime, it is prudent not to supply excess substrates in this setting.

As previously discussed, the increased metabolic demands imposed by overfeeding result in increased glucose production, lipid oxidation, CO_2 production associated with lipogenesis, insulin/glucagon ratio, and lactate and alanine cycling. Although whole body protein synthetic rates increase in some stressed populations, protein breakdown is not substantially decreased in response to overfeeding.[86] These alterations result in increased respiratory work required to remove excess CO_2 and increased hepatic work required to metabolize the excess substrates. Excessive calorie administration augments energy requirements to process the increased substrate load, resulting in further hypermetabolism due to diet-induced thermogenesis. Overfeeding has been documented to increase MEE by 34%

in acutely stressed adult subjects after the initiation of excess protein-calorie delivery.[63]

The effects of calorie overfeeding with carbohydrate were evaluated in postoperative adults retrospectively grouped on the basis of RQ higher than 0.95 (high calorie) versus RQ of less than 0.95 (low calorie).[87] The high calorie group received 150% MEE and the low-calorie group received 100% MEE. Glucose calories were 77% of the total calorie intake in the high calorie group (yielding an average RQ of 1.12), compared with glucose calories of 60.6% (yielding an average RQ of 0.73) in the low-calorie group. Mortality was significantly greater in the high RQ group than in the low RQ group (40% versus 29%; $P < 0.05$). As noted previously, a number of recent studies suggest that hyperglycemia-related mortality may be due to overfeeding.[69, 79,83–85,88]

In a prospective study of septic guinea pigs grouped by calorie intake (100, 125, 150, or 175 kcal/kg/day), there was a significant increase in mortality and decrease in survival time in the animals fed 150 and 175 kcal/kg/day (the mortality rate was 100% in both groups).[89] On the other hand, 175 kcal/kg/day was optimal for guinea pigs subjected to thermal injury.[90] This underscores the differing nutritional requirements based on the nature of the injury insult and the metabolic stress response that it induces. In contrast, data generated in burned children show that pyruvate dehydrogenase activity is not decreased, but, rather, is amplified during this type of acute injury.[44] In sepsis, glucose infusion results in increased levels of lactate and alanine; whereas in thermal stress, increased glucose oxidation occurs, and less lactate and alanine are generated. This may help to explain why the increased nutritional delivery appropriate for burn injury might constitute overfeeding during sepsis in the same animal model.

Another consideration involves the impact of prestress overfeeding on the metabolic stress response. When acute bacterial peritonitis was induced in rats after 6 days of enteral overfeeding (175% of normal intake), the mortality rate increased to 53%, in contrast to the 14% mortality rate observed in animals that were fed normal amounts.[75] These changes were associated with decreased hepatic and whole body protein synthesis, which may reflect a reduced metabolic capability to meet the demands of acute injury in the overfed group.

Precise calorie delivery is best determined during acute injury states by measuring energy expenditure. Owing to substantial inter-patient variability, estimates of energy needs on the basis of disease categories, subject age, or body composition can be misleading and usually result in overfeeding. Overfeeding cannot reverse tissue catabolism until the acute metabolic stress response has resolved. In acutely stressed children, MEE constitutes the total energy requirement, and calorie delivery in excess of this amount should be avoided until metabolic stress parameters indicate resolution of the acute injury state.[55]

Energy Requirements During Metabolic Stress and Growth Recovery

Alterations in the energy requirement of pediatric patients in response to an acute metabolic stress can be dramatic. Additional growth requirements must be met by age and weight-appropriate increases in protein-calorie delivery in the metabolically unstressed (anabolic) pediatric patient.

Acute injury alters energy needs. First, acute injury induces a catabolic response that is proportional to the magnitude, nature, and duration of the injury. Increased serum counterregulatory hormone concentrations induce insulin and growth hormone resistance. This results in the catabolism of endogenous stores of protein, carbohydrate, and fat to provide essential substrate intermediates and energy necessary to support the metabolic stress response. Approximately 30–35% of predicted energy requirements for healthy infants are needed for growth. During the catabolic period, somatic growth cannot occur. Therefore, the calorie allotment for growth, which is substantial during infancy, should *not* be administered. Children treated in the intensive care setting are frequently sedated, and their activity level is reduced. The intensive care environment is temperature controlled and so insensible energy losses are reduced. This is especially true for children who are mechanically ventilated with heated, humidified air, reducing insensible losses by as much as one third. In concert, these factors result in a substantial decrease in energy needs.[15,91,92] If calorie repletion is based on the predicted requirements for healthy infants, substantial overfeeding is likely in critically ill infants.[15]

To account for these alterations in energy metabolism, calories equal to measured energy expenditure values or basal energy requirements should be provided. This therapeutic strategy avoids the provision of excess energy.

The value of indirect calorimetry in the intensive care setting lies in the fact that estimations of energy expenditure based on other clinical criteria are notoriously inaccurate. The actual MEE is frequently much less than predicted values based on clinical grounds. Although average MEE values in large series of patients tend to differentiate various degrees of injury,[37] individual subjects can respond to similar injury states with widely diverse MEE values. One study of critically ill infants found the difference in MEE (adjusted for age and weight) between the lowest and highest inter-patient values to be 3.5 times.[15]

Infant energy expenditure after complication-free surgical procedures does not increase substantially above measured baseline values.[36,93] For surgical stress, the period of injury metabolism is relatively short—generally fewer than 48 hours.[32] Many studies that attempt to evaluate surgically related acute stress changes during later postoperative periods are flawed.[94] The magnitude of the stress response is difficult to predict if a substantial portion of the injury insult results from an additional nonsurgical factor such as burn trauma or sepsis. In a study of infants with a wide variety of stress insults, there was substantial inter-patient variability in MEE relative to the predicted basal metabolic rate.[15] This variability may be attributable to substantial differences in the acute metabolic demands imposed by the underlying disease process.[38]

As the acute phase of metabolic stress resolves, the adaptive anabolic phase ensues, and somatic growth resumes. Recovery is characterized by decreasing serum concentrations of C-reactive protein (CRP).[66] To avoid premature increments in calorie delivery, daily indirect calorimetry measurements are carried out to assess RQ.

Metabolically stressed neonates appear to be particularly susceptible to overfeeding. For this reason, calories should be administered to match only MEE-established needs until acute metabolic stress subsides and anabolic metabolism resumes (CRP < 2 mg/dL),[66] at which time calories can be advanced to promote growth recovery (Figure 6-3). If indirect calorimetry is unavailable, only basal metabolic needs[18] should be delivered until CRP falls below stress levels (Table 6-2).[66] This provides a useful guide to advance calorie delivery and optimize recovery without overfeeding infants during the acute phase of the metabolic response to injury.

Prediction of Energy Expenditure

Some institutions do not have an indirect calorimeter available for clinical use. Because the acute injury response is a dynamic process associated with considerable inter-patient variability, accurate predictive equations are not available.

Harris-Benedict equations are used to calculate basal energy requirements in children. This is inappropriate because the equation was derived from adults. The first important indirect

Table 6-2 Guidelines for infant nutritional support during acute metabolic stress.

Basal metabolic repletion (enteral/parenteral)	
Protein	2.5 g/kg/d
Carbohydrate	8.5 g/kg/d
Lipid	1.0 g/kg/d
Increase caloric intake (enteral route preferred)	
Respiratory quotient (RQ) < 1.0 or decreased × 48 hr and/or CRP </= 2.0 mg/dl	

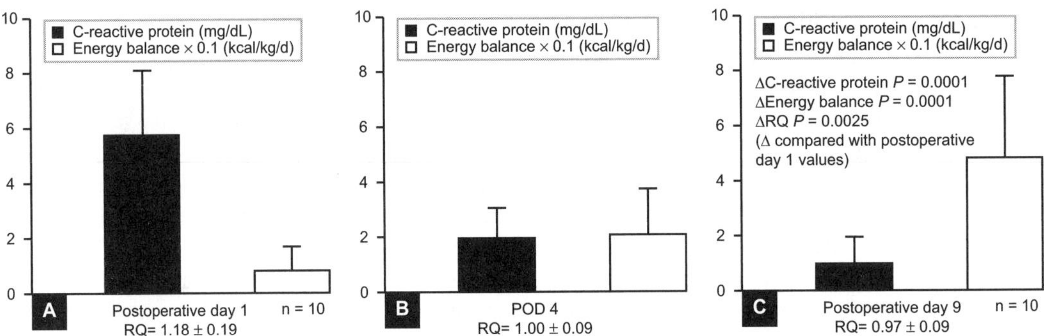

Figure 6-3 Growth and inflammation. **A.** Initial postoperative catabolism. Despite predictably low energy balance associated with basal energy delivery, the respiratory quotient (RQ) is > 1.0 during acute metabolic stress (C-reactive protein > 2.0 mg/dl), suggesting substantial lipogenesis at caloric intake that is moderately in excess of energy expenditure on postoperative day (POD) 1. **B.** Resumption of anabolic metabolism. Twofold increase in energy balance at constant basal energy intake associated with decreasing RQ and decrease of C-reactive protein toward normal serum concentrations, suggesting return of anabolic metabolism as acute metabolic stress resolves. **C.** Normal growth recovery following resolution of metabolic response to acute injury. After gradually increasing energy delivery from POD 4 to POD 9 to caloric intake levels appropriate for adequate growth, RQ remains < 1, reflecting normal nonstress (C-reactive protein < 2 mg/dl) anabolic metabolism. RQ = Respiratory quotient; POD = Postoperative day

calorimetry measurements that were performed in clinically stable, healthy children were during the early part of the 20th century by Fritz Talbot. They serve as the standard for calculating basal metabolic rates.[18] The data from this study group, based on 179 subjects ranging from newborn to 19 years of age, have been analyzed by Schofield,[16] using rigorous criteria to derive simple predictive equations based on weight and height for healthy children under 3 years of age, from 3 to 10 years of age, and from 10 to 18 years of age with excellent correlation ($r^2 = 0.64$ to 0.94). Data on infants is lacking.

It is not surprising that a number of studies involving critically ill children report large differences between measured and predicted energy expenditure, supporting the use of indirect calorimetry rather than predictive formulas, to determine energy requirements.[95–97] Of note is the fact that none of the predictive formulas used an injury-related variable. In contrast, in a more recent study of 100 critically ill children, White and colleagues compared their predictive equation as follows:

$$\text{energy expenditure (kJ/D)} = \{17 \times \text{age(months)}\} + \{48 \times \text{weight(kg)}\} + \{292 \times \text{body temperature °C}\} - 9677$$

against measured calorimetric values and demonstrated an excellent correlation ($r^2 = 0.867$) versus predictive equations based on data from Talbot (Schofield) or Harris-Benedict.[98] The advantage of the White equation in critically ill children is the inclusion of a temperature variable, which reflects the hypermetabolic component of the systemic inflammatory response. Prediction of energy expenditure in critically ill adult patients is similarly improved when a white blood cell count variable is added.[81] However, the White equation is not useful in infants less than 2 months of age. Temperature is much less reliable as an index of injury severity in infants and neonates.[99] Instead, acute phase reactants, such as C-reactive protein, which respond to injury independent of energy reserves, appear to better reflect the systemic inflammatory.[99]

CONCLUSION

The energy needs of infants and children are different from adult requirements and vary with age and clinical setting. Supplying appropriate (neither too much or too little) amounts of substrates is important to outcome. This goal is achievable first by measuring or calculating energy needs and second by ongoing monitoring.

REFERENCES

1. Westenkow DR, Curler CA, Wallace WD. Instrumentation for monitoring gas exchange and metabolic rate in critically ill patients. *Crit Care Med.* 1984;12:183–187.
2. Weir JB De V. New methods for calculating metabolic rate with special reference to protein metabolism. *J Physiol.* 1949 Aug;109 (1–2):1–9.
3. Bursztein S, Saphar P, Singer P, Elwyn DH. A mathematical analysis of indirect calorimetry measurements in acutely ill patients. *Am J Clin Nutr.* 1989;50:227–230.
4. McGilvery RW. *Biochemistry: A Functional Approach.* Philadelphia. PA: WB Saunders; 1979:532.
5. Bursztein S, Elwyn DH, Askanazi J, Kinney JM. *Energy Metabolism, Indirect Calorimetry, and Nutrition.* Baltimore, Md: Williams & Wilkins; 1989:54–64.
6. Schoeller DA. Recent advances from application of doubly labeled water to measurement of human energy expenditure. *J Nutr.* 1999;129:1765–1768.
7. Keshen TH, Miller RG, Jahoor F, Jaksic T. Stable isotope quantitation of protein metabolism and energy expenditure in neonates on- and post-extracorporeal life support. *J Pediatr Surg.* 1997;32:958–962.
8. Gebara BM, Gelmini M, Sarniak A. Oxygen consumption, energy expenditure, and substrate utilization after cardiac surgery in children. *Crit Care Med.* 1992;20:1550–1554.
9. Jequier E. Influence of nutrient administration on energy expenditure in man. *Clin Nutr.* 1986;5:181–186.
10. Rubecz I, Mestyan J. Postprandial thermogenesis in human milk-fed very low birthweight infants. *Biol Neonate.* 1986;49:301–306.
11. Krebs H. The metabolic fate of amino acids. In: Munro HN, Allison JB, eds. *Mammalian Protein Metabolism.* Vol 1. New York, NY: Academic Press; 1964:125–176.
12. Catzeflis C, Schutz Y, Micheli JL, et al. Whole body protein synthesis and energy expenditure in very low birth weight infants. *Pediatr Res.* 1985;19:679–687.
13. Southgate DAT, Durnin JVGA. Calorie conversion factors: an experimental reassessment of the factors used in the energy value of human diets. *Br J Nutr.* 1970;24:517–535.
14. Reichman BL, Chessex P, Putet G. Partition of energy metabolism and energy cost of growth in the very low-birth weight infant. *Pediatrics.* 1982;69:446–445.
15. Chwals WJ, Lally KP, Woolley MM, et al. Measured energy expenditure in critically ill infants and young children. *J Surg Res.* 1988;44:467–472.
16. Schofield WN. Predicting basal metabolic rate: new standards and review of previous work. *Hum Nutr Clin Nutr.* 1985;39(suppl 1):5–41.
17. Holliday MA. Body composition and energy needs during growth. In: Falkner F, Tanner JM, eds. *Human Growth: A Comprehensive Treatise.* 2nd ed. New York, NY: Plenum; 1986;102–104. *Postnatal Growth Neurobiology*; vol 2.
18. Talbot FB. Basal metabolism standards for children. *Am J Dis Child.* 1938;55:455–459.
19. Fomon SJ. Requirements and recommended dietary intakes of protein during infancy. *Pediatr Res.* 1991;30:391–395.
20. Zlotkin SH, Bryan MH, Anderson GH. Intravenous nitrogen and energy intakes required to duplicate in utero nitrogen accretion in prematurely born human infants. *J Pediatr.* 1981;99:115–120.
21. Carlson SE, Barness LA. Macronutrient requirements for growth. In: Walker WA, Watkins JB, eds. *Nutrition in Pediatrics.* Boston, Mass: Little, Brown, & Co; 1985;3–15.
22. Dupont C, Rocchiccioli F, Bougneres PF. Urinary excretion of dicarboxylic acids in term newborns fed with 5% medium-chain triglycerides-enriched formula. *J Pediatr Gastroenteral Nutr.* 1987;6:313–314.
23. Forbes GB. Methods for determining composition of the human body. *Pediatrics.* 1962;29:477–494.
24. Cannon B, Nedergaard J. The biochemistry of an inefficient tissue: brown adipose tissue. *Essays Biochem.* 1985;20:110–164.
25. Nedergaard J, Cannon B. Brown adipose tissue: development and function. In: Polin RA, Fox WW, eds. *Fetal and Neonatal Physiology.* Philadelphia, Pa: WB Saunders; 1992:314–326.
26. Letton RW, Chwals WJ. Endotoxin-induced hepatocyte energy status and metabolic compensation in adult versus neonatal rabbits. *Surg Forum.* 1996;47:683–686.
27. Kinnala A, Nuutila P, Ruotsalainen U, et al. Cerebral metabolic rate for glucose after neonatal hypoglycaemia. *Early Hum Dev.* 1997;49:63–72.
28. Sherman HC. *Chemistry of Food and Nutrition.* 8th ed. New York, NY: MacMillan Company; 1952.
29. Du Bois EF. Energy metabolism. *Ann Rev Physiol.* 1954;16:125–134.
30. Michie HR, Spriggs DR, Manogue KR, et al. Tumor necrosis factor and endotoxin induce similar metabolic responses in human beings. *Surgery.* 1988;104:280–286.

31. Leite HP, Fisberg M, Henriques Vieira JG, De Carvalho WB, Chwals WJ. The role of insulin-like growth hormone and plasma proteins in surgical outcome of children with congenital heart disease. *Pediatr Crit Care Med.* 2001;2:29–35.

32. Anand KJS, Hanson DD, Hickey PR. Hormonal-metabolic stress responses in neonates undergoing cardiac surgery. *Anesthesiology.* 1990;73:661–670.

33. Taylor AF, Lally KP, Chwals WJ, et al. Hormonal response of the premature primate to operative stress. *J Pediatr Surg.* 1993;28:844–846.

34. Khilnani P, Munoz R, Salem M, Gelb C, Todres ID, Chernow B. Hormonal responses to surgical stress in children. *J Pediatr Surg.* 1993;28:1–4.

35. Anand KJS, Aynsley-Green A. Measuring the severity of surgical stress in newborn infants. *J Pediatr Surg.* 1988;23:297–305.

36. Shanbhogue RL, Lloyd DA. Absence of hypermetabolism after operation in the newborn infant. *J Parenter Enteral Nutr.* 1992;16:333–336.

37. Long CL, Schaffel N, Geiger JW, Schiller WR, Blakemore WS. Metabolic response to injury and illness: estimation of energy and protein needs from indirect calorimetry and nitrogen balance. *J Parenter Enteral Nutr.* 1979;3:452–456.

38. Chwals WJ, Letton RW, Jamie A, Charles B. Stratification of injury severity using energy expenditure response in surgical infants. *J Pediatr Surg.* 1995;30:1161–1164.

39. Gump FE, Long C, Killian P, Kinney JM. Studies of glucose intolerance in septic injured patients. *J Trauma.* 1974;14:378–388.

40. Evans EI, Butterfield WJH. The stress response in the severely burned. *Ann Surg.* 1951;134:588–613.

41. Howard JM. Studies of the absorption and metabolism of glucose following injury: the systemic response to injury. *Ann Surg.* 1955;141:321–326.

42. White RH, Frayn KN, Little RA, et al. Hormonal and metabolic responses to glucose infusion in sepsis by the hyperglycaemic glucose clamp technique. *J Parenter Enteral Nutr.* 1987;11:345–353.

43. Long CL, Kinney JN, Geiger JW. Nonsuppressability of gluconeogenesis by glucose in septic patients. *Metabolism.* 1976;25:193–201.

44. Wolfe RR, Jahoor R, Herndon DN, et al. Isotopic evaluation of the metabolism of pyruvate and related substrates in normal adult volunteers and severely burned children: effect of dichloroacetate and glucose infusion. *Surgery.* 1991;110:54–67.

45. Henderson AA, Frayn KN, Galasko CS, et al. Dose-response relationships for the effects of insulin on glucose and fat metabolism in injured patients and control subjects. *Clin Sci (Colch).* 1991;80:25–32.

46. Dahn MS, Jacobs LA, Smith S, et al. The relationship of insulin production to glucose metabolism in severe sepsis. *Arch Surg.* 1985;120:166–172.

47. Vary TC, Siegel JH, Nakatani T, et al. Effects of sepsis on activity of pyruvate dehydrogenase complex in skeletal muscle and liver. *Am J Physiol.* 1987;250: E634–E640.

48. Frayn KN, Little RA, Stoner HB, Galasko CS. Metabolic control in non-septic patients with musculoskeletal injuries. *Injury.* 1984;16:73–79.

49. Brooks DC, Bessey PQ, Black PR, et al. Insulin stimulates branched chain amino acid uptake and diminished nitrogen flux from skeletal muscle of injured patients. *J Surg Res.* 1987;40:395–405.

50. Jahoor F, Shangraw RE, Miyoshi H, et al. Role of insulin and glucose oxidation in mediating the protein catabolism of burns and sepsis. *Am J Physiol.* 1989;257: E323–E331.

51. Sakurai Y, Aarsland A, Herndon DN, et al. Stimulation of muscle protein synthesis by long-term insulin infusion in severely burned patients. *J Parenter Enteral Nutr.* 1994;18:214–218.

52. Valarini R, Sousa MF, Kalil R, Abumrad NN, Riella MC. Anabolic effects of insulin and amino acids in promoting nitrogen accretion in postoperative patients. *J Parenter Enteral Nutr.* 1994;18:214–218.

53. Van den Berghe G, Wouters PJ, Bouillon R, et al. Outcome benefit of intensive insulin therapy in the critically ill: insulin dose versus glycemic control. *Crit Care Med.* 2003;3:359–366.

54. Chwals WJ, Bistrian BF. Role of exogenous growth hormone and insulin-like growth factor I in malnutrition and acute metabolic stress: a hypothesis. *Crit Care Med.* 1991;19:1317–1322.

55. Piedboeuf B, Chessex P, Hazan J, et al. Total parenteral nutrition in the newborn infant: energy substrates and respiratory gas exchange. *J Pediatr.* 1991;118:97–102.

56. Askanazi J, Weissman C, LaSala P, et al. Effect of protein intake on ventilatory drive. *Anesthesiology.* 1984;60:106–110.

57. Bresson JL, Bader B, Rocchiccioli F, et al. Protein-metabolism kinetics and energy-substrate utilization in infants fed parenteral solutions with different glucose-fat ratios. *Am J Clin Nutr.* 1991;54:370–376.

58. Van Aerde JEE, Sauer PJJ, Pencharz PB, et al. Effect of replacing glucose with lipid on the energy metabolism of newborn infants. *Clin Sci.* 1989;76:581–588.

59. Salas-Salvado J, Molina J, Figueras J, et al. Effect of the quality of infused energy on substrate utilization in the newborn receiving total parenteral nutrition. *Pediatr Res.* 1993;33:112–117.

60. Delafosse B, Bouffard Y, Viale JP, et al. Respiratory changes induced by parenteral nutrition in postoperative patients undergoing inspiratory pressure support ventilation. *Anesthesiology.* 1987;66:393–399.

61. Elwyn DH, Kinney JM, Jeevanandam M, et al. Influence of increasing carbohydrate intake on glucose kinetics in injured patients. *Ann Surg.* 1979;190:117–127.

62. Burke JF, Wolfe RR, Mullany CJ. Glucose requirements following burn injury. *Ann Surg.* 1979;190:274–285.
63. Askanazi J, Carpentier YA, Elwyn DH, et al. Influence of total parenteral nutrition on fuel utilization in injury and sepsis. *Ann Surg.* 1980;191:40–46.
64. Askanazi J, Rosenbaum S, Hyman R. Respiratory changes induced by the large glucose loads of total parenteral nutrition. *JAMA.* 1980;243:1444–1447.
65. Van den Berg B, Stam H. Metabolic and respiratory effects of enteral nutrition in patients during mechanical ventilation. *Intensive Care Med.* 1988;14:206–211.
66. Letton RW, Chwals WJ, Jamie A, Charles B. Early postoperative alterations in infant energy use increase the risk of overfeeding. *J Pediatr Surg.* 1995;30:988–993.
67. Cely CM, Arora P, Quartin AA, Kett DH, Schein RMH. Relationship of baseline glucose homeostasis to hyperglycemia during medical critical illness. *Chest.* 2004;126:879–887.
68. Nussbaum MS, Fischer JE. Pathogenesis of hepatic steatosis during total parenteral nutrition. In: Nyhus LM, ed. *Surgery Annual.* Norwalk, Conn: Appleton & Lange; 1991:1–11.
69. Lowry SF, Brennan MF. Abnormal liver function during parenteral nutrition: relation to infusion excess. *J Surg Res.* 1979;26:300–306.
70. Payne-James JJ, Silk DB. Heptobiliary dysfunction associated with total parenteral nutrition. *Dig Dis.* 1992;9:106–124.
71. Freund HR. Abnormalities of liver function and hepatic damage associated with total parenteral nutrition. *Nutrition.* 1991;7:1–6.
72. Das JB, Cosentino CM, Levy MF, et al. Early hepatobiliary dysfunction during total parenteral nutrition: an experimental study. *J Pediatr Surg.* 1993;28:14–18.
73. Bursztein S, Elwyn DH, Askanazi J. Energy metabolism and indirect calorimetry in critically ill and injured patients. *Acute Care.* 1988;15:91–110.
74. Sobrado J, Moldawer LL, Pomposelli JJ, et al. Lipid emulsions and reticuloendothelial system function in healthy and burned guinea pigs. *Am J Clin Nutr.* 1985;42:855–863.
75. Yamazaki K, Maiz A, Moldawer LL, et al. Complications associated with the overfeeding of infected animal. *J Surg Res.* 1987;40:152–158.
76. McMahon MM, Bistrian BR. Host defenses and susceptibility to infection in patients with diabetes mellitus. *Infect Dis Clin North Am.* 1995;9:1–9.
77. Alaedeen DI, Walsh MC, Chwals WJ. Total parenteral nutrition-associated hyperglycemia correlates with prolonged mechanical ventilation and hospital stay in septic infants. *J Pediatr Surg.* 2006;41:239–244; discussion 239–244.
78. Chiaretti A, De Benedictis R, Langer A, et al. Prognostic implications of hyperglycaemia in paediatric head injury. *Child Nerv Syst.* 1998;14:455–459.
79. Hall NJ, Peters M, Eaton S, Pierro A. Hyperglycemia is associated with increased morbidity and mortality rates in neonates with necrotizing enterocolotis. *J Pediatr Surg.* 2004;39:6898–6901.
80. Rosmarin DK, Wardlaw GM, Mirtallo J. Hyperglycemia associated with high, continuous infusion rates of total parenteral nutrition dextrose. *Nutr Clin Pract.* 1996;11:151–157.
81. Hunter DC, Jaksic T, Lewis D, Benotti PN, Blackburn GL, Bistrian BR. Resting energy expenditure in critically ill patients: estimates versus measurement. *Br J Surg.* 1988;75:875–878.
82. McCowen KC, Friel C, Sternberg J, et al. Hypocaloric total parenteral nutrition: effectiveness in prevention of hyperglycemia and infectious complications—a randomized clinical trial. *Crit Care Med.* 2000;28:3606–3611.
83. Veterans Affairs Total Parenteral Nutrition Cooperative Study Group. Perioperative total parenteral nutrition in surgical patients. *N Engl J Med.* 1991;325:525–532.
84. Moore FA, Feliciano DV, Andrassy RJ, et al. *Ann Surg.* 1992;216:172–183.
85. Kudsk KA, Crose MA, Fabian TC, et al. Enteral versus parenteral feeding: effects on septic morbidity after blunt and penetrating abdominal trauma. *Ann Surg.* 1992;215:503–511.
86. Koea JB, Shaw JHF. Total parenteral nutrition in surgical illness: How much? How good? *Nutrition.* 1992;8:275–281.
87. Vo NM, Waycaster M, Acuff RV, et al. Effects of postoperative carbohydrate overfeeding. *Ann Surg.* 1987;53:632–635.
88. Alaedeen DI, Walsh M, Chwals WJ. TPN-associated hyperglycemia correlates with prolonged mechanical ventilation, hospital length of stay, and mortality in septic infants. *J Pediatr Surg.* 2005, in press.
89. Alexander JW, Gonce SJ, Miskell PW, et al. A new model for studying nutrition in peritonitis. *Ann Surg.* 1989;209:334–340.
90. Dominioni L, Trocki O, Fang CH, et al. Enteral feeding in burn hypermetabolism: nutritional and metabolic effects of different levels of calorie and protein intake. *J Parenter Enteral Nutr.* 1985;9:269–279.
91. Garza JJ, Shew SB, Keshen TH, et al. Energy expenditure in ill premature neonates. *J Pediatr Surg.* 2002;37:289–293.
92. Taylor RM, Cheeseman P, Preedy V, et al. Can energy expenditure be predicted in critically ill children? *Pediatr Crit Care Med.* 2003;2:262–263.
93. Jones MO, Pierro A, Hammond P, Lloyd DA. The metabolic response to operative stress in infants. *J Pediatr Surgery.* 1993;28:1258–1263.
94. Billeaud C, Piedboeuf B, Chessex P. Respiratory gas exchange in response to fat-free parenteral nutrition: a comparison after thoracic or abdominal surgery in newborn infants. *J Pediatr Surg.* 1993;28:11–13.

95. Selby AM, McCauley JC, Schell DN, et al. Indirect calorimetry in mechanically ventilated children: a new technique that overcomes the problem of endotracheal tube leak. *Crit Care Med.* 1995;23:365–370.

96. Verhoeven JJ, Hazelzet JA, van der Voort E, et al. Comparison of measured and predicted energy expenditure in mechanically ventilated children. *Intensive Care Med.* 1998;24:464–468.

97. Coss-Bu JA, Jefferson LS, Walding D, et al. Resting energy expenditure in children in a pediatric intensive care unit: comparison of Harris-Benedict and Talbot predictions with indirect calorimetry values. *Am J Clin Nutr.* 1998;67:74–80.

98. White MS, Shepherd RW, McEniery JA. Energy expenditure in 100 ventilated, critically ill children: improving the accuracy of predictive equations. *Crit Care Med.* 2000;28:2307–2312.

99. Chwals WJ, Fernandez ME, Jamie AC, et al. Detection of postoperative sepsis in infants using metabolic stress monitoring. *Arch Surg.* 1994;129:437–442.

CHAPTER 7

Laboratory Assessment

Nancy Nevin-Folino and Robin LeBeouf-Aufdenkampe

INTRODUCTION

Laboratory values are an integral component of nutrition assessment and nutrition therapy. In conjunction with examination of the patient and quantitation of fluid and nutrient intake, laboratory values provide a measure of nutritional status past and present. Detailed information on nutrient availability and stores, biochemical processes, and the effects of nutrition therapy can be derived from laboratory assessment. Results may appear in patterns that are characteristic of specific diseases or in ways that allow us to distinguish between acute and chronic conditions. Serial monitoring provides information on patterns of biochemical status and differences in metabolic function in long term nutrition delivery. Judicious planning should accompany laboratory monitoring. The medical condition, nutritional status, route of nutrient delivery, and drug therapy dictate the schedule for laboratory monitoring. Protocols are helpful for assessing and following disease states and nutrition delivery. Changes in the patient or nutrition prescription warrant laboratory evaluation. Laboratory panels developed by hospitals or testing laboratories are available. They vary from one hospital or laboratory facility to another. This chapter presents laboratory values and discusses tests that may be useful in nutrition support.

BLOOD ANALYSES

Blood is a readily obtained body fluid and should be routinely used to assess fluid, electrolyte, nutrient, and metabolic status. Blood studies are vital for a complete nutrition assessment. Each result should be carefully interpreted in light of the patient's status and nutrition support to determine if it reflects increased need, limited or transient intolerance, or deficit state.

Complete blood count (CBC) is a basic screening and monitoring test panel. The tests quantify number, variety, percentage, concentrations, and quality of blood cells. This information can be used to evaluate the hematological status, provide a prognosis, and measure response to medical nutrition therapy and recovery.

Red blood cell (RBC) count is the number of red cells in a given amount of blood that can be used to evaluate the adequacy of erythrocyte number and production. The measurement is used in the evaluation of anemia or polycythemia. By definition, in all anemias, the RBC is below the normal range. Elevated levels occur in dehydration and in any condition in which the oxygen requirement is increased, such as lung or heart disease, high altitudes, or in genetic polycythemia. Decreased levels occur with blood loss, hemolysis, nutrient deficiencies, or chronic disease. Attributes of RBCs can be determined by counting the number of cells; by assessing hemoglobin (Hgb) concentration, hematocrit, membrane lipid analysis, or fragility studies; by observation of the blood smear; and by a reticulocyte count.

Hemoglobin is the main component of RBCs, and it transports O_2. Hemoglobin is indicated by the grams of Hgb contained in 100 mL of blood. Elevated levels occur in dehydration and any condition in which the oxygen requirement is increased, such as lung or heart disease, high altitudes, or in genetic polycythemia. Decreased levels occur with blood loss, hemolysis, nutrient deficiencies or chronic disease.

Hematocrit (Hct) is a measure of the concentration of RBC in the blood. It is volume of RBC found in 100 mL or 1 liter of blood expressed as a percent. The Hct is about 3 times the value of the Hgb.

RBC indices are useful in the evaluation of anemia, polycythemia, and nutritional disorders. The indices measure the RBC and the Hgb content of RBC. They are calculated from Hgb, RBC, and Hct levels. Mean cell volume (MCV) is an estimate of the average size of RBCs. Abnormally large cells, called macrocytes, occur in B_{12} and folate deficiency. Abnormally small cells are called microcytes; they occur in iron deficiency and chronic lead poisoning. A decrease in MCV occurs in Hgb synthesis abnormalities. Mean cell hemoglobin (MCH) is the percent volume of Hgb per RBC. It indicates the weight of hemoglobin in the RBC, regardless of size. Mean cell hemoglobin concentration (MCHC) is the hemoglobin concentration of individual cells. Falsely elevated levels of MCHC are seen with hyperlipidemia. Decreased levels of MCHC are associated with disorders of Hgb synthesis. However, iron deficiency is the only anemia in which the MCHC is routinely low. Red cell distribution width (RDW) measures variation in the size of the RBC. The RDW, along with MCV, is used in the diagnosis of anemias (see Table 7-1).

Total iron binding capacity (TIBC), transferrin (iron tansport protein), and serum iron values are used in combination to determine the percent of transferrin saturation (calculated as the serum iron × 100 ÷ TIBC). These values help to define the pathophysiology of anemia. Ferritin, which measures body iron stores, is most specific in identifying iron deficiency, but it is an acute phase reactant. Reticulocyte

Table 7-1 Anemia.

Test	*Microcytic hypochromic iron deficiency anemia*	*Macrocytic vitamin B_{12} or folate deficiency*	*Normocytic anemia of chronic disease*
RBC	May be normal	Low	Low
Hemoglobin	Low	Low	Low
Hematocrit	Low	Low	Low
MCV	Low (< 80)	High (> 94)	Normal
MCH	Low	High	Normal
MCHC	Low (< 30%)	Normal (> 30)	Normal (> 30)
TIBC	High	Low	Low
Transferrin saturation percentage	Low	Normal	Low
Iron status	Low	Normal	Normal

count evaluates bone marrow function and distinguishes between anemia caused by blood loss and anemia caused by decreased RBC production. Reticulocyte count can be used to measure the effectiveness of therapy such as iron or B_{12} supplementation. A blood smear, a visual inspection of a smeared drop of blood, is used to evaluate cell morphology.

Values for white blood cells (WBCs) and the percent of different cell types, lymphocytes, monocytes, and polymorphonuclear leukocytes (neutrophils, basophils, eosinophils) vary with a child's age. The WBC and differential count of leukocytes are measured to determine the body's susceptibility and response to infection and inflammation as well as the severity of a disease process.

Platelets are nonnucleated cellular fragments produced by megakaryocytes, large polyploid cells within the bone marrow. Platelets are assessed by quantifying the number of platelets, by assessing platelet aggregation, and by measuring specific platelet functions. Bleeding time can also be used to assess platelet function.

Assays of coagulation quantify each of the factors (I through XII, plasminogen, antithrombin III, prekallikrein, and high molecular weight kininogen). Prothrombin time (PT) and partial prothrombin time (PTT) aid in the overall picture of vitamin K adequacy and blood protein abnormalities.[1]

ELECTROLYTES

Measurement of serum electrolytes gives an overview of fluid and electrolyte status (for more information, see Chapter 23). The frequency with which electrolytes should be measured depends on the stage of nutrition therapy, whether changes in the nutrition prescriptions or the nutrition support are made, and if the patient is stable on long term support. Monitoring electrolyte levels provides information on adequacy of intake and on output.

Sodium is the most abundant cation in extracellular fluid, and it plays a major role in acid base balance. The kidneys are the primary regulatory organ for body sodium and water balance. Sweat and gastrointestinal fluids are major routes of sodium excretion. Sodium is included in the grouping of electrolytes and must be carefully monitored when nutrition support is initiated or changes in therapy are made. Sodium losses are high in patients who have ileostomies. Sodium levels indicate changes in water balance. To determine sodium balance, intake from all sources (oral, parenteral, medications, etc.) is compared to output including urine, stool (especially if diarrhea is present), drains and stoma outputs. Urine sodium is a sensitive marker for sodium homeostasis.[2] Table 7-2 lists some conditions with increased or decreased serum sodium.

There are three types of hyponatremia. Hypo-volemic hyponatremia is caused by sodium loss in excess of water loss. Hypervolemic hyponatremia is caused by water overload as occurs in acute or chronic renal failure, nephrotic syndrome, cirrhosis or congestive heart failure. Normovolemic hyponatremia is caused by inappropriate antidiuretic hormone secretion, severe hyperglycemia, chronic excessive intake of water, or adrenal insufficiency. Hypernatremia or increased serum sodium is caused by increased

Table 7-2 Hypernatremia and urine osmolality.

< 300 mOsm/kg	*300–700 mOsm/kg*	*> 700 mOsm/kg*
Diabetes insipidus; either impaired secretion of antidiuretic hormone (ADH) or the kidneys cannot respond to ADH	Partial defect in ADH release Response to ADH osmotic diuresis	Loss of thirst Insensible loss of water GI loss of hypotonic fluid Excessive sodium intake

water losses, decreased water intake or increased sodium intake. Urine osmolality is increased with extra renal losses of sodium and is low or normal with renal losses of water.[1,3]

Potassium is the major intracellular cation responsible for the regulation of cellular water balance and electrical conduction, and it is important in acid-base balance. Potassium is obtained through dietary intake and excretion is controlled by the kidneys. Daily excretion of potassium is approximately equal to daily intake. The kidneys can adjust quickly to increased potassium intake, but cannot prevent depletion in the absence of intake. Serum potassium is tightly regulated and high or low levels can cause life threatening arrhythmias. Abnormalities in potassium homeostasis are caused by problems with insulin, aldosterone, acid-base balance, renal function, or gastrointestinal and skin losses.[1,3] Although serum potassium is not an accurate indicator of total body potassium, careful continuous monitoring of serum potassium is required at the initiation of nutrition support, when changes in nutrition therapy are made, or when refeeding malnourished individuals. Acidosis is associated with high potassium and alkalosis with low potassium levels.

Chloride is the most abundant anion in the extracellular fluid. Chloride is indirectly regulated through changes in sodium and bicarbonate. Regulation of chloride is primarily by the renal proximal tubules, where it is exchanged for bicarbonate ions. Chloride values are used for acid-base determination or correction and in evaluation of water balance.

Carbon dioxide (CO_2) is a measure of acid base balance. Total CO_2 concentration is determined by acidifying serum to convert bicarbonate to CO_2. Since 95% of total serum CO_2 consists of converted bicarbonate, this value is actually a measure of the bicarbonate concentration. Total CO_2 levels reflect the total amount of CO_2 in the body and are a general guide to the body's buffering capacity. The bicarbonate buffer system, along with the lungs, kidneys, and other buffer systems, helps to maintain the pH of the extracellular fluid. The kidneys regulate CO_2 when it is in the form of bicarbonate. The lungs regulate CO_2 gas. Increased or decreased CO_2 levels indicate an acid-base imbalance.

Calcium plays an important role in all of intermediary metabolism, neuromuscular activity, regulation of endocrine functions, blood coagulation, and bone metabolism. Serum calcium concentration is tightly controlled by parathyroid hormone, serum phosphate, vitamin D, the kidneys, and the gastrointestinal tract. Ionized calcium (ICa) is a measure of unbound calcium that is available for metabolic activity (for more information, see Chapter 25). In nutrition therapy, ICa is the preferred measurement, because serum calcium levels can be affected by serum protein levels. If the serum albumin is low, a correction factor must be applied to the total calcium (corrected Ca = measured Ca + [40 – albumin] × 0.02).[4,5] Table 7-3 lists some causes of hypercalcemia and hypocalcemia.

Table 7-3 Causes of hypercalcemia and hypocalcemia.

Hypercalcemia	*Hypocalcemia*
Acute adrenal insufficiency	Decreased intake
Calcium supplements	Hyperphosphatemia
Chronic immobilization	Hypoalbuminemia
Excessive IV calcium salts	Hypomagnesemia
Excessive vitamin A or D	Hypothyroidism
Hyperthyroidism	Pancreatitis
Malignance	Renal failure
Paget's disease	Vitamin D deficiency
Thyroid hormone increasing intestinal absorption	

Magnesium is the second most abundant intracellular cation, and it is a cofactor in enzymatic reactions involving energy metabolism and protein and nucleic acid synthesis. Serum magnesium is controlled by kidney excretion. Magnesium levels should be obtained when serum calcium levels are decreased. Magnesium supplementation may be required before hypocalcemia and or hypokalemia can be corrected. An increase in serum magnesium levels occurs in decreased kidney function.

Phosphorus, or phosphate, is an intracellular anion that is necessary for energy transfer in intermediary metabolism. It is a component of phospholipids, an acid-base buffer, and it is a principal ion in bone mineral. Phosphorus is controlled by the parathyroid hormone, exists in an inverse relationship with calcium, and is used in assessment of bone metabolism. Serum phosphate levels must be carefully monitored when nutrition support is started, especially in patients who are malnourished. A decrease in serum phosphate levels must be corrected, because uncorrected low serum phosphate can cause cardiac arrthymias.[6]

ACID-BASE BALANCE

Respiratory status can reflect the balance of metabolism, and it is evaluated through arterial blood gas (ABG) measurement. ABGs reflect respiratory and metabolic components of acid-base. The metabolic component depends on the patient's ability to regulate and buffer acids. The hydrogen ion concentration is expressed as pH; PCO_2 measures the respiratory component; PO_2 gives information as to the cause of acid-base imbalance; S_{O2} measures hemoglobin saturation; and the base excess or HCO_3^- measures the amount of buffer in the blood. It is important to note that the serum HCO_3^- indicates the change in the metabolic acid-base balance and should be used in addition to the ABG.[7] Interpretation of ABG occurs in conjunction with other nutrition parameters. Treatment is then based on the cause of an acid-base disorder. The types of acid-base disorders are listed in Table 7-4.

Anion gap (AG) is the difference in concentration between unmeasured cation and anion equivalents, $AG = [Na + K] - [Cl + HCO_3^-]$. Hatherill and colleagues have demonstrated that a correction must be made for albumin (Table 7-5).[8] Table 7-6 lists causes of anion gap imbalance.

KIDNEY FUNCTION

Kidney function tests measure how well the kidneys filter and excrete waste. Evaluation of sodium, potassium, glucose, fluid balance, serum proteins, and urea nitrogen are important measures of renal function.

Blood urea nitrogen (BUN) is the concentration of nitrogen (within urea) in the serum. Along with other laboratory and clinical data, BUN can be used to assess or monitor hydration status, renal function, protein tolerance, dietary intake, and catabolism in some clinical situations. Urea

Table 7-4 Acid-base disorders.

Acid-base disorder	*pH*	*PCO2*	*HCO_3^-*	*Urine pH*
Respiratory acidosis	↓	↑	↑*	
Metabolic acidosis	↓	↓*	↓	↓(< 5.5)
Respiratory alkalosis	↑	↓*	↑	
Metabolic alkalosis	↑	↑	↑*	↑

* compensatory mechanism

Table 7-5 Determining anion gap for therapy.

Steps for interpretation:

1. Determine if the patient has acidemia or alkalemia
2. Use the anion gap (AG) equation to determine if an anion gap is present

   $[Na + K] - [Cl + HCO_3^-] = AG$

3. To account for an albumin deficit, correct the AG equation. For every 1-gram deficit of albumin, there is a 2.5 mEq decrease in the AG.[8]

   $[Na + K] - [Cl + HCO_3^-] - [.25 \times (44 - \text{albumin})] = AG$

4. Compare to the normal AG of 12 ± 2 mEq/L
5. Make corrections in nutrition prescription (volume, etc.)

Example:

A 3-year-old female is lethargic with no oral intake for 8 hours. She had decreased oral intake for 5 days. Weight: 10.5 kg. (Admit weight 11.4kg.)

Labs:

Na: 132; K: 4.3; Cl: 98; HCO_3^-: 14.7; pH: 7.32 BUN: 30; Creatinine: 0.8; Albumin: 3

Steps:

1. Acidemia
2. [132 + 4.3] – [98 + 14.7] = 23.6.
3. AG is 24.
4. Compared to normal (12 ± 2).
5. Patient has metabolic acidosis.
6. Deliver bicarbonate correction; start IV nutrition and fluid to further balance electrolytes.

Table 7-6 Causes of anion gap imbalance.

Increased anion gap:	*Normal anion gap:*
Alcoholic ketoacidosis	Drugs
Diabetic ketoacidosis	GI loss of bicarbonate
Hyperphosphatemia	Hyponatremia
Ketogenic diets	Hyperalimentation
Lactic acidosis	Rapid infusion of sodium
Renal failure	Renal loss of bicarbonate
Starvation or fasting	
Toxins	

is produced in the liver and excreted by the kidneys. Low BUN levels may be observed with malnutrition, fluid overload, protein anabolism, or profound liver disease. High BUN occurs in water and salt depletion, shock or stress, renal disease, urinary tract obstruction, ketoacidosis in diabetes, anabolic steroid use, and excessive protein intake or catabolism.

Serum creatinine is used to estimate glomerular filtration rate (GFR). For children the GFR is calculated using the following equation:

$$\text{GFR} = 0.43 \times \text{height in cm} \div \text{serum creatinine (mg/dL)}.$$

Creatinine clearance for children is calculated with the following equation:

$$\text{Creatinine clearance (mL/min/1.73 m}^2 = 0.55 \times \text{height in cm} \div \text{serum creatinine in mg/dL.}$$ [9]

An online GFR calculator is available from Cornell University.[10] Cystatin C is an endogenous marker for GFR in children and can be used to adjust for height and age.[11] Creatinine height index is a measurement of lean body mass. The index is calculated as the 24-hour excretion of creatinine divided by the 24-hour excretion of creatinine of a normal individual at the same height and sex, expressed as a percent.

A urine analysis is important in the evaluation of kidney function. Urine volume, specific gravity, osmolality, and pH are measured. Agarwal and others showed that there is a statistically significant correlation between spot urine samples and 24-hour collections in the detection of proteinuria.[12] Urine amino acid levels may be helpful in the evaluation of metabolic disease.

LIVER FUNCTION TESTS (LFT)

The liver plays a central role in protein metabolism. Serum levels of albumin, prealbumin, and ammonia are helpful in assessing the effectiveness of nutrition support. Liver function tests (LFTs) are used to evaluate liver function, detect damage to the liver, diagnose and monitor chronic viral hepatitis, and to assess the severity of liver disease. LFTs consist of total (unconjugated) and direct bilirubin (conjugated), aspartate amino transferase (AST), alanine amino transferase (ALT), gamma glutamyl transpeptidase (GGT), and alkaline phosphatase (ALP).

Bilirubin is a measure of liver excretory function. There are two types of bilirubin: indirect, or unconjugated, and direct, or conjugated. Increased levels of indirect bilirubin indicate hemolysis, Gilbert's syndrome, or Cirgler-Najjar type 1 or 2. Elevated levels of direct bilirubin are associated with cholestasis, physiologically defined as a reduction in bile flow. Indirect bilirubin is often elevated during the newborn period.

AST is an enzyme that increases following injury or death of cells and is directly related to the number of damaged cells and the amount of time that passes between tissue injury and the test. The enzyme rises within 12 hours of tissue injury and remains increased for up to 5 days after the injury. Increased levels occur in myocardial infarction, liver disease, traumatic injuries, malnutrition, with refeeding, and after surgery. Decreased levels occur in patients on chronic renal dialysis or who have vitamin B_6 deficiency.

ALT is an enzyme that increases in the blood following injury or death of cells, and as with AST, it is directly related to the number of damaged cells and the amount of time that passes between injury to the tissue and the test. ALT is used to assess liver disease, associated with ongoing liver injury, and to monitor treatment for hepatitis. Increased levels can occur as a result of severe burns, trauma to muscle, shock, malnutrition, or with refeeding or liver damage.

ALP is a zinc-dependent enzyme found in bone, liver, intestine, and placenta. It is less specific for liver disease than GGT. ALP is elevated in cholestasis, liver malignancies, hepatitis, metabolic abnormalities, and toxic liver injury. ALP is also elevated in rickets, provided the patient is not zinc deficient. When the ALP is elevated it may be necessary to fractionate it to identify its source (Liver= AP-1, α_2; Bone= AP-2, β_1; Intestinal= AP-3, β_2; Placental= AP-4).

GGT is an enzyme located in the epithelial lining of the biliary tree. It is increased in most cholestatic disorders including biliary atresia, Alagille syndrome, α-1-antitrypsin deficiency, and idiopathic neonatal hepatitis.

Ammonia (NH_3) is a metabolite of protein catabolism. The liver removes NH_3 from the body by the portal vein and converts NH_3 to urea, which is then excreted. Muscle is also an important site of NH_3 metabolism. A rise in NH_3 affects acid-base balance and brain function. Ammonia is used to evaluate metabolism, the advance of liver disease and in the diagnosis of congenital metabolic abnormalities.

Serum amino acid levels are used to assess liver function, but they are highly dependent on dietary intake. It is assumed that the protein and amino acid intake of the exclusively breastfed infant is optimal and reflected in the aminogram.[13,14] However, postprandial plasma amino acid levels not only represent protein intake, but also synthesis, catabolism, excretion, and tissue utilization. Some researchers are looking at the amino acid profile of placental blood flow to the fetus to identify the ideal amino acid composition for preterm infants.[15] Serum amino acid levels are most often measured to assess the protein status of infants and children with inborn errors of metabolism. Serum amino acid levels vary with age, so it is important that reference values are age appropriate.[16] Methodological issues are important when measuring tryptophan since it is the only amino acid that is primarily bound to plasma albumin (80–90%).[17]

Albumin plays a principal role in the maintenance of plasma oncotic pressure, and it binds hormones, anions, drugs, and fatty acids, and it buffers acids. It is a useful tool to assess protein status and follow rehabilitation of malnourished individuals. Albumin has a half-life of approximately 20 days, but the half-life can be shorter in hypermetabolic conditions. Albumin is decreased in acute infectious or inflammatory states.

Prealbumin, also called transthyretin because it binds thyroxine, is a protein synthesized by the liver; it has a shorter half-life than albumin (2 days). Because of the shorter half-life, prealbumin levels more rapidly reflect changes in nutritional status. Prealbumin is not an important factor in thyroid function because most thyroxine is bound to globulin. Like albumin, prealbumin levels are decreased in liver disease.

Hepatobiliary imaging may be warranted to detect biliary atresia and to assess liver trauma.

INTESTINAL FUNCTION

Secretory Function

Digestion of nutrients requires secretion of digestive substances such as acid, pepsin, bile, and enzymes. In addition, the gastrointestinal tract secretes hormones and paracrine substances that modulate the function of other cells. The secretory function of the gastrointestinal tract can be assessed by quantifying levels of specific secretions such as gastric acid, pepsin, enterokinase, gastrin, cholecystokinin, amylase, trypsin, lipase, motolin, etc., in the lumen or in stool.

For some nutrients, the gastrointestinal tract regulates absorption based on nutrient levels. This regulation is often complex and involves other organs such as the liver and kidney for calcium homeostasis and the bone marrow for iron. To assess this function of the gastrointestinal tract, balance studies are helpful. The levels of specific nutrients in blood or tissue can be also be quantified. Balance studies are difficult to conduct and require hospitalization. Balance studies were initially used for research purposes, but now are commonly used in pediatric small bowel transplantation patients and some intensive care units. Carmine red dye (100 mg/kg) is given with the initial feeding. The red dye colors the stool to mark the duration of the collection but does not affect stool results. Urine is collected. Net retention (or balance) of each nutrient is calculated as the difference between intake and the sum of urine and fecal losses during the 72-hour collection period. Net absorption is defined as the difference between intake and fecal losses.

The pancreas serves as a secretory (exocrine) and hormone (endocrine) producing organ. Exocrine functions are difficult to assess in routine clinical practice, but as noted previously, they can be assessed by directly quantifying lumenal concentrations of enzymes and bicarbonate before and after a stimulus. The stimulus can be a hormone (secretin, cholecystokinin, etc.) or a meal. Indirect tests include assessment of stool for products of pancreatic secretion such as chymotrypsin and elastase or fat, carbohydrate, or protein. The most accurate estimation of pancreatic function is based on the secretin pancreozymin stimulation test. This test requires duodenal intubation and collection of fluid before and after intravenous stimulation of the pancreas.[18] It is invasive, expensive, and time consuming. The most commonly performed test used to assess exocrine pancreatic function is the 72-hour quantitative fecal fat balance study described later. It is not an ideal test. Intake must be carefully recorded during the test period and the stool collection is odious. It does not discriminate among hepatobiliary, mucosal, or pancreatic etiology for fat malabsorption. It is important for interpretation of results that patients not take pancreatic enzyme supplements during the test period. A human pancreatic-specific enzyme-linked immunosorbent assay (ELISA) for stool elastase correlates well with the secretin pancreozymin stimulation test. Exogenous enzyme supplementation, which is porcine, has no effect on the results. The test discriminates between pancreatic and biliary or small bowel causes for malabsorption. Intra-assay and interassay variance of elastase is low.[19]

OTHER NUTRITIONAL MARKERS

Carbohydrate

Glucose is the preferred fuel for the brain, kidneys, and some blood cells. Serum levels are regulated by the hormones insulin and glucagon. Serum glucose levels are affected by the concentration and rate of glucose infusion, inflammatory states, the secretion of insulin and glucagon, and the status of peripheral insulin receptors (for more information, see Chapters 6, 22, and 24). Routine monitoring of serum glucose in nutrition support is important at the initiation of PN, in critical illness, and when PN is being cycled up or down. Long term monitoring is warranted for patients who are at risk for or have diabetes. Glycated serum protein or fructosamine[19] detects acute changes in diabetes treatment and Hgb A_{1C} is used for monitoring of glucose status over a 3-month or longer period of time.

Protein

In addition to serum protein, albumin, and prealbumin, there might be situations in which monitoring, quantifying, and identifying specific serum or urine proteins are warranted. Serum protein electrophoresis (SPE) can be used in the examination of inflammatory states, infection, organ disease, cerebral spinal fluid (CSF) identification, and protein-losing conditions.[1] Urine protein electrophoresis (UPE) is helpful in evaluating the severity of protein loss in clinical situations where kidney damage has occurred.[20] Aminoacidopathies or inborn errors of metabolism are monitored routinely for treatment and assessment of disease management. A complete reference for diagnosis, monitoring, and treatment of inborn errors of metabolism, including amino acid, carbohydrate, lipid, mineral, and nitrogen errors, is available in *Ross Metabolic Formula System: Nutrition Support Protocols*[21] and in Chapter 33 of this book.

Homocysteine synthesis requires cobalamin and folate, so it is often measured in malnutrition or chronic wasting diseases to evaluate vitamin B_{12} and folate states. Retinol binding protein (RBP) levels are important when vitamin A status is assessed. Carnitine levels are followed in long term PN to evaluate adequacy of delivery.[22] C-reactive protein (CRP) is a marker of inflammation, infection, or injury (surgery). In practice, CRP sometimes is measured after surgery, and then serially (daily) to evaluate recovery (see Chapter 6).[1,23]

Alpha-1-antitrypsin (ATT) is a serum protease inhibitor. ATT deficiency causes the release of proteolytic enzymes that cause tissue damage and predominantly affects the lungs and liver. The measurement is a nonspecific marker of inflammation, severe infection, and necrosis. If liver disease is present, ATT measurement is warranted.[1]

SERUM TRACE ELEMENT LEVELS

Trace elements should be measured in infants and children after 1 month of trace-element-free PN. A variety of pediatric trace element packages exist. A complete package includes seven trace elements, zinc, selenium, copper, molybdenum, manganese, iodine, and chromium. If fewer than the seven listed are administered to an infant or child on total PN for longer than 1 month, serum trace element levels should be obtained to identify deficiencies.

LIPID MARKERS

Serum triglycerides are obtained when intravenous fat is started or increased. Samples should be collected between lipid infusions to accurately represent lipid levels. A sudden rise in serum triglycerides suggests the patient is septic. The free fatty acid to serum albumin molar ratio (FA:SA) should be evaluated in infants whose indirect bilirubin is elevated. The FA:SA ratio should be less than 4 to prevent kernicterus. The FA:SA ratio should be less than 4 to prevent kernicterus. The American Academy of Pediatrics recommends that if intravenous lipids are administered over a 24-hour period, lipid infusions do not need to be discontinued in jaundiced infants.[24]

Intravenous lipid is used as a calorie and essential fatty acid source. EFAD can be seen as early as 2 days in neonates. Clinical signs of EFAD include reduced growth; flaky, dry skin; thrombocytopenia; increased susceptibility to infection; and impaired wound healing.[25] EFAD can be prevented by providing 2–4% of total calories as lipid (1–2% linoleic acid). That is an intravenous lipid dose of 0.5 to 1.0 g per kilogram per day. Biochemical assessment of EFAD status includes determination of the ratio of 5, 8, 11-eicosatrienoic to arachidonic acid (triene-to-tetraene ratio). A ratio greater than 0.4 to 1.0 is considered to be an early indicator of EFAD.[26] Not every hospital laboratory performs this test, so samples may be sent to a reference laboratory.

URINE STUDIES

Urine creatinine is measured to evaluate kidney function. Urine protein or albumin may be the first sign of renal disease and may be abnormal before clinical symptoms appear. However, protein substances found in the urine must be used with additional assessment because other physiologic conditions can produce proteinuria.[3] Microalbuminuria is an increase in urine albumin below the detectable range of the normal protein test. This measurement is used for screening, monitoring, and detection of deteriorating renal function in diabetic patients. β2-microglubulin is increased in nonspecific inflammation of active, chronic lymphocyic leukemia, and it may be used to discriminate between tubular and glomerular dysfunction. Urine glucose is measured to assess the renal reabsorption ability. Glucose spills into the urine when the renal threshold is exceeded. In some situations the serum glucose may be normal, but the kidneys cannot process the glucose being ingested or infused.

STOOL STUDIES

Fecal Fat

A quantitative 72-hour stool collection, coupled with a 3-day food record is the gold standard for determining fat malabsorption. Fat intake is maximized to be ≥ 25 g/day in infants and ≥ 100 g/day in school-age children. The coefficient of fat absorption is calculated as follows:

$$\text{Coefficient of fat absorption} = \frac{(\text{Dietary fat intake} - \text{fecal fat excreted})}{\text{Dietary fat intake}} \times 100$$

The normal coefficient of fat malabsorption is estimated at ≈ 7% of intake but may be as high as 14% of intake in healthy subjects who have rapid gut transit because of diarrhea.[27] In premature infants and infants less than 6 months of age, the coefficient of fat absorption is approximately 25% and 15% respectively. Fat excretion can vary daily, and results can be falsely negative or positive.

Polymorphonuclear cells can be found in stool when the colon is inflamed, as occurs in bacterial infections and inflammatory bowel disease. Stool cultures for enteric pathogens, studies for parasites, including *Giardia* and *Cryptosporidium,* are important when diarrhea is present. *Clostridium difficile* should be considered anytime there is persistent diarrhea in patients who have been hospitalized, especially if they have been treated with antibiotics.

A qualitative fecal fat is used to assess for fat malabsorption, but has many confounders and is not recommended. If malabsorption is suspected, the coefficient of fat absorption should be determined.

Fecal electrolyte concentrations are used to differentiate osmotic from secretory diarrhea. A stool sodium of ≥ 90 mEq/L generally indicates a secretory process, while a stool sodium less than 50 mEq/L suggests an osmotic process.[28]

Fecal chymotrypsin, an intestinal proteolytic enzyme secreted by the pancreas, can be measured in the stool to assess pancreatic function. Recently, stool elastase, which measures only human elastase, correlates with pancreatic enzyme concentrations, and can be measured even when patients are taking pancreatic enzymes, has been the stool test of choice to assess exocrine pancreatic function.

Fecal ATT is a measure of gastrointestinal protein loss and is most often assessed if protein-losing enteropathy is suspected. ATT is resistant to gastrointestinal proteolysis and correlates with the excretion of ^{51}Cr in both normal patients and patients with protein-losing enteropathy.

Stool pH is diet dependent; normally it is slightly acidic at about pH 5 to 6. For example, breastfed infants have slightly acidic stools; bottle fed infants have neutral or slightly alkaline stools. Stool pH is increased with protein breakdown and decreased with carbohydrate and fat malabsorption. Reducing substances measure reducing sugars such as glucose, fructose, lactose, galactose and pentose in the stool and are used to indicate carbohydrate malabsorption. For non-reducing sugars such as sucrose, the stool must first be hydrolyzed. Occult blood in the stool can mean the presence of tumors, ulcers, inflammatory bowel disease, arteriovenous malformations, diverticulosis, or hemotobilia. Positive results require examination because hemorrhoids, swallowed blood, and/or some drug therapies could be the cause.

OTHER STUDIES

For children who have suffered malnutrition, have malabsorption, require long term PN, or are at risk for inadequate bone mineralization, dual-energy x-ray absortiometry (DEXA) measures bone density in the spine, hip, and/or forearm.[28] There are 3 major skeletal or bone nutritional diseases. Rickets, or osteomalacia, results from vitamin D deficiency, which leads to the failure of osteoid to calcify, as well as hypertrophy of the epiphyseal cartilages.[1] Osteopenia is usually associated with infants born prematurely and is caused by hypominerialization of the bones due to inadequate intake or medical sequelae that coexists with extreme prematurity (or other disease states such as malabsorption, organ disease, or organ failure). Osteoporosis is an absolute decrease in bone mass resulting from increased bone resorption of multifactorial etiology.

Balance studies compare intake and output of a nutrient. Nitrogen balance (NB) is used to determine the adequacy of dietary protein. Negative nitrogen balance indicates protein catabolism and positive balance indicates protein synthesis. NB can be calculated as follows:

$$NB = N_I - N_O$$

where N_I is nitrogen intake, which is equal to protein intake divided by 6.25; and N_O is nitrogen output and is equal to the urinary urea nitrogen plus 4 or total urinary nitrogen plus 2.

This calculation is most accurate when total urinary nitrogen can be measured. Some diseases, fluid losses, hormones, and body movement affect accuracy. In the critically ill, protein is lost faster than it can be replaced and protein levels must be followed closely. Measurement of NB can help guide nutrition therapy.

Breath Tests

Breath tests can be used to measure carbohydrate, or fat malabsorption, to assess for bacterial overgrowth, gastric emptying time, and *H. pylori* infection.

Sweat Tests

The sweat test is used to diagnosis cystic fibrosis. Sweat is collected, and sodium and chloride are measured. High concentrations are indicative of the disease. Secretin pancreozymin stimulation tests can be used for diagnosis of cystic fibrosis for patients who do not display gastrointestinal symptoms, although as mentioned previously, the tests are arduous. The sweat collection from newborns might not be sufficient for measurement. Serum reactive trypsinogen is used as a screening test of cystic fibrosis but is age specific, so interpretation is necessary. Gene testing is also commercially available.

LIMITATIONS

Laboratory tests provide limited information. However, obtaining blood can be difficult in infants and small children and their small blood volume requires a laboratory that can analyze small samples. Medications can alter expected metabolism and increase or decrease laboratory values. Result errors are possible for a variety of reasons (blood kept at inappropriate temperature or time, hemolyzed sample, etc.). If a lab result is unexpected, it may be prudent to repeat the test before changing medical or nutrition therapy.

CONCLUSION

Laboratory testing in EN and PN is essential to proper patient care; however, tests should be chosen judiciously. The person requesting the test should have a clear idea of the reason for the test, how to interpret the test and what limits the test has. A test result should always be interpreted in the context of the patient's clinical condition and, in pediatrics, taking into account the patients' age.

REFERENCES

1. Fischbach F. *A Manual of Laboratory Diagnostic Tests.* Philadelphia, Pa: Lippincott, Williams & Wilkins; 2004;143–146.
2. Bower TR, Pringle KG, Soper RE. Sodium deficit causing weight gain and metabolic acidosis in infants with ileostomy. *J Pediatr Surg.* 1998;23:567–572.
3. Jacobs D, DeMott W, Oxley DK. *Laboratory Test Handbook.* 5th ed. Cleveland, Ohio: Lexi-Corp Inc; 2001.
4. Slomp J, van der Voort PHJ, Gerritsen RT, Berk JAM, Bakker AJ. Albumin-adjusted calcium is not suitable for diagnosis of hyper and hypocalcemia in the critically ill. *Crit Care Med.* 2003;31:1389–1393.
5. Dickerson RN, Alexander KH, Minard G, Croce MA, Brown RO. Accuracy of methods to estimate ionized and "corrected" serum calcium concentrations in critically ill multiple trauma patients receiving specialized nutrition support. *JPEN.* 2004;28:133–141.
6. Weinsier RL, Krumdiek CL. Death resulting from overzealous total parenteral nutrition: the refeeding syndrome revisited. *Am J Clin Nutr.* 1981;34:393–399.
7. Schwaderer AL, Swartz GJ. Back to basics: Acidosis and alkalosis. *Ped in Review.* 2004. 25(10):350–357.
8. Hatherill M, Waggie Z, Purves L, Reynolds L, Argent A. Correction of the anion gap for albumin in order to detect occult tissue anions in shock. *Arch Dis Child.* 2002;87:526–529.
9. Hogg RJ, Furth S, Lemley KV, et al. National Kidney Foundation's kidney disease outcomes quality initiative clinical practice guidelines for chronic kidney disease in children and adolescents: evaluation, classification, and stratification. *Pediatrics.* 2003;111(6):1416–1421.
10. Cornell University Joan and Sanford I. Weill Medical College. Pediatric Critical Care Medicine Medical

Calculators: Online calculator for creatinine clearance. Available at: http://www-users.med.cornell.edu/~spon/picu/calc/crclcalc.htm. Accessed October 10, 2004.

11. Bokenkamp A, Domamerzki M, Zinck R, et al. Cystatin C-A new marker of glomerular filtration rate in children independent of age and height. *Pediatrics.* 1998;101(5):875–881.
12. Agarwal I, Kirubakaran C, Markandeyulu, Seliakumar. Quantification of proteinuria by spot urine sampling. *Ind J Clin Biochem.* 2004;19(2):45–47. Available at: http://medind.nic.in/iaf/t04/i2/iaft04i2p45.pdf. Accessed September 13, 2004.
13. Bachmann C, Haschke-Becher E. Plasma amino acid concentrations in breast-fed and formula-fed infants and reference intervals. In: Raiha NCR, Rubaltelli FF, eds. *Infant Formula: Closer to the Reference.* Vevey, Switzerland: Lippincott; 2002:121–137.
14. Wu PYK, Edwards N, Storm MC. Plasma amino acid pattern in normal term breast-fed infants. *J Pediatr.* 1986;109:347–349.
15. Bruton JA, Ball RO, Pencharz PB. Current total parenteral nutrition solutions for the neonate are inadequate. *Curr Opin Clin Nutr Metab Care.* 2000;3:299–304.
16. Lepage N, McDonald N, Dallaire L, Lambert M. Age-specific distribution of plasma amino acid concentrations in a healthy pediatric population. *Clin Chem.* 1997;43:2397–2402.
17. Denokla WE, Dewey HH. The determination of tryptophan in plasma, liver, and urine. *J Lab Clin Med.* 1997;69:160–169.
18. Conwell DL, Zuccaro G, Morrow JB, et al. Analysis of duodenal drainage fluid after cholecystokinin (CCK) stimulation in healthy volunteers. *Pancreas.* 2002;25(4):350–354.
19. Wallis C, Leung T, Cubitt D, Reynolds A. Stool elastase as a diagnostic test of pancreatic function in children with cystic fibrosis. *Lancet.* 1997;4:350(9083):1001.
20. American Association for Clinical Chemistry. Lab Tests Online, 2001–2005. Available at: http://www.labtestsonline.org/. Accessed March 5, 2006.
21. Acosta PB, Yannicelli S. *Ross Metabolic Formula System: Nutrition Support Protocols.* 4th ed. Columbus, Ohio: Ross Laboratories; 2001.
22. Vitamin deficiency, dependency, and toxicity. In: Beers MH, Berkow R, eds. *The Merck Manual.* West Point, Pa: Merck and Company; 1999:35–41.
23. Mesters RM, Helterbrand J, Utterback BG, et al. Prognostic value of protein C concentrations in neutropenic patients at high risk of severe septic concentrations. *Crit Care Med.* 2000;28:2209–2216.
24. Nutritional Needs of the Preterm Infant. Oak Brook, Ill. The American Academy of Pediatrics. 5th edition. 2004:44.
25. Kerner JA. Fat requirements. In: Kerner JA, ed. *Manual of Pediatric Parenteral Nutrition.* New York, NY: John Wiley & Sons; 1983:103–127.
26. Kelly DG. Assessment of malabsorption: A tutorial. In: Shils ME, Olsen JA, Shike M, Ross CA, eds. *Modern Nutrition in Health and Disease.* 9th ed. Philadelphia, Pa: Lippincott, Williams Wilkins; 1999:1091–1097.
27. Proujansky R. Protracted diarrhea. In: Wyllie R, Hyams JS, Eds. *Pediatric Gastrointestinal Disease.* Philadelphia, Pa: WB Saunders Company; 1999:288–297.
28. Finberg L. Rickets. *EMedicine.* 2003. Available at: http://www.emedicine.com/ped/topic2014.htm. Accessed June 25, 2005.

Chapter 8

Dietary Reference Intakes in Pediatric Care

Virginia A. Stallings

INTRODUCTION

The Dietary Reference Intakes (DRI) are a series of reports[1–8] that were published between 1997 and 2004; they replaced the periodically revised Recommended Dietary Allowances (RDA) last issued in 1989.[9] DRI reports were developed by panels of food, nutrition, and health experts (Figure 8-1), reviewed by an independent group, and published by the Food and Nutrition Board, Institute of Medicine of the National Academies. The DRI, now jointly endorsed by Canada and the United States, significantly extend the scope of the previous dietary nutrient guidelines. The DRI are quantitative best estimates of nutrient and some nonnutrient intakes used by health care professionals and other groups for assessing and planning the diets of healthy infants, children, and adults. The DRI are used as the starting point from which to modify nutrient intake recommendations for patients with illnesses that affect absorption, storage, metabolism, or excretion of 1 or more nutrients. Nutrient intake information must then be translated into a therapeutic food plan. The DRI are designed for healthy people, consuming typical food orally. They are not appropriate for estimating the nutrient requirements of individuals requiring intravenous nutrition support.

Dietary Reference Intakes

Conceptually, the DRI are different from the RDA in three ways (Table 8-1). First, each nutrient intake value was previously based upon preventing signs of a nutritional deficiency disease. DRI values, where the evidence exists, are based on the concept of preventing chronic degenerative disease, as well as preventing deficiency. Second, the concept of a nutrient value for the maximum or upper level of intake, where evidence exists, was established to reduce the risk of adverse health effects of excessive intake of a nutrient from any source—food, supplementation, or fortification. Third, the DRI system allows evaluation of food components that have health benefits, yet do not meet the usual definition of an essential nutrient. Dietary fiber is one example; adequate data exists and a reference intake was established.

The DRI approach to assessing the dietary intake of individuals or groups of people requires the understanding of a set of four nutrient-based reference values, shown in Table 8-2 and Figure 8-2. If there is sufficient evidence, then a nutrient has an Estimated Average Requirement (EAR)—the average daily intake that meets the requirement of half the healthy individuals. With this information, the RDA is a calculated value designed to meet the nutrient requirements of nearly all (97–98%) of the healthy individuals. If there are inadequate data to calculate the EAR (and therefore the RDA), then an Adequate Intake (AI) is established based on more limited information. The AI comes from a variety of sources, such as observed or experimental approximations of nutrient intake by a group of

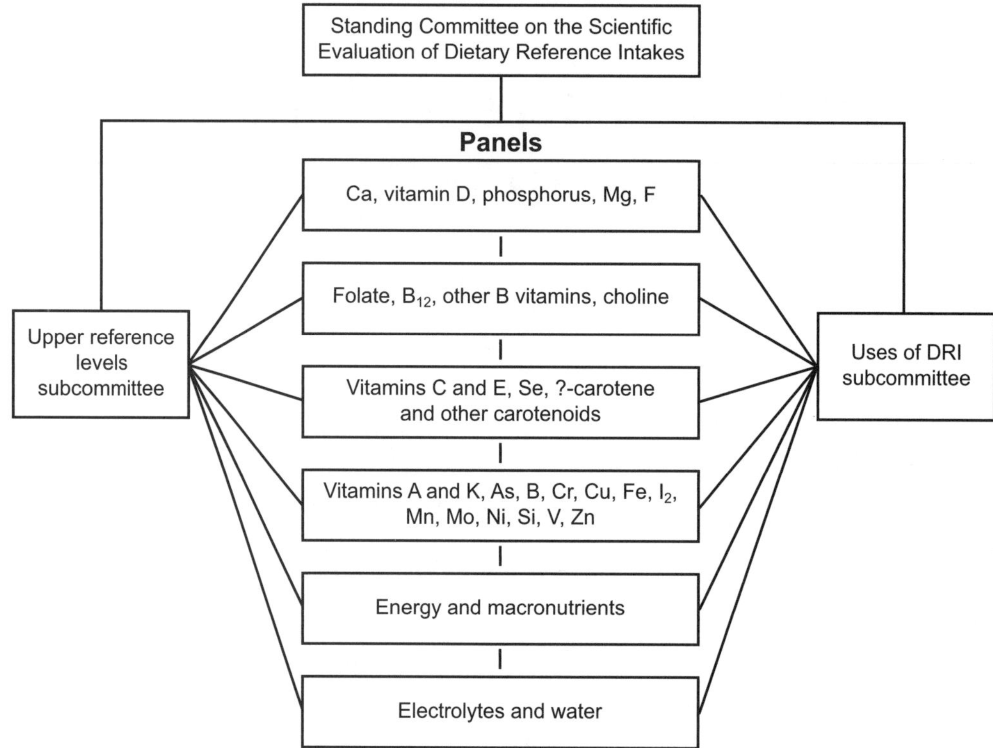

Figure 8-1 Dietary reference intakes project structure. *Source:* Institute of Medicine. *Dietary Reference Intakes: Applications in Dietary Assessment.* Washington, DC: National Academies Press; 2000. Reprinted with permission.

Table 8-1 New concepts underlying the DRI.

- Where specific data on safety and a role in health exist, reduction in the risk of chronic degenerative disease or developmental abnormality, rather than just the absence of signs of deficiency, is included in the formulation of the recommendations.
- The concepts of probability and risk explicitly underpin the determination of the estimated average requirement (EAR), RDA, and tolerable upper intake level (UL) and inform their application in assessment and planning.
- ULs are established where data exist regarding risk of adverse health effects.
- Compounds found naturally in food that may not meet the traditional concept of a nutrient but have potential risk or possible benefit to health are reviewed, and if sufficient data exist, reference intakes are established.

Source: Institute of Medicine. *Dietary Reference Intakes: Applications in Dietary Assessment.* Washington, DC: National Academies Press; 2000. Reprinted with permission.

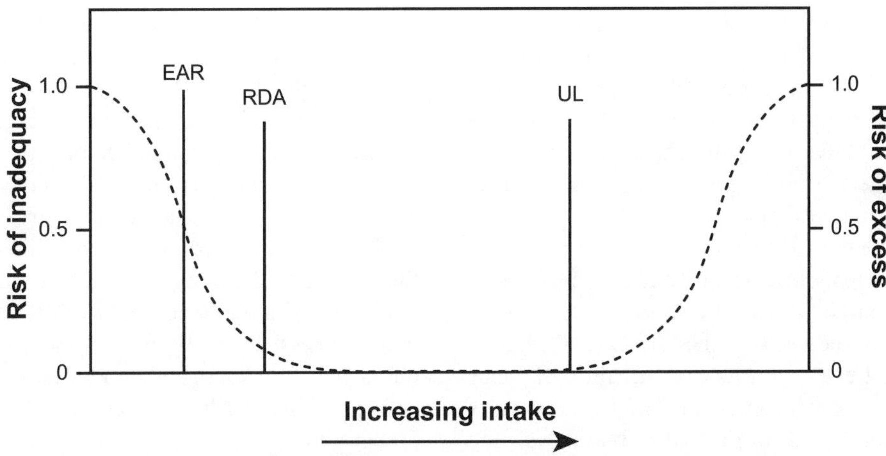

Figure 8-2. Dietary reference intakes. This figure shows that the estimated average requirement (EAR) is the intake at which the risk of adequacy is 0.5 (50%) to an individual. The recommended dietary allowance (RDA) is the intake at which the risk of inadequacy is very small—only 0.02 to 0.03 (2 to 3%).

The adequate intake (AI) does not bear a consistent relationship to the EAR or the RDA because it is set without being able to estimate the requirement. At intakes between the RDA and the tolerable upper intake level (UL), the risks of inadequacy and of excess are both close to 0. At intakes above the UL, the risk of adverse effects increases. *Source:* Institute of Medicine. *Dietary Reference Intakes: Applications in Dietary Assessment.* Washington, DC: National Academies Press; 2000. Reprinted with permission.

Table 8-2 New dietary reference intake definitions.

Estimated Average Requirement (EAR): The average daily nutrient intake level estimated to meet the requirement of half the healthy individuals in a particular life stage and gender group.

Recommended Dietary Allowance (RDA): The average daily nutrient intake level sufficient to meet the nutrient requirement of nearly all (97 to 98 percent healthy individuals in a particular life stage and gender group).

Adequate Intake (AI): A recommended average daily nutrient intake level based on observed or experimentally determined approximations or estimates of nutrient intake by a group (or groups) of apparently healthy people that are assumed to be adequate—used when an RDA cannot be determined.

Tolerable Upper Intake Level (UL): The highest average daily nutrient intake level likely to pose no risk of adverse health effects to almost all individuals in the general population. As intake increases above the UL, the potential risk of adverse effects increases.

Source: Institute of Medicine. *Dietary Reference Intakes: Applications in Dietary Assessment.* Washington, DC: National Academies Press; 2000. Reprinted with permission.

apparently healthy people. The Tolerable Upper Intake Level (UL) is a new concept in the field of nutrient recommendations. The UL is the highest average daily nutrient intake level likely to pose no risk of adverse health effects for almost all healthy people in the general population. Based on evidence available, an intake above the UL has a potential health risk.

Food supply fortification and nutrient supplement use trends of the North American population led to the need for the UL. Over the years, increased use of nutrient fortification of foods has been well documented. The best known is iodination of salt to prevent iodine deficiency diseases and the fluoridation of water to reduce dental caries. Recently in the United States, fortification of bread flour with folate was instituted with an aim to increase the folate consumption in women of childbearing age and thus decrease the incidence of neural tube defects. In North America, much of the food supply is processed, and processed food provides the opportunity for effective fortification. A study of the US food supply evaluated 246 fortified foods found in grocery stores.[10] A large portion was consumed by children 1 to 10 years of age. Of these, 70–80% consumed foods fortified with iron, folate, thiamin, and vitamins A and C. In Germany, a similar study showed children ages 2 to 14 consumed more than 400 different fortified food products.[11] The fortified products most commonly consumed by children are vitamin and mineral fortified breakfast cereal and fruit juices. In addition, infants, children, and adolescents often take daily multivitamin and mineral supplements. Such products designed and marketed for children birth to 4 years of age are regulated by the US Food and Drug Administration (FDA). There are no regulations for combination or single vitamin or mineral products for other age groups. Given this pattern of fortified food and supplement consumption, the UL should be incorporated into clinical care for children. Practitioners can use this method to evaluate typical daily nutrient intake from fresh food, processed food with fortification and enrichment, and vitamin and mineral supplements; and recommend reduced intake when indicated (Table 8-3).

The DRI are presented by age, gender, and physiological status (pregnancy, lactation for younger and older females), reflecting the impact of these factors on nutrient requirements (Table 8-4). For pediatric health care, this approach is essential, because nutrient needs are highly influenced by age and gender-specific pattern of growth (velocity, size) and development (body composition and pubertal development) changes. The assumed normal body weight, length/height, and body mass index (BMI) for infants, children, and young adults used for the DRI are shown in Table 8-5.

In clinical practice, DRI are used to assess the dietary intake of individual patients, and in research settings, they are used to assess individuals or groups of subjects. It is essential that dietary intake and the related DRI comparisons be used in conjunction with the medical history, physical exam, biochemical values, and anthropometric measurements to determine the

Table 8-3 Qualitative interpretation of intakes relative to the tolerable upper intake level (UL).

Intake relative to the UL	*Suggested qualitative interpretation*
Greater than or equal to the UL	Potential risk of adverse effects if observed over a large number of days
Less than the UL	Intake is likely safe if observed over a large number of days

Source: Institute of Medicine. *Dietary Reference Intakes: Applications in Dietary Assessment.* Washington, DC: National Academies Press; 2000. Reprinted with permission.

Table 8-4 The life stage groups for which nutrient recommendations are given.

Life Stage Groups			
Infants	*Males*	*Females*	*Pregnancy*
0–6 mo	9–13 y	9–13 y	< 18 y
7–12 mo	14–18 y	14–18 y	19–30 y
	19–30 y	19–30 y	31–50 y
Children	31–50 y	31–50 y	
1–3 y	51–70 y	51–70 y	*Lactation*
4–8 y	> 70 y	> 70 y	< 18 y
			19–30 y
			31–50 y

Note: Differences in DRI are indicated by gender when warranted by the data.

Source: Institute of Medicine. *Dietary Reference Intakes: Applications in Dietary Assessment.* Washington, DC: National Academies Press; 2000. Reprinted with permission.

Table 8-5 New reference heights and weights for children and adults in the United States.

Sex	*Age*	*Previous median body mass index (BMI) (kg/m²)*	*New median BMI (kg/m²)*	*New median reference height* cm (in)*	*New reference weight† kg (lb)*
Male, Female	2–6 mo	-	-	62 (24)	6 (13)
	7–12 mo	-	-	71 (28)	9 (20)
	1–3 y	-	-	86 (340	12 (27)
	4–8 y	15.8	15.3	115 (45)	20 (44)
	9–13 y	18.5	17.2	144 (57)	36 (79)
	14–18 y	21.3	20.5	174 (68)	61 (134)
	19–30 y	24.4	22.5	177 (70)	70 (154)
Female	9–13 y	18.3	17.4	144 (57)	37 (81)
	14–18 y	21.3	20.4	163 (64)	54 (119)
	19–30 y	22.8	21.5	163 (64)	57 (126)

* Calculated from body mass index and height for ages 4 through 8 y and older.

†*Source:* Institute of Medicine. *Dietary Reference Intakes: Applications in Dietary Assessment.* Washington, DC: National Academies Press; 2000. Reprinted with permission.

individual child's overall nutritional status and nutritional risk. Table 8-6 explains the approach to evaluating the diet of an individual or group using the EAR, RDA, AI, and UL for the DRI. Tables 8-7 to 8-12 are a summary of the DRI recommended energy, macronutrients, vitamin, mineral, and element intakes for individuals by age, gender, and physiological state. The EAR are summarized in Table 8-8 and the UL values are summarized in Tables 8-13 and 8-14.

Table 8-6 Uses of dietary reference intakes for dietary assessment of healthy individuals and groups.

Types of use	*For an individual**	*For a group†*
Assessment	EAR: use to examine the probability that usual intake is adequate (if individual's usual intake is at the EAR, then 50% probability that intake is inadequate).	EAR: use to estimate the prevalence of inadequate intakes within a group (percent in a group whose intakes are inadequate).
	RDA: usual intake at or above this level has a low probability of inadequacy.	RDA: cannot use to assess intakes of groups.
	AI‡: usual intake at or above this level has a low probability of inadequacy.	AI‡: mean usual intake at or above this level implies a low prevalence of inadequate intakes.
	UL: usual intake above this level may place an individual at risk of adverse effects for excessive nutrient intake.	UL: use to estimate the percentage of the population at potential risk of adverse effects from excessive nutrient intake.
Planning	RDA: aim for this intake.	RDA: use to plan an intake distribution with a low prevalence of inadequate intakes.
	AI‡: aim for this intake.	AI‡: use to plan mean intakes.
	UL: use as a guide to limit intake; chronic intake of higher amounts may increase the potential adverse effects.	UL: use to plan intake distributions with a low prevalence of intakes potentially at risk of adverse effects.

RDA = recommended dietary allowance
EAR = estimated average requirement
AI = aequate intake
UL = tolerable upper level

* Evaluation of true status requires clinical, biochemical, and anthropometric data.

† Requires statistically valid approximation of distribution of usual intakes.

‡ For the nutrients in this report, AIs are set for all age groups for water, potassium and sodium (and chloride on an equimolar basis to sodium). The AI may be used as a guide for infants as it reflects the average intake from human milk. Infants consuming formulas with the same nutrient composition as human milk are consuming an adequate amount after adjustments are made for differences in bioavailability. In the context of assessing groups, when the AI for a nutrient is not based on mean intakes of a healthy population, this assessment is made with less confidence.

In the case of energy, an estimated energy requirement (EER) is provided; it is the dietary energy intake that is predicted (with variance) to maintain energy balance in a healthy adult of defined age, gender, weight, height, and level of physical activity, consistent with good health. In children and pregnant and lactating women, the EER is taken to include the needs associated with the deposition of tissues or the secretion of milk at rates consistent with good health.

For individuals, the EER represents the midpoint of a range within which an individual's energy requirements are likely to vary. As such, it is below the needs of half the individuals with specified characteristics, and exceeds the needs of the other half. Body weight should be monitored and energy intake adjusted accordingly.

Source: Institute of Medicine. *Dietary Reference Intakes: Applications in Dietary Assessment.* Washington, DC: National Academies Press; 2000. Reprinted with permission.

Table 8-7 Dietary reference intakes (DRI): estimated energy requirements (EER) for men and women 30 years of age.*

				EER, men§ (kcal/day)		*EER, women§ (kcal/day)*	
Height (m [in])	*PAL†*	*Weight for BMI‡ of 18.5 kg/m²(kg [lb])*	*Weight for BMI of 24.99 kg/m² (kg [lb])*	*BMI of 18.5 kg/m²*	*BMI of 24.99 kg/m²*	*BMI of 18.5 kg/m²*	*BMI of 24.99 kg/m²*
1.50 (59)	Sedentary	41.6 (92)	56.2 (124)	1,848	2,080	1,625	1,762
	Low active			2,009	2,267	1,803	1,956
	Active			2,215	2,506	2,025	2,198
	Very active			2,554	2,898	2,291	2,489
1.65 (65)	Sedentary	50.4 (111)	68.0 (150)	2,068	2,349	1,816	1,982
	Low active			2,254	2,566	2,016	2,202
	Active			2,490	2,842	2,267	2,477
	Very active			2,880	3,296	2,567	2,807
1.80 (71)	Sedentary	59.9 (132)	81.0 (178)	2,301	2,635	2,015	2,211
	Low active			2,513	2,884	2,239	2,459
	Active			2,782	3,200	2,519	2,769
	Very active			3,225	3,720	2,855	3,141

* For each year below 30, add 7 kcal/day for women and 10 kcal/day for men. For each year above 30, subtract 7 kcal/day for women and 10 kcal/day for men.

† PAL = physical activity level.

‡ BMI = body mass index.

§ Derived from the following regression equations based on doubly labeled water data:

Adult man: EER = 662 – 9.53 × age (y) + PA × (15.91 × wt [kg] + 539.6 × ht [m])

Adult woman: EER = 354 – 6.91 × age (y) + PA × (9.36 × wt [kg] + 726 × ht [m])

Where PA refers to coefficient for PAL

PAL = total energy expenditure ÷ basal energy expenditure

PA = 1.0 if PAL ≥ 1.0 < 1.4 (sedentary)

PA = 1.12 if PAL ≥ 1.4 < 1.6 (low active)

PA = 1.27 if PAL ≥ 1.6 < 1.9 (active)

PA = 1.45 if PAL ≥ 1.9 < 2.5 (very active)

Source: Institute of Medicine. *Dietary Reference Intakes: Applications in Dietary Assessment.* Washington, DC: National Academies Press; 2000. Reprinted with permission.

Table 8-8 Dietary reference intakes (DRI): acceptable macronutrient distribution ranges.

	Range (percent of energy)		
Macronutrient	*Children, 1–3 y*	*Children, 4–18 y*	*Adults*
Fat	30–40	25–35	20–35
n-6 polyunsaturated fatty acids* (linoleic acid)	5–10	5–10	5–10
n-3 polyunsaturated fatty acids* (α-linolenic acid)	0.6–1.2	0.6–1.2	0.6–1.2
Carbohydrate	45–65	45–65	45–65
Protein	5–20	10–30	10–35

* Approximately 10% of the total can come from longer-chain *n*-3 or *n*-6 fatty acids.

Sources: Institute of Medicine. *Dietary Reference Intakes for Energy, Carbohydrates, Fiber, Fat, Fatty Acids, Cholesterol, Protein and Amino Acids.* Washington, DC: National Academies Press; 2002/2005. Reprinted with permission.

Table 8-9 Dietary reference intakes (DRI): recommended intakes for individuals, macronutrients.

Life stage group	*Total water† (L/d)*	*Carbohydrate (g/d)*	*Total fiber (g/d)*	*Fat (g/d)*	*Linoleic acid (g/d)*	*α-linolenic acid (g/d)*	*Protein‡ (g/d)*
Infants							
0–6 mo	0.7*	60*	ND	31*	4.4*	0.5*	9.1*
7–12 mo	0.8*	95*	ND	30*	4.6*	0.5*	**13.5**
Children							
1–3 y	1.3*	**130**	19*	ND	7*	0.7*	**13**
4–8 y	1.7*	**130**	25*	ND	10*	0.9*	**19**
Males							
9–13 y	2.4*	**130**	26*	ND	12*	1.2*	**34**
14–18 y	3.3*	**130**	38*	ND	16*	1.6*	**52**
19–30 y	3.7*	**130**	38*	ND	17*	1.6*	**56**
31–50 y	3.7*	**130**	38*	ND	17*	1.6*	**56**
51–70 y	3.7*	**130**	30*	ND	14*	1.6*	**56**
> 70 y	3.7*	**130**	30*	ND	14*	1.6*	**56**
Females							
9–13 y	2.1*	**130**	31*	ND	10*	1.0*	**34**
14–18 y	2.3*	**130**	26*	ND	11*	1.1*	**46**
19–30 y	2.7*	**130**	25*	ND	12*	1.1*	**46**

Table 8-9 continued

Life stage group	*Total water† (L/d)*	*Carbohydrate (g/d)*	*Total fiber (g/d)*	*Fat (g/d)*	*Linoleic acid (g/d)*	*α-linolenic acid (g/d)*	*Protein‡ (g/d)*
Females							
31–50 y	2.7*	**130**	25*	ND	12*	1.1*	**46**
51–70 y	2.7*	**130**	21*	ND	11*	1.1*	**46**
> 70 y	2.7*	**130**	21*	ND	11*	1.1*	**46**
Pregnancy							
14–18 y	3.0*	**175**	28*	ND	13*	1.4*	**71**
19–30 y	3.0*	**175**	28*	ND	13*	1.4*	**71**
31–50 y	3.0*	**175**	28*	ND	13*	1.4*	**71**
Lactation							
14–18 y	3.8*	**210**	29*	ND	13*	1.3*	**71**
19–30 y	3.8*	**210**	29*	ND	13*	1.3*	**71**
31–50 y	3.8*	**210**	29*	ND	13*	1.3*	**71**

Note: This table presents recommended dietary allowances (RDAs) in bold type and adequate intakes (AIs) in ordinary type followed by an asterisk (*). RDAs and AIs may both be used as goals for individual intake. RDAs are set to meet the needs of almost all (97–98%) individuals in a group. For healthy infants fed human milk, the AI is the mean intake. The AI for other life stage and gender groups is believed to cover the needs of all individuals in the group, but lack of data or uncertainty in the data prevent being able to specify with confidence the percentage of individuals covered by this intake.

† Total water includes all water contained in food, beverages, and drinking water.

‡ Based on 0.8 g/kg body weight for the reference body weight.

ND = Not determinable due to lack of data of adverse effects in this age group and concern with regard to lack of ability to handle excess amounts. Source of intake should be from food only to prevent high levels of intake.

Source: Institute of Medicine. *Dietary Reference Intakes: Applications in Dietary Assessment.* Washington, DC: National Academies Press; 2000. Reprinted with permission.

Table 8-10 Dietary reference intakes (DRI): additional macronutrient recommendations.

Macronutrient	*Recommendation*
Dietary cholesterol	As low as possible while consuming a nutritionally adequate diet.
Trans fatty acids	As low as possible while consuming a nutritionally adequate diet.
Saturated fatty acids	As low as possible while consuming a nutritionally adequate diet.
Added sugars	Limit to no more than 25% of total energy.

Sources: Institute of Medicine. *Dietary Reference Intakes for Energy, Carbohydrates, Fiber, Fat, Fatty Acids, Cholesterol, Protein and Amino Acids.* Washington, DC: National Academies Press; 2002/2005. Reprinted with permission.

Table 8-11 Dietary reference intakes (DRI): recommended intakes for individuals, vitamins.

Life stage group	*Vit A (μg/d)†*	*Vit C (mg/d)*	*Vit D (μg/d)‡,§*	*Vit E (mg/d)‖*	*Vit K (μg/d)*	*Thiamin (mg/d)*	*Ribo-flavin (mg/d)*	*Niacin (mg/d)¶*	*Vit B_6 (mg/d)*	*Folate (μg/d)#*	*Vit B_{12} (μg/d)*	*Pantothenic Acid (mg/d)*	*Biotin (μg/d)*	*Choline** (mg/d)*
Infants														
0–6 mo	400*	40*	5*	4*	2.0*	0.2*	0.3*	2*	0.1*	65*	0.4*	1.7*	5*	125*
7–12 mo	500*	50*	5*	5*	2.5*	0.3*	0.4*	4*	0.3*	80*	0.5*	1.8*	6*	150*
Children														
1–3 y	**300**	**15**	5*	**6**	30*	**0.5**	**0.5**	**6**	**0.5**	**150**	**0.9**	2*	8*	200*
4–8 y	**400**	**25**	5*	**7**	55*	**0.6**	**0.6**	**8**	**0.6**	**200**	**1.2**	3*	12*	250*
Males														
9–13 y	**600**	**45**	5*	**11**	60*	**0.9**	**0.9**	**12**	**1.0**	**300**	**1.8**	4*	20*	375*
14–18 y	**900**	**75**	5*	**15**	75*	**1.2**	**1.3**	**16**	**1.3**	**400**	**2.4**	5*	25*	550*
19–30 y	**900**	**90**	5*	**15**	120*	**1.2**	**1.3**	**16**	**1.3**	**400**	**2.4**	5*	30*	550*
31–50 y	**900**	**90**	5*	**15**	120*	**1.2**	**1.3**	**16**	**1.3**	**400**	**2.4**	5*	30*	550*
51–70 y	**900**	**90**	10*	**15**	120*	**1.2**	**1.3**	**16**	**1.7**	**400**	**2.4††**	5*	30*	550*
> 70 y	**900**	**90**	15*	**15**	120*	**1.2**	**1.3**	**16**	**1.7**	**400**	**2.4††**	5*	30*	550*
Females														
9–13 y	**600**	**45**	5*	**11**	60*	**0.9**	**0.9**	**12**	**1.0**	**300**	**1.8**	4*	20*	375*
14–18 y	**700**	**65**	5*	**15**	75*	**1.0**	**1.0**	**14**	**1.2**	**400††**	**2.4**	5*	25*	400*
19–30 y	**700**	**75**	5*	**15**	90*	**1.1**	**1.1**	**14**	**1.3**	**400††**	**2.4**	5*	30*	425*
31–50 y	**700**	**75**		**15**	90*	**1.1**	**1.1**	**14**	**1.3**	**400††**	**2.4**	5*	30*	425*
51–70 y	**700**	**75**	10*	**15**	90*	**1.1**	**1.1**	**14**	**1.5**	**400**	**2.4‡‡**	5*	30*	425*
> 70 y	**700**	**75**	15*	**15**	90*	**1.1**	**1.1**	**14**	**1.5**	**400**	**2.4‡‡**	5*	30*	425*
Pregnancy														
14–18 y	**750**	**80**	5*	**15**	75*	**1.4**	**1.4**	**18**	**1.9**	**600§§**	**2.6**	6*	30*	450*
19–30 y	**770**	**85**	5*	**15**	90*	**1.4**	**1.4**	**18**	**1.9**	**600§§**	**2.6**	6*	30*	450*
31–50 y	**770**	**85**	5*	**15**	90*	**1.4**	**1.4**	**18**	**1.9**	**600§§**	**2.6**	6*	30*	450*

Table 8-11 continued

Life stage group	*Vit A (µg/d)†*	*Vit C (mg/d)*	*Vit D (µg/d)‡,§*	*Vit E (mg/d)‖*	*Vit K (µg/d)*	*Thiamin (mg/d)*	*Ribo-flavin (mg/d)*	*Niacin (mg/d)¶*	*Vit B_6 (mg/d)*	*Folate (µg/d)#*	*Vit B_{12} (µg/d)*	*Pantothenic Acid (mg/d)*	*Biotin (µg/d)*	*Choline** (mg/d)*
Lactation														
14–18 y	**1,200**	**115**	5*	**19**	75*	**1.4**	**1.6**	**17**	**2.0**	**500**	**2.8**	7*	35*	550*
19–30 y	**1,300**	**120**	5*	**19**	90*	**1.4**	**1.6**	**17**	**2.0**	**500**	**2.8**	7*	35*	550*
31–50 y	**1,300**	**120**	5*	**19**	90*	**1.4**	**1.6**	**17**	**2.0**	**500**	**2.8**	7*	35*	550*

Note: This table presents recommended dietary allowances (RDAs) in bold type and adequate intakes (AIs) in ordinary type followed by an asterisk (*). RDAs and AIs may both be used as goals for individual intake. RDAs are set to meet the needs of almost all (97–98%) individuals in a group. For healthy breastfed infants, the AI is the mean intake. The AI for other life stage and gender groups is believed to cover needs of all individuals in the group, but lack of data or uncertainty in the data prevent being able to specify with confidence the percentage of individuals covered by this intake.

† As retinol activity equivalents (RAEs). 1 RAE = 1 µg retinol, 12 µg β-carotene, 24 µg α-carotene, or 24 µg β-cryptoxanthin. The RAE for dietary provitamin A carotenoids is twofold greater than retinol equivalents (RE), whereas the RAE for preformed vitamin A is the same as RE.

‡ As cholecalciferol. 1 µg cholecalciferol = 40 IU vitamin D.

§ In the absence of adequate exposure to sunlight.

‖ As α-tocopherol. α-tocopherol includes RRR-α-tocopherol, the only form of α-tocopherol that occurs naturally in foods, and the 2R-stereoisomeric forms of α-tocopherol (RRR-, RSR-, RRS-, and RSS-α-tocopherol) that occur in fortified foods and supplements. It does not include the 2S-stereoisomeric forms of α-tocopherol (SRR-, SSR-, SRS-, and SSS-α-tocopherol); also found in fortified foods and supplements.

¶ As niacin equivalents (NE). 1 mg of niacin = 60 mg of tryptophan; 0–6 months = preformed niacin (not NE).

As dietary folate equivalents (DFE). 1 DFE = 1 µg food folate = 0.6 µg of folic acid from fortified food or as a supplement consumed with food = 0.5 µg of a supplement taken on an empty stomach.

** Although AIs have been set for choline, there are few data to assess whether a dietary supply of choline is needed at all stages of the life cycle, and it may be that the choline requirement can be met by endogenous synthesis at some of these stages.

‡‡ In view of evidence linking folate intake with neural tube defects in the fetus, it is recommended that all women capable of becoming pregnant consume 400 µg from supplements or fortified foods in addition to intake of food folate from a varied diet.

†† Because 10–30% of older people may malabsorb food-bound B_{12}, it is advisable for those older than 50 years to meet their RDA mainly by consuming foods fortified with B_{12} or a supplement containing B_{12}.

§§ It is assumed that women will continue consuming 400 µg from supplements or fortified food until their pregnancy is confirmed and they enter prenatal care, which ordinarily occurs after the end of the periconceptional period—the critical time for formation of the neural tube.

Source: Institute of Medicine. *Dietary Reference Intakes: Applications in Dietary Assessment.* Washington, DC: National Academies Press; 2000. Reprinted with permission.

Table 8-12 Dietary reference intakes (DRI): recommended intakes for individuals, elements.

Life stage group	*Calcium (mg/d)*	*Chromium (μg/d)*	*Copper (μg/d)*	*Fluoride (mg/d)*	*Iodine (μg/d)*	*Iron (mg/d)*	*Magnesium (mg/d)*	*Manganese (mg/d)*	*Molybdenum (μg/d)*	*Phosphorus (mg/d)*	*Selenium (μg/d)*	*Zinc (mg/d)*	*Potassium (g/d)*	*Sodium (g/d)*	*Chloride (g/d)*
Infants															
0–6 mo	210*	0.2*	200*	0.01*	110*	0.27*	30*	0.003*	2*	100*	15*	2*	0.4*	0.12*	0.18*
7–12 mo	270*	5.5*	220*	0.5*	130*	**11**	75*	0.6*	3*	275*	20*	**3**	0.7*	0.37*	0.57*
Children															
1–3 y	500*	11*	**340**	0.7*	**90**	**7**	**80**	1.2*	**17**	**460**	**20**	**3**	3.0*	1.0*	1.5*
4–8 y	800*	15*	**440**	1*	**90**	**10**	**130**	1.5*	**22**	**500**	**30**	**5**	3.8*	1.2*	1.9*
Males															
9–13 y	1,300*	25*	**700**	2*	**120**	**8**	**240**	1.9*	**34**	**1,250**	**40**	**8**	4.5*	1.5*	2.3*
14–18 y	1,300*	35*	**890**	3*	**150**	**11**	**410**	2.2*	**43**	**1,250**	**55**	**11**	4.7*	1.5*	2.3*
19–30 y	1,000*	35*	**900**	4*	**150**	**8**	**400**	2.3*	**45**	**700**	**55**	**11**	4.7*	1.5*	2.3*
31–50 y	1,000*	35*	**900**	4*	**150**	**8**	**420**	2.3*	**45**	**700**	**55**	**11**	4.7*	1.5*	2.3*
51–70 y	1,200*	30*	**900**	4*	**150**	**8**	**420**	2.3*	**45**	**700**	**55**	**11**	4.7*	1.3*	2.0*
> 70 y	1,200*	30*	**900**	4*	**150**	**8**	**420**	2.3*	**45**	**700**	**55**	**11**	4.7*	1.2*	1.8*
Females															
9–13 y	1,300*	21*	**700**	2*	**120**	**8**	**240**	1.6*	**34**	**1,250**	**40**	**8**	4.5*	1.5*	2.3*
14–18 y	1,300*	24*	**890**	3*	**150**	**15**	**360**	1.6*	**43**	**1,250**	**55**	**9**	4.7*	1.5*	2.3*
19–30 y	1,000*	25*	**900**	3*	**150**	**18**	**310**	1.8*	**45**	**700**	**55**	**8**	4.7*	1.5*	2.3*
31–50 y	1,000*	25*	**900**	3*	**150**	**18**	**320**	1.8*	**45**	**700**	**55**	**8**	4.7*	1.5*	2.3*
51–70 y	1,200*	20*	**900**	3*	**150**	**8**	**320**	1.8*	**45**	**700**	**55**	**8**	4.7*	1.3*	2.0*
> 70 y	1,200*	20*	**900**	3*	**150**	**8**	**320**	1.8*	**45**	**700**	**55**	**8**	4.7*	1.2*	1.8*
Pregnancy															
14–18 y	1,300*	29*	**1,000**	3*	**220**	**27**	**400**	2.0*	**50**	**1,250**	**60**	**13**	4.7*	1.5*	2.3*
19–30 y	1,000*	30*	**1,000**	3*	**220**	**27**	**350**	2.0*	**50**	**700**	**60**	**11**	4.7*	1.5*	2.3*
31–50 y	1,000*	30*	**1,000**	3*	**220**	**27**	**360**	2.0*	**50**	**700**	**60**	**11**	4.7*	1.5*	2.3*

Table 8-12 continued

Life stage group	*Calcium (mg/d)*	*Chromium (µg/d)*	*Copper (µg/d)*	*Fluoride (mg/d)*	*Iodine (µg/d)*	*Iron (mg/d)*	*Magnesium (mg/d)*	*Manganese (mg/d)*	*Molybdenum (µg/d)*	*Phosphorus (mg/d)*	*Selenium (µg/d)*	*Zinc (mg/d)*	*Potassium (g/d)*	*Sodium (g/d)*	*Chloride (g/d)*
Lactation															
14–18 y	1,300*	44*	**1,300**	3*	**290**	**10**	**360**	2.6*	**50**	**1,250**	**70**	**14**	5.1*	1.5*	2.3*
19–30 y	1,000*	45*	**1,300**	3*	**290**	**9**	**310**	2.6*	**50**	**700**	**70**	**12**	5.1*	1.5*	2.3*
31–50 y	1,000*	45*	**1,300**	3*	**290**	**9**	**320**	2.6*	**50**	**700**	**70**	**12**	5.1*	1.5*	2.3*

Note: This table presents recommended dietary allowances (RDAs) in bold type and adequate intakes (AIs) in ordinary type followed by an asterisk (*). RDAs and AIs may both be used as goals for individual intake. RDAs are set to meet the needs of almost all (97–98%) individuals in a group. For healthy breastfed infants, the AI is the mean intake. The AI for other life stage and gender groups is believed to cover needs of all individuals in the group, but lack of data or uncertainty in the data prevent being able to specify with confidence the percentage of individuals covered by this intake.

Sources: Institute of Medicine. *Dietary Reference Intakes for Calcium, Phosphorous, Magnesium, Vitamin D, and Fluoride.* Washington, DC: National Academies Press; 1997. Institute of Medicine. *Dietary Reference Intakes for Thiamin, Riboflavin, Niacin, Vitamin B_6, Folate, Vitamin B_{12}, Pantothenic Acid, Biotin, and Choline.* Washington, DC: National Academies Press; 1998. Institute of Medicine. *Dietary Reference Intakes for Vitamin C, Vitamin E, Selenium, and Carotenoids.* Washington, DC: National Academies Press; 2000. Institute of Medicine. *Dietary Reference Intakes for Vitamin A, Vitamin K, Arsenic, Boron, Chromium, Copper, Iodine, Iron, Manganese, Molybdenum, Nickel, Silicon, Vanadium, and Zinc.* Washington, DC: National Academies Press; 2001. Institute of Medicine. *Dietary Reference Intakes for Water, Potassium, Sodium, Chloride, and Sulfate.* Washington, DC: National Academies Press; 2004. Institute of Medicine. *Dietary Reference Intakes: Applications in Dietary Assessment.* Washington, DC: National Academies Press; 2000. Reprinted with permission.

Table 8-13 Dietary reference intakes (DRI): tolerable upper intake levels (UL*), vitamins.

Life stage group	*Vitamin A (µg/d)†*	*Vitamin C (mg/d)*	*Vitamin D (µg/d)*	*Vitamin E (mg/d)‡,§*	*Vitamin K*	*Thiamin*	*Riboflavin*	*Niacin (mg/d)§*	*Vitamin B_6 (mg/d)*	*Folate (µg/d)§*	*Vitamin B_{12}*	*Pantothenic acid*	*Biotin*	*Choline (g/d)*	*Carotenoids‖*
Infants															
0–6 mo	600	ND	25	ND	ND	ND	ND	ND	ND	ND	ND	ND	ND	ND	ND
7–12 mo	600	ND	25	ND	ND	ND	ND	ND	ND	ND	ND	ND	ND	ND	ND
Children															
1–3 y	600	400	50	200	ND	ND	ND	10	30	300	ND	ND	ND	1.0	ND
4–8 y	900	650	50	300	ND	ND	ND	15	40	400	ND	ND	ND	1.0	ND
Males, Females															
9–13 y	1,700	1,200	50	600	ND	ND	ND	20	60	600	ND	ND	ND	2.0	ND
14–18 y	2,800	1,800	50	800	ND	ND	ND	30	80	800	ND	ND	ND	3.0	ND
19–70 y	3,000	2,000	50	1,000	ND	ND	ND	35	100	1,000	ND	ND	ND	3.5	ND
> 70 y	3,000	2,000	50	1,000	ND	ND	ND	35	100	1,000	ND	ND	ND	3.5	ND
Pregnancy															
14–18 y	2,800	1,800	50	800	ND	ND	ND	30	80	800	ND	ND	ND	3.0	ND
19–50 y	3,000	2,000	50	1,000	ND	ND	ND	35	100	1,000	ND	ND	ND	3.5	ND
Lactation															
14–18 y	2,800	1,800	50	800	ND	ND	ND	30	80	800	ND	ND	ND	3.0	ND
19–50 y	3,000	2,000	50	1,000	ND	ND	ND	35	100	1,000	ND	ND	ND	3.5	ND

* UL = The maximum level of daily nutrient intake that is likely to pose no risk of adverse effects. Unless otherwise specified, the UL represents total intake from food, water, and supplements. Due to lack of suitable data, ULs could not be established for vitamin K, thiamin, riboflavin, vitamin B_{12}, pantothenic acid, biotin, or carotenoids. In the absence of ULs, extra caution may be warranted in consuming levels above recommended intakes.

† As preformed vitamin A only.

‡ As α-tocopherol; applies to any form of supplemental α-tocopherol.

§ The ULs for vitamin E, niacin, and folate apply to synthetic forms obtained from supplements, fortified foods, or a combination of the 2.

‖ β-carotene supplements are advised only to serve as a provitamin A source for individuals at risk of vitamin A deficiency.

ND = Not determinable due to lack of data of adverse effects in this age group and concern with regard to lack of ability to handle excess amounts. Source of intake should be from food only to prevent high levels of intake.

Sources: Institute of Medicine. *Dietary Reference Intakes for Calcium, Phosphorous, Magnesium, Vitamin D, and Fluoride.* Washington, DC: National Academies Press; 1997. Institute of Medicine. *Dietary Reference Intakes for Thiamin, Riboflavin, Niacin, Vitamin B6, Folate, Vitamin B12, Pantothenic Acid, Biotin, and Choline.* Washington, DC: National Academies Press; 1998. Institute of Medicine. *Dietary Reference Intakes for Vitamin C, Vitamin E, Selenium, and Carotenoids.* Washington, DC: National Academies Press; 2000. Institute of Medicine. *Dietary Reference Intakes for Vitamin A, Vitamin K, Arsenic, Boron, Chromium, Copper, Iodine, Iron, Manganese, Molybdenum, Nickel, Silicon, Vanadium, and Zinc.* Washington, DC: National Academies Press; 2001. Institute of Medicine. *Dietary Reference Intakes: Applications in Dietary Assessment.* Washington, DC: National Academies Press; 2000. Reprinted with permission.

Table 8-14 Dietary reference intakes (DRI): tolerable upper intake levels (UL*), elements.

Life stage group	*Arsenic†*	*Boron (mg/d)*	*Calcium (g/d)*	*Chromium*	*Copper (μg/d)*	*Fluoride (mg/d)*	*Iodine (μg/d)*	*Iron (mg/d)*	*Magnesium (mg/d)‡*	*Manganese (mg/d)*	*Molybdenum (μg/d)*	*Nickel (mg/d)*	*Phosphorus (g/d)*	*Potassium*	*Selenium (μg/d)*	*Silicon§*	*Sulfate*	*Vanadium (mg/d)‖*	*Zinc (mg/d)*	*Sodium (g/d)*	*Chloride (g/d)*
Infants																					
0–6 mo	ND	ND	ND	ND	ND	0.7	ND	40	ND	ND	ND	ND	ND	ND	45	ND	ND	ND	4	ND	ND
7–12 mo	ND	ND	ND	ND	ND	0.9	ND	40	ND	ND	ND	ND	ND	ND	60	ND	ND	ND	5	ND	ND
Children																					
1–3 y	ND	3	2.5	ND	1,000	1.3	200	40	65	2	300	0.2	3	ND	90	ND	ND	ND	7	1.5	2.3
4–8 y	ND	6	2.5	ND	3,000	2.2	300	40	110	3	600	0.3	3	ND	150	ND	ND	ND	12	1.9	2.9
Males, Females																					
9–13 y	ND	11	2.5	ND	5,000	10	600	40	350	6	1,100	0.6	4	ND	280	ND	ND	ND	23	2.2	3.4
14–18 y	ND	17	2.5	ND	8,000	10	900	45	350	9	1,700	1.0	4	ND	400	ND	ND	ND	34	2.3	3.6
19–70 y	ND	20	2.5	ND	10,000	10	1,100	45	350	11	2,000	1.0	4	ND	400	ND	ND	1.8	40	2.3	3.6
> 70 y	ND	20	2.5	ND	10,000	10	1,100	45	350	11	2,000	1.0	3	ND	400	ND	ND	1.8	40	2.3	3.6
Pregnancy																					
14–18 y	ND	17	2.5	ND	8,000	10	900	45	350	9	1,700	1.0	3.5	ND	400	ND	ND	ND	34	2.3	3.6
19–50 y	ND	20	2.5	ND	10,000	10	1,100	45	350	11	2,000	1.0	3.5	ND	400	ND	ND	ND	40	2.3	3.6
Lactation																					
14–18 y	ND	17	2.5	ND	8,000	10	900	45	350	9	1,700	1.0	4	ND	400	ND	ND	ND	34	2.3	3.6
19–50 y	ND	20	2.5	ND	10,000	10	1,100	45	350	11	2,000	1.0	4	ND	400	ND	ND	ND	40	2.3	3.6

* UL = The maximum level of daily nutrient intake that is likely to pose no risk of adverse effects. Unless otherwise specified, the UL represents total intake from food, water, and supplements. Due to lack of suitable data, ULs could not be established for arsenic, chromium, silicon, potassium, and sulfate. In the absence of ULs, extra caution may be warranted in consuming levels above recommended intakes.

† Although the UL was not determined for arsenic, there is no justification for adding arsenic to food or supplements.

‡ The ULs for magnesium represent intake from a pharmacological agent only and do not include intake from food and water.

§ Although silicon has not been shown to cause adverse effects in humans, there is no justification for adding silicon to supplements.

‖ Although vanadium in food has not been shown to cause adverse effects in humans, there is no justification for adding vanadium to food and vanadium supplements should be used with caution. The UL is based on adverse effects in laboratory animals and this data could be used to set a UL for adults but not children and adolescents.

ND = Not determinable due to lack of data of adverse effects in this age group and concern with regard to lack of ability to handle excess amounts. Source of intake should be from food only to prevent high levels of intake.

Sources: Institute of Medicine. *Dietary Reference Intakes for Calcium, Phosphorous, Magnesium, Vitamin D, and Fluoride.* Washington, DC: National Academies Press; 1997. Institute of Medicine. *Dietary Reference Intakes for Thiamin, Riboflavin, Niacin, Vitamin B_6, Folate, Vitamin B_{12}, Pantothenic Acid, Biotin, and Choline.* Washington, DC: National Academies Press; 1998. Institute of Medicine. *Dietary Reference Intakes for Vitamin C, Vitamin E, Selenium, and Carotenoids.* Washington, DC: National Academies Press; 2000. Institute of Medicine. *Dietary Reference Intakes for Vitamin A, Vitamin K, Arsenic, Boron, Chromium, Copper, Iodine, Iron, Manganese, Molybdenum, Nickel, Silicon, Vanadium, and Zinc.* Washington, DC: National Academies Press; 2001. Institute of Medicine. *Dietary Reference Intakes for Water, Potassium, Sodium, Chloride, and Sulfate.* Washington, DC: National Academies Press; 2004. Institute of Medicine. *Dietary Reference Intakes: Applications in Dietary Assessment.* Washington, DC: National Academies Press; 2000. Reprinted with permission.

Obtaining accurate information on usual dietary intake is difficult, and patients and their families often under report intake of snack food and beverages. Dietary intake for older children and adolescents may be highly variable, and one day or even several days of diet records may not represent typical dietary intake. Common factors that influence food intake variety are the day of the week, travel from home, restaurant meals, special occasions and the season of the year. In addition, nutrients that are concentrated in only a few foods (calcium in dairy products) may be difficult to evaluate with limited dietary intake information.

CONCLUSION

The DRI are a new approach and system to recommend nutrient intake for healthy people in North America to maintain nutritional health, prevent nutritional deficiencies, and contribute to the prevention of common, chronic diseases. The recommendations are based on currently available evidence and will be revised as new data are published. Nutrient intake evaluation is an essential part of nutritional assessment and care of children with acute and chronic illnesses who are enterally fed or supported. The DRI are not appropriate for the evaluation or planning of intravenous nutrition support.

REFERENCES

1. Institute of Medicine. *Dietary Reference Intakes for Calcium, Phosphorus, Magnesium, Vitamin D and Fluoride*. Washington, DC: National Academies Press; 1997.
2. Institute of Medicine. *Dietary Reference Intakes for Thiamin, Riboflavin, Niacin, Vitamin B6, Folate, Vitamin B12, Pantothenic Acid, Biotin, and Choline*. Washington, DC: National Academies Press; 1998.
3. Institute of Medicine. *Dietary Reference Intakes for Vitamin C, Vitamin E, Selenium, and Carotenoids*. Washington, DC: National Academies Press; 2000.
4. Institute of Medicine. *Dietary Reference Intakes for Vitamin A, Vitamin K, Boron, Chromium, Copper, Iodine, Iron, Manganese, Molybdenum, Nickel, Vanadium, and Zinc*. Washington, DC: National Academies Press; 2001.
5. Institute of Medicine. *Dietary Reference Intakes for Energy, Carbohydrates, Fiber, Fat, Fatty Acids, Cholesterol, Protein, and Amino Acids*. Washington, DC: National Academies Press; 2002/2005.
6. Institute of Medicine. *Dietary Reference Intakes for Water, Potassium, Sodium, Chloride and Sulfate*. Washington, DC: National Academies Press; 2004.
7. Institute of Medicine. *Dietary Reference Intakes: Applications in Dietary Assessment*. Washington, DC: National Academies Press; 2000.
8. Institute of Medicine. *Dietary Reference Intakes: Applications in Dietary Planning*. Washington, DC: National Academies Press; 2003.
9. National Research Council. *Recommended Dietary Allowances*. 10th ed. Washington, DC: National Academies Press; 1989.
10. Berner LA, Clydesdale FM, Douglass JS. Fortification contributed greatly to vitamin and mineral intakes in the United States, 1989–1991. *J Nutr.* 2001;131(8):2177–2183.
11. Sichert-Hellert W, Kersting M, Schoch G. Consumption of fortified food between 1985 and 1996 in 2- to 14-year-old German children and adolescents. *Int J Food Sci Nutr.* 1999;50(1):65–72.

CHAPTER 9

Decision Making in Pediatric Nutrition Support

Aida Miles

INTRODUCTION

Many factors affect how a decision is made for the type of nutrition support (NS), timing of initiation and advancement, amount, formulation, monitoring parameters, and even whether NS is warranted. Nutrition is a science backed by research and clinical experience. As with other clinical sciences, NS lacks evidence-based decision making tools in many important areas. Some areas are not fully investigated, and in other areas the data contains contradictions that constrain decision making. This chapter will cover some of the logistic decisions to be made in NS in order to provide the best type of nutrition intervention at the most appropriate time and for the needed duration. These decisions include how to implement and revise a nutrition risk-screening program, how to develop a nutrition plan of care, and how to monitor for outcomes based on intervention.

NUTRITION SCREENING

Nutrition screening is the process of identifying malnourished patients and those at risk of becoming malnourished. Early identification of these patients is important, because poor nutrition has an impact on outcome in terms of resistance to infection, wound healing, length of hospital stay, and complication rate.[1–4] In children malnutrition is also known to affect growth. Therefore nutrition screening in acute care, chronic care, and ambulatory care settings is important. The purpose of screening is to identify children with more severe problems so that they can be referred to the next level of care, and to provide anticipatory guidance and education to children and their families regarding prevention of nutrition problems.[5]

Since the 1970s, when a high prevalence of malnutrition among hospitalized patients was described,[6–10] many institutions have initiated screening programs to identify and treat patients who are malnourished or are at risk for malnutrition.[11,12] In addition, the Joint Commission on Accreditation of Healthcare Organizations (JCAHO) requires that all health care facilities accredited by them screen patients for nutrition risk. Each JCAHO accredited institution is subject to a survey at least every 3 years, and at that time, nutrition screening, assessment, and the implementation of a nutrition care plan are evaluated.[13,14]

The decision of how to implement or update nutrition screening criteria within an institution should be based on several factors, including: type of facility and patient population served, regulatory and accreditation standards, personnel available to screen, technology available for screening, time frame to complete, available staffing to complete assessments on at risk patients, and budgetary needs. Table 9-1 outlines these factors.

Once the factors related to nutrition screening are determined, the next decision is what parameters to use in nutrition risk screening. Because

Table 9-1 Aspects to consider when implementing or updating nutrition screening.

Type of facility and primary patient population: Is it an ambulatory or acute care facility? What is the primary patient population? What are the most common diagnoses seen at this facility?

Regulatory and accreditation standards: Is the facility accredited by JCAHO? If so, current JCAHO standards (which are updated periodically) need to be followed. Are there state or other agencies that require nutrition screening?

Personnel available to screen: Who will screen? Diet technicians, dietitians, nurses, nursing assistants, unit aides, etc.? The screening form needs to be designed in a way that is easily completed by the person doing the screen and is appropriate for the allotted time and training of the screener.

Technology available for screening: Will the screen be computer based or paper based? This decision affects the length of time it takes to perform the screen, determine risk level, and communicate the information to the registered dietitian or other pertinent personnel.

Time frame to complete: This is a factor of the average number of patients admitted to an institution daily, which personnel group will complete the screen, when and how it will be completed, and the staffing ratios for the institution. When there is a high volume of admissions and a low staffing ratio, the form needs to be short, yet sensitive enough to identify patients at risk.

Available staffing to complete assessments on at risk patients: Once patients are identified as at risk, a complete nutrition assessment and care plan must be completed within a reasonable time. If there is a low ratio of registered dietitians compared to the number of at risk patients, long range plans to increase dietitian staffing and immediate plans to perform assessments in a timely manner need to be put in place. Assessments and care planning can be expedited through the implementation of standard documentation forms with checklists.

Budgetary needs: What resources will be needed to implement or update the nutrition screening program? Budgetary needs can be technological (e.g., laptop computers, personal data assistants, computer programs), material (e.g., preprinted forms), educational (specialized training of personnel), and staffing (e.g., additional staffing to perform the screening and/or assessments).

JCAHO = Joint Commission on Accreditation of Healthcare Organizations

---

nutrition screening must be performed in a relatively short period of time, yet be reliable and valid, careful selection of screening criteria is of utmost importance.

One of the hardest decisions regarding the implementation or evaluation of a nutrition risk screening program is which criteria to use to determine level of nutrition risk. The process of arriving at the best criteria for each individual institution may be lengthy. Many institutions assign points to different screening criteria and establish levels of nutrition intervention needed based on the number of points that each patient received when screened. If a patient is determined to be not at nutritional risk when first screened, a process for rescreening that patient at least 7 days after the initial screen is necessary, since many nutrition related factors can change during hospital admission. For instance, a patient who was identified as not at risk on admission could lose weight, have a new diagnosis, or be unable to eat by mouth during the course of the hospital stay. These new events put the patient at nutritional risk. Some criteria for determining nutrition risk include the following: patients on altered diets or special formulas, multiple food allergies, acute vomiting and/or diarrhea, laboratory parameters related to nutritional status, patients on enteral or parenteral nutrition, diagnoses associated with specific nutrition problems or increased requirements, recent change in body weight or dietary intake, growth failure, or altered weight-for-length or weight-for-height.[15,16] Table 9-2 lists factors that can be used to determine nutrition risk in pediatric patients and Figure 9-1 is an example of a screening form.

Table 9-2 Examples of screening criteria to determine nutrition risk status.

Diagnosis[12,16–19]
Anemia
AIDS
Anorexia nervosa/bulimia nervosa/eating disorder
Bone marrow transplant
Bronchopulmonary dysplasia
Burns
Carcinoma/chemotherapy
Cardiac medicine/cardiac surgery
Cystic fibrosis
Depression, major
Diabetes
Failure to thrive/malnutrition
Gastrointestinal disorder (inflammatory bowel disease, short bowel syndrome, malabsorption, vomiting/diarrhea)
Hepatic disease
Inborn error of metabolism
Prematurity/low birth weight
Respiratory failure
Trauma
Sepsis, severe
Surgery, major
Ventilator dependency

Growth parameters
Points can be assigned depending on the severity of malnutrition as established by these parameters. Not all these parameters are necessary in establishing risk, and each facility should determine which are best suited for its use:
Length or height/age < 5th percentile
Weight/height < 5th percentile
Body mass index < 5th percentile for age (underweight)
Body mass index between 85 and 94th percentile for age (at risk for overweight)
Body mass index ≥ 95th percentile for age (overweight)

Waterlow criteria for classification of protein-energy malnutrition (PEM)[20,21]

	Mild	Moderate	Severe
Acute PEM			
Weight/height (percent of median)	81–90%	70–80%	< 70%
Chronic PEM			
Height/age (percent of median)	90–95%	85–89%	< 85%

Table 9-2 continued

History of weight loss—Blackburn criteria[22]

	Significant weight loss	Severe weight loss
1 week	1-2%	> 2%
1 month	5%	> 5%
3 months	7.5%	> 7.5%
6 months	10%	> 10%

Diet order

The following are examples of diet orders that may be included in nutrition screening and assigned points according to their potential contribution toward malnutrition.

NPO* (if no other risk parameters encountered, consider daily reevaluation and assigning a higher risk if the patient is NPO for > 3 days)

Clear liquid diet (if no other risk parameters encountered, consider daily reevaluation and assigning higher risk if patient is on clear liquids for > 5 days with no other form of nutrition support).

Multiple food allergies

Modified diet (calorie controlled, low sodium, low protein, etc.)

Special formula by mouth (hydrolyzed formula, semielemental, high caloric density, etc.)

Enteral nutrition support

Parenteral nutrition support

Age

Some institutions assign risk points to infants and children younger than 2 or 3 years of age because there is a higher prevalence of malnutrition during periods of rapid growth.[3,18]

Laboratory values

Consider including laboratory parameters only if they are readily available at the time of screening.

Hemoglobin/hematrocrit below standard for age

Total lymphocyte count < 1500 mm^3

Total lymphocyte count < 1000 mm^3

Albumin < 3.0 g/dL

Albumin < 2.5 g/dL

Prealbumin <20 mg/dL[23]

*NPO = Nil per os

Once screening criteria are identified, the screening process should be piloted. This should be done before the full implementation of the screening program, because the pilot may identify limitations and need for alterations. In addition, testing the screening program periodically is important, particularly if there have been changes, for instance alteration in the staffing ratio or changes in the patient population since the program was designed. It must be emphasized that piloting and reassessing the screening program is time consuming and requires careful documentation and effort. It is a step that should not be skipped. Nutrition screening requires time and effort. The process can be expedited and simplified if the screening criteria that is implemented is found to be highly reliable, appropriately uses available resources, and results in benefits. This is important because a given screening program may be the best for one institution, yet not reliable at another, similar facility. Table 9-3 lists recommended steps to follow when piloting a nutrition risk screening program.

Children's Healthcare of Atlanta
PEDIATRIC NUTRITION SCREENING FORM
(Screen to be completed within 24 hours of admission)
Patient's name: ______________________________ Room No.: ____________
Admit date: ___/___/___ Screen date: ___/___/___
Rescreen date: ___/___/___

(Circle all that apply—enter total points and indicate "at risk" or "not at risk")

ADMITTING DIAGNOSIS

Group 1 (2 points)	Group 2 (1 point)
Pancreatic insufficiency	Anemia (nutritional)
Inborn errors of metabolism	Bronchopulmonary dysplasia
Diabetes mellitus (new)	Cerebral palsy
Eating disorders	Cranial-facial surgery
Failure to thrive	Diabetes mellitus (follow-up)
Inflammatory bowel disease	Gastroesophageal reflux
Cystic fibrosis	Encopresis/constipation
Celiac disease	Multiple food allergies
Short bowel syndrome	Congenital heart disease
Malnutrition/malabsorption	Oncologic disease/BMT
Immunodeficiency	Renal or liver disease
Nutritional rickets	Solid organ transplant
Necrotizing enterocolitis	Esophageal atresia
Gastroschisis	Jaundice/hyperbilirubinemia

DIET ORDER

Parenteral or enteral nutrition support	(2 points)
Calculated diet	(2 points)
Clear liquids or NPO (rescreen in 2 days)	(2 points if still NPO/clear liquids at 3 days)

Breastfeeding (notify lactation consultant immediately by telephone for evaluation)

ANTHROPOMETRICS
Wt: ________ kg ________percentile for age
Ht: ________ cm ________percentile for age
HC: ________ cm ________percentile for age
Wt for ht: ________ percentile
BMI: ______kg/m2 ________percentile for age

Wt or ht/age, Wt/ht, BMI/age < 5th percentile	(2 points)
Wt/ht > 95th percentile or BMI > 85th percentile	(0 points)**

**RD to consider outpatient referral for weight counseling

HC < 5th percentile	(1 point)
Excessive weight gain or loss noted on database	(2 points)

TOTAL POINTS: ________

NUTRITIONAL RISK RATING:
____ Patient *at nutritional risk*: ≥ 2 points
(ALL AT-RISK PTS ARE REFERRED TO THE DIETITIAN)
____ Patient ***not at nutritional risk***: < 2 points

__________________Diet technician; Date: ________Rescreened on: ________ by__________________
NUTRITIONAL ASSESSMENT completed: ____________________, RD. Date: __________________

Figure 9-1 Sample pediatric nutrition risk screening form. With permission from Children's Healthcare of Atlanta, Georgia. Note: Screening at Children's Healthcare of Atlanta is now computerized.

Table 9-3 Piloting a nutrition risk-screening program.

- **Pilot the screening program for at least 7–10 days.**
- **Keep careful records on:**
  - How long it takes to complete each nutrition risk screen.
  - When each patient was screened (if not within 24 hours of admission, on which day of admission was the patient screened)
  - How many patients were determined to be at risk and how many not at risk.
  - Which day of admission a nutrition assessment was performed by a registered dietitian (RD) for those deemed at risk.
  - How many of those initially considered to be at risk were considered not at risk once the nutrition assessment was performed (a height measurement could have been erroneous).
  - How many of those rated not at risk were considered at risk but missed by the nutrition screen (i.e., the dietitian or nutrition support team were consulted and/or the patient was identified to be at risk through discussion during interdisciplinary rounds).
  - How many of those considered not at risk were still hospitalized 7 days after the original screen and needed rescreening. (If an institution chooses to rescreen at a different interval, then this would be the interval to document.)
  - How long each individual rescreen took.
  - How many were determined to be at risk and not at risk after being rescreened.
  - How much overtime work was needed to complete screening and assessments.
  - Overall comments from the staff performing nutrition risk screening and the staff performing nutrition assessments and intervention. For instance, their comments might indicate difficulties with the current method; opinion on length of time it takes to perform; deficiencies found within the medical record, e.g., most patients not having heights or lengths available; screening parameters that consistently produced false positive results; responsibilities that were neglected due to the need to perform screening and additional assessments.
- **Communicate with administration regarding any staffing issues that could arise.**
- **Communicate with ancillary departments (e.g., nursing department) regarding deficiencies consistently found in the medical record (e.g., lack of heights, lengths, weights).**
- **Perform in-service workshops to nutrition and ancillary departments on the nutrition screening program and stress the importance of their involvement to assure its success.**
- **Evaluate results and adjust the screening program accordingly.**
- **Once the revised screening program/form is developed, repilot it if at all possible.**

DEVELOPING A NUTRITION PLAN OF CARE

Once a patient has been identified to be at nutritional risk, a comprehensive nutrition assessment is needed (see Chapters 5 and 7). A patient-specific nutrition care plan is then designed. The nutrition care plan involves gathering information from the nutrition assessment to develop a detailed plan of interventions and counseling for each individual patient.[15] The nutrition support team, the patient's physician, other health care providers, nurses, and social workers, as well as the patient and/or caregiver should be involved in the development of the nutrition care plan. The components of a nutrition care plan include the goals of nutrition therapy, hospital discharge planning needs, anticipated length of hospital stay, and educational and training needs. Table 9-4 outlines these components.

Once a care plan is developed and implemented, frequent monitoring is needed to evalu-

Table 9-4 Components of a nutrition care plan.

- Short and long term goals of nutrition support
- Most appropriate route of nutrition administration
- Most appropriate enteral or parenteral feeding formulation
- Anticipated length of therapy
- Educational needs of patient and/or caregiver

Table 9-5 Examples of nutrition goals for patients on nutrition support.

- Attainment of an appropriate caloric intake
- Attainment of an appropriate protein intake
- Adequate average weight gain per day or per month
- Weight maintenance
- Appropriate average weight loss per week or per month
- Serum blood glucose within a target range
- Absence of hypoglycemic episodes
- Serum prealbumin level within a target range or within normal limits
- Patient and/or caregiver demonstrating techniques within a pre-determined percentage of accuracy
- Patient and/or caregiver completing a test after teaching within a pre-determined percentage of accuracy

ate the efficacy of NS, as well as to determine the need for alterations to the care plan (see Figure 9-2 for a sample care plan). It is also important to clearly delineate nutrition goals for each patient. Goals need to be quantifiable, so that an objective evaluation can be made as to whether the goals are reached. Documenting and tracking the attainment of goals can help identify areas that need improvement. Tracking goals can also help determine if the frequency of nutrition follow-up is adequate. For instance, documentation could show that patients advancing on enteral feedings reach their goal faster if followed up daily until the goal rate is achieved (i.e., the NS team can recommend adjustments as soon as any sign of intolerance is noted). Table 9-5 lists examples of nutrition goals that are quantifiable and can be used when establishing short and long term goals for patients on nutrition support.

When developing a nutrition care plan, frequency of patient monitoring should be set. Monitoring by the NS team can be daily, 3 times a week, twice a week, weekly, or even monthly. The frequency of monitoring should be determined based on the patient's level of malnutrition, acuity, type of NS needed, and overall tolerance of the feeding formulation. For patients requiring parenteral nutrition, daily monitoring until the patient reaches and tolerates the established goal is necessary. On the other hand, a patient who has been on the same tube feeding regimen for several days with good tolerance might only need weekly follow-up.

CONCLUSION

Nutrition support in pediatrics requires decision making. Decision making is an interdisciplinary task; however, a clearly delineated method of arriving at decisions for individual patients will facilitate optimal NS. Nutritional decision making is a repetitive process involv-

Patient's name:______________________ M___F___ Age:_____ Admission date:______________
Diagnosis: ____
Significant medical history:____
____

Date									Date	Comments
Weight (kg)										
Total cal/kg										
Prot gm/kg										
Cal TPN										
TF										
PO										
Intake ml/day										
Output/day										
Stool/emesis										
TPN order										
Dextrose gm										
Protein gm										
Na mEq										
K mEq										
Mg mEq										
Ca mEq										
P mM										
Rate ml/hr										
ml/24h										
IV fat gm										
Other										
Other										
Labs										
Glucose										
BUN/creat										
Na										
K										
Cl										
CO2										
Ca/Phos										
Chol/Tg										
Total prot										
Albumin										
Alk phos										
AST/ALT										
T bili/direct										
Mg										
Prealbumin										
Other										
Chart note (RD initials)										

Figure 9-2 Sample pediatric nutrition tracking form and care plan. Adapted and used with permission from Children's Healthcare of Atlanta, Egleston Campus. Atlanta, Georgia. TPN = total parenteral nutrition, TF = tube feeds, PO = per os, AST = aspartate aminotrasferase, ALT = alanine aminotrasferase, Alk phos = alkaline phosphatase

Assessment date: ________ Date of birth: ________ Current age:________ Corrected age: ________

Weight:	Wt/age percentile:	Medications	Diet history
Height:	Ht/age percentile:		
Head circ:	HC/age percentile:		
Wt/ht percentile:			
BMI:	BMI percentile		
IBW:	% IBW:		
Gestational age:	Birth weight:		
Special diet: Calorie goal: Protein goal: TPN goal: Enteral goal: formula/rate			

Outcome goal:________________________ Evaluate (circle): daily twice/week weekly

FORMULA/DIET/FLUIDS	Mode	Interval	Rate	Start	Stop	Advancement/ schedule
Example: Intact protein, lactose-free formula	*G-tube*	*Every 4 h*	*120 cc*	*Oct 25*		*8 am, 12 pm, 4 pm*
Intact protein, lactose-free formula	*G-tube*	*Per hour*	*30cc*	*Oct 25*		*From 8 pm to 6 am*

Figure 9-2 continued

ing: (1) assessing the patient; (2) setting goals; (3) formulating a plan; (4) implementing the plan; (5) reassessing patient, goals, plan, and implementation; (6) reformulating goals and plan; and (7) implementing the reformulated plan. The result of good decision making is providing the best form of NS in the most cost-effective manner.

REFERENCES

1. Redmon HP, Gallagher HJ, Shou J, Daly JM. Antigen presentation in protein-energy malnutrition. *Cell Immunol.* 1995;163:80–87.
2. Grimble RF. Malnutrition and the immune response. Impact of nutrients on cytokine biology of infections. *Trans R Soc Trop Med Hyg*. 1994;88:615–619.
3. Merritt RJ, Suskind RM. Nutritional survey of hospitalized patients. *Am J Clin Nutr.* 1979;32:1320–1325.
4. Tucker NH, Miguel SG. Cost containment through nutrition intervention. *Nutr Rev*. 1996;1:111–121.
5. Taylor Baer M, Bradford Harris A. Pediatric nutrition assessment: identifying children at risk. *J Am Diet Assoc.* 1997;97(suppl 2):S107–S115.
6. Butterworth CE. The skeleton in the hospital closet. *Nutr Today*. 1974;March/April:4.
7. Bristain BR, Blackburn GL, Vitale J, Cochran D, Naylor J. Prevalence of malnutrition in general medical patients. *JAMA*. 1976;253:1567–1570.

8. Hill GL, Pickford I, Young GA, et al. Malnutrition in surgical patients: an unrecognized problem. *Lancet.* 1977;1:689–692.
9. Merritt RJ, Suskind RM. Nutritional survey of hospitalized pediatric patients. *J Clin Nutr.* 1979;32:1320–1325.
10. Parsons HG, Francoeur TE, Howland P, Spengler RF, Pencharz PB. The nutritional status of hospitalized children. *Am J Clin Nutr.* 1980;33:1140–1146.
11. Powers CA. A system for nutrition screening of hospitalized children. *Top Clin Nutr.* 1987;2(4):11–17.
12. Sermet-Gaudelus I, Pisson-Salomon AS, Colomb V, et al. Simple pediatric nutritional risk score to identify children at risk of malnutrition. *Am J Clin Nutr.* 2000;72(1):64–70.
13. Joint Commission on Accreditation of Healthcare Organizations. Web site: http://www.jcaho.org/JointCommission/Templates/GeneralInformation.aspx?NRMODE=Published&NRORIGINALURL=%2fAccreditationPrograms%2fHospitals%2ffaqs%2ehtm&NRNODEGUID=%7b4151AA6B-83CB-4657-8DFF-032B8AAEF99D%7d&NRCACHEHINT=Guest#survey10. Accessed March 9, 2006.
14. Escott-Stump S, Krauss B, Pavlinac J, Robinson G. Joint Commission on Accreditation of Healthcare Organizations: friend, not foe. *J Am Diet Assoc.* 2000;100:839–844.
15. ASPEN Board of Directors. Standards for hospitalized pediatric patients. *Nutrition in Clinical Practice.* 1996;11:217–228.
16. Pediatric Nutrition Practice Group of the American Dietetic Association. In: Nevin-Folino N, ed. *Manual of Pediatric Clinical Dietetics. Nutrition Screening.* Chicago, Ill; 2003:21–34.
17. Mezoff A, Gamm L, Konek S, Beal KG, Hitch D. Validation of a nutritional screen in children with respiratory syncytial virus admitted to an intensive care complex. *Pediatrics.* 1996;97:543–546.
18. Hendricks KM, Duggan C, Gallagher L, et al. Malnutrition in hospitalized pediatric patients. *Arch Pediatr Adolesc Med.* 1995;149:1118–1122.
19. Cameron JW, Rosenthal A, Olson AD. Malnutrition in hospitalized children with congenital heart disease. *Arch Pediatr Adolesc Med.* 1995;149:1098–1102.
20. Waterlow JC. Classification and definition of protein calorie malnutrition. *BMJ.* 1972;3:566–569.
21. Waterlow JC. Some aspects of childhood malnutrition as a public health problem. *BMJ.* 1974;4:88–90.
22. Blackburn GL, et al. Nutritional and metabolic assessment of the hospitalized patient. *JPEN.* 1977;1(1):11.
23. Robinson MK, Trujillo EB, Mogensen KM, Rounds J, McManus K, Jacobs DO. Improving nutritional screening of hospitalized patients: the role of prealbumin. *JPEN.* 2003;27:389–395.

CHAPTER 10

What Is Pediatric Nutrition Support?

Maria R. Mascarenhas and Lori Enriquez

INTRODUCTION

Nutrition support (NS) has been practiced for decades. Enteral nutrition (EN) support, the use of nasogastric tubes, gastrostomies, or enterostomies to provide nutrition, employed blenderized foods until commercial formulas were created.[1] In the 1800s, alternatives for human milk were given to infants who were not breastfed. John Lovett Morse presented his recollections and reflections of artificial infant feeding of the first commercial formula, Synthetic Milk Adapted (SMA), in 1935 in the *Journal of Pediatrics*.[2]

Parenteral nutrition (PN) is a newer form of NS. The first report of PN providing adequate calories, 130 calories per kilogram for 5 days in a 5-month-old white male with Hirschsprung's disease, was published in 1944.[3] The infant received an intravenous mixture of dextrose, protein, and fats that provided total caloric needs and had a desirable composition—58% dextrose, 12% amino acids, and 30% fat achieved by alternating parenteral infusions of a 10% fat emulsion of olive oil and lecithin and a mixture of 50% glucose and 10% amino acids. In 1968, the *Journal of the American Medical Association* published the successful use of PN for 44 days in an infant who had short bowel syndrome.[4]

Several years later, the American Society for Parenteral and Enteral Nutrition (ASPEN) was founded. In 1980, the first report of the placement of percutaneous endoscopic gastrostomy (PEG) tube in children was published.[5] Also in 1980, The Infant Formula Act (IFA) amended the Food, Drug, and Cosmetic Act to ensure safety and quality of infant formulas.[6] Currently, there are hundreds of commercially available EN products and many PN solutions and additives. The practice of pediatric NS continues to evolve as new technology is created and research is completed. In this chapter, we define pediatric NS and discuss who should receive NS, route of administration of NS, the structure of an NS team, and the economics and politics of NS. NS is sometimes known as specialized nutrition support, and in pediatrics, it is the provision of nutrients orally, enterally, and/or parenterally with therapeutic intent.[7] Children have their own set of unique considerations and medical conditions that separate them from adult patients. These considerations include varying nutrition needs for growth and development, and the need for NS initiation earlier than adults. Children may have less fat stores than adults, their organs may be immature and they have medical conditions different from adults. In pediatrics family dynamics must always be taken into consideration. Figure 10-1 is an algorithm for delivery of nutrition support.

ORAL NUTRITION

Oral nutrition (ON) is the preferred route to provide NS. This can be accomplished by modifying the caloric density or nutrient composition, changing consistency of food and fluids, using

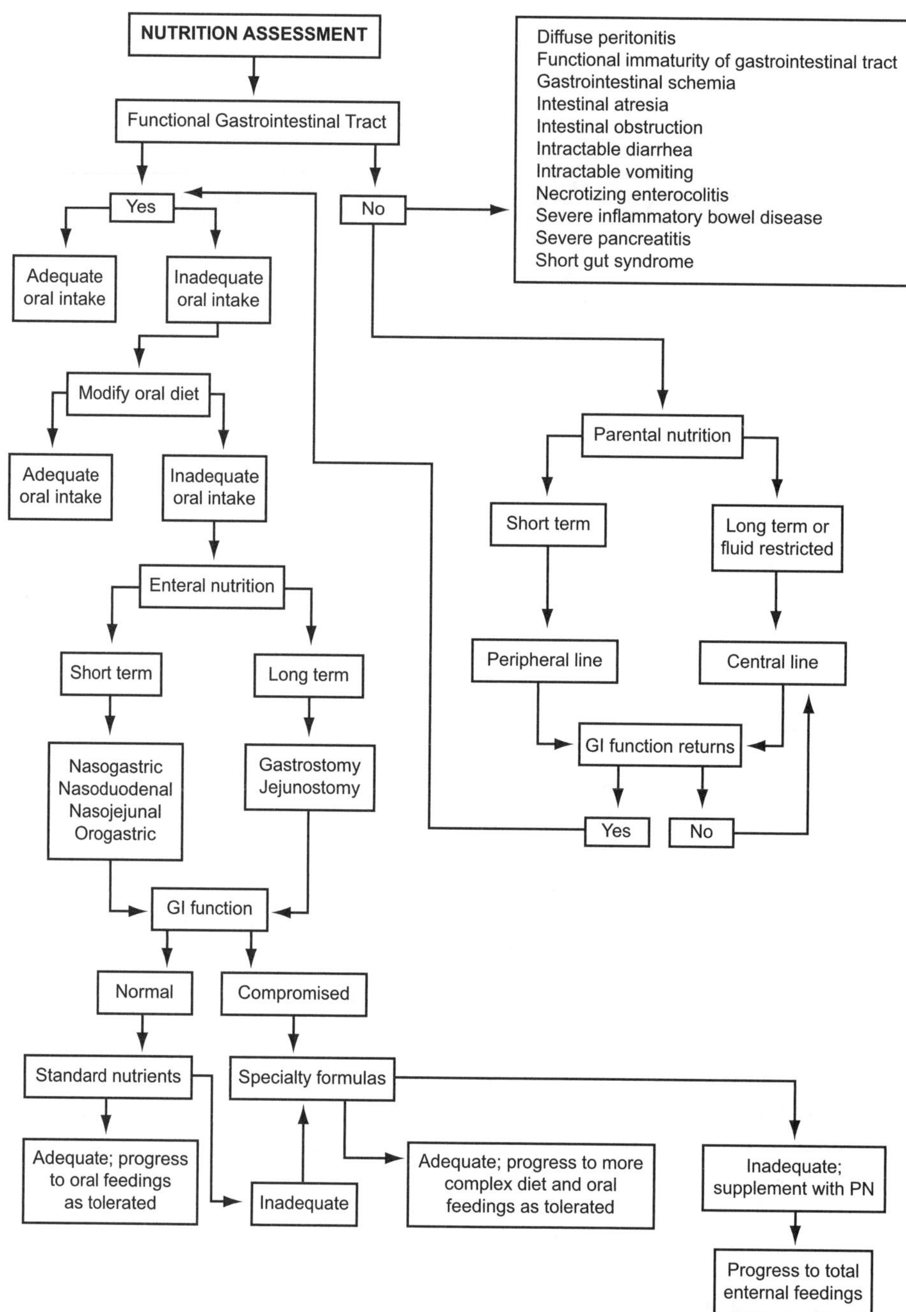

Figure 10-1 Algorithm for Delivery of Nutrition Support. *Source:* Adapted from: ASPEN Board of Directors: *Clinical Pathways and Algorithms for Delivery of Parenteral and Enteral Nutrition Support in Adults.* Silver Spring, Md: American Society for Parenteral and Enteral Nutrition; 1998. With permission from the American Society for Parenteral and Enteral Nutrition (ASPEN). ASPEN does not endorse the use of this material in any form other than its entirety.

adaptive equipment, adding supplements, and/or changing the feeding schedule.

ENTERAL NUTRITION

EN or tube feeding should be used to prevent or correct malnutrition when ON is not sufficient. EN is used when there are functional or structural problems. Functional problems include neurologic and neuromuscular disorders, prematurity, inability to take adequate nutrition, and genetic or metabolic disorders. Structural problems include congenital anomalies (such as tracheoesophageal fistula, esophageal atresia, cleft palate, and Pierre Robin syndrome), obstruction (cancer of head/neck, intubation), injury (caustic ingestions, trauma, sepsis), and surgery.[8] Benefits of EN over PN include lower costs, ease of use, safer administration, more physiologic than PN, maintenance of integrity of the gastrointestinal tract, fewer metabolic and infectious complications, and a more complete range of nutrients.[9,10] Common pediatric conditions where enteral tube feedings may be beneficial are listed in Table 10-1.

When NS is needed, EN is preferable to PN. The most common routes of administration for tube feedings include nasogastric, gastrostomy, nasoduodenal, nasojejunal, gastrojejunal, and jejunostomy (see Chapter 20 for a discussion of these feeding routes). Orogastric feedings are used in the neonatal intensive care setting.

PARENTERAL NUTRITION

PN is the intravenous delivery of nutrients, including fluid, amino acids, lipids, carbohydrates, electrolytes, vitamins, minerals, and trace elements (for information on these nutrients, see Chapters 16 and 22 to 26). When ON is not adequate and EN is not possible or tolerated, then PN can be considered. PN has risks associated with its use and should only be initiated for appropriate indications. Some indications for PN include necrotizing enterocolitis, gastrointestinal obstruction, intestinal atresia, severe inflammatory bowel disease, severe gastrointestinal side effects of cancer therapy, severe acute pancreatitis, and severe malnutrition when EN has failed.[11] PN is not indicated for patients with adequate intestinal function who can tolerate oral or tube feedings. A patient for whom death is imminent may not be a candidate for PN. Infants who require PN for fewer than 3 days are not

Table 10-1 Pediatric conditions that may benefit from enteral feeding.

Biliary atresia
Bone marrow transplant
Burns
Cardiorespiratory illnesses
Cancer
Cerebral palsy
Chronic lung disease
Cleft palate
Congenital heart disease
Cystic fibrosis
Developmental disabilities
Eosinophilic esophagitis
Endocrine disorders
Facial trauma
Failure to thrive
Gastrointestinal disease and dysfunction
Gastrointestinal reflux
Gastroschisis
Human immunodeficiency virus
Immune disorders
Inborn errors of metabolism
Inflammatory bowel disease
Intestinal atresia
Malrotation/volvulus
Multisystem organ failure
Multiple or major trauma
Neocrotizing enterocolitis
Neurologic diseases
Pierre Robin syndrome
Prematurity
Protracted diarrhea of infancy
Pulmonary diseases
Renal disease
Severe inflammatory bowel disease
Severe pancreatitis
Short bowel syndrome
Small bowel ischemia
Stem cell transplant

candidates.[12] ASPEN PN practice guidelines are listed in Table 10-2 and common pediatric conditions in which PN may be necessary are listed in Table 10-3. Peripheral PN is used only when PN is expected to be short term. Central access for PN is necessary for fluid restricted patients or patients requiring PN long term.

WHERE NUTRITION SUPPORT IS ADMINISTERED

NS can be administered in the hospital, rehabilitation centers, long term care settings, or the home. PN requires an interdisciplinary team approach. The team should include patients, parents/caregivers, pediatricians, pharmacists, dietitians, nurses, case managers, subspecialists, social workers, and other therapists as needed.

When PN is used outside a hospital, caregivers must be willing and able to provide care. They also need appropriate community resources to assure a safe environment. Education of patients and caregivers for home NS should begin before hospital discharge and continue in the home. Providing NS in the home is cost effective and supports positive outcomes such as growth and development, and neurologic and intellectual function. Routine monitoring should occur to prevent complications and assess progress of nutrition goals (See Chapter 19 for a discussion of home nutrition support).[13]

HISTORY OF NUTRITION SUPPORT TEAMS

NS teams developed in the late 1970s to early 1980s as a response to the need for treatment standards to decrease complications and improve patient care. Standardized approaches to catheter placement and care, administration of appropriate PN regimens, PN compounding methods, laboratory testing and monitoring, prevention, identification and treatment of complications and the nutritional care of complicated patients were developed. To prevent PN complications, teams developed a system for collecting PN related information. For example, NS teams found that the rate of sepsis was higher than predicted. Protocols for catheter care were established and the rates of sepsis dropped. NS teams also worked to decrease hospital costs by reducing hospital stay and PN complications.[14]

Table 10-2 American Society for Parenteral and Enteral Nutrition (ASPEN) PN practice guidelines.

1. Oral nutrition (ON) or enteral nutrition (EN) is the preferred route to administer nutrition support (NS).
2. Pediatric patients unable to meet their nutrition requirements orally or with EN should receive parenteral nutrition (PN).
3. PN should be initiated within 1 day of birth in neonates and within 5 to 7 days in pediatric patients unable to meet their nutrient requirements with ON or with EN.
4. PN should be initiated in infants when necrotizing enterocolitis is diagnosed.
5. PN should be initiated as soon as possible postoperatively in patients with short bowel syndrome.
6. PN should be used in children with inflammatory bowel disease who are unable to maintain normal growth and development on EN or a standard diet.
7. PN should be initiated for children with intractable diarrhea unable to maintain normal nutrition status with oral intake and EN.
8. PN should be initiated for children on extracorporeal membrane oxygenation (ECMO), using the ECMO circuit for access once hemodynamic stability is achieved.

Source: Developed from August D, Teitelbaum D, Albina J, et al. Guidelines for the use of parenteral and enteral nutrition in adult and pediatric patients. *JPEN.* 2002;26:102SA,1111SA,1113SA,1115SA,1116SA,1118SA,1120SA.

The financial squeeze of the 1990s led hospital administrators to disband teams. In their opinion, teams were expensive and not needed since each member of the team could function independently. This thinking represented a failure to recognize the value of clinical leadership and the team approach to patient care. As a consequence, patient care was transferred from specialized providers to local providers and those at the bedside. Data was no longer collected, analyzed, and used to improve care. In 1982 there were 7,000 hospitals in the United States. Of these, 1,496 could develop NS teams and 521, or 35%, actually had an NS team in place. By 1984, about 56% of the 1,496 hospitals had developed teams but 50 of the 521 teams had disbanded.[15]

The health care industry is in flux. There is a need to contain costs and assure the public that medical institutions provide quality care. Patients have high expectations, staffing of hospitals is streamlined, and the acuity of patients entering the hospital is increased. Despite the evidence that NS teams provide cost savings and improve care, they continue to be cut by hospitals. The success of a team lies in the team's ability to sustain results over a long period of time, to constantly improve itself, and to be effective in spreading change throughout the organization. Teams can achieve this by building on experience and efficiently implementing new concepts.[16]

Table 10-3 Pediatric conditions in which parenteral nutrition may be necessary.

Bone marrow transplant
Severe respiratory disease
Cancer
Cardiac failure
Congenital anomalies of the gastrointestinal tract
Diaphragmatic hernia
Extensive burns
Functional immaturity of the gastrointestinal tract
Gastrointestinal disease and dysfunction
Gastrointestinal fistulas
Intractable chylothorax
Intractable diarrhea
Meconium ileus
Neocrotizing enterocolitis
Obstruction
Protracted diarrhea of infancy
Renal failure
Severe inflammatory bowel disease
Severe malnutrition
Short gut syndrome
Small bowel ischemia
Stem cell transplant
Tracheoesophageal fistula

ESTABLISHING NS TEAMS

Establishing a NS team is difficult. Before any team can be established, a business plan is necessary, and hospital administrators must be convinced of the merits of the team. As will be discussed, clear-cut benefits of NS teams have been shown to include decreased sepsis and metabolic and mechanical complications, reduced costs, and decreased inappropriate use of PN. The NS team can pick a high profile complication that occurs frequently, study the complication, develop a quality improvement initiative, and show how the NS team successfully decreased the complication. The Joint Commission for the Accreditation of Hospitals Organization (JCAHO) set a standard that all patients requiring total PN must have a nutrition assessment performed. This can be useful as a justification for the establishment of an NS team.

The first step in creating an NS team usually happens when a group of interested individuals come together. The makeup of the group varies but can include gastroenterology, medicine, surgery, pediatrics, pharmacy, nursing, and nutrition. The team should consist of at least 1 physician, nurse, dietitian, and pharmacist. Each NS team member should have a role or job description that includes the standards of practice for each discipline, both from ASPEN and from their own professional organization. The team leader is usually, but not necessarily, a physician.

In one survey, 17% of teams did not have the 4 disciplines; others included administrators, education consultants, psychologists, social workers, and researchers. The number of team members ranged from 2 to 31. Most teams had a director and 80–88% of the directors were physicians, but some teams did not have directors.[15] The physician, as leader, assumes overall responsibility for the function of the NS team. The physician must have training in NS and must practice continuing medical education so he or she is knowledgeable about nutrient metabolism, disease pathophysiology, malnutrition, EN, PN, and complications of NS. Additionally, the physician must be able to work with NS team members and other services to help plan nutritional therapy.

The registered dietitian is responsible for performing a complete nutrition and growth assessment and planning the nutrition regimen based on the patient's estimated nutrition needs. Dietitian members assess caloric intake and interpret this for other NS team members. They also help with implementation of PN and EN and make adjustments in the macronutrient and micronutrient content of the prescription.

Pharmacists have varied roles. In addition to being knowledgeable about PN, EN, pharmacokinetics, drug metabolism, and drug interactions, they oversee the technical preparation of solutions. One report indicated that 30% of patients required intervention by a pharmacist. Common interventions included drug information and the expertise to solve drug-related problems. The majority of recommendations were accepted with a positive outcome.[17]

NS nurses provide nursing care around PN and EN; change lines, tubes, and dressings; work toward quality improvement; and perform nutritional assessments and education. Nurse members provide firsthand observation of the patient.

Some teams have data collectors who review charts and collect information on outcomes, complications, and cost containment.

Overlap of team members can occur. Each member should be trained in his or her discipline and pass standard certification. Each team member must be clinically competent. NS team members may belong to their respective departments and remain active in their disciplines. Individual departments provide team members with additional resources, including shared knowledge and experience, educational resources, and financial support. Remaining active in one's discipline allows the practitioner to keep up to date on new research studies, nutrition products, and clinical resources; and it provides an avenue to share and learn from others. Because multifunctional team members are valuable, some NS teams cross train members.

The second task in creating a NS team is to define the role of the team. Will the team provide services for only PN patients, for only EN patients, or for all patients receiving EN or PN? Visiting successful NS teams can be helpful. Not all observed practices are applicable or appropriate in all situations, so team members may need to adapt and modify what they observe. Every NS team must set clinical, teaching, and research goals. The functions of an NS team directly relate to the goals: patient care, teaching, quality improvement, and research. Clinical goals include the provision of safe and effective NS. Teaching goals are directed toward clinicians and NS team members. One goal is to help clinicians identify malnutrition and accurately assess the nutritional status of patients.

Because PN is lifesaving, it can be used indiscriminately. Therefore, it is critical that the NS team guide physicians in the appropriate use of PN. The NS team should educate the clinician as to the optimal route of nutrition, monitor prescriptions for appropriateness, provide bedside teaching and lectures, and develop standards, protocols, handbooks, and ordering forms. Research goals of the NS team include participation in research studies, the evaluation of more effective ways of providing NS, improving PN solutions, and preventing complications.

The NS team members assess anthropometric measurements (see Chapter 5) in conjunction with the nutrition assessment. NS team members are knowledgeable about assessing midarm circumference, triceps skinfolds, and alternative length assessments in patients who have contractures or cannot stand.

NS teams strive to improve efficiency and reduce costs. In the pharmacy, NS teams can reduce PN solution waste by using standard solutions and developing purchasing groups and an enteral and parenteral formulary. Waste can also be reduced by using NS protocols such as ordering time deadlines, allowing changes in PN composition with the next bag, and hanging the next bag when the current one is finished.[18]

NS teams make rounds and communicate their recommendations in the chart using specially created forms or within the progress notes. Some teams make rounds with specific groups such as the intensive care unit or the surgical service and communicate recommendations at that time. Others may seek out the primary care team. All recommendations must be documented in the patient record. It is important for members of the NS team to have visibility within the institution so that hospital administrators can see how the team functions. NS teams might hold walk rounds that make them visible to patients and other health care providers. Finally, teams must become indispensable for patient care.[19]

NS team members are an integral part of hospital nutrition, therapeutic standards, pharmacy, ethics, and infection control committees. This helps the team remain visible, share information, and initiate and participate in hospital projects. NS teams usually have their own business and quality improvement committees.

ASSESSING THE NS TEAM

JCAHO guidelines state that all clinical disciplines must include quality improvement programs, clinical care must be monitored, and problems must be identified and corrected. Thus, outcome monitoring is a function of the NS team. Possible outcomes that can be tracked include mechanical complications (air emboli, subclavian vein thrombosis), septic complications and metabolic complications (fluid, electrolyte, acid base, glucose, lipid, trace element, and vitamins).[20,21]

The components of a successful NS team include "will, ideas and the execution."[22] This translates into the will to change; the ability to draw on the best ideas, which come from front line clinicians; and the need to listen to team members. The team must decide on goals, determine how to measure change, and constantly strive for improvement. It is important that all NS teams have quality improvement programs. The examples in the next section illustrate how NS team members evaluate their goals and functions.

Value of Nutrition Support Team

There is ample evidence that NS improves patient care. For instance, in a report comparing 50 EN patients managed by an NS team to 51 EN patients managed by primary care physicians, more patients managed by the team achieved optimal caloric intake for longer periods and demonstrated positive nitrogen balance. Complication rates were decreased in patients managed by the team. In summary, the NS team provided a more efficient and safe system for nutritional care.[23]

Pace and colleagues followed the appropriate use of NS as the result of an NS team from 1992 to 1996; they showed a reduction in the use of PN by 52%. In 95% of the patients, PN was used appropriately. There was an increase in EN, and this resulted in cost savings of $226,184.[24] Similarly, Maurer and colleagues assessed the appropriate use of PN. They found that 49.7% of PN patient days were avoidable. In order to reduce waste, they developed a formal approval process that required prior authorization by the NS team before PN could be started. This resulted in a significant decrease in the number of days on PN, from 500 per month to 100 per month.[25]

Dalton et al. assessed the use of PN in a group of patients managed by primary care physicians in which NS team consultation was used as needed compared to a group that was jointly managed by the primary physician and NS team. Patients who were jointly managed had fewer mechanical and metabolic complications than the consultation group, and the 2 groups had an equal sepsis complication rate. However when these results were compared to another institution where PN was completely managed by the NS team, the jointly managed group had more mechanical and metabolic complications. The more management the team provides, the better the outcome.[26] Despite this data, primary care physicians still want to manage NS and can prevent NS teams from practicing.

Traeger et al. showed that patients managed by NS teams have fewer catheter complications, better documentation of nutritional status and nutrient requirements, and more frequent nitrogen balance studies. Additionally, nutritional goals for calorie and protein intake were achieved and positive nitrogen balance was seen more frequently in patients managed by NS teams. Nevertheless, primary care physicians opposed the team, so no team was used.[27]

NS teams are beneficial for patients receiving EN. In a prospective study of 102 consecutive hospitalized patients who needed EN over a 3½-month period, Brown and colleagues showed that about half of the patients were managed by an NS team and half by primary care physicians. The patients managed by the NS team received EN for longer periods, and more of them attained caloric requirements. While the total number of pulmonary, mechanical, gastrointestinal, and metabolic abnormalities was similar in both groups, the number of problems per day was lower in the patients managed by the team. Thus the authors showed fewer abnormalities per day and optimization of nutrient delivery by the NS team.[28]

Improvements in patient care by NS teams are clear. Mirtallo et al. showed that septic complications were reduced by using specially trained nurses; 7-day transparent dressings; the deletion of iodophor ointment, heparin, and polyurethane catheters; changing tubing every other day; using Luer lock tubing; eliminating extension sets; and using guidelines for guide wire changes of triple lumen catheters.[18] Spain et al. studied the implementation of an enteral feeding protocol and found that prior to the protocol, critically ill patients received just 52% of their caloric goal because physicians underordered, the feeds were stopped frequently, and they were slowly advanced. Only 58% of eligible patients were placed on the new enteral feeding protocol despite efforts by the NS team to use the protocol for more patients. When the protocol was used, physician ordering, delivery of calories, and advancement of feeds improved. Stopping feeds because of residual volumes, procedures, and patient tolerance still occurred.[29]

In some institutions, all patients receiving PN are automatically seen by the NS team. Anderson et al. assessed the effectiveness of teams by comparing outcomes from 1979 to 1992. They also looked at whether an automatic NS team consult made a difference. The automatic NS team consult did not decrease the complications, but it was associated with lower costs.[30]

There is little doubt that teams save money. It is sometimes difficult to quantify the exact dollar cost of providing NS (see Chapter 18 for a discussion of the economics of NS). In 1987, the costs of PN were estimated to be $3 billion annually and for EN $370 million.[18] In determining the cost of PN, one has to take into account facilities and equipment costs. These include pharmacy, medical supplies, personnel, laboratory testing, and hospital overhead. Pharmacy costs include labor, syringes, additives, dextrose, amino acids, and intralipids. Medical supply costs include gloves, tubing, filters, lines, syringes, dressings, and pumps. Personnel costs include nursing time, dietitian time, and physician time. Other costs are less defined and consist of NS complications, overhead, building depreciation, equipment, housekeeping and maintenance, administration, planned institution expansion, allowance for bad debts, cross subsidization of money losing departments, profit, and adjustment for consensus pricing (rates set to resemble nearby institutions and rates set under pressure by insurance companies). Other factors that influence the cost of PN include the use of high cost products such as albumin or amino acid solutions, PN administration systems, and waste of PN solutions. Costs for EN include the cost of the formula, tubing, nursing time, and personnel costs.[18] EN costs are not as high as those of PN.

It is often cheaper to use a standard formula than to make food in the kitchen. Nasogastric tubes, syringes, bags, and tubing are not expensive.

Factors that can reduce hospital costs include appropriate use of PN, avoiding hospital admissions only for NS, reducing unnecessary laboratory work, direct professional charges, decreasing complications, using standard solutions, and reducing vendor charges for ingredients and supplies.[31] NS team recommendations result in the appropriate use of PN, thereby producing significant savings for the institution. It is sometimes hard to determine what these exact cost savings are. Reducing PN waste results in cost savings to the institution. Eliminating PN waste, establishing order deadlines, and reducing the number of laboratory tests ordered can achieve this. Cost saving measures include the selection of appropriate patients, the use of EN rather than PN, and the use of correct caloric goals. Other ways to reduce the cost of NS are the reduction of complications, the review and justification of the use of high cost products, and the development of computer programs to manage data and patient outcomes. Another way to cut PN-related costs is to use good quality catheters and have protocols for catheter care.

Patient benefits from PN are usually measured by length of stay, complication rate, sepsis, nutritional outcome, nitrogen balance, weight, and growth; but institutional benefits from PN are total patient charges and personnel time workload.[18]

In some institutions, NS teams bill directly. In the current health care climate, this is possible for physicians, but might not be possible for other NS team members. Physician professional fees are not standardized, and they depend on documentation in the patient care record. If NS dietitians work under physician leadership, the physicians can only bill for physician time and not dietitian time. NS team members are generally paid by the hospital. The costs for the pharmacist may be factored into the cost of the PN bag, and those for the dietitian and nurse factored into the daily hospital room charge. In other institutions, a surcharge is added to the PN bag to cover the costs of the NS team. This fee is developed from the salaries of the dietitian, nurse, pharmacist, and secretary, average number of patients per year, and number of bags each patient uses. PN is not always directly reimbursed. Some insurance companies put a cap on reimbursement for PN, while others require justification for PN use. It is important for the NS team to document effectiveness of therapy and positive PN outcomes and to contain costs.[32] The NS team needs to convince insurers that the lack of complications more than makes up for the surcharge. There can be a significant difference between what the insurance company is charged and what the hospital collects.[33]

PN provided in the home is 50–73% less costly than PN in the hospital. Some commercial insurance companies pay for the home management PN team;[34] nevertheless, PN is a costly treatment.

NS teams save money. Their recommendations are usually more economical than those of primary care providers. O'Brien et al. showed in a retrospective study a cost savings of approximately $70,200 for 14 patients, or $5,000 per patient when the recommendations of the NS team were followed.[35] Cost savings can be achieved in the short and long term. In one institution, the NS team started in 1988 and data was collected from 1991 to 1999.[36] The authors showed a 46% decrease in the use of PN in 1991 and a 78.6% reduction in 1999. Simultaneously, the use of EN increased. The authors also looked at wastage of PN bags and found it decreased from 493 in 1991 to 34 bags in 1999. Compliance with recommendations from the NS team increased from 50% in 1991 to 90% in 1999. Additionally, the cost of PN administration decreased from $513,246 in 1991 to $195,176 in 1999. It is hard to estimate the cost savings in nursing time when EN is used instead of PN. With EN there is less laboratory testing, fewer complications, and fewer costs.

In another study, Trujillo et al. showed prospectively the many benefits of an NS team. Justification for appropriate use of PN was seen in 82% of patients managed by the NS team compared to 56% of patients followed by primary care physicians. Metabolic complications were seen in 34% of patients followed by the NS team compared to 66% in patients managed by primary care physicians. Patients who received a NS consultation received fewer days of PN. In this study, more than $500,000 would have been saved had all patients been managed by an NS team.[37]

Experienced NS team members reduce the costs of PN because clinical monitoring by NS team members is less expensive than laboratory assessments commonly used by less experienced clinicians.[38] Goldstein et al. showed that termination of a nurse resulted in an increase in inappropriate PN use, increased risk of line sepsis, and preventable costs. Once the nurse was reinstated, there was a dramatic decrease in costs associated with decreased patient morbidity.[39] Faubion et al. performed a prospective study that assessed infection rates and central venous catheter (CVC) life. CVCs were functional longer on units where the NS team trained nurses (20.4 days versus 14.4 days) and CVC sepsis rates decreased from 24% to 3.5%—a cost savings of $3,700 to $8,900 respectively, for best and worst case scenarios.[40]

CONCLUSION

NS teams improve clinical care, patient outcomes, and reduce hospital costs. They were established because a need existed in the early 1980s and they successfully met the challenge. In the current health care business climate, NS teams are not as robust as they once were. Nutrition research and medical technology are evolving and NS teams provide a needed service.

REFERENCES

1. Dudrick S. Foreword. *JPEN*. 2002;26:S2–S3.
2. Morse JL. Recollections and reflections on forty-five years of artificial infant feeding. *J Pediatr*. 1935;7:303–324.
3. Helfrick FW, Abelson NM. Intravenous feeding of a complete diet in a child. *J Pediatr*. 1944;25:400–403.
4. Wilmore DW, Dudrick SJ. Growth and development of an infant receiving all nutrients exclusively by vein. *J Am Med Assoc*. 1968;203:140–144.
5. Schwenk WF. Specialized nutrition support: the pediatric perspective. *JPEN*. 2003;27:160–167.
6. Mitrallo JM. Introduction to parenteral nutrition. In: Gottschlich MM, Fuhrman MP, Hammond KA, Holcombe BJ, Seidner DL, eds. *The Science and Practice of Nutrition Support*. Dubuque, Iowa: Kendall/Hunt Publishing Company; 2001:212–220.
7. August D, Teitelbaum D, Albina J, et al. Administration of specialized nutrition support. *JPEN*. 2002;26:18SA–21SA.
8. Nevin-Folino N, Miller M. Enteral nutrition. In: Samour PQ, Helm KK, Lang CE, eds. *Handbook of Pediatric Nutrition*. 2nd ed. Gaithersburg, Md: Aspen Publishers, Inc.; 1999:513–549.
9. Kleinman RE, ed. *Pediatric Nutrition Handbook*, 5th ed. Elk Grove Village, Ill: American Academy of Pediatrics; 2004:391–403.
10. Schwenk WF, Olson D. Pediatrics. In: Gottschlich MM, Fuhrman MP, Hammond KA, Holcombe BJ, Seidner DL, eds. *The Science and Practice of Nutrition Support*. Dubuque, Iowa: Kendall/Hunt Publishing Company; 2001:347–372.
11. Cox JH, Melbardis IM. Parenteral nutrition. In: Samour PQ, Helm KK, Lang CE, eds. *Handbook of Pediatric Nutrition*, 2nd ed. Gaithersburg, Md: Aspen Publishers, Inc.; 1999:551–587.
12. Price PT. Parenteral nutrition: Administration and monitoring. In: Groh-Wargo S, Thompson M, Cox JH, Hartline JV, eds. *Nutritional Care for High-Risk Newborns*. Chicago, Ill: Precept Press, Inc.; 2000:91–107.
13. August D, Teitelbaum D, Albina J, et al. Home specialized nutrition support. *JPEN*. 2002;26:137SA–138SA.
14. Wesley JR. Nutrition support teams—Whither thou goest? In: *Nutrition Support Team Anthology*. Silver Springs, Md: Aspen Publishing; 2004:7–8.
15. Hamouii E. Assessing the nutrition support team. *JPEN*. 1987;11(4):4–12.
16. Schneider PJ, Bothe A, Bisognano M. Improving the nutrition support process: assuring that more patients receive optimal nutrition support. *Nutr Clin Pract*. 1999;14:221–226.
17. Cerulli J, Malone M. Assessment of drug-related problems in clinical nutrition problems. *JPEN*. 1999;23:218–221.
18. Mirtallo JM, Powell CR, Campbell SM, et al. Cost-effective nutrition support. *Nutr Clin Pract*. 1987;2(1):42–51.
19. Tougas JG. Starting a nutrition support team: short term pain for long-term gain. *Nutr Clin Pract*. 1994;9 (6):221–225.

20. Nehme AE. Nutritional support of the hospitalized patient. *JAMA.* 1980;243:1906–1908.
21. Mirtallo JM, Jozefzcyck KG, Hale KM, et al. Providing 24-hour nutrient infusions to critically ill patients. *Am J Hosp Pharm.* 1986;43:2205–2208.
22. Schneider PJ, Bothe A, Bisognano M. Improving the nutrition support process: assuring that more patients receive optimal nutrition support. *Nutr Clin Pract.* 1999;14:221–226.
23. Powers DA, Brown RO, Cowan GSM, et al. Nutritional support team versus non-team management of enteral nutritional support in a Veteran's Administration medical center teaching hospital. *JPEN.* 1986;10:635–638.
24. Pace NM, Long JB, Elerding S, et al. Performance model anchors successful nutrition support protocol. *Nutr Clin Pract.* 1997;12:274–279.
25. Maurer J, Weinbaum F, Turner J, et al. Reducing the inappropriate use of parenteral nutrition in an acute care teaching hospital. *JPEN.* 1996;20:272–274.
26. Dalton MJ, Schepers G, Gee JP, et al. Consultative total parenteral nutrition teams: the effect on the incidence of total parenteral nutrition-related complications. *JPEN.* 1984;8:146–152.
27. Traeger SM, Williams GB, Milliren G, et al. Total parenteral nutrition by a nutrition support team: improved quality of care. *JPEN.* 1986;10:408–412.
28. Brown RO, Carlson SD, Cowan GSM, et al. Enteral nutritional support management in a university teaching hospital: team versus non-team. *JPEN.* 1987;11:52–56.
29. Spain DA, McClave SA, Sexton LK, et al. Infusion protocol improves delivery of enteral tube feeding in the critical care unit. *JPEN.* 1999;23:288–292.
30. Anderson DC, Heimburger DC, Morgan SL, et al. Metabolic complications of total parenteral nutrition: Effects of a nutrition support service. *JPEN.* 1996;20:206–210.
31. Twomey PL, Patching SC. Cost-effectiveness of nutritional support. *JPEN.* 1985;9(1):3–10.
32. Cox JH, Melbardis IM. Parenteral nutrition. In: Samour PQ, Helm KK, Lang CE, eds. *Handbook of Parenteral Nutrition.* 2nd ed. Gaithersburg, Mass: Aspen Publishers, Inc.; 1999:551–587.
33. Roberts MF, Levine GM. Nutrition support team recommendations can reduce hospital costs. *Nutr Clin Pract.* 1992;7:227–230.
34. Wesley JR, Khalidi N, Faubian WC, et al. Home parenteral nutrition: a hospital-based program with commercial logistic support. *JPEN.* 1984;8:585–588.
35. O'Brien DD, Hodges RE, Day AT, et al. Recommendations of nutrition support team promote cost containment. *JPEN.* 1986;10(3):300–302.
36. Ochoa JB, Magnuson B, Swintowsky M, et al. Long-term reduction in the cost of nutritional intervention achieved by a nutrition support service. *Nutr Clin Pract.* 2000;15:174–180.
37. Trujillo EB, Young LS, Chertow GM, et al. Metabolic and monetary cost of avoidable parenteral nutrition use. *JPEN.* 1999;23:109–113.
38. Baker JP, Detsky AS, Whitwell J, et al. A comparison of the predictive value of nutritional assessment technique. *Am J Clin Nutr.* 1982;36:233–241.
39. Goldstein M, Braitman LE, Levine GM. The medical and financial costs associated with termination of a nutrition support nurse. *JPEN.* 2000;24:323–327.
40. Faubion WC, Wesley JR, Khalidi N, et al. Total parenteral nutrition catheter sepsis: impact of the team approach. *JPEN.* 1986;10:642–645.

CHAPTER 11

Appetite Regulation in Health and Disease

Lee A. Denson

INTRODUCTION

Under normal conditions, signals originating in the gastrointestinal tract, adipose tissue, and brain combine to closely regulate the balance between energy intake and energy expenditure (Figure 11-1 and Table 11-1). This results in relatively stable body weight over time despite large variations in day-to-day intake. Net energy intake is a function of hunger, or the desire to initiate meals, and satiety, or the desire to terminate meals. It is important to note that the composition and timing of initiation of meals in humans is heavily influenced by multiple environmental factors and learned behaviors, while satiety or meal termination appears to be more strictly biologically controlled. The initial section of this chapter will review regulation of hunger and satiety under basal conditions. Subsequent sections will discuss the dysregulation of these mechanisms that is associated with increased food intake in obesity and reduced intake in anorexia nervosa (AN) and representative chronic diseases.

GASTROINTESTINAL AND HYPOTHALAMIC PEPTIDES THAT STIMULATE INTAKE

Several peptides stimulate intake under basal conditions. Of these, the most significant gastrointestinal factor is ghrelin, a peptide that is produced in the stomach and increases in the circulation immediately before initiation of meals.[1] Ghrelin levels then fall with the completion of meals. Ghrelin was originally identified in a search for endogenous growth hormone (GH) secretagogues. Recent work focused on its role in regulating initiation of meals. In addition to stimulating appetite, ghrelin increases gastric emptying and that contributes to its pronounced stimulatory effect on food intake. Ghrelin regulates the timing of meal initiation throughout the day. Ghrelin levels correlate with fat mass in a longer term, potentially adaptive fashion. Under conditions in which fat mass is reduced, ghrelin levels increase, stimulating energy intake.

Ghrelin stimulates appetite by activating neurons in the arcuate nucleus of the hypothalamus that release neuropeptide Y (NPY) and Agouti-related protein (AgRP). This effect is dependent upon an intact vagal nerve, and therefore is primarily mediated via a peripheral effect of ghrelin. However, ghrelin and the GHs receptor (GHsR) have also been identified on arcuate nucleus neurons that release NPY and AgRP, indicating a direct central effect.[2] Recently, an intracellular energy sensor, adenosine monophosphate-activated protein kinase (AMPK), has been shown to be activated by ghrelin in the hypothalamus.[3] This implicated AMPK in the cellular signaling events that mediate effects of ghrelin. NPY stimulates appetite by activating the Y1 receptor in the paraventricular nucleus.[4] The activated Y1 receptor leads to increased meal size without a change in the overall number of meals.[5] AgRP simulates appetite by inhibiting the activation of melano-

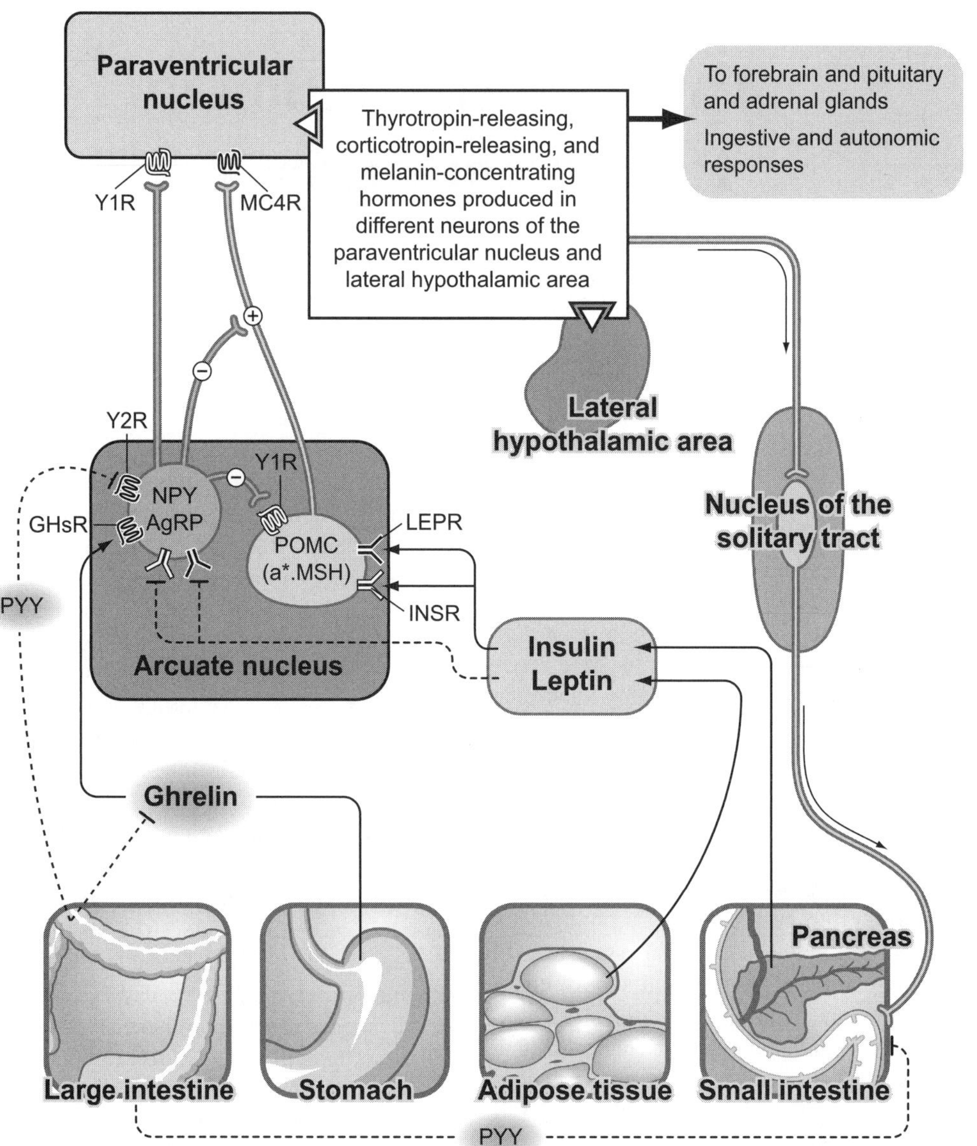

Figure 11-1 Interactions among hormonal and neural pathways that regulate food intake and body-fat mass. In this schematic diagram of the brain, the dashed lines indicate hormonal inhibitory effects, and the solid lines stimulatory effects. The paraventricular and arcuate nuclei each contain neurons that are capable of stimulating or inhibiting food intake. Y1R and Y2R denote the Y1 and Y2 subtypes of the neuropeptide Y (NPY) receptor; MC4R denotes the melanocortin 4 receptor; PYY denotes peptide YY_{3-36}; GHsR denotes growth hormone secretagogue receptor; AgRP denotes agouti-related protein; POMC denotes proopiomelanocortin; α-MSH denotes α-melanocyte-stimulating protein; LEPR denotes leptin receptor; and INSR denotes insulin receptor. *Source:* Korner J, Leibel RL. To eat or not to eat – How the gut talks to the brain. *NEJM*. 2003;349:927. Reproduced by permission.

Table 11-1 Factors that regulate appetite.

Molecules that are produced in the CNS or the periphery and regulate intake are shown, together with their primary source of production and proposed mechanism of action.

Molecule	*Source*	*Mechanism*
Increased intake:		
Ghrelin	Stomach	↑ NPY/AgRP
NPY	CNS	↓ α MSH/CART ↑ NPY receptor 1
AgRP	CNS	↓ MC4R activation
Endocannabinoids	CNS	CB1 receptor ↑ dopaminergic and opioid signaling
Reduced intake:		
CCK	Small intestine	↓ gastric emptying/intake
PYY	Small intestine and colon	↓ NPY/AgRP activity ↓ ghrelin
Leptin	Adipose tissue	↑ α MSH/CART ↓ NPY/AgRP activity
Insulin	Pancreas	↑ α MSH/CART ↓ NPY/AgRP activity
TNF-α	Monocytes	↑ MC4R activity ↑ leptin
IL-1	Monocytes	↑ MC4R activity ↑ serotonin ↑ leptin
α MSH/CART	CNS	↑ MC4R activity
Serotonin	CNS	↑ MC4R activity

NPY: neuropeptide Y; CNS: central nervous system; PVN: paraventricular nucleus; AgRP: agouti-related peptide; α MSH: alpha melanocyte-stimulating hormone; CART: cocaine and amphetamine regulated transcript; MC4R: melanocortin receptor 4; CB1: cannabinoid receptor 1; CCK: cholecystokinin; PYY: peptide YY; TNF-α: tumor necrosis factor-α; IL-1: interleukin 1.

cortin signaling in these regions of the brain. Specifically, it reduces synthesis of 2 potent anorexigenic (appetite suppressing) peptides, α-melanocyte stimulating hormone (α-MSH) and cocaine and amphetamine regulated transcript (CART) in the arcuate nucleus, as well as inhibiting activation of the anorexigenic melanocortin 4 receptor (MC4R) in the paraventricular nucleus. Peripheral short term nutritional signals, specifically low serum glucose, also stimulate central NPY and AgRP activity, as well as the orexigenic (appetite stimulating) neuropeptides orexin A and B and melanin-concentrating hormone (MCH) produced in the lateral hypothalamic area. It is important to note, however, that targeted deletion of either NPY or AgRP in the mouse has not led to a significant reduction in energy intake, indicating that the homeostatic pathways driving food intake are robust and redundant.

Intake of palatable foods (related to sweetness and fat content) is regulated via endogenous opioid receptors, contributing to the increased reward associated with these types of foods.[6] For example, administration of an opioid antagonist will reduce the pleasure associated with consuming foods high in sugar or fat content, and thereby will reduce overall intake. Therefore, it is important to account for regulation of energy intake by reward aspects of eating.[7]

The endocannabinoid system is involved in both hedonic (pleasurable) aspects of energy intake and homeostatic (via leptin) aspects.[6,8] While the relevant reward circuitry is not well understood, it may involve effects on dopaminergic and/or opioid pathways. Central endocannabinoid activity increases as the interval between meals increases, stimulating meal initiation, and it declines with feeding. The stimulatory effect upon intake is particularly potent for sweet and palatable foods. Anandamide was the first endogenous ligand identified for this system; several additional agonists and antagonists have now been characterized. Signaling via the cannabinoid (CB1) receptor stimulates both food intake and lipogenesis. Fat mass might, in turn, regulate cannabinoid activity via alterations in leptin expression, as increased leptin levels have been associated with reduced central cannabinoid and CB1 expression. In contrast to NPY and AgRP, targeted deletion of CB1 in the mouse resulted in reduced intake and fat mass, demonstrating a nonredundant role for endocannabinoid signaling in regulating intake and overall energy balance.[6] This has been associated with increased expression of the anorexigenic factor corticotrophin-releasing hormone (CRH). Specific aspects of ghrelin and endocannabinoid action in disease states, including potential therapeutic applications, will be reviewed in subsequent sections.

GASTROINTESTINAL AND HYPOTHALAMIC PEPTIDES THAT REDUCE INTAKE AND SIGNAL SATIETY

The best characterized gastrointestinal peptide implicated in termination of meals is cholecystokinin (CCK). CCK is a potent immediate satiety signal that is released from the intestine during meals and reduces both gastric emptying and the amount of food intake per meal.[9] This effect of CCK requires an intact vagus nerve. Peptide YY (PYY) also has an effect on food intake. PYY is released from the distal small intestine and colon during meals in proportion to the number of calories ingested, and it acts to decrease intestinal motility and reduce overall food intake.[10] The reduction in food intake is mediated via inhibition of hypothalamic NPY and AgRP signaling, leading to a net increase in anorexic proopiomelanocortin (POMC) expression and MC4R activation. Increases in PYY associated with a meal might also directly inhibit the stimulatory effects of ghrelin on intake. Recently, gastric production of leptin, characterized as a long term regulator of energy balance, has been identified.[11] Meal induced production of gastric leptin suggests that gastric leptin functions as an additional potential short term satiety signal.

Nutritional signals associated with a meal, increasing serum glucose and amino acids in particular, act to favor meal termination.[12] Interestingly, dietary fat and fructose are not as potent in this regard. High serum insulin levels in association with a meal act as a potent short term satiety signal; mechanisms include enhancement of the effects of CCK and PYY, directly activating POMC expression, and possibly reduction of ghrelin expression.

Centrally, increased relative expression of the POMC gene in response to satiety signals results in up-regulation of α-MSH and CART in the arcuate nucleus; the α-MSH and CART then activate MC4R in the paraventricular nucleus. This then leads to increased production of a number of anorexigenic peptides, including thyrotropin-releasing hormone (TRH) and CRH. In contrast to the orexigenic peptides NPY and AgRP, human and murine mutations in POMC and MC4R have resulted in hyperphagia, reduced energy expenditure, and morbid obesity. Several classes of neurotransmitters, including serotonin, which has been shown to reduce intake via activation of MC4R signaling, have also been implicated in regulating food intake.

LONG TERM REGULATION OF ENERGY INTAKE AND FAT MASS

The peptides and nutritional factors summarized in the preceding sections regulate short term meal initiation and termination. Longer term regulation of energy intake in relation to energy stores (fat mass) is primarily mediated by leptin, which is produced in adipose tissue and acts as a potent inhibitor of food intake. Leptin levels increase in direct proportion to both caloric intake and amount of adipose tissue and limit meal size by both activating POMC expression and inhibiting NPY/AgRP expression in the arcuate nucleus. AMPK has also been implicated in the cellular signaling events that mediate central effects of leptin. Hypothalamic AMPK activity is reduced after leptin administration in rodents.[3] There is evidence that leptin may directly reduce additional orexigenic signaling pathways, including those involving ghrelin and CB1. The net effect is activation of anorexigenic/catabolic pathways mediated by the MC4R and associated targets, including TRH and CRH. Conversely, reduced caloric intake and fat mass reduce leptin expression, stimulating appetite and reducing energy expenditure. Insulin functions in a similar manner as a fat mass sensor and long term regulator of intake through mechanisms involving activation of POMC expression and inhibition of NPY/AgRP production. The importance of leptin in this regard has been confirmed in humans and mice. Mutations in the leptin and leptin receptor genes are associated with hyperphagia and morbid obesity. Increased basal levels of leptin enhance the more short term satiety signals such as CCK and PYY, reducing meal size. However, the effect of the leptin/insulin system on meal size may be modified to some extent by the diet itself, as a high fat diet reduces relative insulin/leptin production and contributes to insulin and leptin resistance, leading to greater overall intake and weight gain.

OBESITY

This section briefly summarizes the manner in which mechanisms regulating energy intake may be altered in obesity in terms of both rare primary single gene defects and more common secondary changes in neuropeptide expression and signaling. This section assumes that obesity is due to an imbalance between energy intake and energy expenditure. The significant increase in the proportion of people who are overweight or obese in developed countries indicates that the intrinsic biological mechanisms that would theoretically reduce intake in response to increases in fat mass can be overcome, leading to net weight gain over time.

Recently, a mechanism that might reconcile the biological systems that regulate energy intake and expenditure with the observed overall increase in fat mass in the population has been proposed.[13] In this new model, the insulin/leptin dependent activation of catabolic melanocortin signaling in the arcuate nucleus is predominant relative to tonically inhibited anabolic NPY signaling under basal conditions. Experimental evidence for this includes the observation that destruction of the arcuate nucleus leads to obesity, confirming that catabolic signals are predominant under basal conditions. Moreover, genetic disruption of catabolic melanocortin signaling (e.g., MC4R, POMC, leptin) leads to hyperphagia and obesity, while targeted disruption of anabolic NPY signaling does not, indicating that normal energy balance does not require basal NPY activity.

With an increase in fat mass, leptin expression increases, and this should further activate catabolic signaling, leading to reduced energy intake. However, if catabolic signaling is already highly activated in the basal state by leptin, relative to inhibited anabolic signaling, then additional catabolic signaling may be relatively less robust, and not completely effective in reducing energy intake to a level that will reduce fat mass. Conversely, a loss of fat mass will lead to a reduction in leptin expression, an increase in ghrelin expression, inhibition of tonically active catabolic signaling, and more potent activation of previously inhibited NPY/AgRP anabolic signaling. Anabolic signaling could then increase to a relatively greater degree and will be more effective in protecting against a loss of fat mass than the catabolic system is in protecting against an increase in fat mass. This mechanism is supported by the observation that as ghrelin levels increase and leptin levels fall with diet-induced weight loss, most individuals increase intake and regain lost weight. Conversely, on a population basis, most individuals in developed countries experience net weight gain over time, and are now classified as either overweight or obese. Taken together, this model predicts that interventions that enhance anorexigenic signaling and inhibit orexigenic signaling are most likely to be effective in promoting long term weight loss.

Hedonic (food reward) aspects of the Western diet may also contribute to the relative ineffectiveness of the catabolic systems in protecting against weight gain.[14,15] One practical issue is the easy availability of highly palatable, calorically dense foods that allow for rapid consumption of large amounts of calories. The large amount of calories may temporally overwhelm short term satiety signals including CCK and PYY. Multiple studies have demonstrated increased food intake as palatability (sweetness and fat content) is increased. In addition, over time, diets high in sugar and fat are relatively less effective in stimulating long term leptin/insulin dependent catabolic signals. Moreover, experimental data have demonstrated that consumption of a high fat diet leads directly to the development of resistance to the anorexigenic effects of insulin and perhaps leptin. Therefore, high-fat diets both potently activate food reward centers in the brain, and are less effective in activating homeostatic signals to induce satiety and reduce long term intake. This is clearly demonstrated in rodent studies in which feeding of a high fat (35%) diet leads to obesity, despite circulating leptin.[16] Increased central cannabinoid activity may stimulate ongoing increased intake in this setting. In this respect, antagonists of endocannabinoid action may be useful, and a clinical trial of a CB1 antagonist in obesity is under way.

Most humans with common (polygenic) obesity also exhibit increased circulating leptin, in direct proportion to fat mass. This is consistent with a state of leptin resistance, due to impaired cellular leptin signaling and/or reduced leptin transport across the blood brain barrier.[17] The overall result is that energy intake and expenditure persist at levels that promote ongoing weight gain, rather than weight loss. In addition, there is compelling evidence that once a new level of fat mass is reached efforts to reduce fat mass through voluntary reductions in food intake potently activate ghrelin dependent anabolic signals that stimulate hunger and reduce energy expenditure, leading to restoration of fat mass. The therapeutic implications of this are: (1) exogenous leptin administration is unlikely to promote weight loss in most individuals with obesity, (2) diet-induced weight loss is hindered by the robustness of intrinsic ghrelin-dependent anabolic mechanisms, and (3) ghrelin antagonists may be useful adjuncts to diet in terms of altering energy balance and stimulating long term weight loss in obesity.

Recently, PYY has emerged as a potential therapeutic agent. Under normal conditions, PYY serves as a potent gastrointestinal satiety signal that stimulates meal termination in proportion to the caloric density of the meal. Both basal and meal induced PYY levels are lower in obese individuals than in lean individuals. This, combined with leptin resistance, would be expected to contribute to increased food intake in obese individuals. A recent study demonstrated that a single infusion of PYY significantly reduces food intake at an "all you want to eat" buffet in both obese and lean individuals.[18] This occurred without an increase in nausea or other adverse gastrointestinal symptoms. Animal studies have indicated that chronic PYY administration reduces food intake, raising the possibility that this peptide may be useful in management of obesity.

Hyperphagia and early onset obesity have been linked to single gene defects in a minority of individuals.[19] Of these, the most common to date are mutations in MC4R, which may account for up to 5% of cases associated with early onset of body mass index (BMI) > 40. These patients exhibit significant hyperphagia and binge eating secondary to disruption of anorexigenic melanocortin signaling.[19] Families in which mutations in leptin or the leptin receptor cause obesity have been described. Individuals with leptin deficiency have had a good response to leptin administration, in terms of significant reductions in intake and BMI. Finally, mutations in the POMC gene have been reported in a small number of kindreds with significant obesity. Single gene defects leading to significant reductions in BMI have not been reported, perhaps attesting to either the greater redundancy or evolutionary essentialness of the anabolic systems. Moreover, because of secondary effects on fertility, individuals with single gene defects significantly reducing BMI would be less likely to reproduce.

A number of pharmaceutical agents that suppress appetite have been developed and tested in obesity. For the most part, these agents act via activation of central catecholaminergic, dopaminergic, or serotonergic neurotransmitter pathways. There has been no significant overall success with any one agent, and concerns regarding safety limit the use of several. Serotonin suppresses appetite and increases satiety. The serotonin agonist fenfluramine induces anorexia via activation of central melanocortin pathways.[20] However, fenfluramine was withdrawn from the market because of adverse cardiovascular effects. Nevertheless, this indicated that more specific activation of melanocortin signaling might be a useful approach.[21] Similarly, sibutramine also acts as an appetite suppressant, via inhibition of norepinephrine and serotonin reuptake, and has received FDA approval in the United States as an adjunct to diet and exercise in management of obesity.

Gastric bypass surgery, in carefully selected individuals, results in significant long term reductions in food intake and BMI. This is in part due to mechanical aspects of the procedure, which limit meal size. However, most patients also report and exhibit long term reductions in appetite and intake. These reductions have been linked to persistently reduced levels of ghrelin and increased levels of PYY.[22] The net effect is to reduce hunger and to increase satiety. This has given additional insight into mechanisms to account for the long term success of gastric bypass relative to dieting, which increases ghrelin levels and appetite, and has provided additional support for the therapeutic potential of either ghrelin antagonists or PYY agonists in treatment of obesity.

ANOREXIA NERVOSA

Unlike obesity, single gene defects have not been reported in AN. However, one group has recently described a polymorphism in the AgRP gene that might contribute to enhanced melanocortin signaling and reduced intake in some patients.[23] Complementary studies in a rodent model of anorexia have demonstrated that administration of AgRP reduces melanocortin signaling and increases intake and survival.[24] A number of alterations in neuropeptide pathways regulating food intake have been described; these typically normalize after recovery.[25] These alterations are likely secondary to the primary restriction of food intake and resultant reduction in fat mass, rather than being causative. However, knowledge of these alterations gives insight into the complicated mechanisms involved in this disorder. In particular, some abnormalities that promote reduced food intake, such as enhanced serotoninergic signaling, may persist for a long period of time after intake and BMI have improved, contributing to relapse.

As would be predicted in a state of reduced fat mass, ghrelin levels are increased and leptin and insulin levels are reduced in AN.[26] However, because these changes are not sufficient to restore normal intake and fat mass, the possibility exists that patients with AN develop a relative resistance to ghrelin stimulation of food intake. There is also recent evidence that the expected alterations in ghrelin and insulin levels in response to a glucose load are delayed in patients with restrictive AN relative to controls; this may contribute to chronically reduced intake as well as the higher energy intake required to achieve weight gain in these patients.[27]

Cerebrospinal fluid (CSF) NPY levels are elevated in underweight patients with AN, and they return to normal with recovery. However, as with ghrelin, this is not effective in stimulating appetite. By comparison, CSF PYY levels are normal. Consistent with the stress response to starvation, the anorexigenic factor CRH is elevated in underweight individuals and likely contributes to chronically reduced intake. As previously noted, central serotonergic pathways that suppress appetite via activation of melanocortin signaling are also tonically activated in AN, contributing to reduced intake. Secondary effects of chronic starvation, such as ketosis and reduced gastric emptying, contribute to reduced appetite. Leptin levels normalize during refeeding prior to normalization of body weight and may contribute to ongoing resistance to increased food intake. While these alterations in neuropeptide activity regulating appetite typically correct with refeeding and weight gain, the process may take several months, necessitating long term therapy to prevent relapse.

Some comments are in order regarding potential interventions to modulate appetite and prevent relapse. The antihistamine cyproheptadine, which inhibits central serotonergic signaling, has been used in the past to acutely increase intake, resulting in weight gain in some studies. However, current data do not support the use of pharmacologic agents to acutely increase intake. Once body weight has increased with nutritional rehabilitation, fluoxetine, a selective serotonin reuptake inhibitor, may be considered as an adjunct to prevent relapse. Although patients with AN exhibit increased circulating levels of ghrelin, ghrelin administration in experimental settings has been shown to overcome the anorexia of chronic disease, and will likely also be evaluated in this setting.[28]

APPETITE REGULATION IN DISEASE

Normally, weight loss results in decreased circulating leptin levels, increased ghrelin levels, and a compensatory increase in caloric intake via up-regulation of NPY/AgRP neurons in the arcuate nucleus. However, in chronic diseases such as cancer, inflammatory bowel disease (IBD), AIDS, and chronic liver disease, such adaptive mechanisms may not be effective in maintaining ideal body weight. This may be due to a direct central effect of circulating cytokines, which are increased in these diseases and override the normal adaptive mechanisms involving leptin and ghrelin. Anorexia, which leads to decreased caloric intake relative to an individual's metabolic needs, is common in these conditions, and the malnutrition that results could significantly affect the course of the disease, leading to increased morbidity and mortality. Cachexia, with resultant increased energy expenditure, involuntary weight loss, and loss of fat and skeletal muscle mass, complicates anorexia of chronic disease. The pathophysiology of appetite dysregulation that occurs in chronic diseases will be discussed in the following sections, using cancer and IBD as representative examples.

Anorexia and Cachexia in Cancer

Anorexia is a common complication of cancer, occurring in approximately 50% of patients. The etiology is multifactorial, including disturbances in central mechanisms controlling appetite, altered taste perception, nausea, and altered gastric motility, all of which can combine to decrease caloric intake. Recent evidence suggests that proinflammatory cytokines, specifically tumor necrosis factor-α (TNF-α), interleukin-1 alpha and beta (IL-1α and IL-1β), and interleukin-6 (IL-6), elaborated by the immune system in response to the tumor or produced by the tumor itself, play a critical role in anorexia of cancer. Experimental models examining inflammatory cytokines produced in response to lipopolysaccharide (LPS), a bacterial product, have been critical in elucidating the role of these cytokines in the pathogenesis of anorexia of cancer and other chronic diseases. Intracerebroventicular administration of LPS results in increased mRNA expression of TNF-α and IL-1β in the brain, with the greatest concentrations in the hypothalamus.[29] The preferential expression of TNF-α and IL-1β in brain areas critical in appetite regulation suggests these cytokines are involved in anorexia seen in LPS treated animals. Similarly, in tumor bearing Lobund-Wistar rats, there is an increase in brain IL-1β mRNA expression, corresponding to early anorexia seen in these animals.[30] There is evidence for a role for TNF-α in cancer anorexia. The anorexia seen in tumor bearing rats is in part reversed by TNF-α blockade and results in increased food intake due to both increased meal number and size.[31]

Elevated circulating levels of these cytokines are consistently found in humans with cancer and other inflammatory conditions and correlate with development of anorexia-cachexia. A small study by Mantovani evaluating cytokine and leptin levels in patients with advanced cancer found higher circulating concentrations of TNF-α, IL-1, and IL-6 in patients with advanced cancer compared to healthy controls.[32] These findings provide further evidence for the involvement of cytokines in the pathogenesis of cancer anorexia and more broadly, anorexia of chronic inflammatory conditions, although the exact mechanism has yet to be elucidated. Proposed mechanisms include direct effects on arcuate nucleus neurons, elaboration of central intermediates involved in appetite regulation, and alteration of peripheral signals such as leptin.

Centrally, appetite is regulated through two competing systems located in the arcuate nucleus of the hypothalamus. NPY/AgRP neurons stimulate appetite while simultaneously inhibiting activation of the POMC/CART axis and production of secondary anorexigenic peptides, such as α-melanocyte stimulating hormone. In contrast, activation of POMC/CART neurons results in inhibition of appetite through up-regulation of melanocyte stimulating hormone, cocaine and amphetamine regulated transcript, and corticotropin releasing hormone. Persistent inappropriate inhibition of the NPY/AgRP axis or overactivation of POMC/CART neurons results in overall decreased appetite, and both pathways have been implicated in anorexia of disease and specifically cancer anorexia. Tumor bearing anorectic rats have decreased neuropeptide Y neuron expression within the hypothalamus[33] and significantly decreased concentrations of neuropeptide Y within the paraventricular nucleus.[34] Following tumor resection, neuropeptide Y concentrations return to normal.[34] Similar evidence exists for the role of the POMC/CART axis in cancer anorexia. Melanocortin 3/4 receptors, which are activated by the anorexigenic peptide α-melanocyte, play a critical role in this response. Treatment of anorexic tumor-bearing rats with the melanocortin receptor antagonist SHU9119 leads to normalization of food intake and subsequent weight gain.[35] Additionally, in experimental models, SHU9119 reverses the anorectic effects of IL-1β.[28] Based on these studies, it can be concluded that alteration of central regulatory mechanisms plays a key role in appetite suppression seen in cancer and other inflammatory diseases.

The serotonergic system also plays an important role in appetite regulation. Serotonin inhibits food intake by activation of the melanocortin system in the arcuate nucleus. Direct injection of IL-1β into the anterior hypothalamus results in transient increases in serotonin and its metabolites.[36] In anorexic tumor bearing rats, hypothalamic serotonin levels are elevated, and these levels return to normal after tumor resection.[34] Therefore, in addition to direct actions on the arcuate nucleus, it appears that proinflammatory cytokines indirectly affect these systems by elaboration of central intermediates including serotonin.

Leptin, which normally functions to inhibit overall food intake by activating POMC and inhibiting the NYP/AgRP axis, may also contribute to anorexia seen in chronic diseases. Leptin is induced by proinflammatory cytokines, and in animal models, administration of IL-1 and TNF-α results in increased leptin mRNA expression in adipocytes and increased circulating levels of leptin.[37,38] These findings persist in fasted or anorexic animals, conditions that normally lead to a compensatory decrease in circulating leptin levels. Additionally, leptin induces increased hypothalamic concentrations of IL-1,[39] with further inhibition of food intake via direct actions of IL-1 on arcuate nucleus neurons and up-regulation of central serotonin synthesis. Similar increases in serum leptin levels are seen in cancer patients treated with recombinant human IL-1α[40] or TNF-α,[41] and in the case of IL-1α, treatment is associated with a loss of appetite. However, leptin elevation in human diseases is typically transient, even after continued exposure to proinflammatory cytokines,[40] congruent with the findings of normal or even decreased leptin concentrations in patients with advanced cancer.[32] Therefore, up-regulation of leptin by cytokines including IL-1 may be more important in terms of suppressing appetite in acute inflammatory states, and relatively less important in chronic diseases.

Appetite Regulation in IBD

The principal cause of malnutrition in IBD is reduced caloric intake secondary to decreased appetite and early satiety (see also Chapter 31). While data for IBD are more limited than for cancer, studies have also supported central, cytokine-mediated mechanisms. In experimental colitis, serotonin released from the paraventricular nucleus is significantly higher in animals with colitis than in controls,[42] and central treatment with an IL-1 receptor antagonist significantly attenuates serotonin release, causing partial reversal of the anorexia seen in this model.[43] Leptin over-expression is seen in the early stages of experimentally induced colitis, corresponding to the decreased food intake seen in this animal model.[44] Data in humans is mixed—both elevated and normal leptin levels are reported in IBD. In acute ulcerative colitis, leptin levels are significantly elevated compared to healthy controls.[45] However, plasma leptin levels are reduced and correlate with reduced body fat mass in chronic IBD.[46] This disparity may be caused by tachyphylaxis with respect to cytokine up-regulation of leptin, with regulation primarily by fat mass in chronic disease despite ongoing inflammation. It is therefore likely that leptin's role in anorexia of IBD is limited to the acute phases of disease. Subsequent compensatory mechanisms with chronic weight loss then lead to normalization or depressed leptin expression and elevation of circulating ghrelin levels, which would be expected to stimulate appetite. However, continued impairment of central mechanisms controlling appetite override this compensatory response leading to persistent anorexia and weight loss. These may include primarily central up-regulation of serotonin by IL-1, thereby inhibiting intake via activation of the MC4R.[42]

Therapeutic Approaches to Anorexia of Chronic Disease

As outlined in previous sections, anorexia of chronic disease is a complex process involving both central and peripheral mediators, and so it is not surprising that treatment may be difficult. A variety of appetite stimulants have been used to enhance caloric intake in individuals. Cyproheptadine, which inhibits central serotonergic signaling, has been used for many years for anorexia. Although many individuals with advanced cancer have symptomatic improvement with cyproheptadine therapy, including decreased nausea and vomiting and a subjective increase in appetite, most continue to have progressive weight loss at a rate similar to that seen in placebo treated patients.[47] Other therapies, such as ondansetron, which antagonize serotonergic pathways, have had little success in increasing appetite and weight gain, despite effectively reducing nausea.[48] Treated individuals have enhancement of food enjoyment and improved hedonic scores for food items.

Megestrol acetate, a synthetic progestin, is another pharmacologic agent commonly used to treat anorexia and cachexia of chronic disease. The exact mechanism of action is not known. It is postulated that megestrol acetate has anticytokine effects.[49,50] Several randomized trials of megestrol acetate have demonstrated significant appetite stimulation and weight gain in anorexia associated with AIDS,[51] and it is currently approved by the FDA for this purpose. Megestrol acetate is efficacious for treating cancer anorexia.[50] Two recent systematic reviews of megestrol acetate, one analyzing clinical trials for the treatment of cancer anorexia and the other analyzing clinical trials for the treatment of anorexia-cachexia syndrome (including both cancer anorexia and AIDS anorexia) showed clear benefits of this therapy as measured by increased appetite and weight.[50,52] Quality of life was improved in treated cancer patients.[50] Although megestrol acetate is generally well tolerated, it has serious side effects, including thrombotic complications and adrenal insufficiency. Patients using megestrol acetate must be closely monitored. Patients with chronic inflammatory conditions must be especially carefully monitored because the risk of thrombosis is very high.

Other therapies that target cytokine pathways have had mixed results. Thalidomide suppresses production of TNF-α, a key mediator of anorexia of chronic disease, and preliminary studies of thalidomide in cancer anorexia suggest this agent might increase appetite.[53] However, adverse effects of thalidomide, such as teratogenicity, sedation, and peripheral neuropathy, could limit its widespread use. In contrast to thalidomide, pentoxifylline, a TNF inhibitor, had no benefit for cancer anorexia.[54]

Dronabinol, a cannabinoid derivative, is another FDA-approved therapy for the treatment of AIDS associated anorexia, and it has been shown to enhance appetite and stabilize weight in these patients.[55] Patients with cancer anorexia who are treated with dronabinol report a similar subjective improvement in appetite; however, when compared directly to megestrol acetate therapy, appetite improvement and weight gain are significantly less in patients treated with dronabinol.[56] Combination therapy with megestrol acetate and dronabinol provides no added benefit.[56]

Patients with chronic disease and weight loss typically have elevated circulating levels of ghrelin that are not sufficient to restore caloric intake and weight gain. It is possible that these individuals may be resistant to ghrelin in a manner similar to the leptin resistance observed in obesity. However, recent preclinical and clinical studies showed that ghrelin administration may exert beneficial anti-inflammatory and metabolic effects that promote increased intake and weight gain. Dixit et al. recently reported that ghrelin and the ghrelin receptor are expressed in human T lymphocytes and monocytes, the source for cytokines including TNF-α and IL-1β in chronic diseases.[57] Ghrelin reduced mononuclear cell cytokine production in a dose-dependent manner, and ghrelin administration attenuated LP-induced anorexia in a murine model. Short term studies demonstrated that ghrelin administration improves heart function in subjects with chronic heart failure and cachexia, and acutely increases caloric intake and the pleasure of eating in subjects with cancer and cachexia.[58,59] Importantly, chronic ghrelin administration ameliorates cachexia in animal models of chronic heart failure and cancer.[58,59] If chronic ghrelin administration is well tolerated and effective in patients with cachexia, it may provide an additional treatment option.

CONCLUSION

The regulatory systems that evolved to control intake and body weight are complex and redundant, and overall favor an anabolic state under basal conditions. This, combined with the ready availability of highly palatable calorically dense foods may contribute to the observed increase in obesity in developed countries. However, in chronic disease including cancer, AIDS, IBD, and congestive heart failure, central effects of proinflammatory cytokines can override the adaptive responses that would ordinarily maintain ideal body weight, leading to the anorexia-cachexia syndrome with its associated morbidity and mortality. A better understanding of these mechanisms will hopefully lead to improved therapeutic approaches. Strategies that are being evaluated include CB1 and ghrelin antagonists or PYY administration in obesity, and specific cytokine antagonists or ghrelin administration in anorexia of chronic disease. Currently, however, options for pharmacologic regulation of appetite are limited. Behavioral approaches for obesity and AN and provision of adequate supplemental nutrition for anorexia-cachexia of chronic disease remain the mainstay of therapy.

REFERENCES

1. Asakawa A, Inui A, Kaga T, et al. Ghrelin is an appetite-stimulatory signal from stomach with structural resemblance to motilin. *Gastroenterology.* 2001;120:337–345.
2. Hanada T, Toshinai K, Kajimura N, et al. Anti-cachectic effect of ghrelin in nude mice bearing human melanoma cells. *Biochem Biophys Res Commun.* 2003;301:275–279.
3. Andersson U, Filipsson K, Abbott CR, et al. AMP-activated protein kinase plays a role in the control of food intake. *J Biol Chem.* 2004;279:12005–12008.
4. Kalra SP, Kalra PS. Neuropeptide Y: a physiological orexigen modulated by the feedback action of ghrelin and leptin. *Endocrine.* 2003;22:49–56.
5. Morton GJ, Schwartz MW. The NPY/AgRP neuron and energy homeostasis. *Int J Obes Relat Metab Disord.* 2001;25(suppl 5):S56–62.
6. Cota D, Marsicano G, Lutz B, et al. Endogenous cannabinoid system as a modulator of food intake. *Int J Obes Relat Metab Disord.* 2003;27:289–301.
7. Sorensen LB, Moller P, Flint A, Martens M, Raben A. Effect of sensory perception of foods on appetite and food intake: a review of studies on humans. *Int J Obes Relat Metab Disord.* 2003;27:1152–1166.
8. Harrold JA, Williams G. The cannabinoid system: a role in both the homeostatic and hedonic control of eating? *Br J Nutr.* 2003;90:729–734.
9. Moran TH, Kinzig KP. Gastrointestinal satiety signals II: cholecystokinin. *Am J Physiol Gastrointest Liver Physiol.* 2004;286:G183–188.
10. Batterham RL, Cowley MA, Small CJ, et al. Gut hormone PYY(3-36) physiologically inhibits food intake. *Nature.* 2002;418:650–654.
11. Pico C, Oliver P, Sanchez J, Palou A. Gastric leptin: a putative role in the short-term regulation of food intake. *Br J Nutr.* 2003;90:735–741.
12. Havel PJ. Peripheral signals conveying metabolic information to the brain: short-term and long-term regulation of food intake and energy homeostasis. *Exp Biol Med (Maywood).* 2001;226:963–977.
13. Schwartz MW, Woods SC, Seeley RJ, Barsh GS, Baskin DG, Leibel RL. Is the energy homeostasis system inherently biased toward weight gain? *Diabetes.* 2003;52:232–238.
14. Levine AS, Kotz CM, Gosnell BA. Sugars and fats: the neurobiology of preference. *J Nutr.* 2003;133:831S–834S.
15. Figlewicz DP. Adiposity signals and food reward: expanding the CNS roles of insulin and leptin. *Am J Physiol Regul Integr Comp Physiol.* 2003;284:R882–892.
16. Frederich RC, Hamann A, Anderson S, Lollmann B, Lowell BB, Flier JS. Leptin levels reflect body lipid content in mice: evidence for diet-induced resistance to leptin action. *Nat Med.* 1995;1:1311–1314.
17. Considine RV, Sinha MK, Heiman ML, et al. Serum immunoreactive-leptin concentrations in normal-weight and obese humans. *N Engl J Med.* 1996;334:292–295.
18. Batterham RL, Cohen MA, Ellis SM, et al. Inhibition of food intake in obese subjects by peptide YY3-36. *N Engl J Med.* 2003;349:941–948.
19. Farooqi IS, Keogh JM, Yeo GS, Lank EJ, Cheetham T, O'Rahilly S. Clinical spectrum of obesity and mutations in the melanocortin 4 receptor gene. *N Engl J Med.* 2003;348:1085–1095.
20. Heisler LK, Cowley MA, Tecott LH, et al. Activation of central melanocortin pathways by fenfluramine. *Science.* 2002;297:609–611.
21. Foster AC, Joppa M, Markison S, et al. Body weight regulation by selective MC4 receptor agonists and antagonists. *Ann N Y Acad Sci.* 2003;994:103–110.
22. Cummings DE, Weigle DS, Frayo RS, et al. Plasma ghrelin levels after diet-induced weight loss or gastric bypass surgery. *N Engl J Med.* 2002;346:1623–1630.
23. Vink T, Hinney A, van Elburg AA, et al. Association between an agouti-related protein gene polymorphism and anorexia nervosa. *Mol Psychiatry.* 2001;6:325–328.
24. Kas MJ, van Dijk G, Scheurink AJ, Adan RA. Agouti-related protein prevents self-starvation. *Mol Psychiatry.* 2003;8:235–240.
25. Bailer UF, Kaye WH. A review of neuropeptide and neuroendocrine dysregulation in anorexia and bulimia nervosa. *Curr Drug Targets CNS Neurol Disord.* 2003;2:53–59.
26. Tolle V, Kadem M, Bluet-Pajot MT, et al. Balance in ghrelin and leptin plasma levels in anorexia nervosa patients and constitutionally thin women. *J Clin Endocrinol Metab.* 2003;88:109–116.
27. Tanaka M, Tatebe Y, Nakahara T, et al. Eating pattern and the effect of oral glucose on ghrelin and insulin secretion in patients with anorexia nervosa. *Clin Endocrinol (Oxf).* 2003;59:574–579.
28. Lawrence CB, Rothwell NJ. Anorexic but not pyrogenic actions of interleukin-1 are modulated by central melanocortin-3/4 receptors in the rat. *J Neuroendocrinol.* 2001;13:490–495.
29. Ilyin SE, Gayle D, Flynn MC, Plata-Salaman CR. Interleukin-1 beta system (ligand, receptor type I, receptor accessory protein and receptor antagonist), TNF-alpha, TGF-beta1 and neuropeptide Y mRNAs in specific brain regions during bacterial LPS-induced anorexia. *Brain Res Bull.* 1998;45:507–515.
30. Plata-Salaman CR, Ilyin SE, Gayle D. Brain cytokine mRNAs in anorectic rats bearing prostate adenocarcinoma tumor cells. *Am J Physiol.* 1998;275:R566–573.

31. Torelli GF, Meguid MM, Moldawer LL, et al. Use of recombinant human soluble TNF receptor in anorectic tumor-bearing rats. *Am J Physiol.* 1999;277:R850–855.

32. Mantovani G, Maccio A, Mura L, et al. Serum levels of leptin and proinflammatory cytokines in patients with advanced-stage cancer at different sites. *J Mol Med.* 2000;78:554–561.

33. Makarenko IG, Meguid MM, Gatto L, Chen C, Ugrumov MV. Decreased NPY innervation of the hypothalamic nuclei in rats with cancer anorexia. *Brain Res.* 2003;961:100–108.

34. Meguid MM, Ramos EJ, Laviano A, et al. Tumor anorexia: effects on neuropeptide Y and monoamines in paraventricular nucleus. *Peptides.* 2004;25:261–266.

35. Wisse BE, Frayo RS, Schwartz MW, Cummings DE. Reversal of cancer anorexia by blockade of central melanocortin receptors in rats. *Endocrinology.* 2001;142:3292–3301.

36. Shintani F, Kanba S, Nakaki T, et al. Interleukin-1 beta augments release of norepinephrine, dopamine, and serotonin in the rat anterior hypothalamus. *J Neurosci.* 1993;13:3574–3581.

37. Grunfeld C, Zhao C, Fuller J, et al. Endotoxin and cytokines induce expression of leptin, the ob gene product, in hamsters. *J Clin Invest.* 1996;97:2152–2157.

38. Sarraf P, Frederich RC, Turner EM, et al. Multiple cytokines and acute inflammation raise mouse leptin levels: potential role in inflammatory anorexia. *J Exp Med.* 1997;185:171–175.

39. Luheshi GN, Gardner JD, Rushforth DA, Loudon AS, Rothwell NJ. Leptin actions on food intake and body temperature are mediated by IL-1. *Proc Natl Acad Sci U S A.* 1999;96:7047–7052.

40. Janik JE, Curti BD, Considine RV, et al. Interleukin 1 alpha increases serum leptin concentrations in humans. *J Clin Endocrinol Metab* 1997;82:3084–3086.

41. Zumbach MS, Boehme MW, Wahl P, Stremmel W, Ziegler R, Nawroth PP. Tumor necrosis factor increases serum leptin levels in humans. *J Clin Endocrinol Metab.* 1997;82:4080–4082.

42. Ballinger A, El-Haj T, Perrett D, et al. The role of medial hypothalamic serotonin in the suppression of feeding in a rat model of colitis. *Gastroenterology.* 2000;118:544–553.

43. El-Haj T, Poole S, Farthing MJ, Ballinger AB. Anorexia in a rat model of colitis: interaction of interleukin-1 and hypothalamic serotonin. *Brain Res.* 2002;927:1–7.

44. Barbier M, Cherbut C, Aube AC, Blottiere HM, Galmiche JP. Elevated plasma leptin concentrations in early stages of experimental intestinal inflammation in rats. *Gut.* 1998;43:783–790.

45. Tuzun A, Uygun A, Yesilova Z, et al. Leptin levels in the acute stage of ulcerative colitis. *J Gastroenterol Hepatol.* 2004;19:429–432.

46. Ballinger A, Kelly P, Hallyburton E, Besser R, Farthing M. Plasma leptin in chronic inflammatory bowel disease and HIV: implications for the pathogenesis of anorexia and weight loss. *Clin Sci (Lond).* 1998;94:479–483.

47. Kardinal CG, Loprinzi CL, Schaid DJ, et al. A controlled trial of cyproheptadine in cancer patients with anorexia and/or cachexia. *Cancer.* 1990;65:2657–2662.

48. Edelman MJ, Gandara DR, Meyers FJ, et al. Serotonergic blockade in the treatment of the cancer anorexia-cachexia syndrome. *Cancer.* 1999;86:684–688.

49. Mantovani G, Maccio A, Lai P, Massa E, Ghiani M, Santona MC. Cytokine involvement in cancer anorexia/cachexia: role of megestrol acetate and medroxyprogesterone acetate on cytokine down regulation and improvement of clinical symptoms. *Crit Rev Oncog.* 1998;9:99–106.

50. Pascual Lopez A, Roque i Figuls M, Urrutia Cuchi G, et al. Systematic review of megestrol acetate in the treatment of anorexia-cachexia syndrome. *J Pain Symptom Manage.* 2004;27:360–369.

51. Von Roenn JH. Randomized trials of megestrol acetate for AIDS-associated anorexia and cachexia. *Oncology.* 1994;51(suppl 1):19–24.

52. Maltoni M, Nanni O, Scarpi E, Rossi D, Serra P, Amadori D. High-dose progestins for the treatment of cancer anorexia-cachexia syndrome: a systematic review of randomised clinical trials. *Ann Oncol.* 2001;12:289–300.

53. Bruera E, Neumann CM, Pituskin E, Calder K, Ball G, Hanson J. Thalidomide in patients with cachexia due to terminal cancer: preliminary report. *Ann Oncol.* 1999;10:857–859.

54. Goldberg RM, Loprinzi CL, Mailliard JA, et al. Pentoxifylline for treatment of cancer anorexia and cachexia? A randomized, double-blind, placebo-controlled trial. *J Clin Oncol.* 1995;13:2856–2859.

55. Beal JE, Olson R, Laubenstein L, et al. Dronabinol as a treatment for anorexia associated with weight loss in patients with AIDS. *J Pain Symptom Manage.* 1995;10:89–97.

56. Jatoi A, Windschitl HE, Loprinzi CL, et al. Dronabinol versus megestrol acetate versus combination therapy for cancer-associated anorexia: a north central cancer treatment group study. *J Clin Oncol.* 2002;20:567–573.

57. Dixit VD, Schaffer EM, Pyle RS, et al. Ghrelin inhibits leptin- and activation-induced proinflammatory cytokine expression by human monocytes and T cells. *J Clin Invest.* 2004;114:57–66.

58. Nagaya N, Kangawa K. Ghrelin, a novel growth hormone-releasing peptide, in the treatment of chronic heart failure. *Regul Pept.* 2003;114:71–77.

59. Neary NM, Small CJ, Wren AM, et al. Ghrelin increases energy intake in cancer patients with impaired appetite: acute, randomized, placebo-controlled trial. *J Clin Endocrinol Metab.* 2004;89:2832–2836.

CHAPTER 12

Feeding and Swallowing Issues Relevant to Pediatric Nutrition Support

Joan C. Arvedson and Colin D. Rudolph

INTRODUCTION

Breathing and eating are among the most important functions for survival of all living beings. For humans, breathing should be nearly automatic and usually does not require active effort unless there are complicating factors. Eating does require active effort and exquisite timing and coordination for sucking, swallowing, and breathing in infants. Older children must have adequate protection of the airway, sufficient strength of muscle action, and coordination of the phases of swallowing to prevent aspiration and to take adequate volume of food and liquid to meet nutrition and hydration needs efficiently and safely.

After the establishment of adequate breathing, the highest priority for caregivers is to meet nutritional needs of infants and children. To accomplish this successfully, children require a functional oral sensorimotor system and swallowing mechanism, overall adequate health (including respiratory, gastrointestinal, and neurologic function), central nervous system integration, and musculoskeletal tone. In addition, an often overlooked process, the successful emergence of communication skills depends upon successful feeding and swallowing. Normal feeding patterns reflect the early developmental pathways that are the basis for later communication skills. The interrelationship between feeding (shared by all biological creatures) and complex oral communication (unique to humans) cannot be overstated. The study of comparative anatomy and its implications for human communication are well described.[1] The purposes of this chapter are to provide an overview of (1) development of feeding and swallowing skills to include critical/sensitive periods with implications for behavioral and sensory based feeding problems, (2) impact of taste and smell on oral feeding, (3) clinical assessment of pediatric swallowing and feeding disorders, (4) instrumental examination of such disorders, and (5) management of those disorders.

DEVELOPMENT OF FEEDING AND SWALLOWING SKILLS

Prenatal Swallowing and Suckling

The pharyngeal swallow begins during the 10th to 11th weeks of fetal life. It is one of the first motor responses in the pharynx. Pharyngeal swallows have been observed in delivered fetuses at 12.5 weeks of gestation.[2] A suckling response can be elicited by stroking the lips at this stage.[3] Taste can modify the frequency of suckling motions. Taste buds are evident at 7 weeks of gestation. Distinctively mature receptors are noted at 12 weeks of gestation.[4]

True suckling is not expected to begin until around the 18th to 24th week. A definite backward and forward movement of the tongue characterizes early suckling. Because the tongue fills the oral cavity at this stage of development, this backward and forward movement of the tongue is all that can be expected. The backward movement appears more pronounced than the forward movement, while the tongue protrusion does not extend beyond the border of the lips. Serial ultrasound images show that suckling motions increase in frequency in the later months of fetal life.[5] By 34 weeks of gestation, a healthy preterm infant likely suckles and swallows well enough to sustain nutrition through oral feedings. Some healthy preterm infants have sufficiently coordinated suck, swallow, and breathe patterns to begin oral feeding by 32 to 33 weeks of gestation.[6]

Decreased rates of fetal suckling are associated with digestive tract obstruction or neurologic damage. Intrauterine growth retardation may be a manifestation of neurologic damage.[7] Bosma reported that the fetus swallows about 450–500 mL of amniotic fluid per day (of the total 850 mL) and excretes about the same amount in urine.[8] Lack of regular swallowing by the fetus should lead one to suspect problems that may be related primarily to the fetus or the mother. Maternal polyhydramnios is one such condition that is described as excessive amniotic fluid in the uterus. In about 15% of these cases, a fetal anomaly occurs. As the severity increases, the likelihood of detecting a congenital malformation increases.

Progression of Feeding and Swallowing Skills from Infancy Through Early Childhood

Term infants typically show food seeking behavior through rooting. Preterm infants gradually achieve skills for rooting, suckling, swallowing, and true oral feeding as they advance toward term. Important early developmental milestones are shown in Table 12-1.[9,10]

Feeding and swallowing skill acquisition is critical to infants and young children as they develop self-regulation that eventually leads to independent feeding. Oral sensorimotor skills improve with general neurodevelopment, acquisition of muscle control that includes posture and tone, cognition and language, and psychosocial skills. The development of independent, socially acceptable feeding processes begins at birth and progresses throughout the first few years of childhood[11] (see Table 12-2).

Table 12-1 Gestational ages for swallowing and suckling functions.

Swallowing function	*Gestational age (weeks)*
Pharyngeal swallow	10–12
True suckling	18–24
Sustain nutrition totally oral	34–37

Critical and Sensitive Periods with Implications for Behavioral and Sensory Based Feeding Problems

The concept of critical or sensitive time periods in overall human development is controversial, but well documented in some areas of development and in animal research. Lorenz interpreted findings from embryological studies to imply that there is a period during early development when the organism is primed to receive and perhaps permanently encode important environmental information.[12] These interpretations do not mean that later learning is not important, but they do highlight the possible significance of these early experiences.

Critical or sensitive periods also exist in the development of normal feeding behavior. Critical periods in the development of feeding typically focus on the introduction of chewable textures[13] (Table 12-2). Children develop oral side preferences for chewing that relate to hand preferences in many instances.[14] Chewing skills vary according to food textures. Children develop mature chewing skills for solid foods earlier than for viscous and pureed foods.[15] Yet it is common practice that children who have not mastered the timing and coordination for swallowing purees and other smooth food are often not given experience with appropriate chewable food. Children may also fail to develop the foundations for chewing. Solid foods must be introduced at the most appropriate times or children may experience developmental delays or disabilities. One can assume that children with devel-

Table 12-2 Neurodevelopmental milestones and feeding skills, birth to 36 months.

Age (months)	*Development/posture*	*Feeding/oral sensorimotor*
Birth to 4–6	Balanced flexor and extensor tone of neck and trunk. Visual fixation and tracking. Learning to control body against gravity. Sitting with support near end of this period. Rolling over. Hands to mouth.	Nipple feeding, breast or bottle. Hand on bottle during feeding (2–4 months). Maintains semiflexed posture during feeding. Promotion of infant–parent interaction.
6–9 (transition feeding)	Sitting independently for short time. Oral stimulation by self (mouthing hands and toys). Extended reach with pincer grasp. Visual interest in small objects. Object permanence. Stranger anxiety. Crawling on belly, creeping on all fours.	Feeding in more upright position. Spoon feeding introduced for thin, smooth puree. Suckle pattern initially. Suckle → Suck. Both hands used to hold bottle. Finger feeding introduced. Vertical munching easily dissolvable solids. Parents preferred for feeding.
9–12	Pull to stand. Cruise: walks along furniture. First steps by 12 months. Assisting with spoon; some become independent. Pincer grasp refined.	Cup drinking. Takes lumpy, mashed food. Independent finger feeding with easily dissolvable solids. Chewing with some rotary jaw action.
12–18	Refinement of all gross and fine motor skills. Walking independently. Climbs stairs. Runs. Grasps and releases with precision.	Self-feeding: grasps spoon with whole hand. Holds cup with 2 hands. Drinks with 4–5 consecutive swallows. Holds and tips bottle by self.
18–24	Equilibrium improves with refinement of upper extremity coordination. Increasing attention and persistence in play activities. Parallel or imitative play. Independence from parents. Use of tools.	Swallows with lip closure. Self-feeding predominates. Chewable foods—broad range. Up/down tongue movements precise.
24–36	Refinement of skills. Jumps in place. Pedals tricycle. Uses scissors.	Circulatory jaw rotations. Lip closure with chewing. One-handed cup holding and open cup drinking without spilling. Fills spoon with fingers. Solid foods: wider range. Total self-feeding; uses fork.

Source: Adapted from Rogers B, Campbell J. Pediatric and neurodevelopmental evaluation. In: Arvedson J, Brodsky L, eds. *Pediatric Swallowing and Feeding: Assessment and Management.* San Diego, Calif: Singular Publishing Group, Inc.; 1993:55, and Arvedson JC, Brodsky L, eds. *Pediatric Swallowing and Feeding: Assessment and Management.* 2nd ed. Albany, NY: Singular–Thomson Learning; 2002:62–67.

opmental disabilities or delays not only missed this critical period for chewing, but also missed the foundations for chewing skills that include trunk and neck stability, mobility of limbs and head, and chewing experiences involving hands, fingers, and toys. Physiologic processes that underlie feeding and swallowing ability, including respiratory control, also have critical periods that can impact the feeding process.[16]

Psychosocial development, personality, and environmental factors may also impact feeding issues. Some children demonstrate aversive behaviors toward certain food textures, tastes, or temperatures. They might be hypersensitive to tight clothes or tags on their clothes. They might not like to wear shoes. They might not like to get their hands dirty, so they do not want to do finger painting or put their fingers into pudding or other pureed food. Children may reject solids upon initial presentation if they are introduced after the critical periods. The longer the delay in the introduction of solids, the more difficult it is for many children to accept texture changes. Withholding solids at a time when a child should be able to chew (6 to 7 months developmental level) can result in food refusal and even vomiting.[13] These difficulties are likely to have significant impact on nutrition and hydration status in children.

The concept of critical and sensitive periods can also be applied to the mother in relation to the young infant. A sensitive period in the mother may be an important factor in the potential for efficient feeding and global development of an infant.[17] Maternal early contact with premature and term infants has been shown to have a positive effect on the mother's attachment behavior and ultimately to enhance development of the child.

Preterm infants with major physical and physiologic conditions that prevent them from initiating oral feeding in the expected time periods may demonstrate significant difficulty and delay in getting to oral feeding. There are significant variations in the form and function of the ingestive system when comparing gestational age matched healthy infants with at risk infants. A study by Miller et al. found that fetal swallowing primarily occurred in the presence of concomitant oral facial stimulation. These interrelating factors appear consistent with the concepts of critical and sensitive periods for young infants. Perhaps some infants missed critical periods while still in the womb. Miller and colleagues postulate that prenatal development indices of emerging aerodigestive skills may guide postnatal decisions for feeding readiness and, ultimately, advance the care of the premature, medically fragile neonate.[5]

Studies in mice show that early oral experience may affect the later development of nonoral skills. Postweaning feeding of a soft, powdered diet instead of the usual hard, pelleted diet resulted in the development of fewer synapses in the hippocampus and parietal cortex, as well as subsequent impaired spatial learning ability. Similar deficits could result from the lack of experience and exposure to age-appropriate foods in humans, providing a conceptual framework to explain clinical observations of the challenges encountered in the learning of oral sensorimotor and other skills in children not fed during critical/sensitive periods for oral skill development.[18]

IMPACT OF TASTE AND SMELL ON ORAL FEEDING

Knowledge of infants' sensory world, especially as it relates to flavors, has significant implications for acceptance of new foods of different textures, temperatures, and tastes. There are also implications for physicians and dietitians who guide parents when children are failing to thrive or have a limited range of foods in their diet. Initial experiences with flavors occur prior to birth, since the flavor of amniotic fluid changes as a function of the dietary choices of the mother. Flavors from the mother's diet during pregnancy are transmitted to amniotic fluid, which are not only perceived by the fetus, but enhance the acceptance and enjoyment of that flavor in a food during weaning from the breast.[19] The ability to detect additional tastes and flavors develops after birth. Thus, it is clear that early sensory experiences have an impact on the acceptance of flavors and foods during infancy and childhood.

The human infant possesses a sensory apparatus that can detect sweet tastes. Tatzer and colleagues studied preterm infants who had been fed exclusively via gastric tubes. These infants were presented with minute amounts of either glucose or water solutions intraorally. They exhibited more nonnutritive suckling in response to glucose than to water.[20] Infants have been noted to produce more frequent and stronger suckling responses when offered a sucrose sweetened nipple compared with a latex nipple.[21]

Over the long term, exposure to flavors in breast milk could serve to heighten preferences for these flavors and facilitate the weaning process. Some breastfed infants are more willing to accept a novel vegetable upon first presentation than are formula fed infants.[22] Children who have been breastfed for at least 6 months are also less likely to become picky eaters.[23]

The human newborn is indifferent to and may not detect salt taste. Infants are typically about 4 months of age when they demonstrate the ability to detect and prefer salt.[24] This developmental change may reflect postnatal maturation of central and/or peripheral mechanisms underlying salt taste perception, as has been demonstrated in animal model studies.[25] The preference that emerges at this age appears to be largely unlearned.

An example of the importance of early exposure is found in the acceptance of protein hydrolysate formulas. There appears to be a sensitive period in early infancy when preferences for flavors characteristic of hydrolyzed protein are established as suggested by the finding that infants who are 7 months and older avidly accept these formulas if they experienced them during the first months of life. Infants at 1–2 months of age readily accept protein hydrolysate formula when compared to their regular milk or soy-based formula. However, 7 to 8 month old infants who had no previous experience with hydrolysate formulas strongly rejected them and displayed extreme and immediate facial grimaces, similar to those observed in newborns in response to bitter and sour tastes.[26]

The examples regarding differences in flavor acceptance that occur from breastfed to bottle fed infants and changes over time demonstrate multiple variables that must be considered when professionals make decisions regarding feeding of infants and young children. The sensory factors have to be examined along with motor skills. The interactions of sensory and motor factors are complex.

CLINICAL ASSESSMENT OF PEDIATRIC SWALLOWING AND FEEDING DISORDERS

The clinical evaluation of an infant or child with complex issues related to feeding and swallowing includes a thorough history and physical examination, including oral sensorimotor and feeding observation. Some patients may need instrumental assessments of swallowing (see Instrumental Examination of Swallowing, later in this chapter) in addition to the clinical evaluation. Most children are best served in the context of an interdisciplinary team, but such teams are available only in a limited number of medical centers. This chapter provides information that should be useful for physicians and dietitians who do not have an interdisciplinary team available. Particular attention is paid to factors that are likely to interfere with adequate nutrition and hydration.

The feeding history is critical to decision making. Swallowing and feeding disorders in infants and children are complex and can have multiple etiologies (see Table 12-3).[27] Perceptions of feeding problems differ among reporters. Thus, it is helpful for all examiners to get information from more than one caregiver or professional involved with the child. Questions are best asked in ways to delineate the feeding status as clearly as possible. Table 12-4 lists the questions that can be asked by a professional in any discipline involved with the child.

In most cultures, a child who requires more than 30–40 minutes to feed on a regular basis is considered to have a feeding problem. The prolonged feeding time by itself does not define the nature

Table 12-3 Causes of feeding disorders in children.

- Disorders that affect appetite, food-seeking behavior, and ingestion
  - Depression
  - Deprivation
  - Central nervous system disease (diencephalic syndrome)
  - Metabolic diseases
    - Hereditary fructose intolerance
    - Urea cycle disorders
    - Organic acidemias
  - Sensory defects
    - Anosmia
    - Blindness
  - Neuromuscular disease (see Disorders affecting neuromuscular coordination of swallowing, later in this table)
  - Oral hypersensitivity or aversion resulting from a lack of feeding experience during critical sensitive periods (long term parenteral or enteral feeding)
  - Conditioned dysphagia
    - Aspiration
    - Oral inflammation (see Mucosal infections and inflammatory disorders causing dysphagia)
    - Gastroesophageal reflux
    - Dumping syndrome or gastric bloating after gastric surgery
    - Fatigue (heart disease, lung disease)
  - Poverty
  - Anorexia nervosa
  - Autism (food selectivity)
- Anatomic abnormalities of the oropharynx
  - Cleft lip and/or palate
  - Macroglossia
  - Ankyloglossia
  - Pierre Robin sequence
  - Retropharyngeal mass or abscess
  - Velopharyngeal insufficiency
  - Tonsillar hypertrophy
  - Dental caries
- Anatomic/congenital abnormalities of the larynx and trachea
  - Laryngeal cleft
  - Laryngomalacia
  - Laryngeal cyst
  - Subglottic stenosis
  - Tracheomalacia
  - Tracheoesophageal cleft
  - Tracheoesophageal compression from vascular ring/sling
- Anatomic abnormalities of the esophagus and bowel
  - Tracheoesophageal fistula
  - Congenital esophageal atresia
  - Congenital esophageal stenosis because of tracheobronchial remnants
  - Esophageal stricture, web or ring
  - Esophageal mass or tumor
  - Foreign body
  - Vascular rings and dysphagia lusorum
  - Microgastria
  - Antral webs
  - Intestinal strictures
  - Intestinal malrotation
- Disorders affecting suck-swallow-breathing coordination
  - Choanal atresia
  - Bronchopulmonary dysplasia
  - Cardiac disease
  - Tachypnea (respiratory rates > 60/min
- Disorders affecting neuromuscular coordination of swallowing
  - Cerebral palsy
  - Bulbar atresia or palsy
  - Brain-stem glioma
  - Arnold-Chiari malformation
  - Myelomeningocele
  - Familial dysautonomia
  - Tardive dyskinesia
  - Nitrazepam-induced dysphagia
  - Postdiphtheritic and postpolio paralysis
  - Möbius syndrome (cranial nerve abnormalities)
  - Myasthenia gravis
  - Infant botulism
  - Congenital myotonic dystrophy
  - Oculopharyngeal dystrophy
  - Muscular dystrophies and myopathies
  - Cricopharyngeal achalasia
  - Polymyositis/dermatomyositis
  - Rheumatoid arthritis
- Disorders affecting esophageal peristalsis
  - Achalasia
  - Chagas' disease
  - Diffuse esophageal spasm
  - Pseudo-obstruction
  - Scleroderma
  - Mixed connective tissue disease
  - Systemic lupus erythematosus
  - Polymyositis/dermatomyositis
  - Rheumatoid arthritis
- Mucosal infections and inflammatory disorders causing dysphagia
  - Adenotonsillitis
  - Deep neck space infections
  - Epiglottitis
  - Laryngopharyngeal reflux from gastroesophageal reflux
  - Gastroesophageal reflux (GER)
  - Caustic ingestion
  - Candida pharyngitis or esophagitis
  - Herpes simplex esophagitis
  - Human immunodeficiency virus
  - Cytomegalovirus esophagitis
  - Medication-induced esophagitis
  - Crohn's disease
  - Behcet's disease
  - Chronic graft-versus-host disease
- Other miscellaneous disorders associated with feeding and swallowing difficulties
  - Xerostomia
  - Hypothyroidism
  - Neonatal hyperparathyroidism
  - Trisomy 18 and 21
  - Velocardiofacial syndrome
  - Prader-Willi syndrome
  - Williams syndrome
  - Coffin-Siris syndrome
  - Opitz-G syndrome
  - Cornelia de Lange syndrome
  - Interstitial deletion (13)(q21.3q31)
  - Allergies
  - Lipid and lipoprotein metabolism disorders
  - Neurofibromatosis
  - Globus pharyngeus
  - Epidermolysis bullosa dystrophica

Source: Link DT, Rudolph CD. Feeding and swallowing. In: Rudolph CD, Rudolph AM, eds. *Rudolph's Pediatrics.* 21st ed. New York, NY: McGraw-Hill; 2003:1382. Used with permission.

Table 12-4 Questions to ask in assessing feeding disorders.

How long does it take to feed the child?
Is the child independent for feeding or dependent on others?
Does the child eat entirely by mouth or are supplemental tube feedings necessary?
Does the feeding problem vary with differences in food types, textures, temperature, or tastes?
Does the feeding problem change from beginning to middle to end of the meal?
Does the feeding problem vary with time of day or who is administering the meal?
Does the child maintain midline posture with no additional support? If not, what are the postural problems?
Are there any signs of breathing difficulty during feeding?
Does the child have emesis? If yes, when and how much?
Does the child refuse food? If yes, what are the circumstances?
Does the child get irritable, sleepy, or lethargic during mealtime?
How do the child and the caregiver interact? Are there signs of forced feeding?

---

of the problem. Prolonged meal times may relate to the child's oral sensorimotor deficits, airway issues, risk for aspiration and parent–child interaction or behavior based problems. Independent feeders usually, but not always, have better coordination for functional swallow production than those with neurologic problems that make it difficult to hold the head upright or to produce swallows without delay. Children with cerebral palsy who are dependent feeders often demonstrate reduced oxygen saturation during feeding,[28] and they have a greater probability for silent aspiration.[29]

Many caregivers perceive total oral feeding as a marker of success. However, if the child is at risk for undernutrition, tube feeding allows for nutrition and hydration needs to be met without placing undue risk on the respiratory system and/or the energy levels required for feeding orally.

A child's feeding problem may vary with differences in food textures, temperatures, tastes, or types of food. Aspiration and pharyngeal motility deficits can be texture specific.[30] Children with anatomic abnormalities, such as esophageal webs, strictures, or vascular rings, may have difficulty progressing to solid foods. Children with incoordination of the oral and pharyngeal phases of swallowing or with a delay in initiating a pharyngeal swallow are at greater risk for aspiration with thin liquids than with thicker textures. Some children prefer sour or spicy food over bland food, crunchy versus smooth, cold versus warm, or vice versa. These attributes usually interact and have effects on efficiency and pleasure of feeding.

Children who are orally defensive commonly demonstrate little or no hunger, have poor appetites, have postural problems, have breakdowns in child–parent interactions and show more difficulty before or at the beginning of the mealtime. Children with oral sensorimotor and swallowing deficits may demonstrate more problems as the meal progresses due to fatigue, compromised cardiopulmonary function, and oropharyngeal dysphagia.

Environmental factors that can alter mealtime efficiency need to be explored. They can include differences in feeding methods practiced by different caregivers, possible distractions at mealtimes (e.g., other children, television, pets), appetite suppressants, and fatigue factors.

Body position is important for efficient feeding. Children with cerebral palsy and some other neurologic diagnoses frequently show extensor arching of the trunk and extremities while feeding. The risks for aspiration could be greater for the child with this posture than for the child who sits upright with good head control. At the other extreme is the child with hypotonia who has a "floppy" neck. That child could have increased risk for aspiration because of excessive flexion of the oropharynx.

Changes in respiratory effort and/or rate should be investigated thoroughly. The work of breathing has to take precedence over the work of feeding. Any risks for aspiration with oral feeding must be delineated.

Children with neurogenic dysphagia have a high incidence of gastroesophageal reflux ranging from 15–65%.[31–33] Many of these children have no evidence of emesis.

Food refusal can occur as a result of multiple problems that include, but are not limited to, airway, GI tract, oral sensorimotor, and behavior (e.g., parent–child interaction abnormalities). Infants and young children have limited ways to communicate their stresses. Thus, food refusal may be the way the child can let others know that something is not working well.

Gastrointestinal problems and/or airway problems may present as irritability. Irritability can also represent a behavior. Lethargy at mealtime may relate to excessive fatigue, recurrent seizures, or medications with sedative effects (e.g., anticonvulsants, muscle relaxants).

Parental stress related to feeding can be transmitted to a child, who in turn exacerbates the feeding difficulties. Forced feeding seldom leads to feeding success. Complications are more apt to follow (e.g., food refusal, failure to thrive) and other more global behavior maladaptations.[34,35]

INSTRUMENTAL EXAMINATION OF SWALLOWING

Instrumental examinations may be needed for infants and children, particularly when pharyngeal and esophageal physiology needs to be delineated objectively to answer specific questions related to the safety and efficiency of oral feeding. The decision regarding which examination will be used and when it will be used depends on multiple factors.[36–38] The instrument chosen for each examination depends on which anatomic areas and functional processes need to be assessed. In most cases, infants and children with feeding and swallowing problems require a videofluoroscopic swallow study (VFSS) and/or a fiber optic endoscopic examination of swallowing (FEES). Ultrasound (US) is most helpful in describing oral preparatory and oral phases of swallowing, especially in young infants.[39]

VFSS is the primary technique for detailed dynamic imaging of oral, pharyngeal, and upper esophageal phases of a swallow.[40,41] VFSS is useful for diagnostic purposes; its primary focus is on the pharyngeal phase in relation to the oral phase and the upper esophageal phase. Interpretation is made in light of clinical findings, history, and other health-related issues. At times, a review of normal findings with a child who has a history of a choking event or some other traumatic event related to swallowing will enable that child to return to successful oral feeding. It is common to find that following a traumatic event the child may refuse all solid food.

For infants and children, a pediatric otolaryngologist and speech-language pathologist typically perform the FEES, which can include sensory testing.[42] Findings should help to clarify the oral feeding status, particularly in children with developmental disabilities and neurologic impairments.[43, 44]

MANAGEMENT OF PEDIATRIC FEEDING AND SWALLOWING PROBLEMS

Management decisions are made in light of the total child with consideration for medical/surgical, nutrition, oral sensorimotor, behavioral, and psychosocial factors. There are multiple approaches to intervention when infants and children have primary problems in any of the major areas. All oral sensorimotor and behavioral approaches must take into account the child's airway stability and nutrition/hydration status. Initial efforts to improve caloric intake may include adjustment of texture and increases in caloric density of food. However, assuring intake of adequate fluids may be challenging.

Oral sensorimotor treatment is typically focused on improving function of the structures that are under voluntary neurologic control and are used for bolus formation, i.e., jaw, lips, cheeks, tongue, and palate. Techniques vary widely among therapists. Some children appear to improve function with food varied by textures, tastes, and temperatures. Others require changes in position and postural support. A parent or therapist may tap or stroke the face and inside the mouth believing that this kind of stimulation will "wake up the system," and in turn the child will swallow more quickly and more firmly. Specific exercises may be incorporated with a goal of improved strength and/or coordination.[10]

Placement of a feeding gastrostomy tube often relieves stress on the caregivers by allowing a freedom from fear of malnutrition. More efficient caloric delivery also frees time for other more pleasurable interactions with the child. However, it is important to continue some oral therapy to assure continued experience and maximal development of oral skills over time.

CONCLUSION

As discussed in this chapter, establishing appropriate nutrition involves a functional ingestive system. The development of this system requires a complex interaction of genetic, developmental, environmental, and social factors. We are only beginning to understand how these factors work, alone and together. Science based data are needed. The primary goal of all therapeutic approaches is safe and pleasurable oral feeding, whether for limited quantities and types of food for practice and pleasure or for total oral feeding. However, such interventions must never jeopardize pulmonary and nutritional well-being.

REFERENCES

1. Laitman J, Reidenberg J. Specializations of the human upper respiratory and upper digestive systems as seen through comparative and developmental anatomy. *Dysphagia.* 1993;8:318–325.
2. Humphrey T. Reflex activity in the oral and facial area of the human fetus. In: Bosma JF, ed. *Second Symposium on Oral Sensation and Perception.* 1967. Springfield, Ill: Charles C. Thomas; 1967:195–233.
3. Moore KL. *The Developing Human: Clinically Oriented Embryology.* 4th ed. Philadelphia, Pa: W.B. Saunders; 1998.
4. Miller AJ. Deglutition. *Physiol Rev.* 1982;62:129–184.
5. Miller JL, Sonies BC, Macedonia C. Emergence of oropharyngeal, laryngeal and swallowing activity in the developing fetal upper aerodigestive tract: an ultrasound evaluation. *Ear Hum Dev.* 2003;71(1):61–87.
6. Cagan J. Feeding readiness behavior in preterm infants [Abstract]. *Neonatal Newsweek.*1995; 14:82.
7. Derkay C, Schechter F. Anatomy and physiology of pediatric swallowing disorders. *Dysphagia.* 1998;13:397–404.
8. Bosma JF. Development of feeding. *Clin Nutr.* 1986;5:210–218.
9. Rogers B, Campbell J. Pediatric and neurodevelopmental evaluation. In: Arvedson J, Brodsky L, eds. *Pediatric Swallowing and Feeding: Assessment and Management.* San Diego, Calif: Singular Publishing Group, Inc.; 1993:55–67.
10. Arvedson JC, Brodsky L, eds. *Pediatric Swallowing and Feeding: Assessment and Management.* 2nd ed. Albany, NY: Singular–Thomson Learning; 2002.
11. Pridham KF, Martin R, Sondel S, Tluczek A. Parental issues in feeding young children with bronchopulmonary dysplasia. *J Pediatr Nurs.* 1989;4:177–185.
12. Lorenz K. *Evoluation and Modification of Behavior.* Chicago, Ill: The University of Chicago Press; 1965.
13. Illingworth RS, Lister J. The critical or sensitive period, with special reference to certain feeding problems in infants and children. *J Pediatr.* 1964;65:840–848.
14. Gisel EG. Development of oral side preference during chewing and its relation to hand preference in normal 2- to 8-year-old children. *Am J Occup Ther.* 1988;42:40.
15. Gisel EG. Effect of food texture on the development of chewing of children between six months and two years of age. *Dev Med Child Neurol.* 1991;33:69–79.
16. Carroll JL. Developmental plasticity in respiratory control. *J Appl Physiol.* 2003;94(1):375–389.
17. Kennell JH, Trause MA, Klaus MH. Evidence for a sensitive period in the human mother. *Ciba Found Symp.* 1975;33:87–101.
18. Yamamato T, Hirayama A. Effects of soft-diet feeding on synaptic density in the hippocampus and parietal cortex of senescence-accelerated mice. *Brain Res.* 2001;902:255–263.
19. Mennella JA, Jagnow CP, Beauchamp GK. Prenatal and postnatal flavor learning by human infants. *Pediatrics.* 2001;107:e88.
20. Tatzer E, Schubert MT, Timischl W, Simbruner G. Discrimination of taste and preference for sweet in premature babies. *Ear Hum Dev.* 1985;12:23–30.
21. Maone TR, Mattes RD, Bernbaum JC, Beauchamp GK. A new method for delivering a taste without fluids to preterm and term infants. *Dev Psychobiol.* 1990;23:179–191.

22. Sullivan SA, Birch LL. Infant dietary experience and acceptance of solid foods. *Pediatrics*. 1994;93:271–277.
23. Galloway AT, Lee Y, Birch LL. Predictors and consequences of food neophobia and pickiness in young girls. *J Am Diet Assoc*. 2003;103:692–698.
24. Beauchamp GK, Moran M. Acceptance of sweet and salty tastes in 2-year-old children. *Appetite*. 1984;5:291–305.
25. Hill DL, Mistretta CM. Developmental neurobiology of salt taste sensation. *Trends in Neuroscience*. 1990;13:188–195.
26. Mennella JA. Development of the chemical senses and the programming of flavor preference. Physiologic/immunologic responses to dietary nutrients: role of elemental and hydrolysate formulas in management of the pediatric patient. *Report of the 107th Conference on Pediatric Research*. Columbus, Ohio: Ross Products Division, Abbott Laboratories; 1998:201–208.
27. Link DT, Rudolph CD. Feeding and swallowing. In: Rudolph CD, Rudolph AM, eds. *Rudolph's Pediatrics*. 21st ed. New York, NY: McGraw-Hill; 2003:1385–1386.
28. Rogers B, Arvedson J, Msall M, Demerath R. Hypoxemia during oral feeding of children with severe cerebral palsy. *Dev Med Child Neurol*. 1993;35:3–10.
29. Rogers B, Arvedson J, Buck G, Smart P, Msall M. Characteristics of dysphagia in children with cerebral palsy. *Dysphagia*. 1994;9:69–73.
30. Arvedson J, Rogers B, Buck G, Smart P, Msall M. Silent aspiration prominent in children with dysphagia. *Int J Pediatr Otorhinolaryngol*. 1994;28:173–181.
31. Langer JC, Wesson DA, Ein SH, et al. Feeding gastrostomy in neurologically impaired children: is an antireflux procedure necessary? *J Pediatr Gastroenterol Nutr*. 1998;7:837–841.
32. Mollitt DL, Golladay ES, Seibert JJ. Symptomatic gastroesophageal reflux following gastrostomy in neurologically impaired patients. *Pediatrics*. 1985;75:1124–1126.
33. Wheatley MJ, Wesley JR, Tkach DM, Coran AG. Long-term follow-up of brain-damaged children requiring feeding gastrostomy: should an anti-reflux procedure always be performed. *J Pediatr Surg*. 1991;26:301–305.
34. Arvedson J, Rogers B. Pediatric swallowing and feeding disorders. *J Med Speech-Lang Pathol*. 1993;1(4):203–221.
35. Arvedson JC, Rogers B. Swallowing and feeding in the pediatric patient. In: Perlman AL, Schulze-Delrieu KS, eds. *Deglutition and Its disorders: Anatomy, Physiology, Clinical Diagnosis, and Management*. San Diego, Calif: Singular Publishing Group, Inc.: 1997;419–448.
36. American Speech-Language-Hearing Association. Clinical indicators for instrumental assessment of dysphagia (guidelines). *ASHA Supplement*. Vol 20. Rockville, Md: American Speech-Language-Hearing Association; 2000:18–19.
37. Benson JE, Lefton-Greif MA. (1994). Videofluoroscopy of swallowing in pediatric patients: a component of the total feeding evaluation. In: Tuchman DN, Walter RS, eds. *Disorders of Feeding and Swallowing in Infants and Children: Pathophysiology, Diagnosis, and Treatment*. San Diego, Calif: Singular Publishing Group; 1994: 187–200.
38. Langmore SE, Logemann JA. After the clinical bedside swallowing examination: what next? *Am J of Speech-Lang Pathol*. Sept. 1991:13–19.
39. Bosma JF, Hepburn LG, Josell SD, Baker K. Ultrasound demonstration of tongue motions during suckle feeding. *Dev Med Child Neurol*. 1990;32:223–229.
40. Arvedson JC, Lefton-Greif ML. *Pediatric Videofluoroscopic Swallow Studies: A Professional Manual with Caregiver Guidelines*. San Antonio, Tex: Communication Skill Builders; 1998.
41. Logemann JA. *Manual for the Videofluorographic Study of Swallowing*. 2nd ed. Austin, Tex: PRO-ED;1993.
42. American Speech-Language-Hearing Association. Roles of the speech-language pathologist and otolaryngologist in the performance and interpretation of endoscopic examinations of swallowing (position statement). *ASHA Supplement*. Vol 20. Rockville, Md: American Speech-Language-Hearing Associations; 2000:17.
43. Willging JP. Endoscopic evaluation of swallowing in children. *Int J Pediatr Otorhinolaryngol*. 1995;32: S107–S108.
44. Willging JP, Miller CK, Hogan MJ, Rudolph CD. Fiberoptic endoscopic evaluation of swallowing in children: a preliminary report of 100 procedures. *Dysphagia*. 1996;11:162.

Chapter 13

Dietary Supplements

Christina J. Valentine

INTRODUCTION

Dietary supplements are an integral part of pediatric nutrition support (NS). In the context of NS dietary supplements are nutrients or groups of nutrients that alone cannot be the sole source of nutrition for an infant or child. Dietary supplements can have effects that are separate and distinct from their roles as nutrients.[1] In NS dietary supplements can be used to provide or correct a nutrient deficiency, to enhance the diet, or to meet requirements for specific nutrients that are not achievable with the diet. Most often dietary supplements used in NS are medical foods. For a discussion of medical foods, see Chapter 15.

Dietary supplements are frequently used when NS is unnecessary, and in that sense, the US Congress defines dietary supplements in the Dietary Supplement Health and Education Act (DSHEA)[2] of 1994 as a product (other than tobacco) that is intended to supplement the diet; contains 1 or more dietary ingredients (including vitamins, minerals, herbs or other botanicals, amino acids, and other substances) or their constituents; is intended to be taken by mouth as a pill, capsule, tablet, or liquid; and is labeled on the front panel as being a dietary supplement.[3] Although the US Food and Drug Administration (FDA) regulates dietary supplements as foods, they are regulated differently from other foods and from drugs. Whether a product is classified as a dietary supplement, conventional food, or drug is based on its intended use. Most often, classification as a dietary supplement is determined by the information that the manufacturer provides on the product label or in accompanying literature, although many food and dietary supplement product labels do not include this information.

NS dietary supplements include human milk (mother's own or donor milk), human milk fortifiers, formulas, modular macronutrient additives, functional foods, vitamins, minerals, and trace element supplements. Botanicals and substances designed to enhance athletic or mental performance are rarely prescribed for NS. The decision to use supplements should be based on data that establish efficacy and safety. Dietary supplements are used to augment nutrient intake while keeping the caloric composition appropriate and adequate to support growth and development. Many products used in the clinical setting lack scientific validity.[4] For example, medium chain triglycerides (MCT) are mixed directly with human milk or formulas to boost caloric content, but because the fat is not emulsified, much of it can adhere to tubing and not be available to the infant.[5,6]

Health care providers know little about the prevalence or the characteristics of pediatric dietary supplement use. Ball et al. found that health care providers prescribed 62% of supplements. The kinds of supplements most frequently used, in descending order, are vitamins, minerals, botanicals, and amino acids.[7] There was a high prevalence of use among children with a poor prognosis or for whom there were limited medical treatments. The highest nonprescribed use was among children with cancer, cystic fibrosis, neurobehavioral disorders, and rheumatologic disorders. These are the same children who often require NS. Other factors, including ethnic and cultural background, influence a family's belief in and desire to use integrative therapies such as dietary supplements. Information on efficacy and safety of nonprescribed dietary supplements is lacking, as is information on the interaction among dietary supplements, drugs, and NS products. It is likely that the demand for complementary and alternative medicine (CAM) will increase in pediatrics.[8]

Functional foods are those foods that are shown to affect beneficially 1 or more functions in the body beyond nutritional effects in a way relevant to either the state of well being and health and/or to reduce the risk of a disease.[9] They are used in health promotion and preventative care. In many instances, their mechanism of action is unknown and they can be harmful.[10] This chapter reviews the strategies behind choosing dietary supplements for infants and children on NS. Mixing protocols and safety guidelines will also be presented. Glutamine, prebiotics, and probiotics are considered to be functional foods and are extensively discussed in Chapters 3 and 24. Argnine is also considered to be a functional food.

Human Milk

Human milk is the preferred milk type for infants for approximately the first 6 months of life. From about 4 or 6 to 12 months, human milk alone is insufficient and must be supplemented with foods rich in iron and zinc. If babies cannot suckle, pumped human milk should be provided.[11,12] With clean handling techniques, breast milk can be pumped and stored immediately in glass or hard plastic bottles. The pumped milk must be refrigerated at < 39° F for < 48 hours. Pumped milk can be safely stored frozen at < 0° F for 3 months.[11] Freezing eliminates cytomegalovirus in human milk.[13] This practice is safe and maintains the integrity of the milk.[14,15] It might be possible to boost the caloric content of expressed milk by using hind milk: milk is expressed for about 2 minutes and then stored for later use. The rest of the milk, containing a higher fat content, is fed to the infant to enhance weight gain.[16] Human milk might not be sufficient for preterm infants, infants with increased needs, or infants of women whose milk volume is limited. For these situations, human milk fortifier might be needed.

Human Milk Fortification

Commercial human milk fortifiers should be used for all infants less than < 35 weeks of gestation fed human milk.[17] They are available in powder (Enfamil Human Milk Fortifier by Bristol Myers Squibb, Similac Human Milk Fortifier by Abbott Laboratories), or liquid (Similac Natural Care Advance by Abbott Laboratories) formulations. Both powder and liquid support growth and bone mineralization.[18,19] The powder fortifiers are packaged in small volumes that contain protein, fat, carbohydrate, vitamins, minerals and trace elements. Addition of the powder to human milk increases the osmolality of the milk.[20] In general, 1 packet can be added to 50 mL of human milk and given to the infant once in 24 hours when the infant is on 100 mL/kg body weight. In the next 24 hours, the density is increased to full fortification with 2 packets per 50 mL or 4 packets per 100 mL human milk. Table 13-1 lists the composition of the average mother's milk mixed with 4 packets of human milk fortifier. Liquid fortifier is mixed with human milk at a 1:1 ratio. Depending on which fortifier is used, iron supplementation might be needed to deliver the required iron intake of 2 mg/kg/day for preterm infants. A recent study demonstrated less bacterial inhibition *in vitro* with the fortifier containing iron.[21] *In vivo*, however, there is no difference in infections or sepsis.[22] Furthermore, iron incorporation into red blood cells from the powder fortifier is similar to that seen with iron supplements of 2 mg/kg/day elemental iron.[23] Despite fortification, preterm infants might require volumes of 160–180 mL/kg/day for growth.[24] Volume is a valuable means to increase nutrition without additives. To enhance mother's milk volume, encourage skin-to-skin holding of the infant.[25]

Breast Milk Substitutes

Infants > 35 weeks of gestation might not need as much calcium and phosphorus as human milk fortifiers provide, but they benefit from augmenting human milk if the volume is limited. Standard powder formulas (Enfamil Lipil by Bristol Myers Squibb, Similac Advance by Abbott Laboratories, Store Brands PBM) can be used as human milk fortifiers by adding 1¼ teaspoons per 4 ounces human milk to make a 24 kcal/ounce mixture.[11] For preterm or low birth weight infants, or those who have malabsorption, powder transition formulas might be helpful (Enfacare, Bristol Myers Squibb, Neosure, Abbott Laboratories). These contain a blend of lactose and corn syrup solids and/or maltodextrin, long chain and medium chain triglycerides, and a larger nutrient density per milliliter compared to the standard formulas. Nutrient composition of 1 teaspoon powdered Neosure (Abbott Laboratories) added to 70 mL human milk can be seen in Table 13-2. Nutrient interactions, absorption, and bioavailability of human milk formula combinations are not known and they should only be used in the hospital if no other alternative is available.

Oral and Enteral Supplements

There are more than 100 enteral formulas available for oral NS that are commonly used to wean a child from tube feeding. These formulas are often used as a dietary supplement for children on age-appropriate diets who require additional nutrients. Most of the supplements come in a variety of flavors, taste good, and are sold in grocery stores. The formulas noted below are not meant to represent all formulas in the different categories, but are used only as examples. The formula lists are not inclusive or exhaustive. It is only since the early 1990s that specific supplements designed for children have become available. Adult enteral formulas such as Boost, Ensure, or Nutren can be used for children older than 10 years of age as long as they are not the sole source of nutrition because they might not provide adequate amounts of vitamins (vitamin D) and minerals (calcium, phosphorus, iron, zinc) for this age group. These polymeric formulas are usually lactose free, vary in caloric density from 1.0 to 2.0 kcal/mL, and are available with or without added fiber (soy/oat). In calorically more dense formulas such as Ensure Plus or Two Cal HN, the osmolality is high, 300 to 690 mOsm/kg of water. When high calorie formulas are used, adequate water must be provided and the patient should be monitored for osmotic diarrhea. These formulas are useful in children who cannot tolerate large volumes of fluid.

Pediatric formula supplements have been designed for children less than 10 years of age. They are usually 1.0 kcal/mL such as Pediasure, Nutren Junior, or Kindercal. These formulas are lower in protein, sodium, potassium, chloride, and magnesium than their adult counterparts. Commonly, 100% of a child's caloric, protein, vitamin, and mineral needs can be met with these formulas (950–1100 mL/day) so they can also serve as a sole source of nutrition and are used for tube feeding.

There are specially designed pediatric and adult formulas for specific disease states. Pediatric specialty formulas include predigested, extensively hydrolyzed, and amino acid-based formulas such as: Peptamen Junior EleCare Pediatric Vivonex and Neocate One Plus. Portagen and Lipsorb are formulas with most of the fat from medium chain triglycerides, and they are used in dietary treatment of chylothorax and cystic fibrosis. Other adult specialty formulas designed for stress and trauma, such as Promote, Perative, and Isosource HN, as well as pulmonary and glucose tolerance problems, such as Pulmocare, Nutrivent, and Respalor, are commonly used for children. Children on these formulas must be carefully monitored to be sure they receive adequate water and micronutrients.

Table 13-1 Composition of the average human milk mixed with fortifiers and selected formulas.

Selected nutrients per/100 mL	EBM* (MOM)	FEBM† (MJ)	FEBM‡ (R)	Enf Pre Lipil (MJ)	SSC Adv (R)	Enfacare (MJ)	Neosure (R)	Enf Lipil (MJ)	Sim Adv (R)	Store B§ (W)	Pregestimil (liquid) (MJ)
Kcal/oz	20	24	24	24	24	22	22	20	20	20	20
Kcal/100 mL	67	81	81	81	82	74	74	68	67	67	68
Protein (g)	1	2.1	2	2.4	2.4	2.1	2.1	1.4	1.4	1.5	1.9
Whey/casein	70/30	70/30	60/40	60/40	60/40	60/40	50/50	60/40	48/52	60/40	0/100
(% kcal)	6	10	10	11	12	11	10	8.5	8	8.9	11
Lipid (g)	3.5	4.5	3.9	4.1	4.4	3.9	4	3.6	3.6	3.5	3.8
LCT/MCT	98/2	89/11	89/11	60/40	50/50	80/20	74/25	100/0	100/0	100/0	45/55
DHA	0.2-0.4	0.2-0.4	0.2-0.4	0.33	0.25	0.32	0.15	0.32	0.15	0.2	0
AA	0.5-0.7	0.5-0.7	0.5-0.7	0.68	0.4	0.64	0.4	0.64	0.4	0.35	0
(% kcal)	52	54	43	44	47	47	49	48	49	49	49
CHO (g)	7	7.4	8.8	8.9	8.6	7.7	7.6	7.4	7.3	7.1	6.9
Lactose/polymers	100/0	72/28	80/20	40/60	50/50	40/60	50/50	100/0	100/0	100/0	0/100
(% kcal)	52	36	44	44	42	42	41	44	43	42	41
Calcium (mg)	28	118	145	134	146	89	78	53	52	42	78
Phosphorus (mg)	14	64	81	67	81	49	46	36	28	28	51
Sodium (meq)	0.9	1.6	1.7	2	1.5	1.1	1	0.8	0.7	0.6	1.4
Potassium (meq)	1.3	2	2.9	2	2.6	2	2.7	1.8	1.8	1.8	1.9

Table 13-1 Composition of the average human milk mixed with fortifiers and selected formulas. (continued).

Selected nutrients per/100 mL	EBM* (MOM)	FEBM† (MJ)	FEBM‡ (R)	Enf Pre Lipil (MJ)	SSC Adv (R)	Enfacare (MJ)	Neosure (R)	Enf Lipil (MJ)	Sim Adv (R)	Store B§ (W)	Pregestimil (liquid) (MJ)
Vitamin A (IU)	223	1173	843	1010	1014	330	342	200	202	201	260
Vitamin D (IU)	22	172	142	195	122	59	52	41	40	40	34
Vitamin E (IU)	0.23	4.8	3.4	5	3.3	3	2.7	1.3	1	0.9	2.6
Zinc (mg)	0.12	0.8	1.1	1.2	1.2	0.9	0.9	0.7	0.5	0.5	0.6
Iron (mg)	< 0.1	1.5	0.4	1.4	1.5	1.3	1.3	1.2	1.2	1.2	1.2
Osmolality (mosmol/kg H_2O)	260	295	385	300	280	250	250	300	300	280	280

* (MOM) Mother's own milk—Average term composition.
† (MJ) Mead Johnson (Evansville, Ind)—Fortified mother's own milk w/ 4 packets/100mL.
‡ (R) Ross (Columbus, Ohio)—Fortified mothers own milk with w/ packets/100mL.
§ (W) Wyeth (Philadelphia, Pa)—Multiple store brands available.
EBM = expressed breast milk, FEBM = fortified expressed breast milk, Enf Pre Lipil = Enfamil Premature Lipil, SSC Adv = Similac Special Care Advance, Enf Lipil = Enfamil Lipil, Sim Adv = Similac Advance.

Table 13-2 Human milk mixed with Neosure powder 1tsp/70mL.

Nutrient	*Measure*	*Concentration*
Energy	Kcal	83
Volume	mL	100
Protein	g	1.5
Fat	g	4.7
Carbohydrate	g	8.6
Calcium	mg	44
Phosphorus	mg	24
Magnesium	mg	4.8
Iron	mg	0.32
Zinc	mg	0.31
Manganese	mcg	2
Copper	mcg	44
Iodine	mcg	13
Sodium	mg	23
Potassium	mg	75
Chloride	mg	53
Vitamin A	IU	294
Vitamin D	IU	13
Vitamin E	IU	1
Vitamin K	mcg	2
Thiamin (B_1)	mcg	56
Riboflavin (B_2)	mcg	58
Vitamin B_6	mcg	36
Vitamin B_{12}	mcg	0.11
Niacin	mcg	461
Folic acid	mcg	8.7
Pantothenic acid	mcg	305
Biotin	mcg	1.8
Vitamin C	mg	6
Choline	mg	12
Inositol	mg	20
Potential RSL	mOs	13.6

Source: Reproduced with permission of Melody Thompson, MS, RD, Neonva Abbott Laboratories, 2004.

Modular Nutrients

Nutrient modules are single or multiple nutrients that can be combined with a diet to add nutrients or to change the composition of the diet. Modules exist as food or as medically compounded substances that fulfill a specified need, thus falling within the definition of a medical food (see Chapter 15). Two examples of nutrient modules are margarine, a food, and MCT oil, a medical food. Modular components most often used in NS include carbohydrates, fats, proteins, vitamins, and minerals. The use of modules permits flexible mixing ratios, allowing one module to be combined with another. Studies, however, are needed to validate current use of many supplements and prove efficacy and safety.

For patients maintained on a table food diet, modules can be used to increase specific nutrients. The addition of oil increases calories and the addition of powdered milk to fluid whole milk increases protein. Specific nutrients, such as fat, protein, minerals, vitamins, or trace elements cannot be easily removed from a table food diet, but the addition of a large amount of a single nutrient results in the relative decrease of other nutrients in the final diet.

For patients maintained on enteral feeds, a wide variety of formulas are available. However, if a change in the concentration of single component, the ratio of nutrients, or a specific nutrient not normally found in the formula is required, modules can be used to create the necessary composition. A commonly used indication for the addition of nutrient modules is to increase the caloric content of a diet. In most instances, however, the first step to increase nutrients (calories or protein) in a diet is to increase the concentration of the formula. Concentrating formulas maintains nutrients in the original distribution and decreases the risk of providing a final diet with a single nutrient deficiency (Table 13-3).

Table 13-3 Increasing the caloric density of human milk and infant formula.

Human Milk		
kcal/oz	*Milk volume*	*Powdered standard infant formula*
24	4 oz	1¼ tsp
30	4 oz	1 T
Infant Formula (Powdered)		
kcal/oz	*Amount of powder*	*Volume water*
24	1¼ c	29 oz (32/3 c)
30	1½ c	29 oz (32/3 c)
Infant Formula (Liquid Concentrate)		
Kcal/oz	*Amount of concentrate*	*Volume water*
24	13 oz (1 can)	8 oz (1 c)
28	13 oz (1 can)	5.5 oz (1 c)
30	13 oz (1 can)	4 oz (½ c)

Other additives

Medium-chain triglyceride oil contains 7 kcal/mL; 1 tsp contains 39 kcal.
Vegetable oil contains 40 kcal/tsp.
Polycose liquid contains 60 kcal/oz; Polycose powder contains 8 kcal/tsp.

tsp = teaspoon
T = tablespoon
c = cup

Source: Reprinted with permission, American Academy of Pediatrics. Pediatric Nutrition Handbook, 5th ed. American Academy of Pediatrics, 2004.

CARBOHYDRATES

Carbohydrate, the least expensive of all modules, is available as starch, polysaccharide plus oligosaccharide, disaccharides, glucose polymers, and monosaccharides (Table 13-4).

Carbohydrates are most often used to increase the caloric density of a diet. Carbohydrates combine well with liquid formulas and contribute to the final osmolality of the diet. The smaller the molecular size, the greater the osmolality of the final diet. Long chain glucose polymers have lower osmolality at the same caloric density than smaller carbohydrate molecules. For example, a 5% solution of Polycose with a caloric density of 0.4 kcal/mL has an osmolality of 100 mOsm/kg H_2O. A 5% solution of glucose with a caloric density of 0.2 kcal/mL has an osmolality of 300 mOsm/kg H2O. Maltodextrins and glucose polymers are bland in taste. Disaccharides are sweet in taste and might contribute to taste fatigue in patients on oral diets.[26] For specific carbohydrate malabsorption, carbohydrate modules that do not contain a particular carbohydrate can be selected.

FIBER

Fiber is composed of substances present in plant cell walls that are resistant to human digestion, polysaccharides (cellulose, hemicellulose, pectins, gums, and mucilages) and nonpolysaccharides (mainly lignins). Fiber can be soluble or insoluble. The soluble fibers include hemicelluloses, pectins, gums and mucilages. The insoluble fibers are celluloses, lignins and some hemicelluloses. Soluble fiber is metabolized in the colon and small bowel by anaerobic bacteria. Fiber increases stool size, slows the rate of intestinal transit, gastric emptying, and glucose absorption, and decreases serum cholesterol. Fiber is most often used in NS to help with defecation, either by making stools softer or by decreasing diarrhea. See Table 13-4 for more information on fiber components.

FAT

The American Academy of Pediatrics Committee on Nutrition recommends that children over the age of 2 years receive approximately 30% of dietary intake as fat.[11] In a table food diet, most fat is present as triglyceride, about 2% is phospholipids. MCTs contain fatty acids with a carbon chain length of 6 to 12 carbon atoms. They are found in dairy fat, coconut oil, and palm oil (Table 13-4). MCTs are not reesterified by the enterocyte, but are transported bound to albumin as free fatty acid through the portal circulation. MCTs are not stored in fat depots, but are oxidized to acetic acid. Thus, the efficiency of MCT absorption is estimated to be 4 times that of long chain triglycerides (LCT).[27]

MCT is used for small bowel disease or damage, short small bowel, pancreatic and biliary insufficiency, abetalipoproteinemia, lymphangiectasia, chylous ascites, and chylothorax. Fat increases the caloric content of the diet and adds little to the osmolality of the final diet. However, there are disadvantages to the use of MCT oil. The most important disadvantage for children is that MCT oil does not contain essential fatty acids. When MCTs are used, the fat composition of the final diet must be reviewed to be sure adequate amounts of essential fatty acids are available. Since MCTs do not stimulate chylomicron formation, fat soluble vitamins are not transported out of the enterocyte. Serum levels of fat soluble vitamins should be monitored in children on diets high in MCT oil.

Table 13-4 Modular components.

Carbohydrate				
Ingredients (manufactured by)	*kcal/g*	*Source*	*g/tablespoons*	*Comments*
Dextrose (hydrous)	3.4	Corn sugar	9.5	Monosaccharide added to formulas as a CHO source. Caution: increases osmolality.
Fructose	4	Fruit sugar	12	Monosaccharide added to formulas as a CHO source for infants allergic to corn sugar or intolerant to other sugars. Caution: increases osmolality.
Honey	3	Fructose and glucose	20	40% fructose, 35% glucose, 2% sucrose, 23% water. Contraindicated for infants less than 1 year of age due to the possibility of botulism.
Karo, light (Best Foods)	3	Corn syrup	20	Contains corn syrup, sugar, vanilla, and salt (115 mg Na/100 g).
Moducal (powder) Mead Johnson	3.8	Maltodextrin	8	Consists primarily of glucose polymers produced by the controlled hydrolysis of cornstarch. Added to formulas/foods to increase calories.
Polycose (powder) (liquid) (Ross)	3.8 2 (kcal/ml)	Glucose polymer of corn	6 15mL	Carbohydrate providing low osmolality and minimal sweetness. Added to formulas/ foods to increase calories. Not more than 115 mg sodium/100 g powder.
Dry Infant Rice Cereal (Heinz)	3.57	Rice	3.5	May be added to formula to thicken. 1 tablespoon (dry) = 0.25 g protein, 0.1 g fat, 2.75 g carbohydrate, 12.5 kcal and 2 mg iron.
Dry Infant Rice Cereal (Gerber and Beechnut)	4	Rice	3.75	May be added to formula to thicken. 1 tablespoon (dry) = 0.25 g protein, 0.1 g fat, 3 g carbohydrate, 15 kcal and 2 mg iron.
Sucrose	4	Cane or beet sugar	12	Disaccharide added to formulas as a carbohydrate source. Caution: Increases osmolality.

Protein				
Ingredients (manufactured by)	*kcal/g*	*Source*	*g/tablespoon*	*Comments*
Amino Acid Mixture-Complete (SHS)	3.3	L-amino acids	9.5	Powdered mixture of essential and nonessential amino acids, fat and carbohydrate free. 5% dilution suggested (5 g powder/100 mL water). Not intended as the sole source of nutrition.
Amino Acid Mixture-Essential (SHS)	3.2	L-amino acids	9.04	Powdered mixture of essential amino acids, fat and carbohydrate free. 5% dilution suggested (5 g powder/100 mL water). Not intended as the sole source of nutrition.

Table 13-4 Modular components (continued).

Protein

Ingredients (manufactured by)	*kcal/g*	*Source*	*g/tablespoon*	*Comments*
Instant Nonfat Dry Milk Powder (Bowes and Church)	3.5	Cow's milk	4.3	May be added to foods to increase protein, calcium, and calorie content. 1 tablespoon = 1.5 g protein, 52 mg calcium, 47 mg phosphorus, 24 mg sodium, 73 mg potassium. 1.0 gram = 0.35 g protein, 12 mg calcium, 11 mg phosphorus, 5.5 mg sodium, 17 mg potassium.
Resource Beneprotein Instant Protein Powder (Novartis)	3.6	Whey protein isolate	4.7	1.0 scoop = 1.5 tablespoons = 7 g and contains 25 calories, 6 g protein, 15 mg sodium, 35 mg potassium, 35 mg calcium, 20 mg phosphorous.

Fat

Ingredients (manufactured by)	*kcal/g*	*Source*	*g/tablespoon*	*Comments*
Canola oil	8.8	Canola	14	Contains 19 g linoleic acid and 8.7 g linolenic acid per 100 mL.
Coconut oil	8.8	Coconut	14	Contains 1.6 g linoleic acid and 0 g linolenic acid per 100 mL.
Corn oil	8.8	Corn	14	Contains 53 g linoleic acid and 0.6 g linolenic acid per 100 mL.
Cottonseed oil	8.8	Cottonseed	14	Contains 47 g linoleic acid and 0.2 g linolenic acid per 100 mL.
Linseed oil	8.9	Flaxseed	14	Contains 12 g linoleic acid and 49 g linolenic acid per 100 mL.
MCT oil (Mead Johnson)	8.3	Medium chain fraction of coconut oil	14	Consists primarily of the triglycerides of the C8 and C10 saturated fatty acids. Absorbed directly into portal system. Bile salts and lipase not necessary for digestion and absorption. Does not contain essential fatty acids.
Microlipid (Novartis)	4.5 (kcal/mL)	Safflower oil	15 (7.7 g fat)	A 50% fat emulsion used to increase calories or for treatment or prevention of fatty acid deficiencies. 74% of the fatty acids are provided as linoleic acid.
Olive oil	8.8	Olive	14	Contains 7 g linoleic acid and 0.5 g linolenic acid per 100 mL.
Peanut oil	8.8	Peanuts	14	Contains 29 g linoleic acid and 0 g linolenic acid per 100 mL.
Safflower	8.8	Safflower	14	Contains 68 g linoleic acid and 0 g linolenic acid per 100 mL.
Sesame oil	8.8	Sesame	14	Contains 37 g linoleic acid and 0.3 g linolenic acid per 100 mL.

Table 13-4 Modular components (continued)

Fat

Ingredients (manufactured by)	*kcal/g*	*Source*	*g/tablespoon*	*Comments*
Soy	8.8	Soybeans	14	Contains 46 g linoleic acid and 6 g linolenic acid per 100 mL.
Sunflower	8.8	Sunflower	14	Contains 36 g linoleic acid and 0.1 g linolenic acid per 100 mL.

Combination

Ingredients (manufactured by)	*kcal/g*	*Source*	*g/Tbs.*	*CHO g/Tbs.*	*Pro g/Tbs.*	*Fat g/Tbs.*	*Comments*
Additions (Nestle)	5.2	Carbohydrate—corn syrup solids Protein—sodium caseinate and whey protein isolate Fat-canola oil	8.1	3.9	2.6	2.1	100 calories per scoop can be added to hot foods or hot liquids. 1 scoop = 2 1/3 tablespoons.
Super Soluble Duocal (SHS)	4.92	Carbohydrate—hydrolyzed cornstarch Fat—corn, coconut and MCT oil (35%)	8.5	6.2	0	1.9	Powdered blend of carbohydrate, ideal for protein- and/or electrolyte-restricted diets.
Resource Benecalorie (Novartis)	7/mL	Protein—calcium caseinate Fat—high oleic sunflower oil	—	0	7/1.5 oz	33/1.5 oz	330 calories in each 1.5 oz cup. Contains additional zinc, vitamins C and E.
Scandical (Axcan Pharma)	5.38	Carbohydrate—maltodextrin, corn syrup solids Fat—partially hydrogenated vegetable oil (coconut or soy), medium chain triglyceride (MCT) oil	6.5	4	0	2.5	35 calories per tablespoon, can be added to any food or beverage, hot or cold.

Table 13-5 Modular components (continued).

Thickeners				
Ingredients (manufactured by)	*kcal/g*	*Source*	*g/tablespoon*	*Comments*
Simply Thick (Simply Thick)	0 nectar/packet 5 honey/packet	Xanthan gum	15	Thickening gel that comes in 2 premeasured packets: nectar and honey to be added to a 4-oz serving. For pudding consistency (spoon thick), use 2 honey packets. Also comes in bulk servings of both honey and nectar designed to thicken 32 oz.
THICKIT (Precision Foods)	3.75	Modified cornstarch, maltodextrin	4.8	Instant powdered food thickener for individuals with dysphagia or swallowing impairment. To achieve a consistency of nectar, add 2–3 teaspoons; honey, add 3–5 teaspoons,; pudding, add 5–6 teaspoons and make up to 4 oz by adding water.
Resource ThickenUp (Novartis)	3.75	Food starch modified (corn)	4.0	Powdered food thickener for individuals with dysphagia or swallowing impairment. To achieve a consistency of nectar, add 3–4 teaspoons; honey, add 4–6 teaspoons,; pudding, add 5–6 teaspoons and make up to 4 oz by adding water. Vary amounts to achieve desired thickness.

Fiber				
Ingredients (manufactured by)	*grams fiber*	*Source*	*kcal*	*Comments*
Pectin Certo (Kraft Foods)	1 g/mL	Pectin	0	Liquid fruit pectin. Add to formula in ranges from 1–3% for patients with acute diarrhea and short bowel syndrome.
Fiberbasics (Hormel)	3/tablespoon	Maltodextrin	30/tablespoon	A soluble dietary fiber used to help maintain normal bowel function.
Resource BeneFiber (Novartis)	3/tablespoon	Partially hydrolyzed guar gum	16/tablespoon	A soluble dietary fiber used to help maintain normal bowel function.

Source: Department of Clinical Nutrition Children's Hospital. *Infant Formulas and Selected Nutritional Supplements.* Columbus, Ohio: Department of Clinical Nutrition Children's Hospital; 2003:31–32. Reproduced with permission.

Long term use of high MCT-containing diets was noted to be associated with cirrhosis in abetalipoproteinemia.[28]

Short chain fatty acids (SCFA), defined as fatty acids with less than 7 carbon atoms, are formed in the gastrointestinal tract and are not available as nutrient modules. Of the macronutrient modules, carbohydrate, fat, and protein, fat has the highest caloric density. MCT provides 8.3 kcal/g and LCT 9.0 kcal/g. MCT modules are useful when fat malabsorption or maldigestion exists. Fat modules are generally insoluble, although MCT is more water soluble than LCT. The addition of fats to liquid diets does not require the addition of emulsifiers if the added fat accounts for less than 30% of the energy intake, the fat is added to the liquid preparation at room temperature, and the formula is made daily and not allowed to sit in the tube feeding container for more than 3 to 4 hours. Fat separation and collection on infusion systems occurs in patients on continuous feedings when the fat is mixed with the formula. Fat modules are inexpensive except for MCT oil, and they contribute little to osmolality.

Chapter 24 reviews the long chain polyunsaturated fatty acids (LCPUFA) and their use in pediatric nutrition. Available sources for LCPUFA include egg yolk lipid, phospholipid, triglyceride, fish oils, and oils produced by single cell organisms. Chapter 4 discusses long term outcomes for infants fed on diets to which LCPUFA have been added.

PROTEIN

Protein modules (Table 13-4) are available as intact protein, hydrolyzed protein, and crystalline amino acids. Intact proteins, such as pureed beef, egg white solids, lactalbumin, whey, and sodium or calcium caseinate, require digestion to smaller peptides before absorption. Hydrolyzed proteins are proteins that have been enzymatically or chemically altered to smaller peptides and free amino acids. Intact protein modules are generally thought to be the most palatable, whereas synthetic amino acids have a bitter taste. Although medical indications for the use of protein modules determines the type of protein prescribed, protein quality, osmolality, viscosity, palatability, and patient preference should be considered. Synthetic amino acids contribute to a higher osmolality than intact proteins. Protein contributes to the renal solute load and the protein module must be included in the final dietary estimation of renal solute load (RSL).

$$\begin{aligned} \text{RSL} = {} & 4 \times \text{g protein (final diet)} \\ & + \text{mEq Na (final diet)} \\ & + \text{mEq K (final diet)} \\ & + \text{mEq Cl (final diet)} \end{aligned}$$

Protein modules in powder form are somewhat insoluble and more expensive than either fat or carbohydrate modules.

Dietary protein and energy are intimately related, and before supplementation with a protein module, it is important to assess the adequacy of energy intake. An analysis of the literature by Young and Pelletier suggests diets containing more than 4 mg/kg/d protein offer no growth advantage and are associated with higher plasma amino acid levels.[29]

VITAMINS AND MINERALS

Individual macronutrient modules contain limited or no vitamins, minerals or trace elements. Liquid forms of vitamins and minerals, as opposed to tablets or capsules, combine best with NS feeds. Vitamin modules can be used to deliver 100% of the recommended daily allowance. However, vitamins should have the United States Pharmacopoeia (USP) designation, assuring they meet federal criteria for dissolution and potency (Table 25-4 in Chapter 25).

GENERAL CONCEPTS ABOUT MODULES

Nutrient modules are sold commercially as medical preparations and as over-the-counter products. The patient's nutritional needs dictate the choice of module. Other factors, such as the availability of a particular module, financial constraints, safety, solution design, and the technical knowledge of the prescriber are also important.

Problems are associated with the use of modular nutrients, including infections, metabolic problems, and nutrient incompatibility. Careful attention to potential delivery problems, osmolality, nutrient interactions, and nutrient composition is warranted.

The addition of a single nutrient alters the composition of diets and could result in medical problems. Failure to evaluate the final diet composition can result in clinical problems such as high osmolality and renal solute load, inappropriate ratios of macronutrients, suboptimal nutrient absorption, and physical incompatibility. The diet composition may be altered so that the concentration of a nutrient is diluted or otherwise inadequate in the final diet. For example, a commonly added nutrient module is a calorie source, such as carbohydrate or fat. A 6 kg child with failure to thrive who takes 600 mL of a standard infant formula (20 kcal/oz) per day receives 67 kcal/kg/day. If an additional 10 kcal/oz of carbohydrate is added, the final caloric content of the diet increases to 100 kcal/kg/day, but the protein is 1.5 g/kg/day, calcium 336 mg/day, and the phosphorus 228 mg/day. The protein, calcium, and phosphorus are less than the recommended daily allowance.

Osmolality of the final diet is important. Hyperosmolar feedings and formulas can cause nausea, vomiting, diarrhea, "dumping syndrome," and delayed gastric emptying. Delayed gastric emptying might lead to high gastric residuals and abdominal distention. For example, a 12 kg child with malnutrition and low serum K, Mg, P, and Zn levels who is receiving 120 kcal/kg/d of tube feeds to which K, P, Mg, and Zn are added has a final diet with a high osmolality. The development of diarrhea in this child suggests the osmolality of the final formula should be considered as a possible cause of the diarrhea. Table 13-5 lists the osmolality of some commonly used nutrient modules. Similarly, the addition of a modular nutrient to a diet might change its renal solute load. Electrolyte and/or protein modules contribute to the overall renal solute load, and this could be especially important for children with renal disorders. Thus, it is important to assure adequate free water is supplied to children.

Physical incompatibility can be a problem. Too much powder added to a formula could clog a small-bore feeding tube; poor mixing might lead to separation of diet constituents and result in a bolus of carbohydrate or fat that might be poorly tolerated. The pH of the formula affects both the bioavailability and solubility of the individual nutrients. Casein and soy protein are more soluble in a neutral pH solution. Whey protein is compatible with slightly acidic solutions, such as pH 3.5–7.0.

COMPLEMENTARY AND ALTERNATIVE MEDICINE (CAM)

CAM is defined as "a broad domain of healing resources that encompasses all health systems, modalities, and practices and their accompanying theories and beliefs, other than those intrinsic to the politically dominant health system of a particular society or culture in a given historic period."[30] Dietary supplements as defined by DSHEA can be considered a form of CAM. Nutraceuticals and functional foods are supplements. A nutraceutical is a "diet supplement that delivers a concentrated form of a biologically active component of food in a nonfood matrix in order to enhance health."[31] An example of a nutraceutical is genistein purified from soybeans and delivered in a pill in dosages greater than could be consumed in soy. Dietary supplements and nutraceuticals are different from functional foods that are considered to deliver an active ingredient within the food matrix. An example of a functional food is bread or breakfast cereal with added high dose folic acid. Food additives are substances that enhance flavor or aroma but not the nutritional value of a food. Diet supplements, nutraceuticals and functional foods are designed to supplement the human diet by increasing the intake of bioactive agents that are thought to enhance health and fitness.

Table 13-5 Osmolality of commonly used modular supplements.

Module	*Osmolality*
MgCl (2 mEq/mL)	3000 mOsm/L
NaCl injection (4 mEq/mL)	7090 mOsm/Kg
KCl elixir (10%)	3000–4350 mOsm/Kg
Promix	2 mOsm/tablespoon
Polycose (liquid)	900 mOsm/Kg
Moducal (20 g in 250 mL water)	69 mOsm/Kg
Sumacal (powder)	750 mOsm/Kg
Microlipid	80 mOsm/Kg
MCT oil	N/A (low)
Corn or safflower oil	N/A (very low)
Rice cereal	1.5 mOsm/tablespoon
Calcium glubionate (115 mg/5 mL)	2550–3000 mOsm/Kg
FeSO4 liquid (60 mg/mL)	4700 mOsm/Kg
Multivitamin liquid	5700 mOsm/Kg
Enfamil human milk fortifier	+120 mOsm/packet
Similac natural care fortifier*	280 mOsm/Kg

*1:1 dilution with breast milk = 22 Kcal/oz.

Source: 1992 product information.

Nonmedical food supplements do not need Federal Drug Administration (FDA) approval before they are marketed. They do not need to demonstrate effectiveness or safety. Except in the case of a new dietary ingredient, where premarket review for safety data and other information is required by law, a manufacturer does not need to provide the FDA with the evidence it used to substantiate safety or effectiveness before or after it markets its products. In addition, manufacturers do not need to register themselves or their dietary supplements with the FDA before producing or selling them. Furthermore, the manufacturer is responsible for establishing its own manufacturing practice guidelines to ensure that the dietary supplements it produces are safe and contain the ingredients listed on the label.[3] No mechanism exists to identify or track adverse reactions.

Industry has a great deal of information on who uses dietary supplements, the reasons they are used, kinds of supplements, and areas where development of new products or improved marketing of existing ones would increase use. For example, the main reasons people use dietary supplements are for general health and wellness, to supplement nutrition, to treat ailments such as colds, and to increase energy. Parents give dietary supplements to their children to be a good parent, to control health, to override guilt, and as a substitute for good nutrition. Parents provide herbal products to their children because they used them and were pleased with the experience, the herbals were recommended by a specialist, or the parents had success with vitamins and minerals. Books and magazines are the major sources of information on which people rely. People next look to doctors, friends, and relatives and finally the media for information on dietary supplements. Teenagers use dietary supplements to decrease a deficiency, increase IQ, and for athletic performance.

The importance of product label and product consistency was highlighted when a vitamin D supplement caused toxicity.[32] The investigators found no correlation between product label and content. Depending on the batch, the concentration of the vitamin varied 26 to 430 times the amount listed by the manufacturer. Such products are unsafe for children because the product label does not accurately reflect contents, product consistency may vary from batch to batch, and the FDA does not have the power to set and enforce standards. The United States *Pharmacopoeia*, originally published in 1820, was given legal recognition in 1906 when Congress enacted the first Food and Drug Act. This law recognized drug standards. The objective of the USP is the provision of standards that serve as the basic measures of strength, quality, purity, package, and labeling of drugs to ensure that the American public receives pharmaceutical products of uniform and consistent quality and strength.[33]

BOTANICALS

Botanicals such as teas, infusions, extracts, and plant parts themselves are a form of CAM and are used as dietary supplements (Table 13-6). The medical history should include questions on supplement use.

CONCLUSION

Dietary supplements such as human milk fortifiers, formulas, modular nutrients, and functional foods provide valuable support for patients, but they must be used with close attention to mixing, delivery, and safety. CAM are widely used without prescription or oversight by health care professionals. They cannot be assumed to be safe.

Table 13-6 Commonly used botanicals.

Herbs	*Herbalist classification*	*Typical uses*	*Evidence based on clinical trials*	*Side effects and drug interactions*
Aloe vera	• Anti-inflammatory • Antimicrobial • Laxative • Vulnerary	*External Use:* Applied to treat minor burns, abrasions, insect bites, acne, poison ivy, sunburn, skin irritations, frostbite, and canker sores. *Internal Use:* Gel taken as a peptic ulcer remedy and treatment for digestive disorders. Leaf lining used as a laxative.	• Aloe vera has been an effective topical vulnerary in treating leg ulcers, frostbite, full-face dermabrasions, and partial-thickness burn wounds. In one study of aloe as a treatment for surgical wound healing, the aloe group had delayed healing compared with controls. • A double-blind, placebo-controlled study demonstrated the healing effect of aloe on psoriasis vulgaris. • Experimental trials in human immunodeficiency virus-positive adults have had conflicting results in terms of immunomodulatory effects.	*Side Effects* of leaf lining taken internally: Contact dermatitis, gastric cramping, or diarrhea.* *Pregnancy and Lactation:* † *Drug Interactions* for leaf lining: Might potentiate digitalis and cardiac glycosides due to increased potassium loss. Could enhance potassium loss with corticosteroids and thiazide diuretics. *Other:* Reduced absorption of drugs due to decreased bowel transit time.
Calendula (*Calendula officinalis*)	• Anti-inflammatory • Antiseptic • Antispasmodic • Vulnerary	*External Use:* Skin irritations, rashes, cold sores, eczema, and conjunctivitis.	• A few clinical trials support topical use to accelerate wound healing and ulcers.	*Side Effects:* * *Pregnancy and Lactation:* † *Drug Interactions:* None known.
Catnip (*Nepetia catarua*)	• Antipyretic • Antispasmodic • Calmative • Carminative • Diaphoretic • Digestive aid • Diuretic • Sedative	Low-grade fever, upper respiratory tract infection, colic, headache, nervousness, sleep disorders, indigestion.	• No clinical studies.	*Side Effects:* One case report of central nervous system depression in toddler.* *Pregnancy and Lactation:* † *Drug Interactions:* None known.

Table 13-6 Commonly used botanicals (continued).

Herbs	*Herbalist classification*	*Typical uses*	*Evidence based on clinical trials*	*Side effects and drug interactions*
Chamomile *(Anthemis nobilis)*	• Anti-inflammatory • Antispasmodic • Carminative • Nervine • Sedative • Vulnerary	*External Use:* Skin irritation, prevention and treatment of cracked nipples. *Internal Use:* Colic, peptic ulcer disease, teething, sleep problems, anxiety.	• In controlled trials, chamomile and its constituents have had positive effects on wound healing, as a mild sedative, and in combination with other herbs as a treatment of infant colic. • Mixed results in the efficacy of the treatment of chemotherapy/ radiation-induced mucositis.	*Side Effects:* * *Pregnancy and Lactation:* No known adverse effects in pregnancy, lactation, and childhood. *Drug Interactions:* None known.
Evening primrose oil *(Oenothera biennis)*	• Anti-inflammatory • Sedative • Anticoagulant • Astringent	• Asthmatic coughs, whooping cough, gastrointestinal disorders. • Mastalgia, premenstrual syndrome (PMS). • Atopic eczema, psoriasis, acne. • Rheumatoid arthritis, multiple sclerosis, and other autoimmune diseases. • Diabetic neuropathy, intermittent claudication.	• No studies on asthma or diphtheria. • Effective in treatment of mastalgia; unclear effect in treatment of fibrocystic breast disease. A meta-analysis of 7 placebo-controlled trials found little value in managing PMS, although these studies were small. • Data on effectiveness in treating atopic dermatitis and other dermatologic disorders are mixed. • Preliminary studies appear promising for treatment of rheumatoid arthritis. • Effective in treating diabetic neuropathy in 2 studies.	*Side Effects:* Gastrointestinal disturbances and headaches.* *Pregnancy and Lactation:* † *Drug Interactions:* None known, but caution is suggested for patients taking phenothiazine and other drugs that reduce the seizure threshold.

Table 13-6 Commonly used botanicals (continued).

Herbs	Herbalist classification	Typical uses	Evidence based on clinical trials	Side effects and drug interactions
Fennel (*Foeniculum vulgare*)	• Antimicrobial • Antispasmodic • Carminative • Diuretic • Galactogogue • Expectorant • Mild laxative	• Colic, dyspnea, bloating, fullness, flatulence, and diarrhea in infants. • Cough, bronchitis, upper respiratory tract infection, conjunctivitis.	• One study showed an herbal combination including fennel was helpful in treating colic.	*Side Effects:* * *Pregnancy and Lactation:* † *Drug Interactions:* None known.
Feverfew (*Tanacetum parthenicum*)	• Anti-inflammatory • Antiseptic • Antispasmodic	• Migraine headache, nausea and vomiting, arthritis, fever.	• Clinical research in migraine treatment or prophylaxis shows mixed results, but tends to support feverfew as a prophylactic agent. • Not helpful in one study of treatment of rheumatoid arthritis.	*Side Effects:* Rebound headache, oral ulcers, and gastric disturbances.* *Pregnancy and Lactation:* † *Drug Interactions:* Could potentiate effects of anticoagulants and aspirin.
Garlic (*Allium sativum*)	• Anti-inflammatory • Antimicrobial • Antioxidant • Antispasmodic • Carminative • Diaphoretic • Diuretic • Expectorant • Hypoglycemic • Hypotensive • Lipid-lowering • Stimulant	• Ear infections, upper respiratory tract infection, cough/bronchitis, atherosclerosis, high cholesterol, hypertension, gastrointestinal disorders, menstrual disorders, diabetes mellitus.	• Mild beneficial effect on serum lipids and reducing serum cholesterol, serum triglycerides, and low-density lipoprotein cholesterol. Modest antihypertensive effect. • A randomized, double-blind, placebo-controlled clinical trial found no change in cardiovascular risk factors compared with placebo in children who had familial hyperlipidemia.	*Side Effects:* Flatulence, heartburn, gastric disturbances.* *Pregnancy and Lactation:* Reported emmenagogue in large amounts.† *Drug Interactions:* Inhibits platelet aggregation, prolongs bleeding and clotting times, and has fibrinolytic activity. For patients taking anticoagulants and anti-inflammatory drugs, use large doses with caution.

Table 13-6 Commonly used botanicals (continued).

Herbs	*Herbalist classification*	*Typical uses*	*Evidence based on clinical trials*	*Side effects and drug interactions*
Ginger *(Ziingiber officinale)*	• Antiemetic • Antispasmodic • Antiviral • Carminative • Immune modulator • Stimulates digestion	• Colic, anorexia; indigestion; prevention of vomiting and nausea in motion sickness, morning sickness, and post-operative nausea; upper respiratory tract infection, cough, and bronchitis.	• Mixed results for treatment for motion sickness and post-surgical nausea and vomiting. Helpful in treating hyperemesis gravidarum.	*Side Effects:* Heartburn.* *Contraindications:* Patients with gallstones due to cholagogue effect. *Pregnancy and Lactation:* † *Drug Interactions:* Could potentiate anticoagulants.
Ginkgo biloba	• Anticoagulant at high doses • Vasoactive	• Improving circulation in the brain and periphery. • Arteriosclerosis, cerebral ischemia, claudication. • Alzheimer's disease, dementia, senility. • Arthritic and rheumatic problems. • Lung and bronchial congestion, Raynaud's disease, tinnitus, vertigo, attention-deficit/hyperactivity disorder.	• Controlled trials reported positive results in the treatment of chronic cerebral insufficiency. • Several double-blind, placebo-controlled trials studying patients who have memory loss showed some improvement in memory. • Randomized controlled studies showed promise in treating memory loss and psychopathologic conditions in Alzheimer's disease and dementia. • Controlled studies on intermittent claudication showed favorable results. • No studies on pulmonary problems or attention-deficit/hyperactivity disorder.	*Side Effects:* Headache, dizziness, palpitation, gastrointestinal disorder, dermatitis.* *Pregnancy and Lactation:* † *Drug Interactions:* Could potentiate other anticoagulants, can hinder blood clotting at high doses.

Table 13-6 Commonly used botanicals (continued).

Herbs	*Herbalist classification*	*Typical uses*	*Evidence based on clinical trials*	*Side effects and drug interactions*
Goldenseal *(Hydratis canadensis)*	• Antihemorrhagic • Anti-inflammatory • Antimicrobial • Antiseptic • Astringent • Digestive aid • Oxytocic • Vulnerary	*External Use:* Conjunctivitis, boils, inflammation of gums, hemorrhoids, fungal infections. *Internal Use:* Diarrhea and other digestive disorders, upper respiratory tract infection, postpartum bleeding.	• Randomized, controlled studies demonstrate that berberine, a constituent of goldenseal, is effective in treating diarrhea. • No clinical studies on treatment of conjunctivitis, upper respiratory tract infection, or postpartum bleeding.	*Side Effects:* For large doses, nausea, vomiting, diarrhea, mucocutaneous irritation; increased cardiac and uterine contractility, vasoconstriction, central nervous system stimulation, and neonatal jaundice. *Pregnancy and Lactation:* Avoid in pregnancy and lactation. Not recommended for infants. Berberine displaces bilirubin from albumin. *Drug Interactions:* None known.
Hops *(Humulus lupulus)*	• Antispasmodic • Bitters • Diuretic • Hyponotic • Sedative	• Nervousness, irritability, insomnia, indigestion.	• No clinical studies.	*Side Effects:* *skin irritation. *Pregnancy and Lactation:* † *Drug Interactions:* Sedative activity increases the sleeping time induced by pentobarbital.
Lemon balm *(Melissa officinalis)*	• Antispasmodic • Anxiolytic • Calmative • Digestive aid	• Oral and genital herpes, insomnia, anxiety, depression.	• One study showed a sleep-promoting effect of the combination of valerian and lemon balm.	*Side Effects:* * *Pregnancy and Lactation:* † *Drug Interactions:* None known.

Table 13-6 Commonly used botanicals (continued).

Herbs	*Herbalist classification*	*Typical uses*	*Evidence based on clinical trials*	*Side effects and drug interactions*
Licorice *(Glycyrrhiza glabra)*		• Asthma, cough, sore throat, upper respiratory tract infection, bronchitis, stomach ulcers and digestive disturbances, constipation, colic, cholestatic liver disorders and liver disease, adrenocorticoid insufficiency, hypokalemia, hypertonia, arthritis.	• Licorice, in combination with other herbs, was effective in treating infant colic. • Constituents of licorice have proven effective in treating gastric ulcer in several studies. • Licorice, combined with other Chinese herbs, appears effective in treating severe eczema.	*Side Effects:* Long term use might lead to a mineralocorticoid effect, hypertension, potassium wasting, and arrhythmias.* *Pregnancy and Lactation:* † *Contraindications:* Patients who have hypertension, diabetes, hypokalemia, liver disorders, or kidney disease. *Drug Interactions:* Could potentiate digitalis and cardiac glycosides due to increased potassium loss. Could increase potassium loss in patients taking corticosteroids and thiazide diuretics.
Peppermint *(Mentha piperita)*	• Antimicrobial • Digestive aid • Carminative • Antispasmodic • Cholagogic • Secretolytic • Stimulant	*External Use:* Muscle aches, neuralgia, headache. *Internal Use:* Indigestion, nausea, diarrhea, flatulent colic, anorexia, inflammatory bowel disease, spastic complaints of the gastrointestinal tract, as well as gallbladder and bile ducts, upper respiratory tract infection, cough, tension headache.	• Enteric-coated peppermint oil capsules appear helpful in the treatment of irritable bowel syndrome/spastic colon. Peppermint oil relieves intestinal spasms during barium enema and endoscopy. • Clinical trials have shown a positive role in treating postoperative nausea, nonulcer dyspepsia in combination with caraway oil, and in combination with tension-type headaches.	*Side Effects:* Abdominal pain, heartburn, and perianal burning or hypersensitivity reactions.* *Contraindications:* Biliary duct occlusion, gallbladder inflammation, liver disease, and gastroesophageal reflux disease. Patients who have gallstones could develop colic due to peppermint's cholagogic effect. *Pregnancy and Lactation:* † *Drug Interactions:* None known.

Table 13-6 Commonly used botanicals (continued).

Herbs	Herbalist classification	Typical uses	Evidence based on clinical trials	Side effects and drug interactions
Purple cone flower (*Echinacea angustifolia* or *E purpurea)*	• Anti-inflammatory • Antimicrobial • Antiseptic • Immune modulator • Peripheral vasodilator	*External Use:* Boils, ulcerations, burns, herpes simplex. *Internal Use:* Prevention and supportive therapy for upper respiratory tract infection, urinary tract infection, yeast infection, and other infections.	• Controlled studies for *Echinacea* as an immune modulator to prevent and treat colds and influenza showed mixed results. Several randomized, double-blind, placebo-controlled studies showed a reduction in cold symptoms. However, in one study, *Echinacea* did not significantly decrease the incidence, duration, or severity of colds and respiratory infections compared with placebo.	*Side Effects:* Dermatitis.* *Pregnancy and Lactation:* † *Drug Interactions:* Possible unknown interactions with other immunomodulators.
Slippery elm bark *(Ulmus fulva)*	• Antitussive • Antiviral • Demulcent • Digestive aid • Emollient	*External Use:* Minor skin irritations, cold sores, ulcers, abscesses, and boils. *Internal Use:* Diarrhea, colic, inflammation or ulcerations of stomach or duodenum, urinary tract infections, sore throats, upper respiratory tract infections, abortifacient.	• No clinical studies.	*Side Effects:* Dermatitis.* *Pregnancy and Lactation:* † The whole bark has been used to induce abortions. There are no reported problems with the use of powdered slippery elm. *Drug Interactions:* None known.
St. John's Wort *(Hypericum perforatum)*	• Antidepressant • Anti-inflammatory • Astringent • Antimicrobial • Sedative • Immunomodulator	*External Use:* Wounds, burns, neuralgia, contusions. *Internal Use*: Depression, nervousness, anxiety.	• Double-blind, randomized, controlled trials demonstrate significant effectiveness in the treatment of mild-to-moderate depression. • Pilot case series have shown encouraging effects on immune function in human immunodeficiency virus-positive patients.	*Side Effects:* Gastrointestinal symptoms, sedation, dizziness, and confusion. Photosensitivity is rare but can be severe.* *Pregnancy and Lactation:* † *Drug Interactions:* None known.

Table 13-6 Commonly used botanicals (continued).

Herbs	*Herbalist classification*	*Typical uses*	*Evidence based on clinical trials*	*Side effects and drug interactions*
Thyme *(Thymus vulgaris)*	• Antimicrobial • Antitussive • Astringent • Carminative • Antispasmodic • Antiseptic • Diuretic • Expectorant	• Bronchitis/cough sore throat, upper respiratory tract infection, indigestion, colic, gastritis, dyspepsia, diarrhea, and enuresis.	• No clinical studies specifically on thyme. • An herbal combination that included thyme had positive effects on alopecia.	*Side Effects:* Thyme essential oil can be a mucous membrane irritant.* *Pregnancy and Lactation:* † *Drug Interactions:* None known.
Valerian *(Valeriana officianalis)*	• Anodyne • Antispasmodic • Hypotonic • Hypotensive • Sedative	• Insomnia, restlessness, menstrual cramps, rheumatic pain.	• Randomized, double-blind, placebo-controlled studies showed decreased sleep latency and improved sleep quality.	*Side Effects:* Headaches, insomnia.* *Pregnancy and Lactation:* † *Drug Interactions:* Sedative activity increases the sleeping time induced by pentobarbital.

* Allergic reactions are possible with any natural product.
† Insufficient clinical data on safety during pregnancy and lactation.

Source: Reprinted with permission, American Academy of Pediatrics. Table 2 (in entirety). *Peds in Review,* Vol. 21, No. 2, Feb 2000. Gardiner P, and Kemper KJ, Peripheral Bran: Herbs in Pediatric and Adolescent Medicine.

REFERENCES

1. Koletzko B, Aggettt PJ, Bindels JG, et al. Growth, development and differentiation: a functional food science approach. *Br J Nutr.* 1998;80(suppl):S5–S45.
2. Dietary Supplement Health and Education Act of 1994. Pub L No. 104–17. Available at: http://www.fda.gov/opacom/laws/dshea.html#sec3. Accessed July 2005.
3. National Institutes of Health, Office of Dietary Supplements. Dietary supplements: background information. Available at: http://ods.od.nih.gov/factsheets/dietarysupplements.asp. Accessed July 2005.
4. Valentine CJ, Trombetta A. Mixing practices in neonatal intensive care units. A national survey. *In progress.*
5. Mehta NR, Hamosh M, Bitman J, Wood DL. Adherence of medium-chain fatty acids to feeding tubes during gavage feeding of human milk fortified with medium-chain triglycerides. *J Pediatr.* 1988;112:474–476.
6. Valentine CJ, Schanler RJ. MCT oil added to selected formulas and resultant calorie composition. Unpublished data. 1993.
7. Ball SD, Kertesz D, Moyer-Mileur LJ. Dietary supplement use is prevalent among children with a chronic illness. *JADA.* 2005;105:78–84.
8. Kemper KJ, Wornham WL. Consultations for holistic pediatric services for inpatients and outpatient oncology patients at a children's hospital. *Arch Pediatr Adolesc Med.* 2001;155:449–454.
9. Isolauri E, Ribeiro HC, Gibson G, et al. Functional foods and probiotics: working group report of the first world congress of pediatric gastroenterology, hepatology, and nutrition. *J Pediatr Gastroenterol Nutr.* 2002;35(suppl 2):S106–109.
10. Gardiner P, Kemper KJ. Herbs in pediatric and adolescent medicine. *Pediatr in Rev.* 2000;21:44–57.
11. Committee on Nutrition. *Pediatric Nutrition Handbook.* 5th ed. Elk Grove Village, Il: American Academy of Pediatrics; 2004.
12. American Academy of Pediatrics. [Section on breastfeeding]. Breastfeeding and the use of human milk. *Pediatrics.* 2005;115:496–506.
13. Friis H, Anderson HK. Rate of inactivation of cytomegalovirus in raw banked milk during storage at –20 degrees C and pasteurization. *Br Med J Clin Res.* 1982;285:1604–1605.
14. Jocson MAL, Mason EO, Schanler RJ. The effects of nutrient fortification and varying storage conditions on host defense properties of human milk. *Pediatrics.* 1997;100:240–243.
15. Hamosh M, Ellis LA, Pollock DR, Henderson TR, Hamosh P. Breastfeeding and the working mother: effect of time and temperature of short term storage on proteolysis, lipolysis, and bacterial growth in milk. *Pediatrics.* 1996;97:492–498.
16. Valentine CJ, Hurst NM, Schanler RJ. Hindmilk improves weight gain in low-birth-weight infants fed human milk. *J Pediatr Gastroenterol Nutr.* 1994;18:474–477.
17. Schanler RJ. The role of human milk fortification for premature infants. *Clin Perinatol.* 1998;25:645–657.
18. Moyer-Mileur L, Chan GM, Gill G. Evaluation of liquid or powdered fortification of human milk on growth and bone mineralization status of preterm infants. *J Pediatr Gastroenterol Nutr.* 1992;15:370–374.
19. Raschko PK, Hiller JL, Benda GI, Buist NR, Wilcox K, Reynolds JW. Nutritional balance studies of VLBW infants fed their mothers' milk fortified with a liquid human milk fortifier. *J Pediatr Gastroenterol Nutr.* 1989;9:212–218.
20. Curtis MD, Candusso M, Peltain C, Rigo J. Effect of fortification on the osmolality of human milk. *Arch Dis Child Fetal Neonatal Ed.* 1999;81:F141–F143.
21. Chan GM. Effects of powdered human milk fortifiers on the antibacterial actions of human milk. *J Perinatol.* 2003;23:620–623.
22. Berseth CL, Merkel KL, Harris CL, Hansen JW. Growth, efficacy, and safety of an iron-fortified human milk fortifier. *Pediatr Res.* 2004;56:A2356.
23. Moody GJ, Schanler RJ, Abrams SA. Utilization of supplemental iron by premature infants fed fortified human milk. *Acta Pediatr.* 1999;88:763–767.
24. Schanler RJ, Shulman RJ, Lau C. Feeding strategies for premature infants: beneficial outcome of feeding fortified human milk versus preterm formula. *Pediatrics.* 1999;103:1150–1157.
25. Hurst NM, Valentine CJ, Renfro L, Burns P, Ferlic L. Skin to skin holding in the neonatal intensive care unit influences maternal milk volume. *J Perinatol.* 1997;17:213–217.
26. Smith JL, Heymsfield SB. Enteral nutrition support: formula preparation from modular ingredients. *JPEN.* 1985;60:280–288.
27. Bennett S. Intestinal absorptive capacity and site of absorption of fat under steady state conditions in the unanesthetized rat. *Q J Exp Physiol.* 1964;499:210–218.
28. Partin JS, Partin JC, Schubert WK, et al. Liver ultrastructure in abetalipoproteinemia: evolution of micro nodular cirrhosis. *Gastroenterology.* 1974;67:107–118.
29. Young VR, Pelletier VA. Adaptation to high protein intakes, with particular reference to formula feeding and the healthy, term infant. *J Nutr.* 1989;119:1799–1809.
30. Panel on Definition and Description, CAM Research Methodology Conference; April, 1995. Defining and describing complementary and alternative medicine. *Altern Ther Health Med.* 1997;1995:49–57.

31. Zeisel SH. Regulation of "neutraceuticals." *Science.* 1999;285:1853–1855.

32. Koutkia P, Chen TC, Holick MF Vitamin D intoxication associated with an over-the-counter supplement. *N Eng J Med.* 2001;345:66–67.

33. Gennaro AF, ed. *Remington's Pharmaceutical Sciences.* 17th ed. Easton, Pa: Mack Publishing Company; 1985:52–53.

CHAPTER 14

Drug–Nutrient Interactions: Considerations for Nutrition Support

Beverly W. Henry

INTRODUCTION

Drug–nutrient interactions are key elements in the management of pediatric nutrition support (NS). Interactions vary as to type and strength of effect on drug or nutrient components. Children are at increased risk for poor outcomes from drug–nutrient interactions because they might be unable to take pills or tablets by mouth. Drugs specially compounded at the local pharmacy also add risk. Often the same factors that necessitate enteral or parenteral feeding prompt drug therapy and that can have unexpected outcomes, especially when used in conjunction with a feeding regimen. Chronic diseases can require multiple medications over long periods of time, and children who rely on NS could be at increased risk for metabolic abnormalities or deficiencies. All of these factors can accentuate the negative effects of a drug–nutrient interaction.

Problems commonly associated with drug–nutrient interactions range from feeding intolerance or administration difficulties to metabolic derangements (Appendix A). Gastrointestinal symptoms include appetite changes, nausea, vomiting, and diarrhea, all of which can limit diet or drug efficacy. Incompatibility or instability of solutions complicates delivery. Altered fluid, electrolyte, or acid-base balance, vitamin or mineral status, and hyperglycemia are frequent concerns. Drug–nutrient interactions for common pediatric conditions underscore the importance of monitoring and devising strategies to incorporate drug therapies with NS.

This chapter discusses issues related to drug–nutrient interactions in NS, including basic pharmacy concepts and the types of effects, risk factors in children, interactions in different patient groups, treatment guidelines, and strategies for prevention. Information on drug–nutrient interactions and compatibility with intravenously administered drugs is addressed in the chapter, which also highlights important steps in the care of children receiving NS.

PHARMACY CONCEPTS UNDERLYING DRUG INTERACTIONS

Typically, drug–nutrient interactions involve some element in the administration, metabolism, or efficacy of the drug or NS. An introduction to pharmacy concepts is fundamental to understanding the breadth and potential strength of drug–nutrient interactions. These pharmacy concepts delineate the mechanisms of drug interactions and the responses to various drug and nutrient components. Five basic pharmacy concepts—the physiocochemical, physiologic, pathophysiologic, pharmacokinetic, and pharmacodynamic concepts—serve as the basis for classifying drug–nutrient interaction. Collectively, these processes influence each step in NS: ingestion, digestion, absorption, metabolism, and elimination or excretion. These concepts are discussed in the following paragraphs.

First, physiocochemical reactions concern the physical and chemical changes within specific drug or nutrient components during preparation or delivery. These interactions alter stability and solubility of the products, resulting in changed availability or value. The physiocochemical reactions include absorption, chelation, precipitation, or gel formation. These responses can occur during different phases of delivery. For example, unexpected changes to the drug may happen during compounding, light exposure, exposure to different pH levels or concentrations, and contact with other products or delivery systems. Physiocochemical reactions are the most common drug–nutrient interactions observed in NS patients.[1] Clogged feeding tubes typify the results of a physiocochemical reaction between acidic drugs and enteral formulas. Guidelines for the delivery schedule of intravenous drugs with parenteral nutrition (PN) solutions serve to prevent physiocochemical reactions, such as precipitation due to incompatibility or instability of the medication.[2,3]

Second, physiologic interactions entail functional changes in the body brought about by either a drug or a nutrient, which can influence the actual disposition of a nutrient or a drug. For instance, physiologic effects from a medication on gastric emptying time, either shortened or prolonged, might influence digestion of formulas. Physiologic effects of nutrition components can also affect how the drug is absorbed, as well as other properties. For example, consuming liquid formulas with medications might slow stomach emptying and delay passage of medications that are absorbed in the small intestine. Protein-based products, especially, rely on proteolytic enzymes produced by the pancreas, and physical effects on the transit of drugs or nutrient components can have unintended outcomes.

Third, pathophysiologic changes encompass the effects of drug toxicity on the bioavailability and utilization of nutrients. Adverse drug reactions can occur during treatment or could be caused by overdose. Examples of drug toxicity effects are damage to gastrointestinal cells (nonsteroidal anti-inflammatory drugs), hepatotoxicity (chlorpromazine, isoniazid), and nephrotoxicity (analgesics, antifungal agents).[4] Potential alterations in nutrient metabolism for each effect are absorption, utilization, and excretion, respectively.

The fourth concept, pharmacokinetics, is the study of the characteristic movement of a drug throughout the body and how the drug is altered within the body. The abbreviation ADME reflects the phases of absorption, distribution, metabolism, and excretion. To be of use, the drug must reach the target tissue in target concentration. Changes typically occur in the magnitude and duration of the drug effect. Drugs with a narrow therapeutic range and steep dose response curve are most likely to be influenced by an interaction effect. An example is phenytoin, which has nonlinear pharmacokinetics. Small changes in its absorption significantly impact serum levels and both adherence to polyvinylchloride tubing and interaction with enteral formulas lower absorption.[5,6] An example of drug–nutrient interactions for each pharmacokinetic phase is shown in Table 14-1. Further information about the pharmacokinetics of individual medications is available in pharmacy texts and reports.

The fifth concept, pharmacodynamics, is the study of the action of a drug in the body over a period of time. Drugs act in a general or a specific manner. There can be an overall general effect on body systems or a few organs or systems may be specifically targeted. Specific drug actions are more desirable but not always available. The more general the drug action, the more likely it is that reactions will overlap or that the receptors are shared with other compounds. This can result in a potentiated or synergistic action as compared to an antagonistic or opposing action. For instance, a potassium-rich enteral diet has an additive effect on potassium when taken with drugs prescribed to increase potassium. An example of an opposing action is the decreased anticoagulant effect of warfarin when vitamin K intake is increased. The pharmacodynamic effects of medications include many clinical and physiologic responses. Electrolyte balance is a prime area in which to observe effects. For example, altered sodium homeostasis along with a high sodium content of some medications can cause

Table 14-1 Examples of drug and nutrient interactions by pharmacokinetic activity.

Absorption—bioavailability to reach target tissues
- Nonsteroidal anti-inflammatory drugs are poorly soluble in acidic environments; less effective.
- Cholestyramine binds with bile salts to prevent reabsorption; fecal losses of fat soluble vitamins.
- Theophylline, sustained-release, increased absorption with a high fat meal; dose dumping.

Distribution—affinity for specific tissues (e.g., bloodstream, adipose tissue, CNS)
- β_2-adrenergic agonists induce an intracellular shift of potassium, causing hypokalemia.
- Valproic acid competes for protein binding sites on albumin, causing higher ionized calcium levels.

Metabolism—enzyme induction or inhibition
- Calcium channel blockers and cyclosporine intensified response because of down-regulation of cytochrome P-450 activity caused by grapefruit juice intake (similar effects for ritonavir).

Elimination—renal secretion and absorption functions
- Lithium retention enhanced with a sodium-rich diet.
- Cyclosporine and spironolactone elevate potassium losses in the urine.

---

hypernatremia, or stimulation of antidiuretic hormone by certain medications (β-blockers, angiotensin) can cause water conservation.

These pharmacy concepts characterize drug–nutrient interactions. When drugs are prescribed during the administration of NS, nutritional status must also be considered. As noted previously, drug–nutrient interactions can affect a myriad of factors, from fluid, electrolyte, or acid-base status to nutrient intake and stores. Some general nutrition effects from these interactions include appetite changes, nutrients displaced from protein binding sites, altered enzyme synthesis or regulation, excretion of bound nutrients, inhibited resorption, displacement of nutrients from the body, and decreased protein metabolism or glucose and lipid metabolic effects. The efficacy of the enteral or PN regimen must be monitored in light of drug therapies at each step in the NS process. There are special concerns for infants and children because they handle drugs differently than adults.

RISK FACTORS IN PEDIATRICS

Anatomic and physiologic developmental factors affect drug–nutrient interactions in children.[7] These include maturational changes in enzyme development, body composition, growth rate, and IV access. Also, the delivery of NS and the recent trend for parents to medicate their children with over-the-counter substances increases risk (Chapter 13). A brief look at these issues stresses a higher risk for unintended effects of drug therapy in children compared to adults.[8]

Risk factors in children for drug–nutrient interactions are outlined in Table 14-2. Physiologic considerations in young children, such as gastric volume, pH, and emptying time present challenges that complicate drug and nutrient absorption. Motility issues affect the timing and extent of exposure between compounds and absorbing surface areas.[9] Motility agents, such as metaclopramide, that decrease gastric emptying time and shorten transit time can lessen drug and nutrient contact with absorbing GI surfaces. Also, drug and nutrient compounds may form chelation complexes with antibiotics and metal ions (calcium, magnesium, aluminum, and iron), limiting absorption.[10] Absorption of tetracycline is decreased by half when consumed with food or milk, making the drug less effective.[11] Recommendations to give some medications at least 1 hour before and 2 hours after a meal[12] are intended to prevent such problems. That said, motility issues and stomach capacity could limit the child's tolerance for bolus feedings or larger hourly volumes needed to time drug administration appropriately. Another factor is that some medications significantly increase the osmolarity

Table 14-2 Risk factors and potential effects for drug–nutrient interactions in children.

Immature organ function
- Elevated gastric pH lowers dissolution rate of alkaline medications.
- Prolonged gastric emptying delays contact with gastrointestinal absorbing areas.
- Maturational delay in enzyme activity seen in pancreatic digestive enzymes, hepatic amino acid pathways, and lipoprotein lipase levels.
- Low glomerular filtration rate increases electrolyte losses with diuretics and risk of aluminum toxicity.

High nutrient requirements
- Glucose requirements >6 mg/kg/min, so children are less tolerant of interrupted infusions.
- To meet calorie and protein requirements, children need high energy and nutrient concentration.
- Delivery of high mineral requirements increases likelihood of precipitation.
- Frequent feeding schedule limits drug absorption (slows or binds).

Body composition
- Higher percent body water, so children are more susceptible to dehydration.
- Difficult or limited intravenous access translates to lack of alternative administration sites.

Development
- Lack of chewing or swallowing abilities means drugs must be specially compounded.
- Pills are crushed or capsules opened and given with foods as a delivery vehicle. This is associated with altered drug efficacy.

Delivery systems
- Physical contact by drug with tubing, so compounds adhere to polyvinylchloride.
- Incompatibility of additives puts limits on admixtures to conserve fluids.
- Osmolarity limits, so concentrated dosage forms are poorly tolerated.

---

of the feed and slow gastric emptying. The concentration of the formula may already be high to accommodate nutrient needs within limited fluid tolerance. These factors require a balancing act that demands careful attention from those who care for young children on enteral feedings.

The safe and accurate administration of PN admixtures is reviewed in the 2005 revision of the ASPEN standards of practice.[13] Protocols to prevent physiocochemical interactions should detail appropriate components and compounding sequences. For instance, when calcium gluconate is used as the calcium salt, it should be added near the end of the compounding sequence, following the phosphorus additive(s), when fluid volume is at the highest point.

Another drug–nutrient issue that affects children is the risk of toxicity or deficiency of specific compounds. For example, the risk of aluminum toxicity is higher for young children and those with impaired renal function. The aluminum load is lower in crystalline amino acid solutions but is high in other necessary nutrition substances such as albumin, calcium, heparin, and phosphorus. The FDA set 25 mcg/L as the upper limit for aluminum as of July 2004.[14,15] Alternately, nutrient losses may occur during compounding or delivery of drug–nutrient admixtures. For example, photodegradation and adherence to plastic bags and tubing lowers vitamin A levels. Riboflavin is especially sensitive to light and light can generate peroxides.[16] These examples show that adding vitamins in the final mixing step and protecting the PN bag and tubing from light exposure by using yellow, orange, or darkened bags may limit degradation.[16,17] Careful mixing, storage, and administration safeguard nutrient content of the formula.

The use of dietary supplements in children to improve or maintain health complicates the child's response to drugs and nutrients. Although dietary supplements are intended to improve intake of specific dietary components, herbs, vitamins, and nutritional products can play a role in drug interactions (Chapter 13). Pharmacokinetic and pharmacodynamic interactions appear to be the most common herb drug effects.[18] St. John's wort, garlic, ginkgo biloba, Panex ginseng, milk thistle, licorice, and ephedra (ma huang) can interact with prescribed drugs. Some interactions, outlined in the *Drug-Nutrient Resource*[19] can result in serious health problems. Just to name a few: the risk of nephrotoxicity from amphotericin B is increased with gossypol supplements; valproic acid, hawthorn, ginger, ginseng, and nettle may affect blood glucose levels; St. John's wort decreases blood levels of theophylline. These reactions can mask drug–nutrient interactions and make treatment more difficult. As families follow the trend to self-medicate, careful history taking and monitoring are needed to identify potential drug–nutrient interactions. The risks for ill effects from drug–nutrient interactions are a special concern for young children and those with specific medical conditions that require chronic and complicated care.

PEDIATRIC CONDITIONS LINKED WITH DRUG INTERACTIONS AND NUTRITION SUPPORT

Drug–nutrient interactions are often thought of in the context of a specific condition or medication type. An overview of general pediatric conditions in which drugs and NS coexist contributes to our understanding of how drug–nutrient interactions influence a child's tolerance to both therapies. Five conditions, burn injury, seizure disorders, prematurity, inflammatory bowel disease, and neoplastic disease are briefly described to elucidate familiar types of drug–nutrient problems. Common interactions and outcomes for these pediatric disorders are highlighted in Table 14-3.

Table 14-3 Pediatric conditions with common drug–nutrient interactions.

Condition	*Drug–nutrient effect*	*Outcome*
Burn injury	Acidic drugs and enteral formula	Occluded feeding tube
Seizure disorders	Anticonvulsants and decreased bioavailability of vitamins and minerals	Low absorption, accelerated degradation, increased excretion, and enzyme induction
Prematurity	Steroids and nutrient needs	Catabolism, hyperglycemia, hypertriglyceridemia
	Diuretics and fluid management	Losses of electrolytes, minerals, and bicarbonate
	Low pH of PN solution	Acidosis
	PN amino acid and mineral additives ± lipids	Incompatibility, precipitation, cracked emulsions
	Theophylline with formula, fiber	Enhanced drug absorption
Inflammatory bowel disease	Anti-inflammatory—corticosteroids	Growth stunting and metabolic effects
	Immunosuppressive—methotrexate	Bone marrow, hepatic, pancreatic toxicity
Neoplastic disease	Chemotherapeutic agents	GI effects: inflammation, mouth dryness, altered taste perception
		Nephrotoxicity and mineral losses

Burn Injury

The metabolic response to burn injury, especially in a young, growing child, is complex. Enteral nutrition (EN) delivers nutrients despite pain and therapeutic interventions, and it has the potential to ameliorate catabolism and loss of lean body mass. Nevertheless, burned children experience nutrition-related problems, and some of these are associated with drug therapies. When drugs and formulas are given concurrently, interactions can occur. Drug chelation by minerals limits absorption and efficacy. Physiochemical interactions, such as those between syrups and feeding tubes resulting in tube occlusion, are especially problematic. The enteral tube position dictates which drugs can be given by this route. Antacids and sucralfate act in the stomach and must be delivered directly into the stomach; hypertonic drug solutions can cause diarrhea when delivered directly into the small bowel. Ciprofloxacin is poorly absorbed when delivered into the small bowel or when administered with continuous feedings.[20]

Specific nutrient deficiencies can contribute to poor growth and bone health after injury. Bone health is adversely affected by hypovitaminosis D caused by low vitamin D intake, reduced absorption, and little exposure to sunlight. Low mineral intake and inactivity contribute to poor bone health. Drug–nutrient interactions also play a role. Thyroxine administration is associated with low vitamin D_{25} levels.[21] An interaction between oxandrolone (anabolic agent) and low vitamin D_{25} occurs. Study of drug–nutrient interactions, metabolic changes, and efficacy of vitamin and mineral supplements for burned children is ongoing.

Seizure Disorders

EN is indicated for children with seizure disorders when oral eating is not sufficient to support growth or health. Most drug–nutrient interactions affect peristalsis and alter absorption or utilization.[22] Fiber-containing formulas reduce the absorption of phentoin.[23] Medications can alter gastrointestinal function. Gastrointestinal muscle tone changes that slow peristalsis lead to constipation; antibiotics that alter intestinal flora cause diarrhea. In addition to supplying nutrients, adequate fluid and fiber intake are main objectives with NS.

Anticonvulsant medications are associated with low vitamin status. The drug–drug and drug–nutrient interactions with these medications are complex. For example, phenobarbitol is associated with low levels of vitamins C, B_{12}, and folic acid caused by accelerated degradation, urinary excretion, and reduced absorption.[17,24–26] Phenobarbitol alters vitamin D metabolism by enzyme induction, increases potassium levels, and decreases calcium status.[17] Phenytoin is associated with low vitamins C, B_{12}, D, and folic acid caused by accelerated degradation, urinary excretion, reduced absorption, and inhibited hepatic metabolism.[17,24–27] Calcium levels are low because phenytoin alters vitamin D synthesis. Pyridoxine supplementation could lower phenytoin activity.[17,24,28] Valproic acid increases urinary carnitine excretion.[24] Also, valproic acid exemplifies drug–drug interactions as it displaces phenytoin from protein binding sites and inhibits metabolism of this drug. Supplementation with vitamins, minerals, and carnitine may be needed to compensate for these interactions.

Prematurity

Problems seem to be intensified in infants born prematurely. Low drug or nutrient bioavailability when delivered with EN can lead to poor results in sick infants who have low nutrient reserves. In contrast, theophylline (bronchodilator) absorption is enhanced when given with formula or hemicellulose fiber. Drug-induced metabolic abnormalities include corticosteroid effects on hyperglycemia, increased urinary nitrogen excretion, hypokalemia, hypocalcemia, and hypophosphatemia; dexamethasone and hypertriglyceridemia; furosemide or thiazide's effect and hyperglycemia, hypokalemia, hypercalcemia, and hypomagnesemia; and spironolactone and hyperkalemia and hyponatremia. Loop diuretics cause increased calcium excretion (hypocalcemia) and hypomagnesemia.[18,19]

Management of respiratory and fluid problems (e.g., chronic steroids and diuretic therapy) and prolonged dependence on PN push protein and mineral intake lower and electrolyte losses higher. This contributes to the frequent occurrence of osteopenia (estimated at 30%) in very low birth-weight infants.[29] PN amino acid solutions supplemented with cysteine hydrochloride have a low pH and allow for improved calcium and phosphorus solubility. However, acetate may be needed because of the infant's acid-base status. The higher the acetate, the more limited is the possibility of maximizing protein and mineral intake.[30] Three in one admixtures are avoided in the neonatal intensive care unit because of stability concerns. PN mixes with lipid emulsions can be affected by pH and temperature changes. Also, it is not easy to visually inspect the opaque lipid solution for possible precipitations. Taken together, low enteral absorption, the catabolic effects of corticosteroid therapy, drug effects on electrolyte balance, and stability of concentrated PN admixtures point out the importance of daily monitoring for drug–nutrient interactions.

Inflammatory Bowel Disease

Treatment objectives for children with inflammatory bowel disease include enteral feeding and drug therapy (see Chapter 33). Corticosteroids are commonly used and are associated with fluid retention, hypertension, and metabolic abnormalities such as hyperglycemia. Drug–nutrient effects include the inhibition of calcium absorption and altered protein metabolism. Sulfazine decreases iron levels by chelation and inhibits folate absorption. Immunosuppressive drugs such as azothioprine and methotrexate cause hepatotoxicity, pancreatitis, and bone marrow suppression. Immunomodulating agents, such as cyclosporine, are associated with hyperlipidemia, nephrotoxicity, and hepatotoxicity.[4,18,19]

Neoplastic Disease

There are considerable and varied drug–nutrient interactions for medications used in the treatment of neoplastic disease. Immunotherapies are associated with anorexia, nausea, vomiting, diarrhea, stomatitis, mucositis, xerostomia, and taste perversion. All of these can compromise oral intake. Nutrition effects are also seen with chemotherapeutic agents such as heavy metals. Drug–nutrient interactions with cisplatin, for example, cause low copper, magnesium, potassium, and zinc levels due to renal tubular dysfunction.[24] Plant alkaloids such as vincristine have effects on potassium levels via tumor lysis syndrome.[27] Radiotherapy causes gastrointestinal injury and can negatively impact nutrient intake and exacerbate drug–nutrient interactions.

The discussion of the previous five conditions displays the wide ranging effects and outcomes that can be encountered with drug–drug and drug–nutrient interactions and emphasizes the pharmacy concepts and pediatric risk factors introduced earlier in the chapter.

TREATMENT STRATEGIES FOR DRUG–NUTRIENT INTERACTIONS

To limit the potential effects of drug–nutrient interactions, specific preparation and dosing strategies are necessary for delivery of the medications. In addition to the timing and route of drug administration, the form of the drug, delivery site, and pharmacokinetics must be considered. Drug effects on nutrient intake, absorption, utilization, excretion, and overall status must also be considered. Possible interventions to treat related problems are outlined in Table 14-4. These basic guidelines offer a list of options to consider with different drug therapies.

Information about specific drug–nutrient interactions is available from a variety of sources. Some helpful drug manuals and references are listed in Table 14-5.

When a child experiences alterations in drug effectiveness or nutritional status, the possibility of a drug–nutrient interaction should be

Table 14-4 Treatment of drug–nutrient interactions.

Drug groups	*Interventions*
Anticonvulsants	
Malabsorption	Separate dosing from feeding
Increased turnover	Vitamin and mineral supplementation
Antifungal agents	
Hyperexcretion by the kidneys	Electrolyte supplementation
Anti-inflammatory drugs	
Malabsorption	Alternate drug dosing with food intake
Antiarrhythmics	
GI distress	Take with a small amount of food
Digoxin toxicity with hypokalemia	Maintain potassium levels
Bile acid sequestrants	
Malabsorption	Separate additives of fat-soluble vitamins, bicarbonate
Corticosteroids	
Catabolism	Increase protein delivery
Hyperglycemia, hyperlipidemia	Monitor energy intake and tolerance
Diuretics	
Hyperexcretion by the kidneys	Maintain potassium intake for increased losses
Immunosuppressive	
Pathophysiologic effects	Maintain adequate hydration, nutrient intake
Folate antagonist	Avoid folate supplementation
NSAID	
Poorly water soluble	Delay gastric emptying, allow time for dissolution
Gastric distress	Avoid other GI irritants with use (e.g., caffeine)
Iron-deficiency anemia	Monitor for blood loss

Table 14-5 Helpful drug manuals and references.

- Hardman, JF, Limbird LE, eds. *Goodman and Gilman's the Pharmacological Basis of Therapeutics.* 10th ed. New York, NY: McGraw-Hill; 2001. A classic.
- McCabe BJ, Frankel EH, Wolfe JJ, eds. *Handbook of Food–Drug Interactions.* Boca Raton, Fla: CRC Press; 2003.
- McEvoy GK, ed. *AHFS Drug Information 2003.* Bethesda, Md: American Society of Health-System Pharmacists; 2003. Provides details on usage, stability, and compatibility.
- Taketomo CK, Hodding JH, Kraus DM, eds. *Pediatric Dosage Handbook.* 8th ed. Hudson, Ohio: Lexi-Comp; 2001. A comprehensive list for dosing, administration, and monitoring of medications in children.
- Zucchero FJ, Hogan MJ, Sommer CD, Curran JP, eds. *Evaluations of Drug Interactions.* Vol 1, 2. St. Louis, Mo: First DataBank; 2002. Covers many interactions and alternative therapies.
- *Drug Information for Health Care Professionals (USP-DI, I).* Rockville, Md: U.S. Pharmacopeia Convention, Inc.: 2001. *United States Pharmacopeia*, Vol 1. Information on side effects, dosing, interactions, precautions, and patient counseling guidelines.

explored. If a problem is identified, then alternative drug regimens or nutrition therapy should be implemented. Careful monitoring and delivery of drug therapies is especially important when a child relies on enteral or parenteral support. In some situations, the options for drug or nutrient changes are limited. In these cases, limiting the consequences of side effects is paramount.

PREVENTION OF DRUG–NUTRIENT INTERACTIONS

The incidence of drug–nutrient interactions can be minimized, if not entirely prevented. Several guidelines to limit the occurrence of unexpected responses from drugs and nutrients are listed in Table 14-6. Priorities for minimizing the likelihood of drug–nutrient interactions include careful selection, implementation, and monitoring of the drug treatment. Understanding the risk for an unwanted response from drug–nutrient interactions and the options available to improve clinical efficacy of both are first steps to preventing poor outcomes. Patient education and team communication are necessary for quality care. Careful delivery and monitoring of children receiving nutrition support should be ongoing. It is important to understand the rationale for monitoring protocols and to know how to manage the child's response to treatment. Documentation of drug–nutrient interactions helps to ensure continuing improvements in nutrition support for children.

Table 14-6 Preventing drug–nutrient interactions.

Things to keep in mind:

- Child's prior experience with proposed drug, dose, duration, and reactions.
- Nutritional status affects drug metabolism.
- Knowledge of the mechanisms behind interactions allows one to predict when problems could occur.
- Medications with a narrow range of effectiveness and steep dose-response curve are more likely to have interaction effects.
- Careful tracking of drug doses and duration help to distinguish these effects from the patient's clinical response.
- The site of action and absorption of drugs need to be considered with the route of delivery.
- Serum concentrations of drugs that can be displaced from protein binding sites are not as predictive of the drug action.
- Sorbitol is an osmotic cathartic and can induce osmotic diarrhea.

Things to do:

- Keep detailed records of the child's medication history.
- Review medication dosing with any feeding regimen change.
- For enteral delivery of drugs, keep delivery separate from the feeding and flush the tube before and after each medication.
- Use liquid medication forms for tube administration.
- Limit coadministration of medications with PN solutions according to guidelines.
- When safety information about mixing a drug with PN is not available, separate delivery from PN.
- Periodically inspect every PN solution for signs of particulates.
- Carefully monitor nutrient levels with drug therapies known to cause deficiencies and supplements used to offset drug effects.
- Follow up treatment to identify and communicate the child's response to drug and feeding therapies.

CONCLUSION

Children who suffer from chronic disease or developmental delays are those most likely to receive NS and also to receive multiple medications. The risk of drug-nutrient interaction is high in pediatric care, especially among children on NS. However, knowledge of the issue, vigilance and corrective measures can minimize unwanted complications.

REFERENCES

1. ASPEN. Guidelines for the use of parenteral and enteral nutrition in adult and pediatric patients. Section X; Drug–nutrient interactions. *JPEN*. 2002;26(suppl):42SA-44SA.
2. King JC, Catania PN, eds. *King Guide to Parenteral Admixtures*. Napa, Calif: King Guide Publications, Inc.; 2002.
3. Trissel LA, Gilbert DL, Martinez JF. Compatibility of parenteral nutrition solutions with selected drugs during simulated Y-site administration. *Am J Health-Syst Pharm*. 1997;54:1295–1300.
4. Beers MH, ed. Factors affecting drug responses. In: Beers MH, ed. *Merck Manual of Medical Information*. 2nd home ed. Available at: http://www.merck.com/mrkshared/mmanual/section22/chapter301/301a.jsp. Accessed December 27, 2005.
5. Marvel ME, Bertino JS. Comparative effects of an elemental and a complex enteral feeding formulation on the absorption of phenytoin suspension. *JPEN*. 1991;15:316–318.
6. Doak KK, Haas CE, Dunnigan KJ, et al. Bioavailability of phenytoin acid and phenytoin sodium with enteral feedings. *Pharmacotherapy*.1998;18:637–645.
7. Kearns GL, Abdel-Rahman SM, Alander SW, et al. Developmental pharmacology-drug disposition, action, and therapy in infants and children. *N Engl J Med*. 2003;349(12):1157–1167.
8. ASPEN. Guidelines for the use of parenteral and enteral nutrition in adult and pediatric patients. *JPEN*. 2002;26(suppl):1SA–138SA.
9. Segal S, Kaminski S. Drug–nutrient interactions. *Am Druggist*. 1996;213:42–49.
10. Quinolones. In: McEvoy, GK, ed. *American Hospital Formulary Service Drug Information*. Bethesda, Md: ASH-SP, Inc.; 1999:670–719.
11. Tetracyclines. In: McEvoy, GK, ed. *American Hospital Formulary Service Drug Information*. Bethesda, Md: ASH-SP, Inc.; 1999:438–440.
12. Kirk J. Significant drug–nutrient interactions. *Am Fam Physician*. 1995;51:1175–1182.
13. ASPEN. Standards for specialized nutrition support: hospitalized pediatric patients. *Nutr Clin Pract*. 2005;20:103–116.
14. US Food and Drug Administration Proposed Rule. Aluminum in large and small volume parenterals used in total parenteral nutrition, 63 *Federal Register* 176–185 (1998).
15. Department of Health and Human Services of the Food and Drug Administration. Aluminum in large and small volume parenterals used in total parenteral nutrition; amendment; delay of effective date, 67 *Federal Register* (228):70691–70692 (2002).
16. Laborie S, Laborie J, Pinaeault M, et al. Protecting solutions of parenteral nutrition from perioxidation. *J Parent Enteral Nutr*. 1999;23:104–108.
17. Baumgartner TG, ed. *Clinical Guide to Parenteral Micronutrition*. 3rd ed. Deerfield, Il. Fujisawa USA, Inc.; 1997.
18. McCabe BJ, Frankel EH, Wolfe JJ, eds. *Handbook of Food–Drug Interactions*. Boca Raton, Fla: CRC Press; 2003.
19. Elmes T, Infelise D, Wagner J. *Drug–Nutrient Resource: Part of the Drug–Nutrient Intervention System*. 4th ed. Riverside, Ill: Roche Dietitians, LLC; 2001.
20. Strausberg KM. Drug interactions in nutrition support. In: McCabe BJ, Frankel EH, Wolfe JJ, eds. *Handbook of Food–Drug Interactions*. Boca Raton, Fla: CRC Press; 2003:145–165.
21. Gottschlich MM, Mayes T, Khoury J, et al. Hypovitaminosis D in acutely injured pediatric burn patients. *J Am Diet Assoc*. 2004;104(6):931–941.
22. Lucas BL, Feucht SA, Grieger LE, eds. *Children with Special Health Care Needs: Nutrition Care Handbook*. Chicago, Ill: ADA; 2004.
23. Mayne J, Roe DA. Effects of varied fiber level in enteral formula upon the xenobiotic metabolizing systems of rat intestinal mucosa. *Fed Proc*.1987;46:1168.
24. McEvoy GK, ed. *American Hospital Formulary Service Drug Information*. Bethesda, Md: ASH-SP, Inc.; 2003.
25. Lourenco R. Enteral feeding:drug/nutrient interaction. *Clin Nutr*. 2001;20(2):187–193.
26. Melnick G. Pharmacologic aspects of enteral nutrition. In: Rombeau JL, Caldwell MD, eds. *Clinical Nutrition: Enteral and Tube Feeding*. 2nd ed. Philadelphia, Pa: WB Saunders Co.; 1990.
27. Maka DA, Murphw LK. Drug–nutrient interactions: a review. *AACN Clin Issues*. 2000;11(4):580–589.
28. Sorenson JM. Herb–drug, food–drug, nutrient–drug, and drug–drug interactions: mechanisms involved and their medical implications. *J Alternative Complement Med*. 2002;8(3):293–308.

29. Krug S. Osteopenia of prematurity. In: Groh-Wargo S, Thompson J, Cox T, eds. *Nutritional Care for High Risk Newborns*. 3rd ed. Chicago, Ill: Precept Press; 2000:489–505.

30. Brine E, Ernst JA. Total parenteral nutrition for premature infants. *Newborn Infant Nursing Rev*. 2004;4(3):133–155.

Chapter 15

Regulatory Aspects of Infant Formulas and Medical Foods in the United States

Sue Ann Anderson

INTRODUCTION

Before passage of the 1906 Pure Food and Drug Act, there was no federal regulation of foods in the United States. At the turn of the twentieth century, human milk substitutes (infant formulas) were in the very early stages of development and the first medical foods were not produced until the second half of the century. Development of these products depended on a convergence of scientific discovery, technological advances, and medical practices. Both infant formulas and medical foods are manufactured to meet the nutritional needs of vulnerable populations and regulatory requirements for these product categories are described in this chapter.

INFANT FORMULAS

Infant formulas are products that simulate human milk or are suitable as a complete or partial substitute for human milk and are intended for use by infants (children not more than 12 months old). Like all foods, infant formulas are regulated under the provisions of Chapter IV of the Federal Food, Drug, and Cosmetic Act (FFDCA).[1] Nutritional aspects (nutrient content and production of nutritionally adequate infant formulas) are specifically regulated under the Infant Formula Act of 1980 and its 1986 amendments (see Section 412 of the FFDCA). The legislation was considered necessary to protect the health of infants because formula serves as the sole source of nutrition during early life for many infants, and errors in its composition could lead to adverse effects on growth and development or possibly to death.

Congress enacted the Infant Formula Act in 1980 after an infant formula manufacturer discontinued adding sodium chloride to 2 formulas. Consumption of the chloride-deficient products resulted in development of hypochloremic metabolic alkalosis in more than 140 infants.[2] In 1986, Congress added amendments to strengthen and expand the provisions of the 1980 act and gave the FDA greater regulatory authority over infant formulas.

The FDA has adopted regulations that implement a number of the provisions of the 1980 act and the 1986 amendments. These include regulations for nutrient requirements, quality control procedures, labeling, record and record retention requirements, recall procedures, and exempt infant formulas. These regulations are found in the Code of Federal Regulations (see 21 CFR parts 106 and 107).[3] In 1996, the agency published a proposed rule for current good manufacturing practice, revised quality control procedures, quality factors, notification requirements, and records and reports for the production of infant formulas. This rule has not been finalized (see Food and Drug Administration 1996, 2003).[3,4] Details about current and proposed regulations are provided on the FDA's infant formula web site.[3]

Product Composition

Infant formula must contain all nutrients in amounts that will support growth and development of infants during the time when nutrient requirements, relative to body weight, are higher than at any other time. The Infant Formula Act and FDA regulations specify minimum levels for 29 nutrients in infant formulas. In addition, maximum levels are specified for nine nutrients for which there is scientific evidence of adverse effects at high intakes (see 21 CFR 107.100).[3] Section 412 of the FFDCA provides for revision of nutrient requirements for infant formulas when new scientific evidence supports such adjustments. Specifications for nutrients required in infant formulas are listed in Table 15-1. If an infant formula does not contain these nutrients at the required levels, it is defined by law as an adulterated product.

While the FFDCA and the FDA's implementing regulations specify the nutrient content of infant formulas, they do not require use of particular ingredients to attain the nutrient content. Substances approved for use as food additives in infant formulas and substances generally recognized as safe (GRAS) for this use may be used as ingredients in these products. Regulatory information about food additives and GRAS ingredients may be found on the FDA web sites.[5,6] Evaluation of the safety of ingredients new to infant formulas is discussed in a recent report by the Institute of Medicine.[7]

Current Good Manufacturing Practice and Quality Control

All infant formulas must be manufactured in compliance with current good manufacturing practices for foods (see 21 CFR 110).[3] Manufacture of liquid concentrate and ready-to-feed formulas must also comply with regulations for thermally processed low acid canned foods (see 21 CFR 113).[3] Processing required for liquid infant formulas produces commercially sterile products; however, processing of powdered products does not.

Manufacturers must maintain constant control over the processing of infant formula because a seemingly harmless change in formulation or in a preparation method or exposure to an unanticipated environmental condition could create a health hazard for infants who will consume the product. The FDA has proposed additional regulations for good manufacturing practices specific to infant formula to ensure that these products provide the nutrients required and are manufactured in a manner designed to prevent adulteration (see the FDA's 1996 proposed rule).[3]

FDA quality control regulations require that infant formula manufacturers chemically analyze the nutrient content of each batch of infant formula during production and at the final product stage before distribution. Manufacturers must also analyze infant formulas during product shelf life to confirm that the required nutrient content is maintained throughout the time period when they are intended for consumption by infants (see 21 CFR 106).[3]

Quality Factors

Chemical analysis done for quality control indicates whether infant formulas contain nutrients at the required levels; however, it does not indicate whether the nutrients will reach infants in a usable form and in sufficient quantity to meet their needs for growth and development. For this reason, the Infant Formula Act authorized the Secretary of the Department of Health and Human Services to establish regulations for quality factors, i.e., factors necessary to demonstrate that an infant formula provides nutrients in a form that is bioavailable and safe during the expected shelf life of the product.[1]

Biological quality of protein has been established by FDA regulation as a quality factor for infant formula. As assessed by the protein efficiency ratio (PER) bioassay in growing rats fed the infant formula, the biological quality of the protein must be comparable to that of bovine casein (see 21 CFR 106).[3] The FDA suggested requirements for additional quality factors, specifically for healthy growth and normal physical

Table 15-1 Nutrient requirements for infant formulas (21 CFR 107).[3]

Nutrient	*Minimum level (per 100 kcal)*	*Maximum level (per 100 kcal)*
Protein, g	1.8	4.5
Fat, g (% kcal)	3.3 (30)	6.0 (54)
Linoleic acid, mg (% kcal)	300 (2.7)	—
Vitamin A, IU	250	750
Vitamin D, IU	40	100
Vitamin E, IU	0.7	—
Vitamin K, μg	4	—
Thiamin (vitamin B_1), μg	40	—
Riboflavin (vitamin B_2), μg	60	—
Vitamin B_6, μg	35	—
Vitamin B_{12}, μg	0.15	—
Niacin, μg*	250	—
Folic acid (folacin), μg	4	—
Pantothenic acid, μg	300	—
Biotin, μg†	1.5	—
Vitamin C (ascorbic acid), mg	8	—
Choline, mg†	7	—
Inositol, mg†	4	—
Calcium, mg	60	—
Phosphorus, mg	30	—
Magnesium, mg	6	—
Iron, mg	0.15	3.0
Zinc, mg	0.5	—
Manganese, μg	5	—
Copper, μg	60	—
Iodine, μg	5	75
Sodium, mg	20	60
Potassium, mg	80	200
Chloride	55	150

* Includes niacin (nicotinic acid) and niacinamide (nicotinamide).
† Required only for nonmilk-based formulas.

growth of infants, in its 1996 proposed rule. The FDA proposed the double-blind, randomized, controlled clinical feeding study as the means of providing assurance that a new infant formula would support normal physical growth. All clinical studies that support applications for research or marketing permits for products regulated by the FDA, including infant formulas, must follow regulations for human subject protection, additional safeguards for children as subjects in clinical investigations, and institutional review boards, as required by 21 CFR parts 50 and 56.[3]

Premarket Notifications

Infant formula manufacturers are required to register with the FDA and to submit a notification 90 days before they plan to market any new infant formula, including currently marketed products with major changes (see FFDCA Section 412).[3] The law requires that the notifications contain certain elements, which include:

- the quantitative formulation of the product (i.e., a listing of all ingredients and the quantities of those ingredients needed to produce the given quantity of product),
- assurance that the formula will meet the nutrient content requirements,
- assurance that the formula will meet quality factors, and
- assurances that the formula will be manufactured using current good manufacturing practices, including quality control procedures.

The FDA reviews this information to determine if there is a basis for concern about the marketing of the product. Because this is a premarket notification and not a premarket approval process, FDA approval is not required for a manufacturer to market a new infant formula. However, if a manufacturer does not provide the above assurances in its notification for a new formula, the formula is defined as adulterated under Section 412 of the FFDCA, and the FDA has the authority to take compliance action if the new infant formula is marketed.

Labeling

Certain aspects of labeling requirements for infant formulas differ from those for other food products. For example, concentrations of each of the 29 nutrients required in infant formulas must be listed on the product label. Infant formula labels must provide nutrient information in relation to the energy content of the formula (per 100 kcal), in contrast to labels for other foods that are required to list nutrient content on a per-serving basis.

FDA regulations also require that labels for infant formulas include a use-by date and directions for storage, preparation, and use of the product. Manufacturers select the use-by date based on data or other information showing that the product will contain the quantity of each nutrient listed on the label and will otherwise be of acceptable quality until that date. Labels must also include statements that caution against improper preparation or use and that instruct parents to consult their physician about the use of infant formulas (see 21 CFR 107).[3]

Exempt Infant Formulas

The Infant Formula Act established two regulatory categories for infant formulas. Nonexempt formulas are products for healthy, term infants. Exempt infant formulas are products intended and labeled for use by low birth-weight infants and infants with inborn errors of metabolism or other unusual medical or dietary problems. See Table 15-2 for the types of formulas in each category. While nonexempt products must comply with all provisions of Section 412 of the FFDCA and FDA regulations, exempt products are not required to do so. Deviations from any of the nutrient requirements, quality control procedures, and labeling requirements for nonexempt infant formulas require agency review. Based on its review of the submitted materials and other available information, the FDA may impose additional conditions or require modifications for the quality control procedures, nutrient specifications, or labeling; or it may withdraw a product's exempt status (see 21 CFR 107).[3]

Table 15-2 Regulatory categories for infant formulas.

Nonexempt products
- Cow's milk-based formulas
- Partially hydrolyzed casein and whey protein-based formulas
- Partially hydrolyzed whey protein-based formulas
- Soy-based formulas

Exempt products
- Preterm infant formulas
  - hospital use
  - post discharge use
- Amino acid-based formulas
  - complete mixtures of amino acids
  - modified mixtures for inborn errors of metabolism
- Extensively hydrolyzed casein-based

Formulas regulated as exempt products are listed on the FDA's infant formula web site.[8] Similar products intended for use by children 1 year of age and older are regulated as medical foods, as described later in this chapter.

Manufacturers' Records

Improper formulation and processing of infant formulas are likely to increase the risk of producing an adulterated product that could be harmful to infants. Each manufacturer must maintain records that will allow the FDA to determine whether its infant formula products are being produced as required by section 412 of the FFDCA. The records must contain sufficient information to permit a public health evaluation of any batch of infant formula. Requirements include (1) records pertaining to product manufacture, nutrient content, microbiological quality, and complaints; and (2) records tracking the distribution of infant formulas through any establishment owned or operated by the manufacturer that could be necessary to effect and monitor recalls of a formula (see 21 CFR 107).[3] At least once every year, the FDA inspects each facility producing infant formulas for the US market and examines the required records as part of the inspection procedure.

Product Recalls

The FDA is authorized by law to require an infant formula manufacturer to recall an adulterated or misbranded infant formula when the FDA determines that the product presents a risk to the health of infants. These recalls extend to and include the retail level.

Manufacturers may also initiate voluntary product recalls. For voluntary recalls, the firm must make a written evaluation of the hazard to human health associated with the use of the infant formula, including consideration of any disease, injury, or other adverse physiological effect that has been or could be caused by the infant formula and the seriousness, likelihood, and consequences of such occurrences. In cases of manufacturer-initiated recalls, the FDA also conducts its own health hazard evaluation and is required to promptly notify the recalling firm of the results of that evaluation, if the criteria for an FDA required recall are met (see 21 CFR 107).[3]

MEDICAL FOODS

Medical foods are defined under the Orphan Drugs Amendment of 1988 as foods that are formulated to be consumed or administered enterally under the supervision of a physician and that are intended for the specific dietary management of a disease or condition for which distinctive nutritional requirements, based on recognized scientific principles, are established by medical evaluation.[9]

Medical foods are complex, formulated products that comprise an integral component of the clinical management of patients with certain diseases such as metabolic disorders or renal disease. Products recommended by a health care provider as part of an overall diet designed to reduce the risk of a disease or medical condition, to lose or maintain weight, or to ensure the consumption of a healthy diet are *not* medical foods. For example, medical foods do not include complete liquid nutrition products for use by the general population as supplements to a normal diet or as meal replacements.

Current Regulations

Medical foods must comply with all regulatory requirements for conventional foods, except for nutrition labeling requirements. For example, medical foods must be manufactured in accordance with good manufacturing practices (see 21 CFR 110) and in accordance with low-acid canned food regulations, if applicable (see 21 CFR 113).[3] Like all foods for human consumption, medical foods must be formulated with ingredients that are GRAS or approved food additives.[5,6] Current FDA regulations do not require premarket notification or approval before marketing of a medical food formulation to ensure that it is suitable for the intended patient population.

Exemption from Nutrition Labeling Regulations

The Nutrition Labeling and Education Act of 1990 (see FFDCA Section 403)[1] and FDA labeling regulations include the statutory definition of medical foods as stated above. They exempt medical foods from the nutrition labeling, health claim, and nutrient content claim requirements as applied to most other foods. The FDA has considered that the statutory definition sets narrow limits around the types of products that fall within this exemption. The FDA's labeling regulations provide that a food may claim the medical foods exemption from nutrition labeling only if it meets all of the following criteria specified in 21 CFR 101.9:[10]

- It is a specially formulated and processed product (as opposed to a naturally occurring foodstuff used in its natural state) for the partial or exclusive feeding of a patient by means of oral intake or enteral feeding by tube.
- It is intended for the dietary management of a patient who, because of therapeutic or chronic medical needs has limited or impaired capacity to ingest, digest, absorb, or metabolize ordinary foodstuffs or certain nutrients, or who has other special medically determined nutrient requirements, the dietary management of which cannot be achieved by the modification of the normal diet alone.
- It provides nutritional support specifically modified for the management of the unique nutrient needs that result from the specific disease or condition, as determined by medical evaluation.
- It is intended to be used under medical supervision.
- It is intended only for a patient receiving active and ongoing medical supervision wherein the patient requires medical care on a recurring basis for, among other things, instructions on the use of the medical food.

CONCLUSION

Infant formulas are regulated under provisions of the Infant Formula Act of 1980 and its 1986 amendments. The statute provides the FDA with authority to implement regulations for infant formula in addition to those for other food products. Medical foods must comply with all regulatory requirements for conventional foods but are exempt from certain nutrition labeling regulations.

REFERENCES

1. US Food and Drug Administration. *Laws Enforced by the FDA and Related Statutes*. Available at: http://www.fda.gov/opacom/laws/. Accessed July 6, 2005.
2. Roy S III. The chloride depletion syndrome. *Adv Pediatr.* 1984;31:23–57.
3. US Department of Health and Human Services, US Food and Drug Administration, Center for Food Safety and Applied Nutrition. *Infant Formula: Regulatory/Guidance Documents & Advisory Meetings*. Available at: http://www.cfsan.fda.gov/~dms/inf-ind.html. Accessed December 28, 2005.
4. US Food and Drug Administration. Current good manufacturing practice, quality control procedures, quality factors, notification requirements, and records and reports, for the production of infant formula; reopen-

ing of the comment period. 68 *Federal Register.* 2003; 81:22341–22343. Available at: http://frwebgate.access.gpo.gov/cgi-bin/getpage.cgi?position=page&page=22341&dbname=2003_register. Accessed March 18, 2006.

5. US Food and Drug Administration, Center for Food Safety and Applied Nutrition. Code of Federal Regulations. Title 21–Food and Drugs (parts 170–199). Available at: http://frwebgate.access.gpo.gov/cgi-bin/getpage.cgi. Accessed March 18, 2006.
6. US Department of Health and Human Services, US Food and Drug Administration, Center for Food Safety and Applied Nutrition. *Food Ingredients and Packaging.* Available at: http://www.cfsan.fda.gov/~lrd/foodadd.html. Accessed December 28, 2005.
7. Institute of Medicine, National Academies of Science. *Infant Formula: Evaluating the Safety of New Ingredients.* Washington, DC: The National Academies Press; 2004. Available at: http://www.nap.edu/books/0309091500/html/. Accessed July 6, 2005.
8. US Department of Health and Human Services, US Food and Drug Administration, Center for Food Safety and Applied Nutrition. *Infant Formula: Exempt Infant Formulas Marketed in the United States by Manufacturer and Category.* Available at: http://www.cfsan.fda.gov/~dms/inf-exmp.html. Accessed December 28, 2005.
9. US Food and Drug Administration, Center for Food Safety and Applied Nutrition. Medical foods. Available at: http://www.cfsan.fda.gov/~dms/ds-medfd.html. Accessed March 19, 2006.
10. US Food and Drug Administration, Center for Food Safety and Applied Nutrition. Code of Federal Regulations. Title 21–Food and Drugs (parts 100–169). Available at: http://frwebgate.access.gpo.gov/cgi-bin/get-cfr.cgi. Accessed March 19, 2006.

CHAPTER 16

Physiological Effects of Parenteral Nutrition

Mai Kamal El Mallah and Kathleen J. Motil

INTRODUCTION

The development and maturation of the small intestine during infancy or after surgical resection is characterized by growth of the epithelium, the acquisition of digestive and absorptive functions, the maintenance of gut barrier function with respect to permeability and bacterial translocation, and the enhancement of host defense mechanisms. A variety of trophic factors are suggested to control the development of the gut in response to normal maturation or intestinal resection including genetic programming; luminal factors such as food, bile, pancreatic secretions, and the products of bacterial fermentation; the enteric nervous system; polyamines; systemic hormones such as glucocorticoids, thyroxine, growth hormone, and insulin; enterotrophic hormones such as gastrin, cholecystokinin, enteroglucagon, neurotensin, and peptide YY; and growth factors such as epidermal growth factor (EGF) and insulin-like growth factors (IGF-1, IGF-2).[1] The nutritional mechanisms that promote the maturation and adaptation of the digestive, absorptive, and immunologic function of the gut under clinical conditions where the intestine is immature or where its reserve capacity has been lost is incompletely understood.

Parenteral nutrition (PN) may have profound adverse effects on the maturation and adaptation of the gastrointestinal tract. PN may alter the structural integrity and the functional activity of the intestines, liver, and pancreas. However, the adverse consequences of PN might be species specific and might have fewer implications for humans compared with animal models. The physiological effects of PN on the structure and function of the gastrointestinal tract is most apparent when compared with the physiological effects of enteral feeding alone or in combination with enteral nutrition (EN). This chapter will examine the physiological effects of PN on the structure and function of the intestines, liver, and pancreas in the malnourished and well nourished state, and it will highlight the physiological effects of PN in the context of selected enteral factors that may moderate the adverse outcomes associated with this nutritional modality.

Disclaimer: This chapter is a publication of the United States Department of Agriculture/Agricultural Research Service Children's Nutrition Research Center, Department of Pediatrics, Baylor College of Medicine, Houston, Texas. This project has been funded in part with federal funds from the Agricultural Research Service of the United States Department of Agriculture under cooperative agreement number 58-7MN1-6-100. The contents of this chapter do not necessarily reflect the views or policies of the United States Department of Agriculture, nor does mention of trade names, commercial products, or organizations imply endorsement by the United States government.

PROTEIN-ENERGY MALNUTRITION AND THE GASTROINTESTINAL TRACT

Children who require PN often are critically ill and have a moderate to severe degree of protein-energy malnutrition. As a consequence, it could be difficult to separate the effect of malnutrition itself on the gastrointestinal tract from that which occurs because of the use of PN. Protein-energy malnutrition has long been recognized to have a deleterious effect on the structural integrity and absorptive function of the gastrointestinal tract.[2,3] In severe protein-energy malnutrition, the entire intestinal wall and the mucosal lining are thinner than normal and the villi are blunted in size. The brush border is reduced in height and the mucosal cell becomes more cuboidal than columnar. Mitotic activity is normal in malnourished children with predominantly protein deficient malnutrition (kwashiorkor), but it is reduced when energy deficiency is dominant (marasmus). Cellular proliferation, migration, and maturation along the length of the villi are diminished, and ultrastructural abnormalities occur. The functional consequences of malnutrition include reduced intestinal motility, demonstrated by prolonged total transit time even in the presence of diarrhea; and an overgrowth of facultative and anaerobic bacteria and yeast. At the cellular level, nutrient utilization is impaired because of decreased disaccharidase activity and altered carbohydrate transport, resulting in lactose intolerance and diminished glucose absorption. Fat absorption is diminished because of impaired lipid micelle formation and decreased intraluminal concentrations of conjugated bile salts. Fatty infiltration of the liver, with potential progression to cirrhosis, may occur during malnutrition. The pancreas develops acinar atrophy and fibrosis and secretes reduced amounts of trypsin, chymotrypsin, and lipase. If malnutrition is prolonged, the pancreas develops extensive fibrosis and calcifications.

Clinical experience has shown that PN can prevent progressive malnutrition in patients who cannot be fed enterally.[4] In the 1960s, PN was instrumental in improving the outcome of infants who suffered massive small bowel resection, and consequently, the short bowel syndrome.[5] Clinical observations demonstrated that the use of long term PN in the short bowel syndrome initiates and supports intestinal adaptation and growth. Although the early introduction of trophic feedings is thought to enhance the process of intestinal adaptation,[6,7] the use of PN alone has an enormous impact on initiating and maintaining mucosal hyperplasia and increasing the absorptive and immunologic capacity of the remaining small bowel in this disorder.

PARENTERAL NUTRITION AND THE GASTROINTESTINAL TRACT

Morphology

In the absence of protein-energy malnutrition, PN may have profound effects on the morphology of the gastrointestinal tract. Gut mucosal atrophy occurs when enteral nutrition is totally or partially (< 60% total energy intake) absent in neonatal and adult nonhuman animals,[8] and to a much lesser extent in human infants[9] and adults.[10,11] In adult humans, mucosal atrophy of the intestines has been observed only after 2 to 3 months of complete bowel rest and PN. In infants and young children, mild focal villous atrophy, decreased intestinal disaccharidase activity, and diminished incorporation of thymidine into mucosal tissue occur after 9 months. These observations parallel the hypoplastic effect of PN in animals, but suggest that much longer periods of PN are required to develop adverse outcomes in humans.

In animal models, PN induced mucosal atrophy is characterized by morphological changes, such as reduced villous height, mucosal surface area, and DNA content.[12-15] These changes in morphology are secondary to decreased crypt cell proliferation, diminished protein synthesis, and increased apoptosis.[16] PN reduces the number of enterocytes and is associated with an expansion of mucosal goblet cells and some T lymphocyte subtypes.[17] The increased expression of T lymphocytes is inversely associated with changes in villous height and width.[18] In animals and humans, PN induced activation of lymphocytes may cause mucosal inflammation on the basis of increased intercellular adhesion molecule (ICAM)-1 expression and myeloperoxidase activity.[18,19] In mice, the increased expression of these substances and of the proinflammatory cytokine, interferon-γ (INF-γ), in activated intraepithelial lymphocytes is linked to increased apoptosis and may contribute to the breakdown of epithelial barrier integrity, altering further the structural integrity of the gastrointestinal tract.[20]

Nutrient Absorption

The administration of PN to young animals induces intestinal atrophy and might reduce the digestive and absorptive capacity of the gastrointestinal tract. Premature piglets are less sensitive to PN induced intestinal atrophy than term piglets, the latter of which lose approximately 20% of their intestinal mass and surface area during PN administration.[21] Nevertheless, total intestinal enzymatic and absorptive capacities of PN treated piglets, regardless of gestational age, can be reduced by 50% compared with enterally fed piglets.

PN results in functional defects in lactose digestion and glucose and galactose transport in infant piglets.[22] PN may reduce intestinal brush border hexose transport capacity, resulting in the diminished transport of glucose across the gut mucosa, or it may alter cellular glucose metabolism, resulting in the increased intraluminal metabolism of glucose to lactate and net portal lactate release.[23,24] Total intestinal lactase activity is reduced by 75%, presumably because of reduced villous height and surface area, and it is insufficient to metabolize dietary lactose. These changes in mucosal structure and cellularity in response to PN are mediated by the suppression of lactase phlorizin hydrolase synthesis, total protein synthesis, and crypt cell proliferation, and by the stimulation of villus enterocyte apoptosis.[8,16,25,26]

PN is the primary source of nutrition for preterm infants and other infants who cannot tolerate full enteral feedings. PN alone, in the absence of EN, may lead to suppression of intestinal growth, induce mucosal atrophy, and result in altered digestive capability in infants.[9] Studies conducted in formula fed, preterm infants have shown that their lactose digestion is incomplete. As much as 25% of their dietary lactose intake may be fermented in the colon.[27] Insufficient lactase expression may account for incomplete lactose digestion in preterm infants, and some have linked carbohydrate malabsorption and fermentation to the risk of necrotizing enterocolitis.[28] Because most preterm infants receive some degree of PN before enteral feeding is initiated, PN is thought to be responsible for the suppression of intestinal function, and it might contribute to incomplete lactose digestion and glucose absorption when EN is initiated.[22]

PN has deleterious effects on intestinal protein digestion and amino acid absorption.[29,30] Parenterally fed piglets have increased nitrogen excretion and less body protein deposition than enterally fed piglets. The intestines of parenterally fed piglets are atrophic because of shortened villi and reduced crypt depth, and they have decreased mucosal concentrations of proline and glutamate, both of which serve as precursors for the synthesis of arginine, a conditionally essential amino acid for rapidly growing piglets. PN in piglets is associated with the suppression of the net absorption of several essential or semiessential amino acids, including lysine, threonine, isoleucine, and arginine.[22,31] Net portal appearance of these 4 amino acids can be reduced by 22–67% in parenterally fed piglets compared with enterally fed piglets, possibly because of the high rate of first-pass metabolism for nitric oxide, polyamines, and mucin-glycoprotein synthesis in the intestines.[32,33] PN suppresses leucine oxidation by as much as 50% secondary to the depressed activity of the leucine catabolic enzymes and results in the reduced net portal release of ammonia. Despite these alterations, the adverse effects of PN on protein digestion and amino acid absorption are less significant than those related to carbohydrate digestion and absorption.[22]

The pancreas of the newborn piglet is less sensitive than the small intestine to PN induced changes in structure and function.[21] Nevertheless, PN is associated with lower pancreatic weights than enteral feedings. In addition, the differential regulation of pancreatic enzymes such as amylase, trypsin, and chymotrypsin by PN is present in the newborn pig. Increases in amylase activity and decreases in trypsin and chymotrypsin activities occur after birth, but much less in parenterally fed than in enterally fed piglets.[18]

Infections and Immunity

PN can impair host defense mechanisms and contribute to the pathogenesis of infection in animals and humans. Parenterally fed piglets show a 50% reduction in platelet numbers compared with orally fed piglets.[20] Although circulating white blood cell concentrations remain stable, the proportions of basophils and monocytes are reduced by 50% and 70%, respectively, reflecting a potential compromise in their systemic immune response. Within the gastrointestinal tract, parenterally fed piglets have increased numbers of CD4+ and CD8+ lymphocytes in the jejunum, ileum, and colon. T lymphocyte responses involve the recognition of peptide fragments of antigens bound to cell-surface proteins encoded in the major histocompatibility complex (MHC). MHC class II molecules present bacteria and parasitic antigens to CD4+ lymphocytes. MHC class II expression is higher within the ileum of parenterally fed piglets. Goblet cell numbers are increased in the jejunum and ileum and mast cells are more abundant in the colon of parenterally fed piglets. These findings, taken together, may reflect an altered microbial environment resulting from the lack of EN.[18,34]

PN in mice reduces the size and function of the gut-associated lymphoid tissue (GALT; see Chapter 3) reduces the CD4:CD8 lymphocyte ratio within the lamina propria and impairs intestinal tract immunity by decreasing intestinal secretory IgA levels.[35,36] The production of secretory IgA is regulated by a balance between Th1 (IFN-γ, tumor necrosis factor-α [TNF- α]) and Th2 (interleukin- [IL-] 4, 5, 6, 10, and 13) cytokines.[37-39] PN causes Th2-IgA stimulating cytokines IL-4 and IL-10 to decrease rapidly, while Th1-inhibiting cytokine INF-γ remains normal.[40] As a consequence, INF-γ stimulates ICAM-1 expression on endothelial cells. ICAM-1 binds to selected integrins which, in turn, permit polymorphonuclear cells to attach to the endothelium, migrate into the interstitium, and cause tissue injury.[41]

PN is associated with a high rate of infection and multiple organ failure in infants and adults.[42,43] As many as 37% of infants who receive PN become bacteremic.[44] The most frequently isolated bacterial pathogens are coagulase negative staphylococci.[45] PN impairs systemic bactericidal activity in infants because it contributes to defective phagocytosis,[46] defective intracellular killing of bacteria within neutrophils,[47] diminished proportions of monocytes, and decreased cytokine production, especially TNF-α, IL-6, and IL-1β in monocytes,[48,49] The lipid component of PN is thought to be responsible, in part, for the altered neutrophil function, bactericidal activity, and cytokine production in adults.[50]

Gut Barrier Function

PN is thought to increase paracellular permeability in the gut, although the cellular mechanisms involved have not been established. In parenterally fed mice, increased expression of the proinflammatory cytokine, INF-γ, in activated intraepithelial lymphocytes within the intestinal mucosa, results in increased cellular apoptosis, a factor that may contribute to the breakdown of the gut epithelial barrier integrity.[51] The administration of PN to newborn piglets leads to mucosal atrophy, an inflammatory response, measured by myeloperoxidase activity; and increased paracellular permeability, measured by urinary excretion of mannitol, lactulose, and polyethylene glycol 4000; but it does not increase bacterial translocation when measured by liver, spleen, or mesenteric lymph node cultures.[13] A potential explanation for the increased intestinal permeability could be that it is associated with the disintegration in tight junction integrity, but this hypothesis has not been substantiated. The increased permeability is not associated with down-regulation of tight junction integrity when measured by tight junction proteins such as claudin-1, claudin-2, occludin, and ZO-1, all of which are intimately involved in intercellular adhesion.[13]

The consequence of altered cellular and barrier function of the gastrointestinal tract in neonatal infants is late onset sepsis. Sepsis is the most common cause of morbidity in the preterm infant, and many factors, including PN, have been implicated. The pathogenesis of the increased rate of infection is thought to occur because PN adversely affects the gut mucosal integrity and might compromise gut barrier function. The deterioration in the mucosal epithelial barrier is thought to facilitate the translocation of luminal bacteria and toxins into the blood, the consequence of which is gut derived sepsis.[13] Although PN adversely affects villous architecture and gut permeability in animals, studies in adults do not show an association between PN induced changes in barrier function and bacterial translocation.[52]

PARENTERAL NUTRITION AND NUTRIENT DEFICIENCY

Glutamine

In recent years, there has been an increasing interest in the nutritional role of glutamine supplementation in PN. See Chapter 24 for more discussion on glutamine supplementation. Glutamine is not an essential amino acid because it can be synthesized adequately in the brain and skeletal muscle from glutamate and ammonia via glutamine synthetase. Under normal conditions, glutamine is the preferred respiratory fuel for rapidly proliferating cells such as enterocytes and lymphocytes. The benefits of glutamine as a supplement in PN are controversial.[53]

The addition of glutamine to PN has variable effects on small intestinal mucosa morphology. In piglets, parenteral glutamine supplementation does not confer a trophic effect on the intestinal mucosa.[29,54,55] The total mucosal weight, villous height, crypt depth, mucosal nitrogen content, and dissaccharidase activities of the small intestines are nearly identical in piglets receiving glutamine supplemented PN to those receiving PN without glutamine. Glutamine has some effects on the mitotic activity of the colon, but these effects are modest and unlikely to have much impact in the young animal.

It is postulated that the trophic effects of glutamine may be more evident when animals are under gut stress such as bowel resection or diarrhea.[29,54]

In rats subjected to 75% intestinal resection, glutamine supplemented PN reverses the jejunal mucosal atrophy observed with the use of unsupplemented PN.[12] Improvement in mucosal architecture is due to a proportional increase in mucosal thickness, villous height, crypt depth, and villous surface area. Mucosal glutaminase and jejunal and ileal mucosal IGF-1 mRNA increase twofold to threefold in treated animals compared with untreated animals, suggesting that glutamine is used for intestinal growth and adaptation after resection.[56]

Glutamine supplementation also has variable effects on bacterial translocation. In one study in which rats underwent a 60% small bowel resection, glutamine supplemented PN was associated with culture positive lymph nodes in 20% of the treated animals compared with 70% culture positive lymph nodes in the untreated animals.[56] On the other hand, glutamine supplemented PN did not influence gut bacterial translocation to the blood or the mesenteric lymph nodes in rats that received colonic radiation and surgical intervention.[57]

It has been suggested that glutamine confers a protective effect on intestinal tract mucosal immunity by positively influencing GALT. In mice, PN without glutamine causes atrophy in GALT and reduces intestinal secretory IgA levels, thereby impairing intestinal tract immunity.[35,36] PN is associated with a decrease in 2 IgA-stimulating cytokines, IL-4 and IL-10, both of which suppress endothelial ICAM-1 expression. In the absence of IgA stimulating cytokines, ICAM-1 expression increases and polymorphonuclear cells accumulate and migrate into tissues, causing tissue injury. The administration of PN supplemented with glutamine prevents GALT atrophy in Peyer's patches, the lamina propria, and intraepithelial cell populations.[19] Glutamine supplemented PN also normalizes IL-4 levels and ICAM-1 expression and maintains IgA levels in the supernatants of small intestine homogenates.[58-60] Glutamine appears to reverse the deleterious effects of PN by maintaining mRNA expression of these IgA stimulating cytokines, thereby promoting mucosal immunity.[19]

Clinical outcomes of glutamine supplemented PN on rates of infection in preterm infants are controversial. Premature infants uniformly tolerate glutamine supplemented PN.[61-63] One study reported that the time to full enteral feedings was shorter in a glutamine supplemented group.[53] In several studies, weight gain, length of hospital stay, and rates of infection did not differ between infants given glutamine supplemented PN and those given standard formulations.[53,61,62] One study, however, reported a decreased incidence of sepsis in a glutamine supplemented group.[62] Although the subject of glutamine supplemented PN is popular, the consensus is that glutamine supplemented PN provides negligible benefit in animals and infants.[29,53,54,61,62]

PARENTERAL NUTRITION AND INTRALUMINAL FACTORS

The adverse effects of PN on the maturation and adaptation of the gut are thought to reflect the absence of luminal factors. Luminal factors include biliary and pancreatic secretions, nutrients, hormones, and growth factors normally found in enteral feedings such as human milk. The presence of these intraluminal factors is necessary to maintain the structural integrity of the intestinal mucosa and functional development of the gut.

Biliary and Pancreatic Secretions

In the animal model, diversion of bile acids results in duodenal and jejunal hypoplasia, suggesting that bile secretion is one of the most important mucosal trophic factors. These findings emphasize the importance of EN, particularly in the context of their stimulatory effect on pancreatic and biliary secretions.[64] PN alone results in decreased gallbladder contraction and may be associated with the formation of gallstones.

Dietary Nutrients

Dietary factors alone may be the sole identifiable cause of the accelerated growth and maturation of the small intestine in artificially fed rats. In infant rats fed their mothers' milk or rat's milk substitute (cow milk based formula), small intestinal overgrowth in length and weight and precocious functional maturation occurred in the artificially fed group.[6] Growth factors such as IGF-1 and IGF-2, EGF, or transforming growth factor-α (TGF-α) were not associated with this trophic effect because they are absent in cow milk based formulas. Other milk-borne trophic factors, as yet unidentified in the rat's milk substitute formula, could contribute to accelerated maturation. The accelerated intestinal growth of rats fed artificial formula is thought to reflect the functional demands of the gut for the digestion and absorption of individual nutrient components such as whey protein in the cow's milk-based formula.[65]

Hormones

Prolactin

Prolactin, a polypeptide hormone found in amniotic fluid and human milk, could promote gut growth and maturation. In rats, prolactin induces both alkaline phosphatase and maltase activity by twofold to threefold, and it stimulates thymidine incorporation into intestinal explants after incubation.[66] EGF has similar effects on these two hydrolases, but neither EGF nor prolactin has an effect on lactase. These observations suggest that prolactin could promote intestinal growth and maturation in the infant.

Glucagon-like Peptide-2

Glucagon-like peptide-2 (GLP-2), an amino acid peptide released from the enteroendocrine L cells of the small and large intestine, is a potent trophic factor in neonatal and adult animals.[67] Intestinal GLP-2 secretion is stimulated by EN intake. Piglets that receive PN have decreased circulating GLP-2 concentrations.[8] GLP-2 increases small intestine mucosal mass, colonic mass, villous height, and crypt depth, and it reverses the gut atrophy associated with PN.[16,67,68] GLP-2 increases intestinal growth by decreasing proteolysis and apoptosis, whereas EN acts by increasing protein synthesis and cell proliferation as well as decreasing apoptosis.

Growth Factors

Insulin-like Growth Factor-1

Human milk contains growth factors not found in formula that promote gut development. One of these factors, IGF-1, is found in the milk of many animals, including pigs, cows, rats, and humans. The concentration of IGF-1 is usually high in colostrum. The oral treatment of newborn rats with IGF-1 leads to intestinal epithelial cell maturation.[69] The effect of oral IGF-1 on the intestinal tract is region specific. Orally administered IGF-1 stimulates brush border enzyme activity at the proximal region of the small intestine, but not the distal region. The reason for this effect is thought to be a result of the gradient effect in as much as the proximal region of the intestine has a better chance of exposure to orally administered growth factors.[69]

Epidermal Growth Factor

EGF, another growth factor found in the milk of animals and humans, has trophic effects on the gut, including stimulation of mucosal cell proliferation. EGF increases crypt depth, villous height, and mucosal thickness throughout the small intestine with maximal effect on the colon.[70] EGF also reverses the PN induced reduction in brush border enzyme activity.[71] In the rat, the addition of EGF to PN reduces gut mucosal atrophy, bacterial translocation to the mesenteric lymph nodes, and the frequency of blood and catheter infections.[70]

Transforming Growth Factor-α

Another growth factor in human milk, TGF-α, is a member of the EGF family. TGF-α is thought to play a major role in postnatal gut maturation by activating the EGF receptor. TGF-α is derived from the mammary myoepithelial cells and the macrophages in colostrum and mature milk. Human milk macrophages in the small intestine provide a potentially continuous interaction between the epithelial cells of the gut with EGF receptors and TGF-α.[72] Culturing human fetal small intestine cell lines with human milk macrophages or human milk macrophage-conditioned media leads to increased proliferation of the small intestinal cell line. This data suggests that TGF-α derived from human milk macrophages could enhance gut epithelial proliferation.[72]

Pectin

Pectin is a water soluble dietary fiber that some consider a prebiotic (see Chapter 3). It is completely fermented by colonic bacteria. A pectin supplemented elemental diet has been shown to promote intestinal adaptation following small and large bowel resection in adult rats and enhance colonic mucosal cell proliferation in rats with colonic anastomosis.[73] Pectin decreases gastric emptying time and increases small and large bowel intestinal transit time.[74] Fermentation of pectin in the large bowel produces short chain fatty acids that stimulate colonic mucosal proliferation and increase intestinal blood flow, a factor that may facilitate intestinal adaptation following resection.[75] One case study of a 3-year-old child showed that pectin supplementation was associated with greater nitrogen absorption and the maintenance of electrolyte balance.[76]

PARENTERAL AND ENTERAL NUTRITION COMBINED

Minimal EN is an approach to feeding that involves the early initiation of low volume, low energy density feedings in young animals and infants after birth in conjunction with the provision of PN. The practice of providing minimal EN developed as a strategy to facilitate gastrointestinal maturation in a way that safely improves feeding tolerance and decreases the time to reach full feedings. Although minimal EN provides insufficient dietary energy to promote growth, it is thought to confer a protective advantage because it exerts a trophic effect on the development and maturation of the intestines, particularly the gut mucosal barrier.

The gut mucosal barrier consists of mechanical components, primarily the epithelial cell layer and intermediate junctions (tight junctions, zonula adherens, and desmosomes), and immunological components, including secretory IgA and GALT. Minimal EN, in conjunction with PN, protects the gut mucosal barrier better than PN alone. Minimal EN, administered to rats in amounts that approximate 10% of their total daily energy intake, maintains the macromorphological structure of the gut and prevents gut mucosal atrophy, measured by increased villous height and crypt depth.[34] Trophic feedings administered to rats in amounts of at least 15% of their total daily energy intake are necessary to prevent the disruption of the micromorphological structures and the immunological function of the gut. This increased amount of trophic EN decreases the excretion rate of phenolsulfonphthalein, a marker of intestinal macromolecular permeability, increases villous heights and depths of intestinal crypts in the jejunum and ileum, and it increases the number of IgA positive cells in the intestinal lamina propria of rats, measured by biopsy and immunohistochemical staining.[34] The addition of trophic feedings that corresponds to 15% of total energy intake prevents increases in intestinal permeability and bacterial translocation in stressed rats.[77]

During the first few weeks of life, nutritional support of preterm infants often is limited to PN when these infants are clinically unstable and require ventilator support. EN may be withheld because of concerns of an increased risk of necrotizing enterocolitis during the early neonatal period. However, withholding EN from these infants could limit intestinal mucosal growth and delay the maturation of digestive enzymes, enteric hormone release, and gut motility.[78–80] EN benefits the premature infant by preventing starvation catabolism, maintaining immunocompetence, and promoting wound healing. EN is considered to reduce septic complications, shorten hospital stay, and reduce the risk of death.[78] To provide a minimal stimulus to the gut, while minimizing the risk of necrotizing enterocolitis, infants are given small EN feedings during the first 2 weeks of life. Infants who are given milk volumes comprising 1–10% of daily fluid intake have more mature small intestinal motor patterns and higher plasma gastrin and motilin concentrations than infants who have not been given any feedings.[81,82] The small amount of EN may trigger maturation of intestinal function by stimulating the release of enteric hormones, neurotransmitters, and other gastrointestinal peptides. Infants given early, small, enteral feedings experience fewer complications when full EN volumes are later introduced during the second or third postnatal week.[83,84]

PARENTERAL NUTRITION ASSOCIATED CHOLESTASIS

PN associated cholestasis is a persistent problem that causes morbidity and mortality in young infants. PN associated cholestasis is defined as a conjugated bilirubin greater than 2.0 mg/dL that occurs in conjunction with a prolonged (usually greater than 3 weeks) course of PN in the absence of other identifiable causes. The development of PN associated cholestasis is associated with several risk factors.[85] The younger the infant, the lower the birth weight, the earlier in life that PN is administered, and the longer its use, the more likely the infant will develop cholestasis. Septic episodes are associated with a 30% increase in bilirubin, further complicating the clinical course of cholestasis.[85] The etiology of PN associated cholestasis has not been established, although several possibilities have been proposed.[86–88] Some investigators have postulated that bacterial translocation with subsequent formation of endotoxins and release of cytokines injure the liver and lead to cholestasis. Others have suggested that a deficiency in selected amino acids such as taurine may be responsible for cholestasis. In the absence of EN, cholecystokinin release is impeded, resulting in the lack of gallbladder contraction, biliary stasis, and subsequent cholestatic injury. In addition, a lack of EN may lead to diminished expression of the multidrug resistant-2 P-glycoprotein gene which is responsible for the secretion of phospholipid into bile, further impeding normal bile flow.[89] The early initiation of trophic feedings, cycling the administration of PN, and the use of ursodeoxycholic acid constitute the current approach to therapy.[90] Prophylactic cholecystokinin therapy has been proposed as an alternative approach with some success to reduce the severity of cholestasis, but an effective cure has not been found.[91]

CONCLUSION

PN may have profound effects on the maturation and adaptation of the gastrointestinal tract. PN may alter the structural integrity and the functional activity of the intestines, liver, and pancreas. However, the adverse consequences of PN may be species specific and may have fewer implications for humans compared with animal models. The adverse effects of PN on the maturation and adaptation of the gut are thought to reflect the absence of luminal factors such as biliary and pancreatic secretions, individual nutrients, hormones, and growth factors, even if PN is maintained. Nevertheless, PN is the mainstay of treatment for premature infants and infants with massive bowel resection who cannot be fed enterally. In the final analysis, PN prevents progressive malnutrition, initiates mucosal hyperplasia, and supports the absorptive and immunologic capacity of the small bowel in children with special nutritional needs.

REFERENCES

1. Thiesen A, Wild G, Keelan MT, et al. Ontogeny of intestinal nutrient transport. *Can J Physiol Pharmacol.* 2000;78:513–527.
2. Suskind RM. Gastrointestinal changes in the malnourished child. *Pediatr Clin North Am.* 1975;22:873–883.
3. Viteri FE, Schneider RE. Gastrointestinal alterations in protein-calorie malnutrition. *Med Clin North Am.* 1974;58:1487–1505.
4. Quiros-Tejeira RE, Ament ME, Reyen L, et al. Long-term parenteral nutritional support and intestinal adaptation in children with short bowel syndrome: a 25-year experience. *J Pediatr.* 2004;145:157–163.
5. Dudrick SJ, Wilmore DW, Vars HM, Rhoads JE. Long-term total parenteral nutrition with growth, development, and positive nitrogen balance. *Surgery.* 1968;64:134–142.
6. Andorsky DJ, Lund DP, Lillehei CW, et al. Nutritional and other postoperative management of neonates with short bowel syndrome correlates with clinical outcomes. *J Pediatr.* 2001;139:27–33.
7. Sondheimer JM, Cadnapaphornchai M, Sontag M, Zerbe GO. Predicting the duration of dependence on parenteral nutrition after neonatal intestinal resection. *J Pediatr.* 1998;132:80–84.
8. Burrin DG, Stoll B, Jiang R, et al. Minimal enteral nutrient requirements for intestinal growth in neonatal piglets: how much is enough? *Am J Clin Nutr.* 2000;71:1603–1610.
9. Rossi TM, Lee PC, Young C, Tjota A. Small intestinal mucosa changes, including epithelial cell proliferative activity, of children receiving total parenteral nutrition (TPN). *Dig Dis Sci.* 1993;38:1608–1613.
10. Guedon C, Schmitz J, Lerebours E, et al. Decreased brush border hydrolase activities without gross morphological changes in human intestinal mucosa after prolonged total parenteral nutrition of adults. *Gastroenterology.* 1986;90:373–378.
11. Jeejeebhoy KN. Enteral and parenteral nutrition: evidence-based approach. *Proc Nutr Soc.* 2001;60:399–402.
12. Gu Y, Wu ZH, Xie JX, Jin DY, Zhuo HC. Effects of growth hormone (rhGH) and glutamine supplemented parenteral nutrition on intestinal adaptation in short bowel rats. *Clin Nutr.* 2001;20:159–166.
13. Kansagra K, Stoll B, Rognerud C, et al. Total parenteral nutrition adversely affects gut barrier function in neonatal piglets. *Am J Physiol Gastrointest Liver Physiol.* 2003;285:G1162–G1170.
14. Park YK, Monaco MM, Donovan SM. Delivery of total parenteral nutrition (TPN) via umbilical catheterization: development of a piglet model to investigate therapies to

improve gastrointestinal structure and enzyme activity during TPN. *Biol Neonate.* 1998;73:295–305.

15. Gall DG, Chung M, O'Loughlin EV, Zahavi I, Opeleta K. Effects of parenteral and enteral nutrition on postnatal development of the small intestine and pancreas in the rabbit. *Biol Neonate.* 1987;51:286–296.
16. Burrin DG, Stoll B, Jiang R, et al. GLP-2 stimulates intestinal growth in TPN-fed pigs by suppressing proteolysis and apoptosis. *Am J Physiol Gastrointest Liver Physiol.* 2000;279:G1249–G1256.
17. Conour JE, Ganessunker D, Tappenden KA, Donovan SM, Gaskins HR. Acidomucin goblet cell expansion induced by parenteral nutrition in the small intestine of piglets. *Am J Physiol Gastrointest Liver Physiol.* 2002;283:G1185–G1196.
18. Ganessunker D, Gaskins HR, Zuckermann FA, Donovan SM. Total parenteral nutrition alters molecular and cellular indices of intestinal inflammation in neonatal piglets. *J Parenter Enteral Nutr.* 1999;23:337–344.
19. Fukatsu K, Kudsk KA, Zarzaur BL, Wu Y, Hanna MK, DeWitt RC. TPN decreases IL-4 and IL-10 mRNA expression in lipopolysaccharide stimulated intestinal lamina propria cells but glutamine supplementation preserves the expression. *Shock.* 2001;15:318–322.
20. Kiristioglu I, Teitelbaum DH. Alteration of the intestinal intraepithelial lymphocytes during total parenteral nutrition. *J Surg Res.* 1998;79:91–96.
21. Sangild PT, Petersen YM, Schmidt M, et al. Preterm birth affects the intestinal response to parenteral and enteral nutrition in newborn pigs. *J Nutr.* 2002;132:2673–2681.
22. Burrin DG, Stoll B, Chang X, et al. Parenteral nutrition results in impaired lactose digestion and hexose absorption when enteral feeding is initiated in infant pigs. *Am J Clin Nutr.* 2003;78:461–470.
23. Miura S, Tanaka S, Yoshioka M, et al. Changes in intestinal absorption of nutrients and brush border glycoproteins after total parenteral nutrition in rats. *Gut.* 1992;23:484–489.
24. Inoue Y, Espat NJ, Frohnapple DJ, Epstein H, Copeland EM, Souba WW. Effect of total parenteral nutrition on amino acid and glucose transport by the human small intestine. *Ann Surg.* 1993;217:604–612.
25. Dudley MA, Jahoor F, Burrin DG, Reeds PJ. Brush-border disaccharidase synthesis in infant pigs measured in vivo with [$^2H_3$]leucine. *Am J Physiol.* 1994;267: G1128–G1134.
26. Stoll B, Chang X, Fan MZ, Reeds PJ, Burrin DG. Enteral nutrient intake level determines intestinal protein synthesis and accretion rates in neonatal pigs. *Am J Physiol Gastrointest Liver Physiol.* 2000;279:G288–G294.
27. Kien CL, McClead RE, Cordero L Jr. In vivo lactose digestion in preterm infants. *Am J Clin Nutr.* 1996;64:700–705.
28. Kien CL. Digestion, absorption, and fermentation of carbohydrates in the newborn. *Clin Perinatol.* 1996;23:211–228.
29. Bertolo RF, Pencharz PB, Ball RO. A comparison of parenteral and enteral feeding in neonatal piglets, including an assessment of the utilization of a glutamine-rich, pediatric elemental diet. *J Parenter Enteral Nutr.* 1999;23:47–55.
30. Dudley MA, Wykes LJ, Dudley AW Jr, et al. Parenteral nutrition selectively decreases protein synthesis in the small intestine. *Am J Physiol.* 1998;274:G131–G137.
31. Bertolo RF, Chen CZ, Law GP, Pencharz PB, Ball RO. Threonine requirement of neonatal piglets receiving total parenteral nutrition is considerably lower than that of piglets receiving an identical diet intragastrically. *J Nutr.* 1998;128:1752–1759.
32. Bertolo RF, Chen CZ, Pencharz PB, Ball RO. Intestinal atrophy has a greater impact on nitrogen metabolism than liver bypass in piglets fed identical diets via gastric, central venous or portal venous routes. *J Nutr.* 1999;129:1045–1052.
33. Fogg FJ, Hutton DA, Jumel K, Pearson JP, Harding SE, Allen A. Characterization of pig colonic mucins. *Biochem J.* 1996;316:937–942.
34. Ohta K, Omura K, Hirano K, et al. The effects of an additive small amount of a low residual diet against total parenteral nutrition-induced gut mucosal barrier. *Am J Surg.* 2003;185:79–85.
35. Li J, Kudsk KA, Gocinski B, Dent D, Glezer J, Langkamp-Henken B. Effects of parenteral and enteral nutrition on gut-associated lymphoid tissue. *J Trauma.* 1995;39:44–51.
36. King BK, Li J, Kudsk KA. A temporal study of TPN-induced changes in gut-associated lymphoid tissue and mucosal immunity. *Arch Surg.* 1997;132:1303–1309.
37. Kramer DR, Sutherland RM, Bao S, Husband AJ. Cytokine mediated effects in mucosal immunity. *Immunol Cell Biol.* 1995;73:389–396.
38. Ramsay AJ. Genetic approaches to the study of cytokine regulation of mucosal immunity. *Immunol Cell Biol.* 1995;73:484–488.
39. Lebman DA, Coffman RL. The effects of IL-4 and IL-5 on the IgA response by murine Peyer's patch B cell subpopulations. *J Immunol.* 1988;141:2050–2056.
40. Wu Y, Kudsk KA, DeWitt RC, Tolley EA, Li J. Route and type of nutrition influence IgA-mediating intestinal cytokines. *Ann Surg.* 1999;229:662–667.
41. Fukatsu K, Lundberg AH, Hanna MK, et al. Route of nutrition influences intercellular adhesion molecule-1 expression and neutrophil accumulation in intestine. *Arch Surg.* 1999;134:1055–1060.
42. Kudsk KA, Croce MA, Fabian TC, et al. Enteral versus parenteral feeding: effects on septic morbidity after blunt and penetrating abdominal trauma. *Ann Surg.* 1992;215:503–511.

43. Moore FA, Feliciano DV, Andrassy RJ, et al. Early enteral feeding, compared with parenteral, reduces postoperative septic complications. The results of a meta-analysis. *Ann Surg.* 1992;216:172–183.
44. Wesley JR, Coran AG. Intravenous nutrition for the pediatric patient. *Semin Pediatr Surg.* 1992;1:212–230.
45. Pierro A, van Saene HK, Donnell SC, et al. Microbial translocation in neonates and infants receiving long-term parenteral nutrition. *Arch Surg.* 1996;131:176–179.
46. Okada Y, Klein NJ, van Saene HK, Webb G, Holzel H, Peirro A. Bactericidal activity against coagulase-negative staphylococci is impaired in infants receiving long-term parenteral nutrition. *Ann Surg.* 2000;231:276–281.
47. Okada Y, Klein NJ, Pierro A. Peter Paul Rickham Prize—1998: neutrophil dysfunction the cellular mechanism of impaired immunity during total parenteral nutrition in infancy. *J Pediatr Surg.* 1999;34:242–245.
48. Okada Y, Papp E, Klein NJ, Pierro A. Total parenteral nutrition directly impairs cytokine production after bacterial challenge. *J Pediatr Surg.* 1999;34:277–280.
49. Cruccetti A, Pierro A, Uronen H, Klein N. Surgical infants on total parenteral nutrition have impaired cytokine responses to microbial challenge. *J Pediatr Surg.* 2003;38:138–142.
50. Sedman PC, Somers SS, Ramsden CW, Brennan TG, Guillou PJ. Effects of different lipid emulsions on lymphocyte function during total parenteral nutrition. *Br J Surg.* 1991;78:1396–1399.
51. Kiristioglu I, Antony P, Fan Y, et al. Total parenteral nutrition-associated changes in mouse intestinal intraepithelial lymphocytes. *Dig Dis Sci.* 2002;47:1147–1157.
52. Sedman PC, MacFie J, Palmer MD, Mitchell CJ, Sagar PM. Preoperative total parenteral nutrition is not associated with mucosal atrophy or bacterial translocation in humans. *Br J Surg.* 1995;82:1663–1667.
53. Thompson SW, McClure BG, Tubman TR. A randomized, controlled trial of parenteral glutamine in ill, very low birth-weight neonates. *J Pediatr Gastroenterol Nutr.* 2003;37:550–553.
54. Mandir N, Goodland RA. The effects of glutamine on intestinal epithelial cell proliferation in parenterally fed rats. *Gut.* 1999;44:608–614.
55. Burrin DG, Shulman RJ, Storm MC, Reeds PJ. Glutamine or glutamic acid effects on intestinal growth and disaccharidase activity in infant piglets receiving total parenteral nutrition. *J Parenter Enteral Nutr.* 1991;15:262–266.
56. Zhuming J, Yuewu L, Yongxian M, et al. Alteration in enterocyte gene expression may explain structural and functional changes following glutamine supplemented parenteral nutrition. *Chin Med Sci J.* 1999;14:112–116.
57. El-Malt M, Ceelen W, Boterberg T, et al. Does the addition of glutamine to total parenteral nutrition have beneficial effect on the healing of colon anastomosis and bacterial translocation after preoperative ratiotherapy? *Am J Clin Oncol.* 2003;26:e54–e59.
58. Li J, Kudsk KA, Janu P, Renegar KB. Effect of glutamine-enriched total parenteral nutrition on small intestinal gut-associated lymphoid tissue and upper respiratory tract immunity. *Surgery.* 1997;121:542–549.
59. DeWitt RC, Wu Y, Renegar KB, Kudsk KA. Glutamine-enriched total parenteral nutrition preserves respiratory immunity and improves survival to a pseudomonas pneumonia. *J Surg Res.* 1999;84:13–18.
60. Kudsk KA, Wu Y, Fukatsu K, et al. Glutamine-enriched TPN maintains intestinal interleukin-4 and mucosal immunoglobulin A levels. *J Parenter Enteral Nutr.* 2000;24:270–274.
61. Lacey JM, Crouch JB, Benfell K, et al. The effects of glutamine-supplemented parenteral nutrition in premature infants. *J Parenter Enteral Nutr.* 1996;20(1):74–80.
62. Neu J, Roig JC, Meetze WH, et al. Enteral glutamine supplementation for very low birth weight infants decreases morbidity. *J Pediatr.* 1997;131(5):691–699.
63. Poindexter BB, Ehrenkranz RA, Stoll BJ, et al. Effect of parenteral glutamine supplementation on plasma amino acid concentrations in extremely low-birth-weight infants. *Am J Clin Nutr.* 2003;77:737–743.
64. Gelinas MD, Morin CL. Effects of bile and pancreatic secretions on intestinal mucosa after proximal small bowel resection in rats. *Can J Physiol Pharmacol.* 1980;58:1117–1123.
65. Dvorak B, McWilliam DL, Williams CS, et al. Artificial formula induces precocious maturation of the small intestine of artificially reared suckling rats. *J Pediatr Gastroenterol Nutr.* 2000;31:162–169.
66. Bujanover Y, Wollman Y, Reif S, Golander A. A possible role of prolactin on growth and maturation of the gut during development in the rat. *J Pediatr Endocrinol Metab.* 2002;15:789–794.
67. Litvak DA, Hellmich MR, Evers BM, Banker NA, Townsend CM Jr. Glucagon-like peptide 2 is a potent growth factor for small intestine and colon. *J Gastrointest Surg.* 1998;2:146–150.
68. Kato Y, Yu D, Schwartz MZ. Glucagon like peptide-2 enhances small intestinal absorptive function and mucosal mass in vivo. *J Pediatr Surg.* 1999;34:18–20.
69. Ma L, Xu RJ. Oral insulin-like growth factor-I stimulates intestinal enzyme maturation in newborn rats. *Life Sci.* 1997;61:51–58.
70. McAndrew HF, Lloyd DA, Rintala R, van Saene HK. The effects of intravenous epidermal growth factor on bacterial translocation and central venous catheter infection in the rat total parenteral nutrition model. *Pediatr Surg Int.* 2000;16:169–173.
71. Goodlad RA, Raja KB, Peters TJ, Wright NA. Effects of urogastrone-epidermal growth factor on intestinal brush border

enzymes and mitotic activity. *Gut.* 1991;32:994–998.

72. Wagner CL, Forsythe DW, Pittard WB. Variation in the biochemical forms of transforming growth factor-α present in human milk and secreted by human milk macrophages. *Biol Neonate.* 1995;68:325–333.
73. Rolandelli RH, Koruda MJ, Settle RG, Rombeau JL. The effect of enteral feedings supplemented with pectin on the healing of colonic anastomoses in the rat. *Surgery.* 1986;99:703–707.
74. Spiller GA, Chernoff MC, Hill RA, Gates JE, Nassar JJ, Shipley EA. Effect of purified cellulose, pectin, and a low-residue diet on fecal volatile fatty acids, transit time, and fecal weight in humans. *Am J Clin Nutr.* 1980;33:754–759.
75. Goodlad RA, Lenton W, Ghatei MA, Adrian TE, Bloom SR, Wright NA. Effects of an elemental diet, inert bulk and different types of dietary fibre on the response of the intestinal epithelium to refeeding in the rat and relationship to plasma gastrin, enteroglucagon, and PYY concentrations. *Gut.* 1987;28:171–180.
76. Finkel Y, Brown G, Smith HL, Buchanan E, Booth IW. The effects of a pectin-supplemented elemental diet in a boy with short gut syndrome. *Acta Paediatr Scand.* 1990;79:983–986.
77. Omura K, Hirano K, Kanehira E, et al. Small amount of low-residue diet with parenteral nutrition can prevent decreases in intestinal mucosal integrity. *Ann Surg.* 2000;231:112–118.
78. McClure RJ, Newell SJ. Randomised controlled study of clinical outcome following trophic feeding. *Arch Dis Child Fetal Neonatal Ed.* 2000;82:F29–F33.
79. McClure RJ, Newell SJ. Randomised controlled trial of trophic feeding and gut motility. *Arch Dis Child Fetal Neonatal Ed.* 1999;80:F54–F58.
80. McClure RJ, Newell SJ. Randomized controlled study of digestive enzyme activity following trophic feeding. *Acta Paediatr.* 2002;91:292–296.
81. Berseth CL. Effect of early feeding on maturation of the preterm infant's small intestine. *J Pediatr.* 1992;120:947–953.
82. Shulman DI, Kanarek K. Gastrin, motilin, insulin, and insulin-like growth factor-I concentrations in very-low-birth-weight infants receiving enteral or parenteral nutrition. *J Parenter Enteral Nutr.* 1993;17:130–133.
83. Dunn L, Hulman S, Weiner J, Kliegman R. Beneficial effects of early hypocaloric enteral feeding on neonatal gastrointestinal function: preliminary report of a randomized trial. *J Pediatr.* 1988;112:622–629.
84. Slagle TA, Gross SJ. Effect of early low-volume enteral substrate on subsequent feeding tolerance in very low birth weight infants. *J Pediatr.* 1988;113:526–531.
85. Beath SV, Davies P, Papadopoulou A, et al. Parenteral nutrition-related cholestasis in postsurgical neonates: multivariate analysis of risk factors. *J Pediatr Surg.* 1996;31:604–606.
86. Kaufman SS, Gondolesi GE, Fishbein TM. Parenteral nutrition associated liver disease. *Semin Neonatol.* 2003;8:375–381.
87. Forchielli ML, Walker WA. Nutritional factors contributing to the development of cholestasis during total parenteral nutrition. *Adv Pediatr.* 2003;50:245–267.
88. Kelly DA. Liver complications of pediatric parenteral nutrition—epidemiology. *Nutrition.* 1998;14:153–157.
89. Smit JJ, Schinkel AH, Oude Elferink RP, et al. Homozygous disruption of the murine mdr2 P-glycoprotein gene leads to a complete absence of phospholipid from bile and to liver disease. *Cell.* 1993;75:451–462.
90. Chen CY, Tsao PN, Chen HL, Chou HC, Hsieh WS, Chang MH. Ursodeoxycholic acid (UDCA) therapy in very-low-birth-weight infants with parenteral nutrition-associated cholestasis. *J Pediatr.* 2004;145:317–321.
91. Teitelbaum DH, Han-Markey T, Drongowski RA, et al. Use of cholecystokinin to prevent the development of parenteral nutrition-associated cholestasis. *J Parenter Enteral Nutr.* 1997;21:100–103.

Chapter 17

Ethical and Quality of Life Issues

Beth L. Leonberg

INTRODUCTION

Nutrition and hydration are unique as life sustaining therapy. For both parents and health care providers, individual beliefs and attitudes play a significant role in the moral consideration of withholding or withdrawing therapy. Advances in medical technology raise ethical questions about appropriate use of nutrition and fluids to extend or improve the life of infants and children. As life sustaining therapies, enteral and parenteral nutrition are often at the center of these discussions. Those who provide nutrition play an important role in helping to guide and expand this discussion, as well as in helping families and other health care providers work through complicated questions that determine the fate of children and their families. An understanding of the history and evolution of thought and American case law, as well as the principles of bioethics, provides a basis from which providers can think through these complex issues. It is especially important to consider the duration and the quality of life of the child sustained by nutrition support as well as the impact it has on the family.

HISTORICAL PERSPECTIVE

An almost 60% decrease in the infant death rate in the United States between 1940 and 1970 contributed to a period of great personal and legal debate about the use of life sustaining therapies in children, especially newborns. Technologic advances made it possible to sustain life, sometimes at great expense, regardless of the long term prognosis. In 1973, Duff and Campbell reported that health care providers and parents were routinely challenged in newborn intensive care nurseries to make decisions about the use of life sustaining therapies.[1] Although it wasn't clear how decisions to withhold or withdraw therapy should be made, it was the opinion of the authors that the decision belonged to the parents. Simultaneously, rapid advances in the delivery of enteral and parenteral nutrition made these therapies routinely available in the hospital and at home, for short and long term treatment.

In the spring of 1982, an infant later to become known as "Baby Doe" was born in Bloomington, Indiana. Baby Doe was born with Down's syndrome and tracheal esophageal fistula. Although the baby's pediatrician advocated for transferring the child to a pediatric facility to undergo surgery, the parents, with the advice and support of their obstetrician, decided to forgo treatment and allow the child to die untreated.[2] Three court challenges, including 1 before the Indiana Supreme Court, upheld the parents' decision. But the subsequent media attention and public outcry caused President Reagan to send a memo to the Department of Health and Human Services (DHHS) secretary, resulting in the issuance of a notice to health care providers in May 1982, which became known as the Baby Doe regulations.[3] This memo notified hospitals that they risked losing federal funds if they withheld treatment, nutrition, or hydration from children on the basis of their handicap. In contradiction to the President's own Commission for the Study of Ethical Problems in Medicine and Biomedical and Behavioral Research,[4] the memo appeared to promote the use of life sustaining treatment at all costs and in all situations. The following year, DHHS issued its interim final rule, which required hospitals receiving federal funds to post warning signs to staff, reading "Discriminatory failure to feed and care for handicapped infants in this facility is prohibited by federal law. Failure to feed and care for infants may also violate the criminal and civil laws of your state" and established a toll free hotline to facilitate reporting of parents, physicians, and hospitals who were noncompliant.[5] Within a short time, the American Academy of Pediatrics, the National Association of Children's Hospitals and Related Institutions, and Children's Hospital National Medical Center brought suit in U.S. District Court to challenge the memo. The presiding judge found the DHHS rule invalid because affected parties had not been granted appropriate time for comment. The presiding judge called the rule "arbitrary and capricious."[6] As a result, amendments to the Child Abuse Protection Act were published the following year. The amendments remain in effect today.[7] While the impact of noncompliance is solely on the award of federal grants for child abuse and neglect programs and carries no civil or criminal penalty for physicians, the amendments have continued to influence care decisions over the last 20 years.[8] Their explicit exclusion of "appropriate nutrition and hydration" from care that may be withheld has served as fodder for ongoing debate about withholding/withdrawing nutrition from infants and children.

The Baby Doe incident became the catalyst for a 20-year ethics discussion of the question eloquently posed by Angell, "Do we have the right to inflict a life of suffering on a helpless newborn just because we have the technology to do so and despite the fact that we ourselves would have the legal right to reject such a life?"[9] Baby Doe elevated the principle of "best interest" for consideration of the treatment of infants and children and advocated for institutional ethics committees to be established and develop processes for consideration of ethical dilemmas.[10] Subsequent case law has supported the right of parents to make decisions based on the best interest of their child over either the rights of physicians or society (as represented by the government).[11] Specific cases related to nutrition and hydration resulted in the opinion that it should be viewed no differently than other life sustaining therapies. As such, the decision to forgo the use of nutrition and hydration, by either withholding or withdrawing support, may be made under appropriate circumstances.

PRINCIPLES OF BIOETHICS

The fundamental principle in the application of bioethics in the United States is the principle of *autonomy*. Autonomy refers to self-determination, or the right of the individual to make choices related to his medical treatment. Assuming the patient or his responsible caregiver is competent and informed, this right generally supersedes the rights or wishes of health care providers or society. In the case of an incompetent individual, a *surrogate* acting on behalf of the individual may make decisions for the individual based on the individual's previously expressed wishes or consistent with how the appropriate surrogate interprets the wishes of the individual. The clearly expressed views of a child should be given great weight in decision making and parents should be seen as the best surrogate decision makers only when children are unable to express their wishes to forgo life sustaining medical treatment.[12]

Decisions made for the never autonomous individual, specifically the infant or child who has never had the ability to develop views, call into play the *best interests* standard.[13] Under this standard, the benefits of treatment must be weighed against the burdens that will accompany treatment. Determination of the best interest of the child must be the goal, separate from the interests of either the parents or the health care providers.[13–15] Over the last 20 years, opinion has generally shifted to support this as the guiding principle for making decisions for neonates, rather than sustaining life at all costs and regardless of prognosis.

Additional principles that guide ethical decision making include *beneficence, nonmaleficence,* and *justice.*[12,16] *Beneficence* is the concept that the course of action recommended or taken should bring about the most good for the individual, or be most beneficial. *Nonmaleficence* refers to doing no harm to the patient and guides consideration of whether a therapy or intervention will do more harm than good. *Justice* guides consideration of fairness of treatment of an individual in comparison to similar individuals in similar situations. This principle could come into play when considering whether limited health care resources are overused in life sustaining medical treatments. The American Academy of Pediatrics Committee on Bioethics has recommended "Decisions to forego critical care services on the grounds of resource limitations, generally speaking, are not clinical decisions and physicians should avoid such 'bedside rationing.' "[16]

Recent discussions of the *family's interest* introduce a new principle for ethical decision making about care for children, and such discussions are likely to increase in the future, particularly in light of the movement toward family centered care. Hardart argues that the interests of the family and those of the patient cannot be considered separately, and he raises the question of how much weight should be given to each.[17]

Informed consent is a key part of any decision to forgo life sustaining care. True informed consent by children, including appropriate decision making capability and legal empowerment, occurs on occasion. However, most often in pediatrics, the process involves *informed permission* on the part of parents or another surrogate, and *assent* on the part of the child whenever appropriate.[18] The American Academy of Pediatrics Committee on Bioethics outlines four key elements of informed consent: provision of information; assessment of the patient's understanding; assessment of the capacity of the patient or surrogate to make the decision; and assurance that the patient has the freedom to choose without coercion or manipulation.

FORGOING NUTRITION AND HYDRATION

While the Baby Doe regulations stipulate the provision of "appropriate nutrition and hydration" in all cases, there is debate over the interpretation of this phraseology. The use of the word "appropriate" has variously been interpreted to mean either the use of *appropriate technology* to deliver nutrition and hydration, or the delivery of nutrition and hydration as *appropriate to the patient's medical condition.*[19,20] At least eight judicial decisions have been issued on the legality of stopping medically provided nutrition and hydration to children. In seven cases the right of the parent or surrogate to discontinue treatment was upheld. While state law varies in regard to forgoing nutrition and hydration for children, at least six states specifically address the issue, and only one, Louisiana, prohibits forgoing food and nutrients and defines nutrition as comfort care which must always be provided.

The decision to forgo nutrition and hydration for infants and children must be given careful consideration. Nelson et al. outlined three generally accepted circumstances when this decision is ethically permissible and legally justifiable.[19] They included neurologic devastation, irreversible total intestinal failure, and proximate death from any pathologic cause. More recently, Johnson and Mitchell have outlined at least four circumstances in which they believe forgoing nutrition and hydration is ethically permissible.[20] They include: (1) Provision causes harm, such as providing parenteral nutrition to a child with fulminate liver failure. (2) Dying children who would experience the provision as painful, burdensome, or decreasing their quality of life. In these instances they recommend that palliative food and fluid for pleasure and comfort might be more appropriate. (3) Permanently unconscious infants and children if the parents have requested that nutrition and hydration be stopped. (4) In limited circumstances for patients not permanently unconscious but who have profound and irreversible neurologic damage. They acknowledge the extreme difficulty in establishing this fourth group and suggest criteria for inclusion in this group. The criteria include: the patient cannot suck or swallow effectively; expresses no desire to be fed; does not suffer from the absence of nutrition and hydration; and the diagnosis can be made with a high degree of certainty. When circumstances arise where some but not all of these criteria are present, a moral uncertainty is present. In these cases, the authors argue it is better to override the wishes of the parents if they choose to forgo nutrition and hydration. Similarly, it should be noted in cases where there is disagreement on this issue between the child's parents, the usual course of action is to provide the treatment rather than forgo it.

The concept of *futility* is central to the discussion of circumstances when nutrition and hydration may be forgone. It is important to note that an ethical dilemma could also be present when health care providers believe providing care is futile but parents insist on the continued treatment of their child. This situation can create a strain on the therapeutic relationship between provider and parent, especially since the majority of legal challenges in these cases have given little importance to the views of the health care providers. Because of the difficulties it engenders, Children's Hospital in Boston has developed a policy on the withdrawal of treatment against the wishes of the family that requires support and endorsement at all levels in the institution, from the bedside clinicians to the legal and administrative officers.[21] A key part of the process is giving staff the opportunity to express their views and opt out of caring for the child if necessary. In general, the predominant opinion stated by the American Medical Association is that "judgments of futility cannot be made by reference to rules or definitions, but must be determined on a case by case basis."[22]

Finally, the issues might present themselves at any stage of the feeding or refeeding process. The ethics of force-feeding an orally aversive child was raised by Kelly Justus, a pediatric nurse disturbed by causing what appeared to be pain while trying to orally feed an infant previously maintained on parenteral and enteral nutrition as a result of severe gastroesophageal reflux.[23,24] While teaching the child to feed by mouth was felt to be in the child's best long term interest, as with the consideration of providing care in a futile situation, this scenario raises strong emotions in health care providers.

ATTITUDES OF HEALTH CARE PROVIDERS

The attitudes of health care providers about forgoing nutrition and hydration play an important role in how scenarios play out. In the Baby Doe case, the diametrically opposed views of the obstetrician and pediatrician were reported to cause a dramatic showdown at the infant's bedside.[2] While case law has established that medically provided nutrition and hydration are viewed as any other medical treatment, and as such can be withheld or withdrawn, there are unique psychological attributes given to providing food and water. For some they are viewed as the most basic of human needs and must be provided in all circumstances and at all times. For others, they are central to the concept of caring or nurturing, especially of a parent for an infant or child. Carter and Leuthner outlined the considerations brought into play by the concept of starving and the issue of time.[25] The concepts of hunger pains and starving could connote lack of nutrition and suffering to some, in spite of physiologic evidence that there is no pain experienced. The issue of the amount of time between the withdrawal of treatment and when the patient expires is uncomfortable for some. Whereas a patient withdrawn from mechanical ventilation expires within minutes or hours, it could take up to 2–3 weeks for an infant to die following the withdrawal of nutrition and hydration.

Attributes given to nutrition and hydration lead many people, including physicians, nurses, and dietitians, to be uncomfortable with forgoing these treatments. Levi reported his experience with a premature infant who had severe neurologic disease while he was a medical resident.[11] The circumstances were such that discontinuing nutrition support was a reasonable consideration. However, differences in opinion existed between the neurologist and neonatologist. The neonatologist maintained that withholding nutrition and hydration was an option only considered once in her 20-year career, and that was with great angst. Levi describes how difficult it was to be caught between differing opinions despite 20 years of case law supporting the right to forgo this treatment.

Rubenstein et al. reported on the willingness of second and third year pediatric residents to withdraw intravenous fluid (41%) or nutrition (35%) in a hypothetical pediatric patient in a persistent vegetative state, and they contrasted these results with the residents' willingness to withdraw mechanical ventilation (97%).[26] Residents were strongly influenced by parental input, but were more likely, in theory, to modify their care plan to continue therapies at parents' request than to recommend withdrawal of treatment. The difference between the theory and practice of withdrawing nutrition and hydration was presented in the context of a case report by Richard Lin, a physician in the pediatric intensive care unit of a pediatric tertiary care center.[27] He reflects on the experience and comments on the importance of the family obtaining a court order allowing the withdrawal as a means to forestall challenges to carrying out their wishes.

Langdon et al. reported on opinions of dietitians in Louisiana on nutrition support at the end of life.[28] As mentioned earlier, Louisiana is the only state that specifically prohibits the withdrawal of nutrition and hydration from children. While at least 60% of respondents agreed with forgoing nutrition support at the end of life and 95% agreed dietitians should be involved in the decision making process, only 50% felt well qualified to help a patient or family make the decision. Dietitians over the age of 45 or in practice more than 20 years were more likely to disagree with withdrawal of nutrition support than younger dietitians or those practicing less than 10 years. The American Dietetic Association's position on ethical and legal issues in nutrition, hydration and feeding indicates that dietitians have the responsibility to offer a sound, technical judgment on a feeding strategy to achieve the desired goals.[29] Dietitians should become informed of what is wanted by the patient, educate them on the options, and advocate for an adequate deliberation of various options.

ROLE OF THE ETHICS COMMITTEE

Institutional ethics committees should be organized to provide structure to the discussion to forgo medical nutrition and hydration.[30] Johnson and Mitchell make 3 recommendations key to the decision making process.[20] First, they suggest that each decision requires careful deliberation and discussion among all clinical staff and the family, with attention to both the privacy of the family and moral responsibilities of the staff. Second, they characterize the clinical facts about an infant's neurologic status as elusive, and as such recommend consideration of a second opinion and a waiting period for the neurological picture to evolve and stabilize. Third, they express the need to acknowledge the profound moral dilemma and distress for all those involved, including staff and parents. The 3 central roles of an institutional ethics committee were delineated by the Committee on Bioethics of the American Academy of Pediatrics as case consultation, policy development, and ethics education.[31] The value of case consultation is in providing a forum for frank discussion of the complex legal, moral and medical issues that might be involved. They advocate that recommendations resulting from an ethics consult are advisory only; all parties involved bear responsibility for their own actions. Policy should be developed and placed in operation to standardize and guide care throughout a facility. Policies provide a framework for discussion prior to precipitating events. Ethics committees should implement proactive and ongoing education to all staff. In addition, continuous professional development of committee members should be a priority.

QUALITY OF LIFE CONSIDERATIONS

The extensive technical skill required to provide enteral and parenteral nutrition to a child at home has been outlined.[32] See Chapter 19 for a discussion of home nutrition support. As life sustaining medical treatments become standard therapies now routinely delivered at home, their impact on long term quality of life must be considered. Quality of life is defined as "the ability to develop and maintain meaningful human relationships"[33] or as "a multidimensional concept referring to a person's total well being including his or her psychological, social, and physical health status."[34] Quality of life must be considered in the context of the individual, since individuals with severe disabilities could find a rewarding quality of life in what might seem intolerable to those without disabilities.[35] The difficulties encountered in assessing health related quality of life for children with chronic disease are described.[36,37]

Little has been written about the quality of life of children at home on enteral or parenteral nutrition; however, quality of life has been measured for maternal caregivers. Studies in the 1990s found significantly higher levels of stress, depression, or impact on the family among those caring for enterally fed and/or parenterally fed children compared to those caring for children with other disabilities or receiving other high tech therapies.[38,39] More recently, however, Heyman et al. compared children's functional status, as well as caregivers' depression and life satisfaction for 51 children enterally fed via gastrostomy tube (GT) to 50 children with similar chronic illness not being fed by GT, from 3 sites around the nation.[40] Measurement instruments included: the Functional Status II Revised (FSIIR) to measure children's functional status (in which health is the capacity to perform age-appropriate roles and tasks);[41] the Center for Epidemiologic Studies Depression Scale (CES-D) to measure maternal depression;[42] and the Quality of Life Enjoyment and Satisfaction Questionnaire (Q-LES-Q) to measure maternal satisfaction with life.[43] The authors found no differences in the children's functional status, or in maternal caregivers' depressive mood or life satisfaction between the groups studied. This was in spite of caregivers of children with a GT spending 8 hours daily providing care compared to only 3 hours daily for caregivers of the non-GT group. The authors propose that this could be the result of GT placement improving quality of life compared with treatment before GT placement and might lead to more stability in the home environment. Both GT and non-GT caregivers had significantly increased depressive mood and lower levels of life satisfaction than caregivers of healthy children.

In a report on caregiver coping strategies used by those caring for children with long term gastrostomies, Thorne et al. discussed "maintaining normalcy" as an important strategy.[44] This was done to preserve or create a life that was as normal as possible for both the child and the family. Three key elements described as maintaining normalcy were providing oral stimulation, fostering social stimulation, and maintaining a personal life. Oral stimulation included offering the child tastes and mouthfuls of food and drink as appropriate to skill level, most often based on the caregiver's assessment of ability rather than on guidelines or limits prescribed by health care providers. Fostering social stimulation varied from devising a way to make the gastrostomy feeding time a social interaction by making it story time, to sending a lunch to school with a child so she could participate in the activity with the other children, in spite of her inability to actually ingest anything. Finally, maintaining a personal life for the caregiver fell largely into the categories of finding appropriate respite care on a regular basis or coping by relinquishing the need for time away from the child and enjoying noncare giving time with the child as a way to reenergize.

The American Academy of Pediatrics Guidelines for Home Care of Infants, Children, and Adolescents with Chronic Disease recommend the development of an individualized health care plan.[45] The plan should include consideration of how having a sick child at home affects both the child and the other family members. It recommends assessment of the impact on family dynamics, activities, and schedules, along with social and financial burdens. Clearly, maintaining a child at home on enteral or parenteral nutrition requires careful consideration of the impact on quality of life of all those involved.

CONCLUSION

Providing enteral and parenteral nutrition to infants and children necessitates consideration of the ethics of providing or forgoing treatment. A quarter century of case law confirms the right of parents to make these decisions in the best interest of their child. But practical reality causes decision making to be complicated and difficult for parents, health care providers, and others. Increasingly, the quality of life of the child and the family are a central part of the discussion. The significant moral, ethical, and legal implications of decisions to forgo nutrition and hydration mandate that the discussion continue to evolve.

REFERENCES

1. Duff RS, Campbell AGM. Moral and ethical dilemmas in the special-care nursery. *N Engl J Med.* 1973;289:890–894.
2. Lyon J. "Baby Doe," two children and a White House crusade. In: Lyon J *Playing God in the Nursery*. New York, NY: W.W. Norton; 1985:21–58.
3. Dotson ML. Notice to health care providers. *Letter from the Department of Health and Human Services.* Washington, DC: Government Printing Office; May 18, 1982.
4. President's Commission for the Study of Ethical Problems in Medicine and Bioethical and Behavioral Research. *Deciding to forego life-sustaining treatment.* Washington, DC: Government Printing Office; March 1983.
5. Nondiscrimination on the basis of handicap. 48 *Federal Register* 9630–9632 (1983).
6. *American Academy of Pediatrics vs. Heckler*. US District Court No. 83-0774 (April 14, 1983).
7. Child Abuse and Prevention Act of 1984. 50 *Federal Register* 14878–14901 (1984).
8. Kopelman LM, Irons TG, Kopelman AE. Neonatologists judge the "Baby Doe" regulations. *N Engl J Med.* 1988;318:677–683.
9. Angell M. Handicapped children: Baby Doe and Uncle Sam. *N Engl J Med.* 1983;309:659–661.
10. Weir RF. The government and selective nontreatment of handicapped infants. *N Engl J Med.* 1983;309:661–663.
11. Levi BH. Withdrawing nutrition and hydration from children: legal, ethical, and professional issues. *Clin Pediatrics*. 2003;42:139–145.
12. American Academy of Pediatrics, Committee on Bioethics. Guidelines for forgoing life-sustaining medical treatment. *Pediatrics*. 1994;93:532–536.
13. American Academy of Pediatrics, Committee on Fetus and Newborn. The initiation or withdrawal of treatment for high-risk newborns. *Pediatrics.* 1995;96:362–363.
14. Paris JJ, Ferranti J, Reardon F. From the Johns Hopkins baby to Baby Miller: what have we learned from four decades of reflection on neonatal cases? *J Clin Ethics.* 2001;12:207–214.
15. Spence K. The best interest principle as a standard for decision making in the care of neonates. *J Adv Nurs.* 2000;31:1286–1292.
16. American Academy of Pediatrics, Committee on Bioethics. Ethics and the care of critically ill infants and children. *Pediatrics.* 1996;98:149–152.
17. Hardart G. Including the family's interests in medical decision making in pediatrics. *J Clin Ethics.* 2000;11:164–168.
18. American Academy of Pediatrics, Committee on Bioethics. Informed consent, parental permission, and assent in pediatric practice. *Pediatrics.* 1995;95:314–317.
19. Nelson LJ, Rushton CH, Cranford RE, Nelson RM, Glover JJ, Troug RD. Forgoing medically provided nutrition and hydration in pediatric patients. *J Law, Med Ethics.* 1995;23:33–46.
20. Johnson J, Mitchell C. Responding to parental requests to forego pediatric nutrition and hydration. *J Clin Ethics.* 2000;11:128–135.
21. Troug RD. Futility in pediatrics: from case to policy. *J Clin Ethics*. 2000;11:136–141.
22. American Medical Association, Council on Ethical and Judicial Affairs. Medical futility in end-of-life care. *J Am Med Assoc.* 1999;281:937–941.
23. Justus K. Oral aversion: a case and discussion. *Pediatr Nurs.* 1998;23:474,478.
24. Palmer MM. Weaning from gastrostomy tube feeding: Commentary on oral aversion. *Pediatr Nurs.* 1998;23:475–478.
25. Carter BS, Leuthner SR. The ethics of withholding/withdrawing nutrition in the newborn. *Sem in Perinatol.* 2003;27:480–487.
26. Rubenstein JS, Unti SM, Winter RJ. Pediatric resident attitudes about technologic support of vegetative patients and the effects of parental input: a longitudinal study. *Pediatrics*. 1994;94:8–12.

27. Lin RJ. Withdrawing life-sustaining medical treatment: a physician's personal reflection. *MRRD Res Rev.* 2003;9:10–15.

28. Langdon DS, Hunt A, Pope J, Hackes B. Nutrition support at the end of life: opinions of Louisiana dietitians. *J Amer Diet Assoc.* 2002;102:837–841.

29. American Dietetic Association. Position of the American Dietetic Association: ethical and legal issues in nutrition, hydration, and feeding. *J Amer Diet Assoc.* 2002;102:716–726.

30. Mitchell C, Troug RD. From the files of a pediatric ethics committee. *J Clin Ethics.* 2000;11:112–120.

31. American Academy of Pediatrics, Committee on Bioethics. Institutional ethics committees. *Pediatrics.* 2001;107:205–209.

32. George DE. Home parenteral and enteral nutrition. In: McConnell MS, ed. *Guidelines for Pediatric Home Health Care.* Elk Grove, Ill: American Academy of Pediatrics; 2002:113–123.

33. Stanley AL. Withholding artificially provided nutrition and hydration from disabled children: assessing their quality of life. *Clin Pediatr.* 2000;39:575–579.

34. Schron EB, Schumaker SA. The integration of health quality of life in clinical research: experiences from cardiovascular clinical trials. *Prog Cardiovasc Nurs.* 1992;7:21–28.

35. Campbell M, McHaffie H. Prolonging life and allowing death: infants. *J Med Ethics.* 1995;21:339–344.

36. Marra CA, Levine M, McKerrow R, Carleton BC. Overview of health-related quality-of-life measures for pediatric patients: application in the assessment of pharmacotherapeutic and pharmacoeconomic outcomes. *Pharmacotherapy.* 1996;16:879–888.

37. Nathan PC, Furlong W, Barr RD. Challenges to the measurement of health-related quality of life in children receiving cancer therapy. *Pediatr Blood Cancer.* 2004;43:215–223.

38. Fleming J, Challela M, Eland J, et al. Impact on the family of children who are technology dependent and cared for in the home. *Pediatr Nurs.* 1994;20:379–388.

39. Adams RA, Gordon C, Spangler AA. Maternal stress in caring for children with feeding disabilities: implications for health care providers. *J Amer Diet Assoc.* 1999;99:962–966.

40. Heyman MB, Harmatz P, Acree M, et al. Economic and psychologic costs for maternal caregivers of gastrostomy-dependent children. *J Pediatr.* 2004;145:511–516.

41. Stein REK, Jessop DJ. Functional Status II®: a measure of child health status. *Med Care.* 1990;28:1041–1055.

42. Radloff L. The CES-D scale: a self-report depression scale for research in the general population. *Appl Psychol Meas.* 1977;3:385–401.

43. Endicott J, Nee J, Harrison W, Blumenthal R. Quality of life enjoyment and satisfaction questionnaire: a new measure. *Psychopharmacol Bull.* 1993;29:321–326.

44. Thorne SE, Radford MJ, Armstrong E. Long-term gastrostomy in children: caregiver coping. *Gastroenterol Nurs.* 1997;20:46–53.

45. American Academy of Pediatrics. Committee on Children with Disabilities. Guidelines for home care of infants, children and adolescents with chronic disease. *Pediatrics.* 1995;96:161–164.

CHAPTER 18

Economics of Nutrition Support

Jacqueline Jones Wessel

INTRODUCTION

The economics of nutrition support are complicated, difficult to figure, and are based on the questions asked and the variables considered. For example, to answer the question, What constitutes the cost of nutrition support? decisions must be made about what to include. Is only the cost of the bag of parenteral nutrition (PN) solutions considered, or are the costs of the tubing and the pumps included? Are the costs of a nutrition support team factored into all estimates? Do we include the costs of feeding therapy by speech pathology and occupational therapy for the child who missed out on the normal developmental feeding milestones? How many children have special needs? How many have insurance? When do children qualify for Medicaid? This chapter will discuss some of the costs of nutrition therapies and some methods of payment for these costs.

The most current position paper of the American Dietetic Association on cost effectiveness of medical nutrition therapy (MNT) describes cost savings of medical nutrition therapy throughout the life cycle.[1] MNT saves money by providing the most appropriate therapy at the lowest possible cost for the patient and family (Table 18-1).

The literature details cost savings and improved care with the use of a multidisciplinary nutrition support team (NST) for the management of PN.[2–12] Financial benefits were also noted in a study examining the effect of NST management of enteral nutrition (EN). A cost benefit analysis revealed that for every $1 invested in NST management of EN, a benefit of $4.20 was realized.[13] One study showed greater cost ranging from $38,148 to $194,285 (depending on the estimate for sepsis) and more complications when the nutrition support nurse was terminated in a cost-cutting move, as well as decreased costs ranging from $34,485 to $156,654 (again depending on the estimate for sepsis) when the nurse was reinstated.[12]

Table 18-1 Hierarchy of the costs of nutrition therapy.

Cost of nutrition therapy, from most expensive to least expensive.
Parenteral nutrition using specialized ingredients.
Parenteral nutrition without special ingredients.
Continuous enteral nutrition using specialized product (tube feeding using a pump).
Continuous enteral nutrition (tube feeding using a pump).
Tube feeding—enteral nutrition using specialized product.
Tube feeding—enteral nutrition.
Feedings by mouth with specialized supplements.
Feedings by mouth including supplements.
Feedings by mouth, normal diet.

In computing the cost of nutrition support, which costs should be used, the cost to the hospital using a group buying contract or the cost to the parent at home? There is a difference between the costs negotiated by insurance companies and large buying groups and those costs assumed by parents. Similarly, enteral products have different prices depending on where and when the formula is purchased, if it is on sale, if coupons are used, etc.

What are the costs of feeding a child? The US Department of Agriculture (USDA), Center for Nutrition Policy and Promotion (CNPP), with assistance from the USDA Economic Research Service and the USDA Food and Nutrition Service, has established and continues to revise food plans described as thrifty, low-cost, moderate-cost, and liberal. They reflect current dietary recommendations, food consumption patterns, food composition data, and the previous plan's cost levels.[14] The recommendations incorporate the serving guidelines for the food pyramid and each age gender group meets at least 100% of the age group's recommended dietary allowances (RDA) for 15 essential nutrients. The thrifty food plan is used as the basis for food stamp allotments for the USDA. These plans, at different levels, are also used to set state child support guidelines, foster care payments, and Department of Defense allotments.[14] For our purposes, these plans can be used as a frame of reference to compare typical costs of feeding children of various ages to the cost of nutrition support (Table 18-2).

What are the specific costs of each therapy? Tables 18-3 and 18-4 list 2004 costs for nutrition therapy billed by a Midwestern hospital, and Table 18-5 lists costs for the formulas themselves.[15–18] Each center's costs vary depending on protocols and individual practices; for example, 4-hour enteral product hang time in a newborn intensive care unit generates more costs than a 24 hour hang time because 6 feeding sets are used in each 24-hour period instead of one.. Some costs, such as nursing time, are hard to measure. Some of this is captured in the patient acuity rating for each patient.

What is billed for nutrition support and the payment received could be entirely different. Some hospitals bill for every item and procedure and receive reimbursement, often a portion of what is billed. Some hospitals operate on a capitated system in which they are given a nego-

Table 18-2 Official USDA food plans: cost of food at home at four levels; US average January 2004.

Age groups	*Weekly cost*			
Children	*Thrifty plan*	*Low-cost plan*	*Moderate-cost plan*	*Liberal plan*
1 year	$17.50	$21.70	$25.50	$31.30
2 years	$17.40	$21.40	$25.40	$30.80
3–5 years	$19.00	$23.50	$29.10	$35.20
6–8 years	$23.80	$31.70	$39.10	$45.50
9–11 years	$27.90	$35.60	$45.50	$53.00
Males:12–14 years	$29.00	$40.20	$49.70	$58.70
15–19 years	$29.90	$41.40	$51.70	$60.10
Females: 12–19 years	$29.00	$34.80	$42.20	$51.00

Source: United States Department of Agriculture Center for Nutrition Policy and Promotion. Official USDA food plans: cost of food at home at four levels, US average, September 2004. USDA: Alexandria, Va; 2004. Available at: http://www.cnpp.usda.gov/using3.html. Accessed February 21, 2006.

Table 18-3 Costs of parenteral nutrition.

Product/therapy	*Inpatient*	*Outpatient*
Parenteral nutrition, dextrose, amino acids, electrolytes, minerals, vitamins	250 ml, $266.15 500 ml, $291.15 1,000 ml, $341.15	500 ml, $230 1,000 ml, $450
Additives:		
Ranitidine	25 mg, 1 ml, $19.74	Similar
Carnitine	5 ml vial, $339.48	
Albumin	25%, up to 50 ml, $458.27	
Lipids	100 ml, $140.89 250 ml, $166.46 500 ml, $319.72	$100–$200
Pumps	Included in cost of above	Included in cost of above
Tubing	$10–$30	$10–$30
Nursing charges	NA	Skilled RN visit $185/hr billed; Medicaid reimbursement $55/hr
PICC insertion	$505 billed	Same
Central venous catheter insertion	Tunneled $1,055 if pt is < 5 years, if pt is > 5 years, $1,003	Same
Lab monitoring	TPN labs $232.92 Including prealbumin pkg, $254.92	Same
Clinic visits	NA	High complexity, $235
Other: oral motor therapy, etc.	OT evaluation, $221, treatment, $38/15 minutes	

OT = occupational therapy.
NA = not applicable.

Source: Data provided from billing office, Cincinnati Children's Hospital Medical Center, 2005.CHMC.

Table 18-4 Costs of enteral therapy.

Product/Therapy	*Inpatient*	*Outpatient*
Products	$22 charge to prepare special formula	Same
Tube insertion GT	$959	Same
Monitoring	NA	Skilled nurse visit $185/hr billed; Medicaid reimbursement $55/hr
Disposable sets	Changed every 4 hours × 6 = $60 – $180 Changed every 8 hours = $30 – $90	Changed every 24 hours $10–$30
Optional gastric pop-off (Farrell bag)	Changed with feeding set	Changed every 24 hours, part of above charge
Pumps		Some rent, some buy

NA = not applicable.

Source: Data provided from billing office, Cincinnati Children's Hospital Medical CenterCHMC.

Table 18-5 Relative costs of infant and pediatric formulas.

Type of formula	*Cost per oz*	*Dispersed as*
Preterm infant 24 cal	$0.53–$0.83	2 or 3 oz* RTF bottles
Human milk fortifier†	Per packet $0.99–$1.10	Box of 50 packets
Preterm follow-up	$0.24–$0.52	RTF*,‡ or powder
Term formula with DHA ARA	$0.18–0.24	‡Concentrate, RTF, powder
Protein hydrolysate	$0.20–$0.24	RTF, powder‡
Amino acid 20 cal/oz	$0.32–$0.52	Powder
Amino acid 30 cal/oz	$0.48–$1.19	Powder
Pediatric polymeric	$0.23–$0.32	RTF 8 oz
Pediatric hydrolyzed	$0.85	RTF 8 oz

* RTF denotes ready to feed.
† 1 packet to 25 ml human milk = 24 calorie.
‡ Type used in price comparison. Prices obtained from a survey of formula companies' online stores accessed in April 2005.

Sources: Data provided from billing office, Cincinnati Children's Hospital Medical Center; Ross web site. Available at: http//www.Ross.com. Accessed January 2, 2006; Mead Johnson web site. Available at: http://www.MeadJohnson.com. Accessed January 2, 2006; SHS North America web site. Available at: http://www.SHSNA.com. Accessed January 2, 2006.

tiated amount for each medical diagnosis. In that case, increased billing does not generate more income; it just documents greater costs.

Data from a recent Agency for Healthcare Research and Quality (AHRQ) report found that 65% of US children were privately insured, 22% were insured through public resources, and 14% were uninsured. The report also showed that the parents of children without health insurance were less likely to use health care services for their children. Publicly insured children were the most likely to use hospital inpatient and emergency room care. Eighty percent of all children's health care expenditures are attributed to 20% of children.[19, 20]

How many US children require nutrition support? That number is difficult to determine. However, an AHRQ report provides estimates of the number of children in the United States with special health care needs (SHCN).[21] These children were identified by the Maternal and Child Health Program's broad definition as "Children with special health care needs are those who have or are at increased risk for a chronic physical, developmental, behavioral, or emotional condition and who also require health and related services of a type or amount beyond that required by children generally."[22] Not all children thus described require specialized nutrition support; however, this definition includes all children who do require nutrition support. In 2000, according to parent reported data, approximately 16.2% of children under 18 (11.7 million children in the US civilian noninstitutionalized population) were estimated to have special health care needs. The average yearly medical expense for children with SHCN was $2,497.84, and 10.7% of families of children with SCHN spend at least 2% of the family income on medical care.[21] Another analysis of the data found that parents with very high out-of-pocket expenses, greater than 5% of income, were 11 times more likely to be from families with incomes less than 200% of the federal poverty level.[23] A less recognized expense could stem from the use of alternative therapies such as herbal supplements in children with SCHN.[24]

REIMBURSEMENT

In the United States, children are covered by private health insurance or public health insurance or have no health insurance coverage. Insurance policies vary widely in terms of coverage for nutrition therapy. Some common items not covered are disposables such as feeding sets. Sometimes infant or pediatric formulas are not covered unless specified as "exempt infant formulas" or, for children over 1 year, "medical food." The federal definitions are provided in Tables 18-6 and 18-7. Sometimes infant and pediatric formulas are covered by Medicaid if they

Table 18-6 Federal definition of exempt formula.

Food and Drug Administration, HHS 21 CFR Ch. 1 (4-1-97 Edition) § 107.50

Subpart C–Exempt Infant Formulas

Infant formulas not generally available at the retail level. These exempt infant formulas are not generally found on retail shelves for general consumer purchase. Such formulas typically are prescribed by a physician, and must be requested from a pharmacist, or are distributed directly to institutions such as hospitals, clinics, and State or Federal agencies. Such formulas are also generally represented and labeled solely to provide dietary management for specific diseases or conditions that are clinically serious or life-threatening and generally are required for prolonged periods of time.

Sources: From the Office of the Federal Register, National Archives and Records Administration; Available at: http://www.shsna.com/insurance/SHS_insurance/Exempt_infant.htm. Accessed .

Table 18-7 Federal definition of medical food.

Food and Drug Administration, HHS 21 CFR Ch. 1 (4-1-95 Edition) § 101.9

(8) Medical foods are defined in section 5(b) of the Orphan Drug Act (21 U.S.C. 360ee(b) (3)): A medical food is a food which is formulated to be consumed or administered enterally under the supervision of a physician and which is intended for the specific dietary management of a disease or condition for which distinctive nutritional requirements, based on recognized scientific principles, are established by medical evaluation. A food is subject to this exemption only if:

- (i) It is a specially formulated and processed product (as opposed to a naturally occurring foodstuff used in its natural state) for the partial or exclusive feeding of a patient by means of oral intake or enteral feeding by tube;
- (ii) It is intended for the dietary management of a patient who, because of therapeutic or chronic medical needs, has limited or impaired capacity to ingest, digest, absorb, or metabolize ordinary foodstuffs or certain nutrients, or who has other special medically determined nutrient requirements, the dietary management of which cannot be achieved by the modification of the normal diet alone;
- (iii) It provides nutritional support specifically modified for the management of the unique nutrient needs that result from the specific disease or condition, as determined by medical evaluation;
- (iv) It is intended to be used under medical supervision; and
- (v) It is intended only for a patient receiving active and ongoing medical supervision wherein the patient requires medical care on a recurring basis for, among other things, instructions on the use of the medical food.

Source: From the Office of the Federal Register, National Archives and RecordsAccessed Available at: www.shsna.com/pages/exempt_infant.htm. Accessed May 24, 2006.

are not fed by mouth and exclusively used for tube feedings (Table 18-8). Many of the formula manufacturers have letters of medical necessity already written and available for health care providers to use, including the reimbursement coding.[25,26]

There are 4 major forms of private insurance in the United States:

- Fee-for-service (or traditional health insurance).
- Health maintenance organizations (or HMOs).
- Preferred provider organizations (or PPOs).
- Point of service plans (or POSs).

Fee-for-service plans will be discussed in the next section; health maintenance organizations, preferred provider organizations, and point of service plans will be discussed in the section called Managed Care Plans.

Fee-for-Service Plans

In fee-for-service reimbursement plans, the medical provider (usually a doctor or hospital) will be paid a fee for each service rendered to the patient who is covered under the policy. With fee-for-service insurance, patients are allowed to go to the doctor of their choice, and the patients or their doctors or hospitals submit claims to their insurance company for reimbursement. Patients will only receive reimbursement for covered medical expenses, which are the items listed in the benefits summary.

Table 18-8 Medicaid state coverage for enteral nutrition.

<table>
<tr><th>Type of enteral nutrition support</th><th>Coverage for children</th><th>Prior authorization required</th><th>Payment rates</th><th>Coding used</th></tr>
<tr><td>Tube feeding</td><td>All states except West Virginia</td><td>Varies by state</td><td rowspan="3">Some rates are based on Medicare part B; some rates are based on states' unique formula for payment, including an estimate of the average wholesale price and a multiplier.</td><td rowspan="3">HCPCS, NDC, other combinations using average wholesale price + formula to add or subtract.
Adding BO on HCPCS means orally administered.</td></tr>
<tr><td>Oral formula as sole source of nutrition</td><td>Yes except for Utah and West Virginia, must be strongly justified in South Carolina.</td><td>Varies by state</td></tr>
<tr><td>Oral supplement</td><td>Yes except for Kansas, Maine, Maryland, Montana, North Carolina, South Carolina, Tennessee, Utah, West Virginia, or Texas—any oral use evaluated case by case.</td><td>Varies by state</td></tr>
</table>

HCPSC = health care common procedure coding system.
NDC = national drug code.

Source: Ross Products. Reimbursement. Available at: http://www.ross.com/reimbursement/medicaid.asp. Accessed January 3, 2006.

When a service is covered, reimbursement is provided for some, but generally not all of the cost. How much is paid depends on the provisions of the policy regarding coinsurance and deductibles. The portion of the medical expenses the patient pays is the coinsurance. Although there are variations, fee-for-service policies often reimburse doctor bills at 80 percent of the reasonable and customary charge. Reasonable and customary charge is the prevailing cost of a medical service in a given geographic area. The patient pays the other 20 percent, the coinsurance. However, if a medical provider charges more than the reasonable and customary fee, the patient pays the difference.[27,28]

Some fee-for-service plans pay hospital expenses in full; some reimburse at the 80/20 level. Deductibles are the amount of the covered expenses a patient must pay each year before the insurer reimbursement starts. These range from $100 to $300 per year per individual, or $500 or more per family. Generally, the higher the deductible the policy has, the lower the premiums the insured pays for the insurance. Policies typically have an out-of-pocket maximum. This means that once expenses reach a certain amount in a given calendar year, the reasonable and customary fee for covered benefits is paid in full by the insurer. If the hospital or doctor bills are more than the reasonable and customary charge, the patient might have to pay a portion of the bill. There could be lifetime limits on benefits paid under the policy. Most experts recommend a policy with a lifetime limit of at least $1 million.[27,28]

Managed Care Plans

The 3 major types of managed care plans are health maintenance organizations (HMOs), preferred provider organizations (PPOs), and point-of-service (POS) plans. Managed care plans generally provide comprehensive health services to their members and offer financial incentives for patients to use providers who belong to the plan. In managed care plans, providers are paid a set amount in advance. Premiums are the same whether the plan member uses services or not. The plan may charge a co-payment for some services, such as $10 for an office visit. As long as doctors or hospitals that participate in or are part of the HMO are used for service, there are few out-of-pocket expenses; there are only the small co-payments. Typically, managed care plans do not have deductibles or coinsurance. With an HMO, all medical care is managed through a coordinating primary care physician plan member. Primary care physicians may be pediatricians or other physicians. The primary care physician is responsible for referral to specialists when needed. Specialists must be participating providers in the HMO.

PPOs and POS plans are also categorized as managed care plans. POS plans are often called an HMO with a point of service option. These plans combine features of fee-for-service plans and HMOs. They offer more flexibility than HMOs, but premiums are usually higher. With a PPO or a POS plan, unlike most HMOs, there is some reimbursement for a covered service from a provider who is not in the plan. Choosing a provider outside the plan's network costs more than choosing a provider in the network. These plans act like fee-for-service plans and charge coinsurance for visits outside the network. The difference between a PPO and a POS plan is that a POS plan has primary care physicians who coordinate patient care; and in general, PPO plans do not.[27,28]

COBRA

A federal law known as the Consolidated Omnibus Budget Reconciliation Act of 1985, or COBRA, stipulates that group health plans sponsored by employers with 20 or more employees are required to offer continued coverage for the employee and the employee's dependents for 18 months after the employee terminates employment. Under the same law, following an employee's death or divorce, the worker's family has the right to continue coverage for up to 3 years. The employer must be notified with in 60 days. The entire premium, up to 102 percent of the cost of the coverage, must be paid. If COBRA does not apply because an employer has fewer than 20 employees, the employee might be able to convert the group policy to individual coverage. The advantage of that option is that it is not necessary to pass a medical examination, although exclusion based on a preexisting condition might apply, depending on the medical and insurance history.[29]

PREEXISTING CONDITIONS

Many people worry about coverage for preexisting conditions, especially when they change jobs. The Health Insurance Portability and Accountability Act (HIPAA) helps assure continued health insurance coverage for employees and their dependents. As of July 1, 1997, insurers could impose only one 12-month waiting period for any preexisting condition treated or diagnosed in the previous 6 months. Prior health insurance coverage is credited toward the preexisting condition exclusion period as long as continuous coverage is maintained without a break of more than 62 days. Pregnancy is not considered a preexisting condition, and newborns and adopted children who are covered within 30 days are not subject to the 12-month waiting period.[29]

FLEXIBLE SPENDING ACCOUNTS

A flexible spending account (FSA) is a plan in which individuals put aside a certain percent of their salary each year to reimburse themselves for out-of-pocket expenses not covered by insurance or other plans. The dollars that go into an FSA are pretax dollars, meaning the contributions to the FSA are deducted from a paycheck before federal and Social Security taxes are withheld (FSA contributions are sometimes exempted from state and local taxes as well). Using pretax money results in lower taxes overall and an increase in disposable income. Money contributed to an FSA must be spent in the course of a given calendar year, since unspent funds are forfeited at year's end.

WOMEN, INFANTS, AND CHILDREN PROGRAM

The Women, Infants, and Children (WIC) program is a federal grant program administered at the federal level by the Food and Nutrition Service, which provides funds to the WIC state agencies. WIC is available in every state, 33 American Indian tribal organizations, the District of Columbia, Puerto Rico, American Samoa, Guam, and thc Virgin Islands. To be eligible, family income must be at or below 185 percent of the federal poverty rate, which is about $33,485 for a family of 4, meet state residency requirements, be individually assessed as at nutritional risk by a health professional, or already qualify for certain other low income programs, such as Medicaid. About 54% of all babies born in the United States participate in WIC. WIC is available for pregnant women, breastfeeding women, and infants determined to be at nutritional risk. Children up to 5 years of age are eligible if they have serious medical problems. WIC provides food for pregnant and lactating women. Infant and pediatric formulas are provided when prescribed by a physician for a medical problem. Each of the 88 agencies is required to have a competitively bid rebate contract with an infant formula manufacturer; therefore each WIC agency has a contract formula line of products. Some noncontract formulas might be available with a physician's prescription for valid medical reasons.[30,31]

MEDICAID AND SOCIAL SECURITY INCOME

Medicaid provides health care coverage for some low income people who cannot afford insurance. Medicaid covers those who are eligible because they are aged, blind, disabled, or are in families with dependent children. Medicaid is a federal program that is operated by the states. Each state decides who is eligible and the scope of health services offered.[29]

In most states, children who get supplemental Social Security Income (SSI) benefits qualify for Medicaid. In many states, Medicaid comes automatically with SSI eligibility. In other states, it requires a separate application. Some children qualify for Medicaid coverage even if they do not qualify for SSI. Medicare is a federal health insurance program for people 65 or older and for people who have been getting Social Security disability benefits for 2 years. Because children, even those with disabilities, do not get Social Security disability benefits until they turn 18, ordinarily, no child can get Medicare coverage until he or she is 20 years old. The only exception to this rule is for children with chronic renal disease who need a kidney transplant or maintenance dialysis. Children with chronic renal disease can get Medicare if a parent is getting Social Security or has worked enough to be covered by Social Security (SSI).[30]

SSI is a program that pays monthly benefits to people with low incomes and limited assets who are 65 or older, blind, or disabled. Children can qualify if they meet Social Security's definition of disability and if their income and assets fall within the eligibility limits. SSI benefits for children are benefits payable to disabled children under age 18 who have limited income and resources or who come from homes with limited income and resources.[31]

State Children's Health Insurance Program (SCHIP)

Legislation passed in 1997 created a new Title XXI of the Social Security Act, known as SCHIP. This program enables states to insure children from working families with incomes too high to qualify for Medicaid, but too low to afford private health insurance. The program provides for prescription drugs, vision, hearing, and mental health services and is available in all 50 states and the District of Columbia.[32] A study found that children with special health care needs (SHCN) were more likely to be eligible for this program than children without special needs. Children with SHCN had higher rates of participation in the program than those children without special needs.[33]

Medicaid has a confusing assortment of rules to cover nutritional products. Each state administers its program differently. HMOs have also entered the state system and some states have as many as 12 different methods of reimbursement based on a particular plan. Ross Laboratories has an excellent section on reimbursement on its web site. It includes the state-by-state rules for enteral reimbursement.[34] Table 18-8 includes data from that site as well as information from individual states' Medicaid web sites. The state of Washington has well thought-out policies. The Washington State Medical Nutrition Program reimburses when the client is unable to meet daily nutritional requirements using traditional foods alone due to injury or illness. The claim must include the following:

1. Estimation of the total nutritional requirements,
2. Estimation of the number of supplemental calories,
3. The client's weight or description of body build,
4. The client's height, and
5. Determination of why meeting an individual's nutritional requirements cannot be part of the daily diet.

Nutritional assessments by a certified dietitian must be made for all clients 20 years and younger within 30 days of initiation of medical nutrition, and periodically as needed while on medical nutrition. A handbook with case studies is available to explain the process of obtaining enteral products using this system, as well as information about nutrition for special needs children.[35–37]

The federal Healthcare Common Procedure Coding System (HCPCS) for nutrition billing is used by some states. New coding is being added every year. The list in Table 18-9 includes the 2004 pediatric enteral/parenteral nutrition related coding obtained from the Center for Medicare and Medicaid. NDC is the national drug code, used for reimbursement coding in some states.[38]

Table 18-9 HCPCS coding for nutrition.

Product category	*HCPCS code*	*Item description*
Enteral	B4034	Enteral feeding supply kit; syringe, per day.
Enteral	B4035	Enteral feeding supply kit; pump fed, per day.
Enteral	B4036	Enteral feeding supply kit; gravity fed, per day.
Enteral	B4081	Nasogastric tubing with stylet.
Enteral	B4082	Nasogastric tubing without stylet.
Enteral	B4083	Stomach tube—levine type.
Enteral	B4084	Gastrostomy/jejunostomy tubing.
Enteral	B4085	Gastrostomy tube, silicone with sliding ring, each.
Enteral	B4103	Enteral formulae, pediatric fluid and electrolyte 500 ml = 1 unit.
Enteral	B4104	Additive for enteral formula.
Enteral	B4149	Enteral formulae blenderized foods.
Enteral	B4150	Enteral formulae; category I: semi-synthetic intact protein/protein isolates, 100 calo-
Enteral	B4151	Enteral formulae; category I: natural intact protein/protein isolates, 100 calories = 1
Enteral	B4152	Enteral formulae; category II: intact protein/protein isolates (calorically dense), 100
Enteral	B4153	Enteral formulae; category III: hydrolyzed protein/amino acids; 100 calories = 1 unit.
Enteral	B4154	Enteral formulae; category IV: defined formula for special metabolic need, 100 calo-
Enteral	B4155	Enteral formulae; category V: modular components (protein, carbohydrates, fat), 100
Enteral	B4156	Enteral formulae; category VI: standardized nutrients, 100 calories = 1 unit.
Enteral	B4157	Enteral formulae; special metabolic inherit 100 cal = 1 unit.
Enteral	B4158	Enteral formulae; pediatric complete intact nut 100 cal = 1 unit.
Enteral	B4159	Enteral formulae; pediatric complete soy based 100 cal = 1 unit.
Enteral	B4160	Enteral formulae; pediatric caloric dense >/= 0.7 100 cal = 1 unit.
Enteral	B4161	Enteral formulae; pediatric hydrolyzed/amino acid 100 cal = 1 unit.
Enteral	B4162	Enteral formulae; pediatric spec metabolic inherit 100 cal = 1 unit.
Enteral	B9000	Enteral nutrition infusion pump; without alarm.
Enteral	B9002	Enteral nutrition infusion pump; with alarm.
Enteral	E0776	IV pole.
Parenteral	B9004, 6	TPN infusion pump.
Parenteral	B4220,	PN supply kit.
Parenteral	B4224	PN administration kit.
Parenteral	B4189	Parenteral nutrition 10–51 gm of protein, electrolytes, trace elements, vitamins, pre-
Parenteral	B4193	As above 52–73 gm protein
Parenteral	B4197	As above 74–100 gm protein
Parenteral	B4199	As above > 100 gm protein

Source: Centers for Medicare and Medicaid Services web site. Available at: http://www.cms.hhs.gov. Accessed January 3, 2006.

CONCLUSION

The provision of nutrition for infants and children costs money. There is evidence that thoughtful multidisciplinary care is cost-effective. Evidence based outcomes research for specialized nutrition support in pediatrics is needed. Reimbursement for nutrition support varies by state in public financing and in private insurance from policy to policy. Thoughtful consideration should be made for simplification of the rules and regulations regarding the provision of nutrition and the inclusion of necessary nutrition support for all children.

REFERENCES

1. Carey M, Gillespie S. Position of the American Dietetic Association cost-effectiveness of medical nutrition therapy. *JADA.* 95:88–91;1995.
2. Naylor CJ, Griffiths RD, Fernandez RS. Does a multidisciplinary total parenteral nutrition team improve patient outcomes? A systematic review. *J Parenter Enteral Nutr.* 2004;28:251–258.
3. Higashiguchi T. The roles of a nutrition support team. *Nippon Geka Gakkai Zasshi.* 2004;105:206–212.
4. Gianino MS, Brunt LM, Eisenberg PG. The impact of a nutritional support team on the cost and management of multilumen central venous catheters. *J Intraven Nurs.* 1992;15:327–332.
5. Anderson CD, Heimburger DC, Morgan SL, et al. Metabolic complications of total parenteral nutrition: effects of a nutrition support service. *J Parenter Enteral Nutr.* 1996;20:206–210.
6. Roberts MF, Levine GM. Nutrition support team recommendations can reduce hospital costs. *Nutr Clin Pract.* 1992;7:227–230.
7. O'Brien DD, Hodges RE, Day AT, et al. Recommendations of nutrition support team promote cost containment. *J Parenter Enteral Nutr.*1986;10:300–302.
8. Saalwachter AR, Evans HL, Willcutts KF, et al. A nutrition support team led by general surgeons decreases inappropriate use of total parenteral nutrition on a surgical service. *Ann Surg.* 2004;70:1107–1111.
9. Gales RJ, Riley DG. Improved total parenteral nutrition therapy management by a nutritional support team. *Hosp Pharm.* 1994;29:469–470.
10. Oakes L. Anseline M. Carlton J. Reduction of complications associated with total parenteral nutrition by introduction of a clinical monitoring team. The Total Parenteral Nutrition Committee. *Australian Clinical Review. 1991;11(4):138–42, 1991.*
11. Oliveira Fuster G, Mancha Dobles I, Gonzalez-Romero S, et al. The quality of care in parenteral nutrition: the benefits after the incorporation of a nutritional support nurse. *Nutr Hosp.* 2000;15:118–121.
12. Goldstein M, Braitman LE, Levine GM. The medical and financial costs associated with termination of a nutrition support nurse. *J Parenter Enteral Nutr.* 2000;24:323–327.
13. Hassell JT, Games AD, Shaffer B, et al. Nutrition support team management of enterally fed patients in a community hospital is cost beneficial. *J Am Diet Assoc.* 1994;94:993–998.
14. United States Department of Agriculture Center for Nutrition Policy and Promotion. Official USDA food plans: cost of food at home at four levels, US average, September 2004. USDA: Alexandria, Va; 2004. Available at:http://www.cnpp.usda.gov/FoodPlans/Update/foodmar06.pdf. Accessed May 22, 2006 .
15. Data provided from billing office, Cincinnati Children's Hospital Medical Center.December 1, 2005
16. Ross web site:. Nutritional Products; http://www.ross.com/library/2005%20medicare%20part%20b%20rates.pdf accessed May 24, 2006
17. Mead Johnson web site. Available at: http://. http://www.meadjohnson.com/products_store.html Accessed May 22, 2006.
18. Nutricia North America web site. Available at: http://www.SHSNA.com/pages/ordering.html. Accessed May 22, 2006.
19. Novartis web site. Available at: http://www.Novartisnutrition.com/us/products. Accessed May 22,, 2006.
20. Elixhauser A, Machlin SR, Zodel MW, et al. Health care for children and youth in the United States: 2001 annual report on access, utilization, quality, and expenditures. *Ambulatory Pediatr.* 2002;2:419–437.
21. Chevarley FM. Utilization and expenditures for children with special health care needs. Agency for Healthcare Research and Quality working paper no. 05010, February 2005. Available at:.www.meps.ahrq.gov/papers/rf24/rf24.pdf. Accessed May24, 2006.
22. McPherson M, Arango P, Fox H, et al. A new definition of children with special health care needs. *Pediatrics.* 1998;102:137–140.
23. Newacheck PW, Kim SE. A national profile of health care utilization and expenditures for children with special health care needs. *Arch Pediatr Adolesc Med.* 2005;159:10–17.
24. Harris AB. Evidence of increasing dietary supplement use in children with special health care needs: strategies for improving parent and professional communication. *J Am Diet Assoc.* 2005;105:34–37.
25. Ross metabolic formula letter. In: Accosta P. *Ross Metabolic Handbook.* Ross Labs: Columbus, Ohio; 2002; v–viii.

26. Sample insurance letters, Nutricia North America, Available at:. http://www.shsna.com/pages/insurance_info.htm. Accessed May 22, 2006
27. Health Insurance Association of America. A guide to health insurance. Washington, DC; 2003. Available at: http://www.ahip.org/content/default.aspx?bc=41|329|. Accessed May 24,2006.
28. Health Care Financing Administration. Baltimore, Md: Health Care Financing Administration; . Publications N1-26-27.,Checkup on Health Insurance Choices.
29. US Social Security Administration web site. Available at: http://www.socialsecurity.gov. Accessed January 3, 2006.
30. Nutrition program facts, Food and Nutrition service. Available at: http://. www.fns.gov/wic/WIC-Fact-Sheet.pdf Accessed May 24, 2006
31. United States Department of Agriculture, Food and Nutrition Service web site. Available at: http://www.fns.usda.gov. Accessed January 3, 2006.
32. Centers for Medicare and Medicaid Services web site. Available at: http://www.cms.hhs.gov/schip/. Accessed January 3, 2006.
33. Davidoff AJ, Yemane A, Hill T. Public insurance eligibility and enrollment for special health care needs children. *Health Care Financ Rev.* 2004;26:119–135.
34. Ross Laboratories. Reimbursement. Available at: http://www.ross.com/reimbursement/medicaid.asp. Accessed January 3, 2006.
35. Washington State Department of Health, Maternal and Child Health Programs. Children with Special Health Care Needs Program. Available at: http:www.doh.wa.gov/cfh/mch/CSHCNhome2.htm. Accessed January 3, 2006.
36. Washington State Department of Health, Children with Special Health Care Needs Program. Medicaid reimbursement for medical nutrition products and nutrition services for children with special health care needs: a Washington state case studies report. Publication 970-109. Olympia, Wash: Washington State Department of Health; March, 2004. Available at: http://www.doh.wa.gov/cfh/mch/documents/nutr_case-studies_web.pdf. Accessed January 3, 2006.
37. Nutrition interventions for children with special health care needs, 2002. Available at: http://www.doh.wa.gov/cfh/mch/documents/nutrition_interventions.pdf. Accessed .May 22, 2006
38. Centers for Medicare and Medicaid Services web site. Available at: http://www.cms.hhs.gov/medhcpcsgeninfo/01_overview.asp. Accessed May 22,, 2006.

CHAPTER 19

Home Nutrition Support

Jay A. Perman and Anjali Malkani

INTRODUCTION

The objective of nutrition support in the pediatric population is to promote growth. In some cases, nutrition support treats the underlying medical condition, for example glycogen storage disease, or is an adjunct to primary therapy for a medical condition, as with inflammatory bowel disease.

With the recognition that improved nutritional status positively influences treatment outcomes, there has been a renewed interest in home nutrition support (HNS). Home enteral nutrition (HEN), tube feeding, has been underused in the past. Recent increased interest in HEN is the result of ongoing advances in technology and growth of support structures in the community. Home parenteral nutrition (HPN), together with intestinal transplantation, has revolutionized the approach to and treatment of patients with intestinal failure.

As with HPN, HEN may be used to reverse growth failure associated with chronic illnesses or maintain growth during a disease state of high energy requirements. A retrospective study of 78 children on HEN in Canada showed a positive effect on their nutritional status. Children in 3 nutritional groups—one group appropriately nourished, another wasted, and the third stunted—at the time of entry into the study, showed significant improvement in their weight-for-age z-scores in the mean follow-up period of 9 months.[1] HEN and HPN are effective also in maintaining weight in children undergoing chemotherapy.[2,3]

PREVALENCE OF HNS

In the United States, national and state agencies monitor the prevalence of HNS. These agencies could underestimate the prevalence of HNS because reporting is not mandatory and HNS is initiated, managed, and monitored by various local and hospital-based programs. Medicare data show there were 73,000 patients on HEN in 1992, a 25% increase from 1982. This corresponds to Medicare HEN prevalence of 200 per million population.[4] The estimated prevalence of HPN in 1992 was 40,000 patients. Data in the literature on children receiving HEN in the United States is limited, and hence more difficult to estimate.

There is a significant increase in HNS on a global basis. In the United Kingdom, the 1999 BANS (British Artificial Nutrition Survey) report showed an annual increase in HEN of 20%, with 26% of the 10,864 registered HEN patients being children. The most common indication for HEN in children was failure to thrive (51%). Cerebral palsy was the primary diagnostic category, comprising 19% of those younger than 15 years.[5] In a prospective community study in the East Anglia community of Cambridge, UK over 5 years (1988–1993), Parker described a yearly prevalence of 110 HEN patients per million population in 1992, which had doubled over the study period.[6] In this study, 20% of the patients were between 1 and 10 years of age and were receiving HEN because of failure to thrive. A study from the West of Scotland reported a 23% increase in the number of children receiving HEN in 1995.[7] There are limited data on the use and outcome of HEN in Australia. The report of the Ministerial Working Party on HEN in the state of Victoria reported 631 patients receiving HEN in 1996. Over 6 years, there was a 428% increase in the number of percutaneous gastrostomy and jejunostomy procedures performed. Of these HEN patients, 41% were children and half had an underlying neurological disease.[8]

The BANS from the United Kingdom reported a 5% annual increase in the number of patients receiving HPN over a 3-year period. Of these patients, 81 were children, and almost half the children were under a year of age. Short bowel syndrome was the most common diagnosis in children receiving HPN.[5]

BENEFITS OF HNS

Enteral nutrition (EN) is commonly used in hospitalized children who are unable to meet their nutritional needs orally. When their underlying medical condition does not require ongoing hospitalization, this benefit can be transferred to a home setting. Parents have stated that their children are happier and more active at home, and being at home provides a sense of freedom.[9] HNS also reduces health care costs. For the health care institution and payer, HNS is cost effective because it reduces the length of hospitalization. It is estimated that HPN costs are 25–50% less than in-hospital costs for adults.[10,11] HNS also frees beds for other patients and allows for the development and growth of home care programs. These benefits are summarized in Table 19-1.

Table 19-1 Benefits of home nutrition support.

Patient
- Physiological
  - Repletion of nutritional status
  - Maintenance of nutritional status
- Psychosocial
  - Return to home, work, or school
  - Return to family, friends
  - Return of independence
- Financial
  - Reduced health care costs
  - Reduced loss of work days
  - More stable family budget

Health care institutions
- Financial
  - Reduced length of stay
  - Fewer potential complications than with parenteral nutrition
- Program development
  - Potential for establishment of profitable home care programs
  - Potential growth of profitable home care programs

PATIENT SELECTION FOR HNS

Not all patients who receive nutrition support (NS) in the hospital setting are candidates for HNS (Table 19-2). In addition to the medical indication for HNS, the underlying disease state must be stable and not require ongoing hospitalization. Appropriate enteral or parenteral access should be in place, and the patient should tolerate the planned home regimen prior to discharge. The patient and caregiver should be willing to perform care at home with adequate support from the family, and if necessary, a visiting nurse. The caregiver should be able to understand and perform HNS and monitor for complications. Prior to discharge, financial reimbursement issues must be addressed. Finally, a plan for appropriate follow-up must be agreed upon by the patient, the caregiver, and the health care team.

Management of patients in the hospital, coordination of discharge planning, and follow-up of the patient on HNS requires a multidisciplinary approach involving the physician, dietitian, social worker, nurse, coordinator, pharmacist, and psychologist. All should have experience in pediatrics.[12] This team develops a nutrition care plan, defines the goals of nutrition therapy, an-

Table 19-2 Criteria for patient selection for home nutrition support.

Medical	Functional impairment of the gastrointestinal tract or inability to deliver adequate nutrients to the gastrointestinal tract using the oral route.
	Underlying disease state stable; continued hospitalization not needed.
	Underlying condition not adversely affected by HNS.
Nutritional	Appropriate access in place and functioning.
	Ability to tolerate home regimen prior to hospital discharge.
Psychosocial	Willingness to perform HNS.
	Adequate support of caregiver.
Educational	Ability to understand and perform HNS therapy.
Financial	Availability of affordable HNS supplies.
Other	Resources to provide in-home monitoring and troubleshooting.

Source: Adapted from JCAHO Board of Directors. *Comprehensive Accreditation Manual for Hospitals.* Oakbrook, Ill: JCAHO; 1996.

ticipates duration of nutrition therapy, provides for caregiver education, and performs the discharge planning. If criteria for HNS cannot be met, ongoing hospitalization or placement in an extended care facility should be considered.

HOME ENTERAL NUTRITION (HEN)

EN as defined by the American Society for Parenteral and Enteral Nutrition,[13] is the nonvolitional delivery of nutrients by tube into the gastrointestinal tract. There are few randomized, controlled, prospective studies comparing matched patients receiving EN versus parenteral nutrition (PN). However, the proposed benefits of EN include safety, reduced cost, simpler skills required for administration, fewer infectious and metabolic complications, and promotion of the physiological and immunological integrity of the gut.

INDICATIONS FOR HEN IN PEDIATRICS

Table 19-3 lists some indications for HEN in childhood. Irrespective of underlying diagnosis, these include the inability to ingest adequate calories orally, impaired digestion and absorption, and growth failure associated with high metabolic needs. However, a functioning gastrointestinal tract with adequate length and absorptive capacity is necessary for the use of EN.

Table 19-3 Indications for home enteral nutrition in childhood.

A. Impaired ingestion of oral nutrients
    1. Failure to thrive
    2. Neurological impairment, e.g., cerebral palsy
    3. Oral effects of chemotherapy and radiation
    4. Tracheo-esophageal fistula
    5. Anorexia nervosa
    6. Feeding disorder
    7. Metabolic disease requiring special diets
    8. Mucositis
B. Impaired digestion and absorption
    1. Cystic fibrosis
    2. Inflammatory bowel disease
    3. Short bowel syndrome
    4. AIDS
    5. Enteric fistulas
C. Hypermetabolic states
    1. Malignancy
    2. Congenital heart disease
    3. Liver disease
    4. Chronic pulmonary disease
    5. Renal disease

Enteral Access

There are several factors to consider when determining the appropriate route of administration of enteral nutrients. These include the underlying medical condition, anticipated duration of home therapy, risk for aspiration, and patient preference. Generally, a nasogastric or nasoenteric tube can be placed if the intended therapy is short term. If HEN is expected to last more than 4–6 weeks, a more permanent access such as tube enterostomy (gastrostomy or jejunostomy) is preferred.[1]

Enteral access for delivering HEN includes (1) nasogastric tubes, (2) nasojejunal tubes, (3) gastrostomy tubes, (4) gastrojejunal tubes, and (5) jejunal tubes. These methods of accessing the gastrointestinal tract are discussed in detail in Chapter 20.

HEN IN NEUROLOGICALLY IMPAIRED CHILDREN

The major population for HEN in pediatrics are neurologically impaired children. The 10-year survival rate of neurologically impaired children residing in skilled nursing homes is better if fed via gastrostomy as compared to the nasogastric route (78% versus 41%), independent of other medical illness.[14] The need for an antireflux procedure at the time of gastrostomy tube placement for the long term nutritional management of neurologically impaired children is controversial. Generally, if a trial of nasogastric feeds for 4 weeks results in adequate weight gain with no exacerbation of reflux disease, an antireflux procedure at the time of percutaneous endoscopic gastrostomy (PEG) tube placement might not be necessary.[15,16,17] Other authors have recommended a pH probe study to help determine the need for an antireflux procedure at the time of gastrostomy tube placement.[18,19] Parents of children with neurodevelopmental disabilities requiring gastrostomy feeding need support because of their concerns about the loss of oral feeding, despite the expected nutritional benefit of tube feeding.[20]

Method of Administration

There are 3 ways to administer enteral feeds: bolus, timed intermittent, and continuous. The method of delivery depends on the type of enteral access, patient tolerance, and lifestyle of the patient. Prior to discharge, it is necessary to ensure that the patient tolerates the proposed home feeding schedule. Bolus feeds are given over 20–30 minutes through a gastrostomy tube via gravity using a syringe or bolus feeding set. This mimics mealtime and does not require a pump.

Timed intermittent feeds are bolus feeds that are administered through a gastrostomy but on a pump over a specified time (usually 30–60 minutes). This allows for improved tolerance but requires the patient to be hooked up to a pump. Lightweight portable pumps with extended battery life make this method of administration acceptable to families. In a prospective, randomized, crossover study of 100 adults receiving pump assisted bolus feeds compared to gravity controlled PEG feeding, pump assisted bolus feeds were associated with a lower rate of regurgitation and vomiting. By the end of the study, 96% of the patients initially using gravity controlled feeds changed to pump assisted feeds.[21] Continuous pump assisted feeds can be administered around the clock or at night while the child is asleep, allowing for oral feeding and normal activities during the day.

Schedules for feeding children requiring HEN can be creative and depend on the child's needs and schedule. A child may receive continuous feeds at night with a combination of oral and bolus feeds during the day. In some instances a child could get supplemental nightly feeding 6 nights per week, allowing a free night for sleepovers.

To minimize complications and maximize patient comfort and compliance, appropriate equipment must be chosen. Bolus feeding requires only a syringe with administration tubing. Those on timed intermittent and continuous feeds require an infusion pump, container or bag for the feeds, tubing, and a pole from which to hang the feeding bag. A wide array of feeding containers and tubing varying in design, ease of use, and cost are available for home use, and should be compatible with the pump that will be used at home. The distal tubing should fit the enteral access device. Clean technique is essential to minimize the risk of bacterial contamination. Tubes should be flushed with water before and after every use and every 4 hours during continuous feeds to prevent clogging.[16]

Enteral infusion pumps for home use should be safe, simple to use, and accurate in delivering a constant flow rate. They should have an alarm system (visual and/or audible) that will automatically shut off in case of occlusion, inadvertent rate change, or low battery. In the pediatric population, the pump should be able to advance preset rates in small increments. Newer pumps have an automatic water flush system that decreases clogging of tubes.[22] Children can carry lightweight, portable pumps with extended battery life in a backpack. This allows children to be mobile and develop appropriate motor skills while receiving needed nutrition.

Formula Selection

There are more than 100 infant and pediatric formulas available in the United States (Appendix A).[23] The choice of formula depends on the patient's nutrient needs, caloric and fluid requirements, digestive and absorptive capacity, route of administration, cost, and availability (Table 19-4).

The needs of most HEN patients can be met with one of the complete formulas. Rarely, modular additives are necessary. If they must be used, the caregiver needs to learn how to use the modular additive before discharge and the patient must be able to tolerate the planned home feeding formula and regime prior to discharge. See Chapter 20.

HOME PARENTERAL NUTRITION (HPN)

HPN is an indispensable option for children with gut failure who are unable to tolerate enteral feeds necessary to promote growth, or whose underlying medical condition precludes the long term use of EN. Table 19-5 lists common indications for HPN.

Appropriate permanent and secure vascular access is necessary for the administration of PN at home (Chapters 22 and 26). The catheter must be in a large central vein, typically the superior vena cava, to avoid chemical phlebitis from hyperosmolar nutrient solutions. Commonly used lines are the subcutaneously tunneled central lines (Broviac, Hickman) or lines with an implanted subcutaneous port. Peripherally inserted central venous catheters (PICC) are used frequently because they are easily inserted at the bedside.[24]

Broviac and Hickman lines are tunneled subcutaneously away from the site of venous access to exit near the axilla. There is a Dacron cuff under the skin, which promotes the development of scar tissue at the cutaneous exit site. This prevents bacteria from traveling up

Table 19-4 Factors to consider when selecting an enteral formula.

Patient-related factors	*Formula-related factors*
Age	Caloric density
Underlying diagnosis	Osmolality
Digestive and absorptive capacity of the GI tract	Ease of preparation
Fluid, nutrient, and caloric needs	Cost
Food allergies	Insurance coverage
Route of administration	Availability at home

Table 19-5 Indications for home parenteral nutrition in pediatrics.

1. Postsurgical conditions
   a. Short bowel syndrome
   b. Enterocutaneous fistula
2. Motility disorders, e.g., pseudoobstruction
3. Cancer related conditions
   a. Radiation enteritis
   b. Graft versus host disease
   c. Mucositis
4. Chronic malabsorptive states, e.g., microvillous inclusion disease
5. Inflammatory bowel disease

the outside of the catheter. The catheters are made of silicone or polyurethane and come with single, double, or triple lumens. The exit site needs to be dressed daily and the catheter flushed daily with heparin to prevent occlusion. Catheters with a subcutaneous implantable access device do not require daily dressing, but need to be flushed daily. Since they require a skin puncture for access, they are not frequently used in children. Although PICC lines have a higher incidence of local complications—including phlebitis and malposition—there is no increase in the rate of infection, dislodgement, or occlusion. This makes them a suitable alternative for long term venous access.[25,26]

Line related complications include infection and mechanical problems. In adults, central venous catheter related line infections are reportedly 5–8 per 1,000 patient days.[27] A study in children reported the mean incidence of infection of 2.1 per 1,000 HPN days, with early infection after initiation of HPN being a worse predictor for repeated line infection. There was no difference in the number of line infections relating to underlying diagnosis, presence of an ostomy, or pathogen isolated.[28] A study from a tertiary pediatric gastroenterology center in the United Kingdom reported a significant reduction in the rate of line infection at home compared with the hospital.[29] A UCLA study group reported an incidence of 1.66 catheter related infections for 1,000 days of inpatient catheter use compared to 1.13 infections per 1,000 days of home use.[30] The Centers for Disease Control defines infection at the exit site or tunnel as a localized infection, and it defines systemic infection as a positive culture from the line and peripheral blood or from the catheter tip.[31] The goal of treatment is to salvage the line and avoid systemic symptoms. Treatment is controversial and includes systemic antibiotics for site and systemic infections and line removal for tunnel infections or persistence of infection after treatment with appropriate antibiotics.[13]

Although there is no specific test to monitor for line infection, a high index of suspicion along with subtle signs (biochemical changes or vague systemic symptoms) is the key to early recognition of line sepsis. Meticulous aseptic technique during all aspects of line use is necessary to prevent infection. There is no difference in the rate of infection with clear film versus gauze dressing at the exit site.[32] Frequent manipulation of the catheter hub and multilumen catheters is associated with a higher incidence of infection.[33]

NUTRIENT SOLUTIONS

The fluid, energy, macro- and micronutrient prescription should be tailored to each child's specific needs. This is dependent on age, nutritional status, underlying medical condition, and whether parenteral support is total or partial. In pediatrics, most solutions are 2-in-1, protein and dextrose are mixed in the bag and the lipid infusion is piggybacked onto the protein and dextrose. A 3-in-1 solution (with dextrose, protein, and lipid mixed together) is associated with a higher incidence of line occlusion.[34] Vitamins and minerals are added to the bag by the pharmacy. The caregiver occasionally must add medications just prior to administration. In countries where HPN solutions are not manufactured, caregivers have successfully compounded the nutrients at home for infusion.[35]

METHOD OF ADMINISTRATION

It could take a few days to reach the desired concentration of dextrose in the solution. Once the goal for nutrient composition has been reached, and tolerance for lipid and glucose are documented on a 24-hour infusion, the infusion is then cycled so that the entire daily volume is administered over 8–16 hours. This allows time off the pump for normal daily activity. Since reactive hypoglycemia can occur with abrupt discontinuation of the infusion, the rate of fluid administered is decreased during the final hour of the infusion. The cycling process takes 5–7 days as the infusion time is decreased in increments of 2–4 hours/day. It is necessary to monitor for hyperglycemia during the infusion, and for hypoglycemia when off the infusion.

DISCHARGE PLANNING

Planning for home care should begin once it is evident that a patient will need nutrition support after discharge. Discharge planning involves the coordinated efforts of physician, nurse, dietitian, case manager, vendor for supplies and home services, and the payer/insurance company. There are 2 broad categories of HNS patient preparation: patient/caregiver training, and arrangement for supplies and services at home.

Patient/Caregiver Training

The first step to discharge planning should be a family meeting to explain the rationale for HNS therapy, goals for therapy, possible length of therapy, role of each team member, plans for obtaining supplies, follow-up after discharge, and the financial responsibilities for the parent. Parents are often unaware of the health insurance coverage benefits and deductibles for HNS. Care managers can take a proactive role in assisting parents to identify additional options for HNS coverage. The caregiver's questions and concerns must be addressed. Parents should be reassured that every effort will be made to meet their lifestyle within what is medically possible.

The instructor should be able to communicate effectively with the caregiver and determine whether the caregiver understands his role in HNS. The willingness and capability of the caregiver to provide HNS should be assessed. The caregiver needs to understand the purpose, function, use, and care of all the equipment, methods for formula mixing, administration of feeds and medications, and line care. The patient and caregiver should be able to demonstrate all aspects of nutrition support with 100% accuracy to the staff, and be given ample opportunity for asking questions. A backup person should also be trained to provide relief for the primary caregiver. Tables 19-6 and 19-7 outline the teaching requirements for HPN and HEN[36] and Tables 19-8 and 19-9 list some of the problems caregivers might encounter in the home.

Many members of the health care team, including the hospital dietitians, floor nurses, home care nurses, and outpatient dietitians provide teaching to the patient/caregiver. A checklist is helpful to be sure all aspects of the education are completed and the caregiver can demonstrate competence. In one study, the dietitian spent an average of 2 hours and 35 minutes on tube feeding education over an average of 3.7 days.[37] In a large pediatric study, the average parent required approximately 10 days of teaching to become independent in all aspects of care for HPN.[38] The technique for teaching includes a combination of live demonstration, verbal instruction, simple written instructions and videotape. Training is intended to enable the caregiver to provide HNS safely and effectively with minimal complications. Caregivers should also be able to recognize complications and manage them. They should have appropriate contact numbers and clear instructions on whom to call in an emergency.

A 12–24 hour trial run with the patient and caregiver assuming full responsibility for HEN or HPN administration in the hospital setting is often beneficial for the caregiver and staff, reassuring the staff that HNS is safe and giving the caregiver confidence. Any unrecognized questions or problems that were not addressed during teaching can be addressed in the hospital setting prior to discharge. Although this is ideal, the current environment of reimbursement favors short hospitalizations, which makes provision of home services extremely critical in the continuum of therapy.

Arrangement for Supplies and Services at Home

Although some hospitals have their own home care teams that provide all the supplies and support needed at home, most institutions require the services of a commercial vendor. Selection of the vendor is the choice of the patient/caregiver. However, from a practical point of view, the HNS team is often in a position to suggest vendors. Having a list of acceptable vendors enables the HNS team to aid in the selection in an unbiased way. The vendor should be capable of providing all needed services, including nurses with pediatric experience, home delivery of all supplies and nutrients, full time availability for problem solving, financial management with direct billing to the carrier, and frequent communication with the physician. Proper vendor selection is crucial to safe home nutrition therapy.

Table 19-6 Teaching requirements for HEN.

A. General principles
   1. Disease process and why HEN is needed
   2. Formula type and feeding schedule
   3. Clean technique, hand washing, cleaning utensils
   4. Preparation and storage of formula
      a. Measuring formula and additives
      b. Mixing formula
B. Specific feeding techniques
   1. Preparation of each feeding
      a. Setting up and filling feeding set
      b. Checking tube placement and gastric residuals
   2. Operation of pump
   3. Administration of feeding
      a. Patient position
      b. Flushing the tube
      c. Care of tube and equipment
      d. Skin care
C. Problem solving, monitoring, and complications
   1. Pump, alarms, feeding set
   2. Gastrointestinal symptoms
   3. Clogged tube
   4. Displaced tube, aspiration, peritonitis
   5. Nutritional status
   6. Blood sugar increase or decrease
   7. Fluid balance, intake and output, weight
   8. Assessment of skin at tube site
   9. When to call nurse, nutritionist, and/or physician

HEN = Home enteral nutrition.

Source: Lifshitz F, Finch N, Lifshitz J. *Children's Nutrition.* Sudbury, Mass: Jones and Bartlett Publishers; 1991. Reprinted with permission.

FOLLOW-UP

Follow-up of patients discharged on HNS is essential to monitor for tolerance, adjust for

Table 19-7 Teaching requirements for HPN.

A. General principles
   1. Disease process
   2. Intravenous nutrition
   3. Aseptic and clean technique
   4. Intravenous catheter
B. Specific feeding techniques
   1. Catheter care
   2. Pump operation
   3. Starting, monitoring, and stopping the infusion
   4. Flushing the catheter
   5. Making additions to nutrition solutions
C. Problem solving, monitoring, and complications
   1. Pump, administration set, filter
   2. Catheter occlusion, kink, position, infection, repair
   3. Hypoglycemia, hyperglycemia, urine testing
   4. Fluid balance, intake and output, weight
   5. Signs and symptoms of infection
   6. When to call nurse and/or physician

HPN = home parenteral nutrition.

Source: Lifshitz F, Finch N, Lifshitz J. *Children's Nutrition.* Sudbury, Mass: Jones and Bartlett Publishers; 1991. Reprinted with permission.

Table 19-8 Problems associated with home enteral nutrition.

Complications	*Possible causes*
Tube related	
Site redness, irritation	Leakage of gastric acid, infection
Occlusion	Inadequate flushing Administration of crushed medications
Displacement/removal	Trauma, coughing, vomiting
Equipment	
Pump alarm	Malfunction Occlusion Low battery
Gastrointestinal	
Vomiting	Tube misplacement High fat intake Rapid infusion rate
Diarrhea	Medications Rapid infusion rate Carbohydrate malabsorption Infection/bacterial contamination Inappropriate formula preparation
Constipation	Low residue formula Dehydration Medication Inactivity
Pulmonary	
Regurgitation/aspiration	Tube misplacement Neurological impairment Improper patient positioning
Developmental	
Food refusal	Lack of oral stimulation Overfeeding Medication
Service related	
Difficulty obtaining formula and equipment	Inadequate discharge planning
Point of contact logistics	Inadequate discharge planning

Table 19-9 Problems associated with home parenteral nutrition.

Complications	*Possible causes*
Catheter related	
Site redness, irritation	Infection
Occlusion, slow return	Inadequate flushing
Displacement/cracking	Trauma
Equipment	
Pump alarm	Malfunction Occlusion Air in system
Metabolic	
Hypoglycemia	Interruption of infusion Too rapid cycling down Sepsis
Hyperglycemia	Medications Rapid infusion rate Sepsis Inappropriate formula preparation
Electrolyte imbalances	Diarrhea
Cholestasis	Excess calories or protein Sepsis
Systemic	
Fever	Sepsis
Dehydration	Hyperglycemia
Developmental	
Food refusal	Lack of oral stimulation Overfeeding Medication

changing nutritional and medical needs, and transition to oral feeding.[39] Appropriate follow up for oromotor therapy is essential to prevent the development of a feeding disorder and to allow for developmentally appropriate feeding skills.[40]

For patients on HEN, the intensity and frequency of follow-up depends on individual needs. Follow-up can be in the form of scheduled telephone calls, communication regarding in-home visits by a home health care nurse, and return office visits. In Australia, dietitians saw 95% of all HEN patients in follow-up an average of 7 times/year, while doctors saw 65% of the HEN patients an average of 15 times/year.[8]

Patients on HPN should be seen a week after discharge and subsequently every 2–4 weeks, depending on their age, the underlying medical illness, and when changes are made in their care. Monitoring includes evaluation of clinical status, anthropometrics, and laboratory data. Electrolytes should be checked at every visit, liver function monthly to quarterly, and trace elements and vitamins every 3–6 months in a stable patient or more frequently if changes are made to the nutrition support solutions. It is beneficial to have a liaison physician in the community who is comfortable assisting in management, so families do not have to return to the tertiary center for minor issues. Even though children may ultimately be weaned off PN, it is essential to have long term, broad-based nutritional assessment as they are at risk for abnormalities in growth and nutritional status due to their underlying medical problems.[41]

CONCLUSION

While there is an increasing trend to treat children with HNS in a way that meets the needs of patients, caregivers, hospitals, and third party payers, much needs to be done to ensure that the standard of care remains consistent in the community. Significant resources, support, and funding are required to transition a technology dependent child into nonhome-based educational and child care settings. There are several legislative initiatives under way that will serve to monitor states' compliance with provision of skilled care and ensure access to appropriate public education. The provision of nutrition support in the community requires continuous improvement so there is a consistent, seamless, and satisfactory transition from the hospital to the home.[39,42]

REFERENCES

1. Kang A, Zamora S, Scott R, Parsons H. Catch-up growth in children treated with home enteral nutrition; part 1 of 2. *Pediatrics*. October 1998;102(4):951–955.
2. Papadopoulou A, Holden C, Paul L, et al. The nutritional response to home enteral nutrition in childhood. *Acta Paediatr.* 1995;84:528–531.
3. Forchielli ML, Paolucci G, Lo CW. Total parenteral nutrition and home parenteral nutrition: an effective combination to sustain malnourished children with cancer. *Nutr Rev.* 1999;57(1):15–20.
4. Howard L, Ament M, Fleming CR, Shike M, Steiger E. Current use and clinical outcome of home parenteral and enteral nutrition therapies in the United States. *Gastroenterology.* 1995;109(2):355–365.
5. British Association of Parenteral and Enteral Nutrition. *Report of the British Artificial Nutrition Survey (BANS) August 1999.* Maidenhead, England: British Association Parenteral and Enteral Nutrition; 1999.
6. Parker T, Neal G, Cotte S, Elia M. Management of artificial nutrition in East Anglia: a community study. *J Royal Coll Physicians, London*. 1996;30(1):27–32.
7. McCarey D, Buchannan E, Gregory M, Clark B, Weaver LT. Home enteral feeding in the West of Scotland. *Scottish Med J.* 1996;41:147–149.
8. Department of Human Services, Acute Health Division. Report of The Ministerial Working Party on Home Enteral Nutrition. Available at: http://www.dhs.vic.gov.au/ahs/archive/hen/index.html. Accessed February, 2006.
9. Holden C, Puntis J, Charlton C, Booth I. Nasogastric feeding at home: acceptability and safety. *Arch Dis Child*. 1991;66:148–151.
10. Puntis J. The economics of home parenteral nutrition. *Nutrition*. 1998;14(10):809–812.
11. Richards D, Irving M. Cost-utility analysis of home parenteral nutrition. *Br J Surg*. 1996;83(9):1226–1229.
12. JCAHO Board of Directors. *Comprehensive Accreditation Manual for Hospitals*. Oakbrook, Ill: JCAHO; 1996.
13. ASPEN Board of Directors and the Clinical Guidelines Task Force. Guidelines for the use of parenteral and enteral nutrition in adult and pediatric patients. *JPEN*. Jan–Feb 2002;26(1):S1SA–138SA
14. Plioplys A, Kasnicka I, Shelley L, et al. Survival rates among children with severe neurological disabilities. *South Med J*. 1998;91(2):161–173.
15. Boyle J. Nutritional management of the developmentally disabled child. *Pediatr Surg Int*. 1991;6:76–81.
16. Puntis J, Thwaites R, Abel G, et al. Children with neurological disorders do not always need fundoplication concomitant with PEG. *Dev Med Child Neurol.* 2000;42:97–99.
17. Wheatley M, Wesley J, Tkach D, et al. Long term follow-up of brain damaged children requiring feeding gastrostomy: should an anti-reflux procedure always be performed? *J Pediatr Surg*. 1991;26:301–305.
18. Sulaeman E, Udall J, Brown R, et al. Gastroesophageal reflux and Nissen fundoplication following percutaneous endoscopic gastrostomy in children. *J Pediatr Gastroenterol Nutr*. 1998;26:269–273.
19. Schwarz S, Corredor J, Fisher-Medina J, et al. Diagnosis and treatment of feeding disorders in children with developmental disabilities. *Pediatrics*. 2001;108:671–676.
20. Craig G, Scambler G, Spitz L. Why parents of children with neurodevelopmental disabilities requiring gastrostomy feeding need more support. *Dev Med and Child Neurol*. 2003;45:183–188.
21. Shang E, Geiger N, Sturm J, et al. Pump-assisted versus gravity controlled enteral nutrition in long-term percu-

taneous endoscopic gastrostomy patients: a prospective controlled trial. *JPEN.* 2003;27(3):216–219.

22. Jones S, Günter P. Automatic flush feeding pumps: a move forward in enteral nutrition. *Nursing.* 1997;27:56–58.
23. Kleinman R, ed. Appendix O. *Pediatric Nutrition Handbook.* 5th ed. American Academy of Pediatrics;Elk Grove Village, Ill; 2003–2004:1032–1057.
24. Chung DH, Ziegler MM. Central venous catheter access. *Nutrition.* 1998;14:119–123.
25. Duerksen DR, Papineau N, Siemens J, et al. Peripherally inserted catheters for parenteral nutrition: a comparison with centrally inserted catheters. *JPEN.* 1999;223:85–89.
26. Smith JR, Friedell ML, Cheatham ML, et al. Peripherally inserted central catheters revisited. *Am J Surg.* 1998;176:208–211.
27. Gosbell IB, Duggan D, Breust M, Mulholland K, Gottlieb T, Bradbury R. Infection associated with central venous catheters: a prospective survey. *Med J Aust.* 1995;162(4):210–213.
28. Colomb V, Fabiero M, Dabbas M, Goulet O, Merckx J, Ricour C. Central venous catheter-related infections in children on long-term home parenteral nutrition: incidence and risk factors. *Clin Nutr.* 2000;19(5):355–359.
29. Melville CA, Bisset WM, Long S, Milla PJ. Counting the cost: hospital versus home central venous catheter survival. *J Hosp Infect.* 1997;35(3):197–205.
30. Moukarzel AA, Haddad I, Ament ME, et al. 230 patient years of experience with home long-term parenteral nutrition in childhood: natural history and life of central venous catheters. *J Pediatr Surg.* 1994;29:1323.
31. Hospital Infection Control Advisory Committee, Centers for Disease Control and Prevention: Guidelines for prevention of intravascular device related infections. *Infect Control Hosp Epidemiol.* 1996;17:438–473.
32. Mermel LA. Prevention of intravascular catheter-related infections. *Ann Intern Med.* 2000;132:391–402.
33. McCarthy MC, Shives JK, Robison RJ, Broadie TA. Prospective evaluation of single and triple lumen catheters in total parenteral nutrition. *JPEN.* 1987;11:259.
34. Erdman SH, McLee CL, Kramer JM, Zupan CW, White JJ, Grill BB. Central line occlusion with 3-in-1 nutrition admixture administration at home. *JPEN.* 1994;18:177.
35. Ksiazyk J, Lyszkowska M, Kierkus J, Bogucki K, Ratynska A, Tondys B, Socha J. Home parenteral nutrition in children: the Polish experience. *J Pediatr Gastroenterol Nutr.* 1999;28(2):152–156.
36. Lifshitz F, Finch N, Lifshitz J. *Children's Nutrition.* Sudbury, Mass: Jones and Bartlett Publishers;1991.
37. McNamara EP, Flood P, Kennedy NP. Home tube feeding: an integrated multidisciplinary approach. *J Hum Nutr Dietet.* 2001;14(1):13–19.
38. Moukarzel AA, Ament ME. Home parenteral nutrition in infants and children. In: Rombeau J, Rolandelli R, eds. *Clinical Nutrition: Parenteral Nutrition.* Philadelphia, Pa: WB Saunders; 1993:791–813.
39. Puntis J. Nutritional support at home and in the community. *Arch Dis Child.* 2001;84:295–298.
40. Tuchman DN. Oropharyngeal and esophageal complications of enteral tube feeding. In: Baker SB, Baker RD, Davis A, eds. *Pediatric Enteral Nutrition.* New York, N.Y.: Chapman and Hall; 1994:179–191.
41. Leonberg B, Chuang E, Eicher P, Tershakovec A, Leonard L, Stallings V. Long-term growth and development in children after home parenteral nutrition. *J Pediatr.* 1998;132(3):461–466.
42. Howard P, Bowen N. The challenges of innovation in the organization of home enteral nutrition. *J Hum Nutr Diet.* 2001;14(1):3–11.

CHAPTER 20

Enteral Nutrition Tube Feedings

Valérie Marchand

INTRODUCTION

Adequacy of growth is perhaps the most valuable indicator of nutritional status in children. Deviation from the expected growth rate requires prompt evaluation and intervention since the timing, duration, and severity of the nutritional insult may influence the potential for catch-up growth. It is important that all children be provided with sufficient calories and nutrients to ensure adequate growth. Growing children may require up to 3 times more energy and protein per unit of body weight than adults. Appetite and self-regulation usually result in sufficient intake. However, while most normal children have the ability to ingest enough nutrients to meet their needs, children with chronic medical conditions or prolonged illnesses might not be able to achieve that goal and could develop chronic or acute malnutrition. Such patients are candidates for nutrition support.

Nutrition support can be either enteral or parenteral. Enteral nutrition (EN) is considered safer, more physiologic, and less expensive than parenteral nutrition (PN). A recent meta-analysis showed that EN was cheaper than PN but did not find that EN led to better outcomes, improved intestinal function, or decreased bacterial translocation.[1] See also Chapter 16. A second meta-analysis showed fewer infections with EN compared with PN.[2] EN can be easily administered at home and should be the preferred mode of nutrition for patients with a functional or even partly functional gastrointestinal tract.

This chapter discusses the indications and contraindications for EN, how to select the appropriate means of enteral access, as well as methods of initiating and administrating EN.

INDICATIONS

Children who will not or cannot safely ingest enough nutrients to sustain their needs but who have a functional gastrointestinal tract are candidates for EN. Some children require EN for management of their primary disease. Table 20-1 summarizes indications for EN. Figure 20-1 illustrates the decision process for initiation of tube feedings.

CONTRAINDICATIONS

EN is contraindicated in conditions where the gastrointestinal tract is anatomically or functionally impaired, as indicated in Table 20-2. Despite popular belief that the gut cannot be used in the postoperative period, EN can be started early after surgery. Small bowel motility returns within 6–8 hours, stomach motility return follows after 24–48 hours, and the colon regains normal motility after 48–72 hours. If the stomach can be decompressed while feeding the patient directly into the small bowel, EN can be started almost immediately after surgery.

CHOICE OF ENTERAL ACCESS

The difficulty of choosing the best enteral access for a patient should not be underestimated. Previously, only nasogastric tubes and surgical gastrostomy or jejunostomy were available, but since newer and less invasive endoscopic and radiological techniques have emerged, the medical team has more from which to choose.

Table 20-1 Indications for enteral nutrition.

1. Insufficient oral intake
   - Anorexia
     - Anorexia nervosa
     - Anorexia secondary to chronic medical condition
     - Anorexia secondary to medication (chemotherapy)
     - Food aversion
   - Malabsorption
     - Cystic fibrosis
     - Short bowel syndrome
     - Pancreatic insufficiency
     - Cholestatic liver disease
   - Increased needs
     - Bronchopulmonary dysplasia
     - Congenital heart disease
     - Recovering from malnutrition
     - Infections
2. As a primary therapy
   - Metabolic diseases
   - Intolerance to fasting
   - Unpalatable or monotonous diet
   - Inflammatory bowel disease
3. Oral motor dysfunction
   - Prematurity
   - Neuromuscular disorder
   - Neurological impairment (cerebral palsy)
4. Structural or functional abnormality of the gastrointestinal tract
   - Congenital malformation
   - Oesophageal stenosis (tumor, caustic stenosis, iatrogenic stenosis)
   - Intestinal pseudoobstruction
5. Injury/critical illness
   - Burn
   - Trauma
   - Surgery

Once the indication for EN is clear, the patient should be evaluated carefully by a multidisciplinary team that includes a gastroenterologist, a nurse, a speech therapist, an occupational therapist, a surgeon, and a radiologist, to ensure the patient has the best enteral access possible. Special attention should be paid to neurologically impaired patients who require long term enteral access, because they are often challenging and usually require more extensive evaluation.

The choice of the enteral access route will be determined by several factors shown in Table 20-3. Chronically ill children with various diseases (cerebral palsy, cystic fibrosis, congenital heart disease, bronchopulmonary dysplasia, etc.) often require long term EN. These children often have gastroesophageal reflux and/or chronic respiratory symptoms. The potential risk of aspiration should be carefully evaluated before choosing the type of enteral access.

One who takes a careful history will look for signs of aspiration such as chronic respiratory symptoms or recurrent pneumonia. Aspiration may be secondary to gastroesophageal reflux or

Table 20-2 Conditions that contraindicate enteral feeds.

- Gastrointestinal obstruction
- Prolonged ileus
- Enterocolitis
- Digestive fistula
- Severe pancreatitis
- Intestinal ischemia
- Severe flare of inflammatory bowel disease

Table 20-3 Choice of optimal enteral access.

1. Indication for tube feeds
2. Duration of tube feeds
3. Anatomical integrity of the gastrointestinal tract
4. Functional integrity of the gastrointestinal tract
5. Risk of aspiration

dysfunctional swallowing. Choking or coughing during meals is suggestive of aspiration due to dysfunctional swallowing. It may be useful to observe the patient during a meal and perform a swallowing study under fluoroscopy using food with different textures to document swallowing dysfunction and aspiration.

Respiratory symptoms may also result from aspiration of gastric contents in patients with gastroesophageal reflux. An upper gastrointestinal series will exclude an anatomical cause for reflux such as superior mesenteric artery syndrome. Scintigraphy should be performed to evaluate gastric emptying, to detect preexisting gastroparesis, and, to some extent, reflux and pulmonary aspiration of gastric contents. Finally, 24-hour esophageal pH monitoring is the best available test to detect and quantify gastroesophageal reflux. An upper gastrointestinal endoscopy might also be performed in specific cases. Despite careful evaluation, it could still be difficult to choose the best enteral access for a particular patient. With difficult patients, the least invasive approach should be used. If unsuccessful, more invasive options can be explored. Figure 20-2 summarizes the decision process for choosing optimal enteral access.

The different available types of enteral accesses are oro-gastric, naso-gastric or naso-enteric, gastrostomy, gastrojejunostomy or jejunostomy.

GASTRIC FEEDS

Whenever possible, gastric feedings should be chosen over intestinal feedings. Gastric feeds

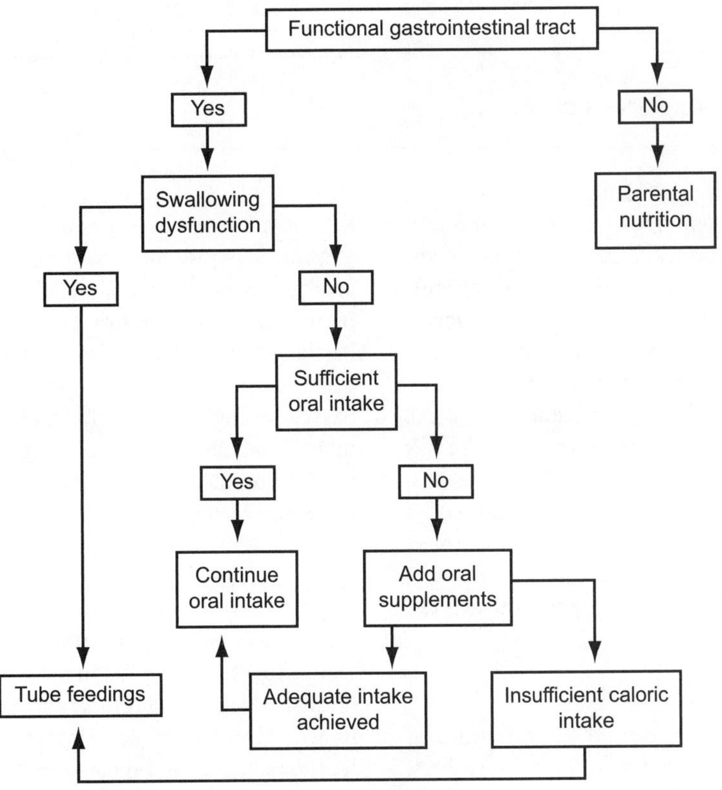

Figure 20-1 Decision tree for tube-feeding support.

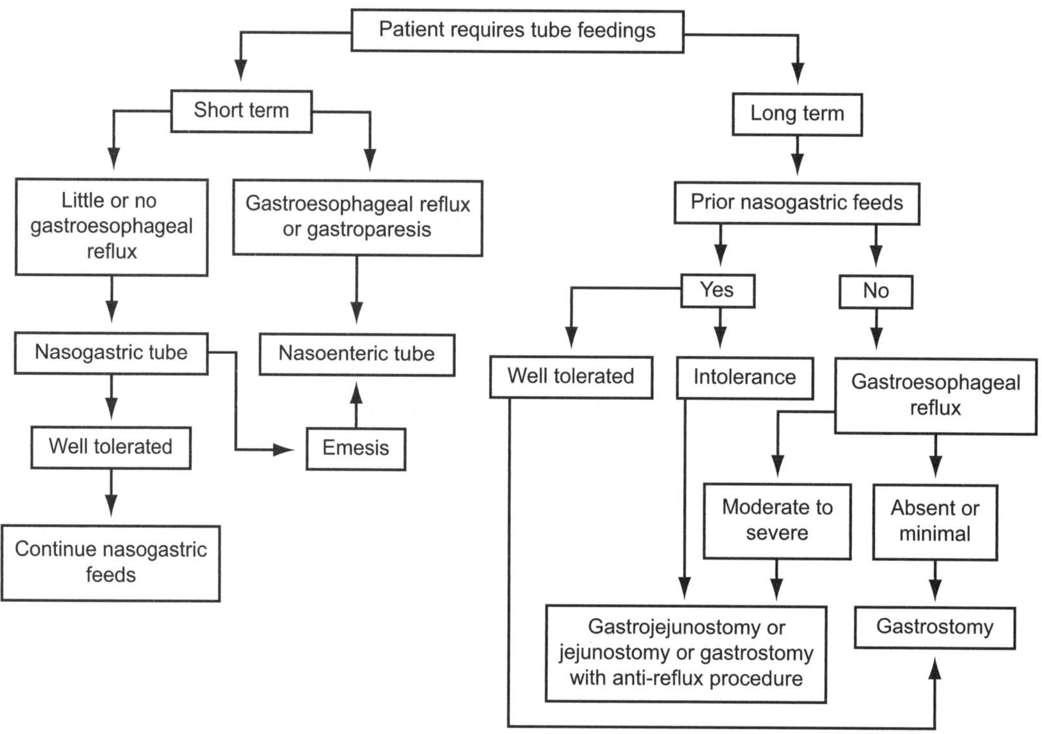

Figure 20-2 Decision tree for enteral access.

allow a more normal digestive process and hormonal response to meals than intestinal feeds. The stomach serves as a reservoir and permits a higher infusion rate and the use of bolus feeds. This allows for a more flexible feeding schedule, which is particularly important in ambulatory patients. Solutions with a higher osmotic load can also be infused in the stomach with less of a risk of dumping. However, patients with severe gastroesophageal reflux, aspiration, gastroparesis, or persistent emesis, and patients who cannot protect their airways should be fed into the stomach with caution, and another route might be advised.

Oro-gastric Feeds

Oro-gastric feeds are used in premature or small infants who are obligatory nose breathers, to avoid obstructing the nostrils. These feedings are usually well tolerated in premature infants less than 34 weeks of gestational age when no gag reflex is present. Oro-gastric feeds are also useful in patients with choanal atresia. They are preferred over nasogastric feeds in children with basilar skull fractures who cannot be fed orally, because a nasogastric tube could be inadvertently passed through the cribriform plate into the cranium. Long term nocturnal orogastric tube feeds with 8 French (Fr) silastic tube have been successful in teenage cystic fibrosis patients.[3]

Naso-gastric Feeds

The naso-gastric (NG) route is the method of choice for short term EN in patients with little or no gastroesophageal reflux, normal gastric function, and low risk of aspiration. It is the simplest, least expensive, and most widely used mode of EN. No invasive procedure is required. The tube is easy to insert and allows aspiration of air or gastric contents if needed. On the other hand, it is easily dislodged, uncomfortable, and aesthetically displeasing. Besides skin and mucosal irritation, local complications include sinusitis, nasal obstruction, and otitis media. Care should be taken in patients with thrombocytopenia, as inserting the tube could cause epistaxis. NG feeds are generally used for short term nutrition support, although some patients use NG tubes at home on a long term basis, inserting the tube every evening for night feeds and removing it in the morning.

Taking into account the patient's size and the volume and viscosity of the formula, the tube should be the smallest diameter possible. The length of the tube to be inserted is estimated by measuring the distance between the tip of the patient's nose to the earlobe and from the earlobe to the xiphoid process. Proper position in the stomach should be checked by aspirating gastric contents or confirmed radiologically.

Gastrostomy

For long term EN (> 3 months), a gastrostomy is preferred. A gastrostomy will not obstruct the airway, and when converted to a low profile device, is more aesthetic and carries a lesser risk of dislodgement than an NG tube. However, it is more invasive. There is a risk of local complications (granulation, local infection, skin irritation) and more serious complications such as peritonitis, intra-abdominal abscesses, colonic perforation, and bleeding. There is also a potential risk of inducing or of exacerbating gastroesophageal reflux. A gastrostomy can be placed surgically or percutaneously (endoscopically or under fluoroscopy).

Twenty-five years ago, surgical gastrostomy was the only option. Often, a fundoplication was performed along with the gastrostomy. The literature comparing surgical gastrostomy alone with surgical gastrostomy with antireflux procedure in neurologically impaired children shows that between 11.5 and 50% of patients with no clinical reflux before the gastrostomy ultimately require an antireflux procedure.[4–7] However, a fundoplication is not without complications, especially in neurologically impaired patients for whom the incidence of major complications after fundoplication varies between 10 and 29% and for whom the recurrence of gastroesophageal reflux occurs in 10–28% of cases. A redo of the fundoplication is often necessary (3.8–19% of cases).[4,5,8–15] In neurologically impaired patients, Nissen fundoplication can induce inappropriate activation of the emetic reflex, resulting in retching, which can be particularly disturbing.[14]

If a surgical gastrostomy is to be performed, the literature does not support the need for a prophylactic antireflux procedure in patients with no clinical reflux. In addition, surgical gastrostomy should now be reserved for patients with anatomic abnormalities such as esophageal stenosis, previous extensive abdominal surgeries, or severe gastroesophageal reflux requiring fundoplication and/or pyloroplasty. Otherwise a percutaneous gastrostomy, which carries a lesser risk of morbidity and mortality, should be performed.

Percutaneous endoscopic gastrostomy (PEG) has been performed since 1980.[15] This technique is less invasive than surgical gastrostomy. It may be performed under conscious sedation, involves less discomfort in the post-operative period, and can be used for feedings within a few hours. Four hours after the procedure, if medical evaluation is reassuring, tube feeds can be initiated with formula.[16] Prior abdominal surgery is not a contraindication for PEG. However, a PEG should not be performed in patients with ascites or massive splenomegaly, or hepatomegaly. PEG procedure can sometimes be performed in patients with portal hypertension when the benefits outweigh the risks.

Minor complications with PEG placement in the pediatric population have been reported in 3.6–22.5% of cases and major complications in 2–17.5%.[16–18] Post-PEG gastroesophageal reflux occurs in 25–60% of neurologically impaired children without prior symptoms, and various series report the need for fundoplication after PEG in 5–16.6% of cases, mostly in neurologically impaired patients.[16,19–21] However, these studies are inconsistent in terms of pre-PEG evaluation and patient selection since some relied solely on clinical symptoms of gastroesophageal reflux, and others included further investigation. One study involving primarily neurologically impaired patients undergoing PEG placement showed that 29% of those with an abnormal pH probe study before the procedure versus 5% of those with a normal pH probe study eventually required a fundoplication.[16] In neurologically impaired patients without prior clinical reflux, there was a lower incidence of symptomatic gastroesophageal reflux requiring fundoplication after PEG as compared to surgical gastrostomy (10% versus 39%).[22]

After the tract has healed (2–3 months), a gastrostomy can be converted to a low profile device. The gastrostomy also allows the option of being converted to a gastrojejunostomy if needed.

Jejunal Feeds

Jejunal feeds are useful in patients with gastroesophageal reflux and/or gastroparesis and in patients at high risk for aspiration. Patients with frequent emesis, particularly those receiving chemotherapy, are also good candidates for jejunal feeds.

Jejunal feeds have the advantage of bypassing a dysmotile stomach, but in doing so, they also bypass the gastric part of the digestive process and the bactericidal activity of the stomach. Jejunal feeds need to be administered by continuous drip, which is not convenient for ambulatory patients. Hyperosmolar formulas might not be well tolerated. Malabsorption has been described in healthy low birth weight infants given jejunal feeds.[23] Jejunal tubes can migrate back into the stomach in some patients and X-rays are needed when the tube is replaced to verify position. Finally, jejunal tubes are usually long and have a small diameter, increasing the risk of clogging.

Naso-jejunal Feeds

Naso-jejunal (NJ) feeds are used primarily for short term nutritional support in patients requiring temporary bypass of their stomach. They may also be used as a long term method of feedings for mechanically ventilated patients or patients with medical problems that make them poor candidates for anesthesia or surgical procedures.

NJ tubes are difficult to position properly and are easily dislodged. Radiological confirmation of the tube's position is necessary before initiating feeds. There are different methods for placement of an NJ tube. They can be inserted in the stomach and allowed to progress into the small bowel with gastric peristalsis. Using a weighted versus nonweighted tube does not seem to increase the rate of spontaneous passage into the duodenum. Erythromycin could help migration of the tube into the small bowel.[24–27] However, one study showed that erythromycin failed to facilitate transpyloric passage of feeding tubes in critically ill pediatric patients.[28–30] A Cochrane review concluded that metaclopramide administered intramuscularly or intravenously was ineffective in facilitating transpyloric intubation.[31] Using pH-assisted tube placement showed promising results. An additional benefit gained when using these tubes is that the pH will drop if the tube migrates back in the stomach.[32,33] Rapid placement of transpyloric feeding tubes using a pH probe was successful in 97% of patients in less than 6 minutes.[32,33] A pH > 5.6 was predictive of adequate position 97% of the time. This allowed earlier institution of feeds and less use of X-rays.[32] After 2 unsuccessful attempts of nonfluoroscopic placement, fluoroscopic placement should be considered.[34] Placement of the tube under fluoroscopy is very effective but radiation exposure for the patient is not negligible.[35,36] Another option is endoscopic placement of the tube. This can be done by inserting the gastroscope into the small bowel and pushing a guide wire in the biopsy channel, then slowly removing the scope while pushing the guide wire. The feeding tube is then fed on the guide wire to the small bowel. Another endoscopic placement technique is to attach a suture to the end of the feeding tube and to endoscopically drag it into the small bowel with a biopsy forceps. However, there is a risk that the feeding tube will migrate back into the stomach while pulling back the endoscope. The endoscopic technique may be combined with fluoroscopy to position the tube further in the jejunum.

Gastrojejunal Feeds

Gastrojejunal feeds can be used for long term EN in patients with severe gastroesophageal reflux who are poor candidates for an antireflux procedure. They can also be used short term in patients who have a gastrostomy and who temporarily do not tolerate gastric feeds. Some tubes allow simultaneous jejunal feeds and drainage of the stomach. Gastrojejunostomy can be installed under fluoroscopy or endoscopically. Like NJ tubes, they can be difficult to position properly and might migrate back into the stomach. Unlike gastrostomies, which can be converted to a low profile device, gastrojejunal tubes are difficult to convert to a low profile device, since most commercially available tubes are too long for pediatric patients.

A comparison between radiologic gastrojejunostomy and surgical gastrostomy with antireflux procedure in neurologically impaired children with gastroesophageal reflux showed no difference in infections, aspiration pneumonia, esophagitis, and hospital admissions for gastroesophageal reflux between the 2 groups. Thirty-six percent of patients in the surgical group experienced retching, 12.7% had dysphagia, 14.3% had wrap failure, and 11.1% required a revision of the fundoplication. In the radiologic group, 85% of patients had technical problems (broken tube, dislodgement, and/or clogging), and they needed an average of 1.68 manipulations per year. Only 8.3% eventually required a fundoplication, and 14.5% improved enough to have the gastrojejunal tube removed. One patient died from aspiration in the radiologic group and 5 patients died in the surgical group (3 due to aspiration 1 due to small bowel obstruction, 1 due to postgastrostomy change).[37]

Surgical Jejunostomy

Surgical jejunostomy may be used in patients requiring jejunal feeds for at least 6 months. This method should be used as a last resort, since it is technically more difficult and carries a higher risk of complications (volvulus, leak, intussusception). Percutaneous endoscopic jejunostomy could be an option, although the pediatric literature on this technique is scarce.

CHOICE OF TUBE

Feeding tubes come in a variety of sizes and lengths. Diameters vary between 5 and 12 Fr. Some have a weighted tip, and some have a stylet to facilitate insertion. Large bore tubes (> 14 Fr) are used mostly for decompression. Small bore tubes are used for feedings; they are more comfortable for the patient but are more difficult to insert (often requiring a stylet). They are also more prone to clogging and do not allow aspiration of gastric contents. Previously, polyethylene or PVC tubes were used, but because they stiffened, they had to be replaced every 3–4 days to prevent intestinal perforation. Tubes are now made of Silastic or polyurethane, and they are soft and pliable. They can be kept in place longer because they are nonreactive and will not stiffen. For the same external diameter, polyurethane tubes have a larger internal diameter than Silastic tubes, and therefore they could have a lower risk of occlusion.

The use of a small bore tube combined with a viscous formula or medication and inadequate flushing promotes tube clogging. The tube should be irrigated before and after each feed or medication administration. Prophylactic use of pancreatic enzymes every 4 hours to prevent clogging has led to fewer occlusions and longer intervals before occlusion[38] and may be considered in specific cases. Before changing an obstructed tube, pancreatic enzymes should be used. Viokase (1 tablet) mixed with sodium bicarbonate (324 mg) and 5 cc of lukewarm water was successful in 72% of cases, and it was 96% successful if formula was the cause of the obstruction.[39,40]

PEGs are made of silicone or polyurethane. They also come in different sizes and shapes. Most commonly used PEGs have a diameter between 16 and 20 Fr, but smaller (12 Fr) and larger PEGs are available. There are different shapes of internal bumpers; most allow external nonendoscopic removal (traction). However, positive identification (either endoscopic or radiologic) of intragastric position of the replacement gastrostomy tube is advisable when removing a PEG. This will avoid accidental intraperitoneal placement and subsequent peritonitis. Certain types of PEGs are compatible with a jejunal tube. Radiologically inserted tubes are usually 8 to 12 Fr. They do not have an internal bumper, but after insertion, the tip of the catheter curls up, preventing it from being pulled out.

CHOICE OF PUMP

For pediatric use, the feeding pump should be light and compact. Portable pumps are available. The pump should allow accurate administration of small volumes (5cc/h), and it should allow the infusion rate tube to be changed in small increments (0.5–1cc/h). It should be tamper proof.

CHOICE OF FORMULA

The choice of formula depends on the patient's age, needs, and underlying condition as well as the type of enteral access (gastric versus jejunal). Infant formula should be used for children less than 1 year old. Cow milk based, soy based, casein hydrolysate, and elemental formulas are available. They can be concentrated, and if needed, modular nutrients can be added to increase the caloric density. After the child reaches the age of 1 year, a pediatric formula can be used. Polymeric, semielemental, elemental, fiber containing, high caloric and disease-specific formulas are available. When modifications are made to the formula (concentration, addition of modular nutrients), a dietician should be involved to ensure that the proportion of calories from proteins, carbohydrates, and lipids is adequate and to determine that osmolality is not too high. The renal solute load should be verified. Fluid needs should be assessed as carefully as caloric needs, and the patient should receive an adequate amount of free water. Overhydration can occur when refeeding patients with severe malnutrition. Dehydration can occur when losses (emesis, diarrhea) are underestimated or when hyperosmolar formula is used. Excessive calories combined with insufficient fluid intake will result in increase blood urea nitrogen or the so-called tube feeding syndrome, where too little free water is available to allow excretion of the solution's solute load.[41]

METHOD OF NUTRIENT DELIVERY

Feeds can be administered as a continuous or intermittent drip, boluses, or a combination of continuous drip and boluses. The preferred method will depend on the many factors listed in Table 20-4.

Bolus Feeds

Bolus feeds are the most physiologic way to administer tube feeds, as they mimic meals. They can be given by gravity or over a certain period of time with a pump. They are convenient in ambulatory patients, since they allow a more flexible schedule. They should be reserved for patients who are fed in the stomach, as the jejunum generally does not tolerate large volumes. Bolus feeds might not be the best option for patients with gastroesophageal reflux or gastroparesis or in patients requiring a large volume of feeds. Dumping syndrome or emesis could limit the use of bolus feeds.

Continuous Feeds

Continuous feeds require an infusion pump. They are mandatory in patients with jejunal enteral access but are also widely used in patients with a gastrostomy or an NG tube. They are particularly useful in malnourished patients who

Table 20-4 Factors to consider when deciding upon feeding schedule.

- Location of the tube (gastric or jejunal)
- Type of patient (ambulatory or not)
- Feeding schedule (nocturnal or not)
- Tolerance to feeds
- Specific underlying disease (intolerance to fasting)
- Specific problems
  - Emesis
  - Gastroparesis
  - Dumping syndrome

temporarily require a considerable amount of calories for catch-up growth and who do not tolerate large boluses. Nocturnal continuous feeds are often used as a supplement in ambulatory patients who require additional calories to complement their regular diet. Critically ill patients in the intensive care unit are also good candidates for continuous feeds. Patients with malabsorption or intestinal disease with decreased absorptive surface such as short bowel syndrome often benefit from a continuous infusion. Energy requirements seem to be lower during continuous feeds as compared to intermittent feeds, suggesting better absorption.[42]

When using continuous feeds, one should keep in mind that nonemulsified fat (breast milk, meat based formula and some modular nutrients such as medium chain triglycerides oil) can precipitate in the tube, resulting in a significant energy loss for the patient. On the other hand, a large lipid bolus might be inadvertently administered to the patient when flushing the tube at the end of the feedings, leading to abdominal discomfort.

Combination Feeds

A combination of nocturnal continuous feeds and daytime boluses is ideal for patients who require a considerable amount of calories. This regimen can be used in ambulatory patients who do not tolerate large volumes.

INITIATION OF TUBE FEEDS

Usually, EN is initiated in the hospital or in a day hospital. This allows close monitoring of the patient's tolerance and clinical response. A 3- to 5-day hospitalization may be necessary. The family can then meet the dietician, the physician, the home EN nurse, and the rest of the nutrition support team if needed. The patient and/or the parents are taught to care for the enteral access device, to handle the formula, and to use the feeding pump if needed. The family should also be taught to detect and handle problems correctly (Chapter 19).

Bolus feeds are initiated with an isotonic solution in most cases. There is no need to dilute the formula. A small volume of full strength isotonic formula is usually tolerated. Twenty-five percent of the patient's caloric needs are given the first day. The total volume can be divided into 6 to 8 boluses. According to the patient's tolerance, volume is increased by 25% each day so the caloric goal is obtained in about 4 days. Another way to initiate bolus feeds is to give 5 to 8 boluses of 2.5–5 cc/kg and to increase by 2.5–5 cc/kg/bolus until nutritional requirements are met. With both methods, once caloric needs are met, the number of boluses can be decreased to 3–5 per day while increasing the volume of each bolus according to the patient's desired schedule and tolerance.

For continuous feeds, an isotonic solution at full strength is also used. The initial drip should be 1–2 cc/kg/h, and this can be increased by 0.5–1 cc/kg/h every 8 to 24 hours, according to the patient's tolerance. Initially, gastric residual volumes can be checked. If they exceed twice the hourly rate, the rate should be reduced. Once the caloric goal has been reached, the rate can be slowly increased to shorten the duration of feeds while maintaining the same caloric intake.

GASTROESOPHAGEAL REFLUX IN TUBE-FED PATIENTS

Emesis is a problem frequently encountered in tube fed patients and could result in frank aspiration or chronic respiratory problems. Ideally, the patient's head should be elevated 30° when fed to prevent emesis and aspiration.

Gastroesophageal reflux can occur after initiating NG feeds or after a gastrostomy. However, the NG tube or the gastrostomy might not be the only factors causing reflux. Worsening of the underlying disease or an intercurrent infection can cause reflux. When tube feedings are initiated, the patient's diet undergoes major changes. The patient will often go from an oral diet consisting of thickened fluids and pureed food or solids to an enteral liquid diet, and the volume of formula administered through the tube could exceed what the patient was previously ingesting, thus promoting reflux.

In the event of increased or new onset reflux after initiation of EN, a conservative approach is usually adequate. A good clinical evaluation and the appropriate paraclinical investigation (UGI and/or pH probe and/or radionuclide scan) are important. Often a change in the feeding schedule, such as changing from bolus to continuous feeds or giving the total amount of formula over a longer period of time will help. If symptoms persist, concentrating the formula to reduce the volume of feeds should be attempted. If this approach fails, medical treatment should be attempted. Moderate reflux might respond to treatment with H2 blockers or proton pump inhibitors. Prokinetic agents may be added if necessary. If medical treatment fails, an attempt to use a naso-jejunal tube or to convert the gastrostomy into a gastrojejunostomy can be made. An antireflux procedure should be reserved for those who fail this conservative approach or for those who improve when fed jejunally but for whom a jejunal tube cannot be used long term due to frequent dislodgement or clogging.

SOCIAL CONSIDERATIONS

The decision to initiate EN may be a difficult one for the medical team, but it is often an even more difficult decision for the patient and his/her family. Parents might see the need for tube feeds as a failure on their part to adequately feed their child and might feel threatened by the idea of tube feedings. Once initiated, tube feedings are often stressful for the family and can interfere with sleep, work, and familial activities. An NG tube can lead to undesired attention from strangers in public places. In one study, parents reported an improvement in weight gain, ease and time to feed the child, and a decrease in stress associated with meals, but they reported it was more difficult to get respite care and mobility was restricted.[43] Other parents reported mostly sleeping problems but considered that the benefits outweighed the disadvantages.[44] It is therefore important to adequately prepare the child and the family for the realities of tube feeds and to provide them with adequate support.

Whenever possible, oral intake should be preserved; if not possible, oral stimulation during tube feeds should be promoted to avoid food aversion. Early referral to occupational or speech therapy is suggested in tube fed patients.

Tube feedings should have excellent results in well selected patients and with good medical supervision. When a patient fails to gain weight despite adequate caloric intake, a careful reassessment of caloric needs and intake should be performed. Increased losses from emesis and diarrhea should be excluded and compliance should be assessed. Further investigation might be necessary to look for underlying pathology.

CONCLUSION

Adequate nutrition is extremely important for the growing child. A child who will not or cannot safely ingest enough nutrients to meet his or her needs should receive adequate nutritional support. Children who require tube feedings should be carefully evaluated to ensure that they have the best enteral access to administer nutrients in a safe and efficient manner.

REFERENCES

1. Lipman TO. Grains or veins: is enteral nutrition really better than parenteral nutrition? A look at the evidence. *JPEN*. 1998;22:167–182.

2. Braunschwieg CL, Levy P, Sheean PM, Wang X. Enteral compared with parenteral nutrition: a meta-analysis. *Am J Clin Nutr*. 2001;74:534–542.
3. Asfaw M, Miles A, Caplan DB. Orogastric enteral feedings: an alternative feeding access. *Nutr Clin Pract*. 2000;15:91–93.
4. Mollitt DL, Golladay ES, Seibert JJ. Symptomatic gastroesophageal reflux following gastrostomy in neurologically impaired patients. *Pediatrics*. 1985;75:1124–1126.
5. Wheatley MJ, Wesley JR, Tkach DM, Coran AG. Long-term follow-up of brain-damaged children requiring feeding gastrostomy: should an antireflux procedure always be performed? *J Pediatr Surg*. 1991;26:301–304.
6. Langer JC, Wesson DE, Ein SH, et al. Feeding gastrostomy in neurologically impaired children: is an antireflux procedure necessary? *J Pediatr Gastroenterol Nutr*. 1988;7:837–841.
7. Jolley SG, Smith EI, Tunell WP. Protective antireflux operation with feeding gastrostomy. Experience with children. *Ann Surg*. 1985;201:736–740.
8. Martinez DA, Ginn-Pease ME, Caniano DA. Sequelae of antireflux surgery in profoundly disabled children. *J Pediatr Surg*. 1992;27:267–271.
9. Pearl RH, Robie DK, Ein SH, et al. Complications of gastroesophageal anti-reflux surgery in neurologically impaired versus neurologically normal children. *J Pediatr Surg*. 1990;25:1169–1173.
10. Vane DW, Harmel RPJ, King DR, Boles ET Jr. The effectiveness of Nissen fundoplication in neurologically impaired children with gastroesophageal reflux. *Surgery*. 1985;98:662–667.
11. Spitz L, Roth K, Kiely EM, Brereton RJ, Drake DP, Milla, PJ. Operation for gastro-oesophageal reflux associated with severe mental retardation. *Arch Dis Child*. 1993;68:347–351.
12. Smith CD, Othersen HBJ, Gogan NJ, Walker JD. Nissen fundoplication in children with profound neurologic disability. *Ann Surg*. 1992;215:654–658.
13. Dedinsky GK, Vane DW, Black T, Turner MK, West KW, Grosfeld JL. Complications and reoperation after Nissen fundoplication in childhood. *Am J Surg*. 1987;153:177–183.
14. Richards CA, Andrews PL, Spitz L, Milla PJ. Nissen fundoplication may induce gastric myoelectrical disturbance in children. *J Pediatr Surg*. 1998;33:1801–1805.
15. Gauderer MW. Percutaneous endoscopic gastrostomy: a 10-year experience with 220 children. *J Pediatr Surg*. 1991;26:288–292.
16. Sulaeman E, Udall JNJ, Brown RF, et al. Gastroesophageal reflux and Nissen fundoplication following percutaneous endoscopic gastrostomy in children. *J Pediatr Gastroenterol Nutr*. 1998;26:269–273.
17. Khattak IU, Kimber C, Kiely EM, Spitz L. Percutaneous endoscopic gastrostomy in paediatric practice: complications and outcome. *J Pediatr Surg*. 1998;33:67–72.
18. Behrens R, Lang T, Muschweck H, Richter T, Hofbeck M. Percutaneous endoscopic gastrostomy in children and adolescents. *J Pediatr Gastroenterol Nutr*. 1997;25:487–491.
19. Heine RG, Reddihough DS, Catto-Smith AG. Gastro-oesophageal reflux and feeding problems after gastrostomy in children with severe neurological impairment. *Dev Med Child Neurol*. 1995;37:320–329.
20. Isch JA, Rescorla FJ, Scherer LR, West KW, Grosfeld JL. The development of gastroesophageal reflux after percutaneous endoscopic gastrostomy. *J Pediatr Surg*. 1997;32:321–322.
21. Grunow JE, al-Hafidh A, Tunell WP. Gastroesophageal reflux following percutaneous endoscopic gastrostomy in children. *J Pediatr Surg*. 1989;24:42–44.
22. Cameron BH, Blair GK, Murphy JJ, Fraser GC. Morbidity in neurologically impaired children after percutaneous endoscopic versus Stamm gastrostomy. *Gastroint Endosc*. 1995;42:41–44.
23. Roy RN, Pollnitz RB, Hamilton JR, Chance GW. Impaired assimilation of nasojejunal feeds in healthy low-birth-weight newborn infants. *J Pediatr*. 1977;90:431–434.
24. Rees RG, Payne-James JJ, King C. Spontaneous transpyloric passage and performance of "fine-bore" polyurethane feeding tubes: a controlled clinical trial. *JPEN*. 1988;12:469–472.
25. Levenson R, Turner WW, Dyson A. Do weighted nasoenteric feeding tubes facilitate duodenal intubation? *JPEN*. 1988;12:135–137.
26. Lord LM, Weiser-Maimone A, Pulhamus M. Comparison of weighted vs unweighted enteral feeding tubes for efficacy of transpyloric intubation. *JPEN*. 1993;17:271–273.
27. Taylor B, Schallom L. Bedside small bowel feeding tube placement in critically ill patients utilizing a dietician/nurse approach. *Nutr Clin Pract*. 2001;16:258–262.
28. Kalliafas S, Choban PS, Ziegler D, Drago S, Flancbaum L. Erythromycin facilitates postpyloric placement of nasoduodenal feeding tubes in intensive care unit patients: randomized, double-blinded, placebo-controlled trial. *JPEN*. 2004;20:385–388.
29. Stern MA, Wolf DC. Erythromycin as a prokinetic agent: a prospective randomized controlled study of efficacy in nasoenteric tube placement. *Am J Gastroenterol*. 1994;89:2011–2013.
30. Gharpure V, Meert KL, Sarnaik AP. Efficacy of erythromycin for post pyloric placement of feeding tubes in critically ill children: a randomized, double-blind placebo controlled study. *JPEN*. 2001;25:160–165.

31. Silva, CCR, Saconato H, Atallah AN. Metoclopramide for migration of naso-enteral tube. *Cochrane Database of Systematic Reviews. 1, 2006.*
32. Krafte-Jacobs B, Persinger M, Carver J, Moore L, Brilli R. Rapid placement of transpyloric feeding tubes: a comparison of pH-assisted and standard insertion techniques in children. *Pediatrics.* 1996;98:242–248.
33. Dimand RJ, Veereman-Waters G, Braner DA. Bedside placement of pH-guided transpyloric small bowel feeding tubes in critically ill infants and small children. *JPEN.* 1997;21:112–114.
34. Chen MY, Ott DJ, Gelfand DW. Nonfluoroscopic, post-pyloric feeding tube placement: number and cost of plain films for determining position. *Nutr Clin Pract.* 2000;15:40–44.
35. Hoffer F, Sandler RH, Kaplan LC. Fluoroscopic placement of jejunal feeding tubes. *Pediatr Radiol.* 1992;22:287–289.
36. Pobiel RS, Bisset GS, Pobiel MS. Nasojejunal feeding tube placement in children: four year cumulative experience. *Radiology.* 1994;190(1):127–129.
37. Wales PW, Diamond IR, Dutta S, et al. Fundoplication and gastrostomy versus image-guided gastrojejunal tube for enteral feedings in neurologically impaired children with gastroesophageal reflux. *J Pediatr Surg.* 2002;37:407–412.
38. Bourgeault AM, Heyland DK, Drover JW, Keefe L, Newman P, Day AG. Prophylactic pancreatic enzymes to reduce feeding tube occlusion. *Nutr Clin Pract.* 2003;18:398–401.
39. Marcuard SP, Stegall KL, Trogdon S. Clearing obstructed feeding tubes. *JPEN.* 1989;13:81–83.
40. Marcuard SP, Stegall KS. Unclogging feeding tubes with pancreatic enzyme. *JPEN.* 1990;14:198–200.
41. Pardoe EM. Tube feeding syndrome revisited. *Nutr Clin Pract.* 2001;16:144–146.
42. Heymsfield SB, Casper K, Grossman GD. Bioenergetic and metabolic response to continuous vs intermittent nasoenteric feeding. *Metabol Clin Exp.* 1987;36:570–575.
43. Smith SW, Camfield C, Camfield P. Living with cerebral palsy and tube feedings: a population-based follow-up study. *J Pediatr.*1999;135:307–310.
44. Holden CE, Puntis JW, Charlton CP, Booth IW. Nasogastric feeding at home: acceptability and safety. *Arch Dis Child.* 1991;66:148–151.

Chapter 21

Transitional and Combination Feeding

Anne M. Davis

INTRODUCTION

As ill or premature infants and children move toward health, they tolerate more physiologically normal feeds. As this process occurs, a need to change methods of feeding arises. How this change is accomplished is the topic of this chapter.

TRANSITIONAL AND COMBINATION FEEDING

Transitional nutrition support (NS) represents a change from one method of delivering nutrients to another. The goal of transition NS is to link an infant or child's feeding methods with as little compromise in nutrient intake as possible. Transitional and combined NS provides an overlapping of feeding methods so the infant or child has an opportunity to adjust to the new feeding mode with no net loss in nutrient intake. Possible feeding methods are parenteral, transpyloric, intragastric, and oral. Each of these methods includes various strategies such as continuous and cycled parenteral nutrition (PN), bolus and continuous intragastric feeds, and solid and liquid oral feeds (Table 21-1). Changing from one feeding method to another usually requires a period of time when more than 1 method is used simultaneously. The simultaneous use of feeding methods is termed "combination feeds." While transitional feeds usually include the simultaneous use of feeding methods, combination feeding can be used outside the context of transitional feeds as a permanent strategy for delivering adequate nutrition. One route of delivery might not be sufficient to supply all the nutrient needs of an infant or child. For instance, in multisystem organ failure, the patient's need for dextrose might be greater than can be delivered via the parenteral route. In protein energy malnutrition, absorption is impaired and tube feeding can induce diarrhea.[1] Extreme nutrient stress conditions might require more than 1 mode of nutrition support simultaneously. Examples of such conditions include cystic fibrosis, burns, and short bowel syndrome. In these high caloric requirement conditions, combination feeds are essential. Table 21-2 lists combination feeds and their possible uses.

TRANSITIONAL NUTRITION SUPPORT

It can be difficult to determine when a child or infant is ready to begin transition feeds (Table 21-3). Factors to consider in making this determination include: stable clinical condition, developmental or neurologic status, gastrointestinal motor function, digestive function, mucosal function, adequacy of elimination, emotional readiness, and the environment.

Stable Clinical Condition

Transitional feeding requires multiple, stepped manipulations. Each step depends on successful attainment of the previous step. In order to move from one step to the next, monitoring the clinical status and thus determining the efficacy of the each step is necessary (Figure 21-1). Documenting this kind of incremental progression is not possible in the face of an ill or unstable child. If many changes other than nutritional manipulations are taking place, the effect of the nutritional change cannot be determined. Thus a clinically stable child is a prerequisite for beginning transition feeds.

Developmental or Neurological Status

Sucking and swallowing begin *in utero* at about 10 weeks of gestation; however, effective sucking and swallowing enabling oral feeding are not present until approximately 34–35 weeks' gesta-

Table 21-1 Possible transitional feeding.

Previous method	*New method*	*Condition*
1. Parenteral nutrition	Oral intake	Prematurity
2. Parenteral nutrition	Tube feeding (TF)	Trophic feeding Short gut syndrome
3. Parenteral nutrition	Parenteral nutrition (PN) Continuous PN → cyclic PN Continuous PN → intermittent PN	 Cancer-chemotherapy
4. Tube feeding	Tube feeding Predigested TF → intact TF formula Increasing caloric density Continuous TF → cyclic TF Continuous TF → bolus TF	 Failure to thrive Cerebral palsy
5. Tube feeding	Oral intake	Breastfeeding Protracted diarrhea

TF = tube feeding.

Table 21-2 Combined feeding.

Methods	*Condition*
1. Parenteral nutrition and oral intake	Nonnutritive feeding and sensory development
2. Parenteral nutrition and tube feeds	Burns Severe protein-energy malnutrition
3. Overnight cyclic tube feeds and daytime bolus tube feeds	Neurological impairment, cerebral palsy
4. Tube feeds and oral intake	Cystic fibrosis
5. Parenteral nutrition and tube feeds and oral intake	Post-small bowel transplantation Prematurity

Date									
Wt (change)									
Parenteral nutrition									
Volume/hrs per day									
Protein									
Dextrose									
Lipid									
Total Kcal									
NaCl/Na acetate									
KCl/K acetate									
Total K									
Total Na									
$NaPO_4/KPO_4$ P_{Total}									
Ca gluconate									
$MgSO_4$									
MVI/trace									
IV									
D5W									
Volume									
Tube feeding									
Volume/hrs per day									
H_2O flushes									
Kcal									
Protein									
CHO									
% DRI vitamins/minerals									
Oral intake									
Volume									
Kcal									
Protein									
Meds/supplements									
H_2O flushes									
Output—total									
Urine									
Stool									
Ostomy									
TOTAL BALANCE									
Volume									
Kcal									
Protein									
Fat									
CHO									
Vitamins/minerals									

Figure 21-1 Flow sheet for combined and transitional nutrition support.

Table 21-3 Readiness factors for transitioning feeding techniques.

Feeding mode/factor	*Parenteral nutrition →*	*Tube feeding →*	*Oral intake*
1. Stabilized or resolved original condition for nutrition support	Stabilized	Stabilized	Resolved
2. Nutritional status	Stabilized	Improved	Adequate
3. Oral motor skills	In progress	In progress	Improved
4. Swallowing	Stabilized	Stabilized	Adequate
5. Critical sensitive period and development	Assessed	Assessed	Resolved
6. Parental motivation	Assessed	Improved	Adequate
7. Child's eagerness	Assessed	Assessed	Improved
8. Environment	Assessed	Improved	Adequate
9. Potential barriers	Assessed	Improved	Resolved
10. Behavioral intervention	Assessed	Improved	Improved

tion. In a neurologically impaired child, assessment of the swallowing mechanism by a speech therapist might be necessary to determine the safety of oral feeds. The consistency of the feeding changes the safety profile. When aspiration occurs with swallowing, intragastric or transpyloric feeding might be necessary.

Gastrointestinal (GI) Motor Function

Premature infants do not develop normal GI motor activity until about 30–32 weeks' gestation. Until an infant has close to normal GI motility, the enteral route cannot be relied on to deliver the bulk of needed nutrition. There appear to be clear advantages to trophic feeds in terms of accelerated GI maturation and long term nutritional outcomes, even though this method does not supply nutritionally significant quantities (Chapter 16). After surgery, the presence or absence of bowel sounds is not indicative of a functional or nonfunctional GI tract. Because infants and children have low body energy reserves, it is important not only to restart nutrition as soon as possible following surgery, but to advance directly to full liquids (breast milk, infant formula, etc.). Clear liquids have a much higher osmolality (Table 21-4) and can induce osmotic diarrhea. The caloric density of clear liquids is typically much lower than that of full liquids.

Digestive Function

To sustain enteral nutrition (EN), a fully functioning GI tract is not needed, since feeding can be provided as predigested formulas, and exogenous enzymes can also be used. Feedings can be delivered at a slow rate, so that the digestive capacity of a compromised GI tract is not exceeded. Digestive enzymes are down-regulated in PN when compared to EN.[2] In the premature infant, the changes associated with the deprivation of enteral feeding are reversible with the introduction of EN.[3] Fang and colleagues described a significant correlation between increase in mean blood flow velocity in the mesenteric artery and tolerance of EN in premature infants.[4]

Table 21-4 Osmolality of selected oral liquids and medications.

Product	*Osmolality mOsm/kg water*	*Product*	*Osmolality mOsm/kg water*
Enteral formulas		**Oral beverages**	
Term human milk	290	Whole milk	285
Preterm human milk (HM)	290	Carnation Instant Breakfast	661–747
Preterm HM + Enfamil HM Fortifier—2 pkt/50 mL	410–440	Apple juice	705
Similac Special Care with Iron 24	280	Ginger ale	565
Enfamil Premature with Iron 24	310	Diet ginger ale	53
Similac with Iron	300	Flavored ice	1,064
Similac with Iron 24	340	Orange juice	601
Enfamil with Iron	300	Gelatin	735
Enfamil with Iron 24	320	Low-calorie gelatin	57
Generic store brand (formerly SMA, Wyeth)	300	Cranberry juice	836
Enfamil LactoFree	200	Low-calorie cranberry juice	287
Similac Lactose Free	230	Pedialyte	250
Isomil	240	Infalyte	200
ProSobee	200	**Medications (concentration)**	
Carnation Alsoy	296	Calcium glubionate (115 mg/5 mL)	2,550–3,000
Generic store brand (formerly Nursoy, Wyeth)	296	Calcium carbonate (500 mg/5 mL)	3,140
Similac PM 60/40	280	Dexamethasone (1 mg/1 mL)	10,737
Carnation Good Start	265	Digoxin elixir (50 mg/liter)	1,350–3,000
Similac NeoSure	290	Ergocalciferol (8,000 IU/1 mL)	16,277
Enfamil 22	230	Ferrous sulfate liquid (60 mg/mL)	4,700
Alimentum	370	Multivitamin liquid	5,700
Nutramigen	320	Lactulose syrup (0.67 g/mL)	3,600
Pregestimil	320	Lasix, oral (10 mg/5 mL)	3,938
Neocate	342	Phenobarbitol (4 mg/1 mL)	7,417
Neocate One +	835	Ranitidine (15 mg/ 1 mL)	2,360
Pediasure	310	Theophylline elixir (80 mg/15 mL)	3,000
EleCare	596	Vitamin E drops (50 mg/1 mL)	4,083

Mucosal Function

Mucosal handling of nutrients, fats, carbohydrates, amino acids, vitamins, and minerals can be affected by immaturity, disease, or surgery. As the final common pathway of absorption, mucosal function is critical to establish EN.

Adequacy of Elimination

Both fecal elimination and renal excretion are necessary to establish and maintain GI nutrition. In renal failure, kidney function can be replaced by dialysis. Fecal elimination can be assisted by various medical and mechanical means. In the case of a bowel obstruction, surgery is needed to allow elimination to proceed.

Emotional Readiness

For the young infant and child, emotional readiness refers to the readiness of the caregivers. Cooperation and teamwork between the medical staff and the child's immediate caregiver is all important. This is especially true if the transition is to occur at home; unless there is willingness to make it work, the process will be fraught with difficulty and more than likely will fail. For the older child, a similar situation is true; however, the emotional readiness of the child also comes into play. Older children are more likely to be invested in making progress.

The Environment

Transitional NS needs to take place where there is knowledge and experience. This can be in an intensive care setting, on a pediatric floor in the hospital, or at home. If the transition is to occur at home, the medical staff needs to be familiar with the process, the child and the family. It must also be able to steer through the multiple challenges of home care (see Chapter 19).

CYCLED PARENTERAL NUTRITION

There are physiologic and psychological advantages to cycling PN administration. Cycling PN refers to infusing the PN solution in less than 24 hours. For the older child, time without the infusion apparatus allows freedom for greater activity, more social interaction, and school attendance. Continuous PN infusion leads to unrelentingly high insulin levels. The hyperinsulinemia is thought to cause hepatic lipid deposition and increased hepatic lipogenesis. Essential fatty acid deficiency could occur because insulin inhibits the release of free fatty acids from adipose tissue. These physiologic effects of continuous PN are reversed by cycling.[5]

Cycling PN is often the first step in the transition to a more physiologic feeding regimen. Sudden discontinuation of a high glucose infusion can cause hypoglycemia, especially in children less than 3 years of age.[6,7] Blood glucose levels should be monitored following cessation of high glucose infusions. To avoid hypoglycemia, PN should be tapered by decreasing to one half the rate for an hour, and one fourth the original rate for a second hour. Then PN can be discontinued. This strategy for tapering PN and monitoring blood sugars should be followed whenever cycling PN. It can also be used whenever stopping PN. Most infants and children can tolerate 1–4 hours off PN depending on their age, clinical condition, and quantity of EN they are receiving.[8] Increasing the time off of PN is usually tolerated in increments of 1–4 hours, again depending on the individual. Infants not receiving EN should not be off PN for more than 4–6 hours due to the risk of hypoglycemia.

MULTIPLE CYCLE PARENTERAL NUTRITION

Two or more cycles of PN within a 24-hour period are used when there is limited IV access and the infant or child needs PN as well as other intravenous therapies not compatible with PN. This technique is most often reserved for the hospital setting since close monitoring is required, and it should only be used when the infant or child is metabolically stable. The number of PN cycles depends on the total volume of PN desired and the number of daily infusions. Ideally, the infant or child should be receiving cycled PN that is tapered before attempting more than 1 cycle per 24-hour period (Table 21-5).

TROPHIC FEEDS

Trophic feeding, also known as minimal enteral feeding, gut priming, or early hypocaloric feeding, is used to prevent the negative effects of enteral starvation. Trophic feeds deliver nutritionally insignificant volumes of enteral fluids to directly stimulate the gastrointestinal tract. A systematic review of clinical outcomes after trophic feeding revealed that time to full EN, number of days that feedings were withheld, and total hospital stay were significantly reduced.[9,10] McClure and Newell conducted a prospective,

Table 21-5 Example of multiple PN cycles.

Patient:	5-yr-old female with leukemia, malnutrition, and intolerance to tube feeding Weight: 12.1 kg (< 5th percentile for age)
Chemotherapy:	500 mL b.i.d. @ 150 mL/hr. (8 am and 8 pm)
PN solution:	1,000 mL @ 2 cycles of 500 mL b.i.d.
Total fluid:	2,000 mL/d (= 1.8 × fluid maintenance)
PN order:	2.5% amino acids (2.1 g protein/kg/day) 25% dextrose (250 g) 120 mL 20% lipid (2 g fat/kg/day) Split into 2 bags
Calories:	99 kcal/kg/day

Chemotherapy cycles:	8–12 am and pm daily
PN cycles:	1–5 am and pm daily
1–5 am:	55 mL/hr × 1 hr 130 mL/hr × 3 hrs 55 mL/hr × 1 hr
1–5 pm:	55 mL/hr × 1 hr 130 mL/hr × 3 hrs 55 mL/hr × 1 hr

Blood glucose should be checked using same technique when cycling PN.

randomized study of trophic feeding and clinical outcomes in 100 high risk, preterm infants receiving intensive care. Preterm infants were randomized on the third day of life to receive either PN alone or PN and trophic feeds (0.5–1.0 mL/hr). Groups were matched for birth weight, gestation, and clinical acuity. The trophic feeding group demonstrated significantly higher energy intake, weight gain, and head circumference gain, as well as fewer episodes of culture confirmed sepsis, less PN, earlier tolerance of full EN, reduced supplemental oxygen requirements, and earlier home discharge.[11]

TRANSITION FROM PARENTERAL TO ORAL NUTRITION

It is unusual in nutrition support to go directly from PN to oral feeds. This circumstance occurs in an otherwise normal child who is recovering from a serious illness and in the well premature infant who has been developmentally unable to tolerate EN, but who has matured so that oral feeds are possible. Even in the well premature infant, an interim period of tube feeding might be advisable. Kliethermes and colleagues compared nasogastric tube and bottle supplementation as two methods of transitioning preterm infants to breastfeeding. After adjusting for confounding variables, infants who were nasogastric tube fed were more likely to be breastfeeding at discharge and at 3 days, 3 months, and 6 months following discharge.[12] A new technique known as a self-paced flow system[13,14] delivers milk to a nipple chamber from an open reservoir. The reservoir is continuously adjusted so that the level of milk is maintained at the level of the infant's mouth. At the base of the nipple, a catheter is inserted into the nipple chamber and connected to a graduated reservoir containing the milk. With this hydrostatic pressure system, milk only flows when the infant is sucking. Elimination of the vacuum build-up that occurs in bottles improved feeding performance in infants born at less than 30 weeks' gestational age.[13]

Oral feeds should begin with small, frequent volumes of full strength breast milk or formula. In the older child, initial oral feeds should be isotonic and then advance to full liquid. Commercially available liquid supplements are helpful during this transition. PN can be decreased by 10–25% when full liquids are tolerated. Daily enteral intake must meet all nutrient requirements before PN can be discontinued. PN can eliminate a child's appetite. DeSonnery and Hansen conducted a monkey study and found that for every 1 day of administered PN, it took 20 days for appetite to be reestablished.[15] Another study, however, showed that in children aged 8 to 16 years with orthopedic problems but no GI or neurological disease, PN did not affect oral intake.[16]

TRANSITION FROM PARENTERAL TO ENTERAL FEEDING

Special care should be exercised for patients who have impaired digestion or absorption, in those who have been without EN for longer than 7 days, in short bowel syndrome, in those fed transpylorically, and after bowel transplant. In such patients, an isotonic, predigested, elemental formula should initially be infused continuously at a slow rate. Continuous infusion allows for maximum absorption.[10] In infants, infusion rate should begin at about 1–2 mL/kg/hour and advance at 10–20 mL/kg/day as tolerated. In the older child, initial rates are approximately the same; however, advances should be slower at 3–6 mL/kg/day (see Table 21-6). When EN reaches 35% of calculated enteral caloric requirements, PN can be tapered. Patients being fed transpylorically should remain on an isotonic formula. Others may have their formula concentrated after isotonic formula is supplying approximately 50% of caloric needs. When the process of converting PN to EN is prolonged (longer than 1 month), the intake of intravenous and enteral vitamins, minerals, and trace elements should be assessed.

CHANGING ENTERAL FEEDS

Changing from Elemental to Polymeric Formula

The transition from a predigested enteral formula to an intact protein formula, especially in short bowel syndrome and small bowel transplantation, could take several days to weeks, depending on individual tolerance. It might even require the mixing of the two enteral formulas in a gradual, stepped approach such as one fourth

Table 21-6 Continuous tube feedings.

Category/age	*Starting point*	*Incremental increases*	*Goal rate*	*Total volume/d*
ELBW	0.5 mL/kg/hr	0.2–0.5 mL/kg/hr q 8 hr shift	4–5 mL/kg/hr/d	120 mL/kg/d
VLBW	1 mL/kg/hr	0.5–1 mL/kg/hr q 8 hr shift	6–7 mL/kg/hr/d	150 mL/kg/d
LBW	1–2mL/kg/hr	1 mL/kg/hr q 8 hr shift	7–8 mL/kg/hr/d	175 mL/kg/d
Neonate	1–2 mL/kg/hr	1–2 mL/kg/hr q 8 hr shift	6 mL/kg/hr/d	540–720 mL/d
Up to 12 months	1–2 mL/kg/hr	1–2 mL/kg/hr q 8 hr shift	5–6 mL/kg/hr/d	750–900 mL/d
1 to 3 years	1 mL/kg/hr	1 mL/kg/hr q 8 hr shift	4–5 mL/kg/hr/d	900–1,080 mL/d
4 to 10 years	20–30 mL/hr	20–30 mL/hr q 8 hr shift	3–4 mL/kg/hr/d	1,050–1,260 mL/d
11 to 18 years	30–60 mL/hr	30 mL/hr q 8 hr shift	100–150 mL/hr/d	2,400–3,600 mL/d

ELBW = extremely low birth weight; VLBW = very low birth weight; LBW = low birth weight.

intact and three fourths predigested; half intact and half predigested; three fourths intact and one fourth predigested; and finally to full strength intact protein formula. If this transition is prolonged (greater than 1 month), micronutrient adequacy should be evaluated.

Increasing Caloric Density

There is no advantage to prescribing dilute feeds; however, concentrating feeds above isotonicity should proceed gradually. Even small changes could exceed the capacity of the GI tract to adapt.

Continuous to Cycled Tube Feeds

Cycled tube feeds refer to the administration of continuous EN via a pump but delivered over less than 24 hours. Continuous feeding should be used for transpyloric feeds because the small bowel cannot tolerate large volumes. Usual time for cycled EN is 8–18 hours, depending on individual tolerance. Cycled feeds are more energy efficient and are associated with less abdominal discomfort than continuous feeds.[17] Cycled EN might not be tolerated in critically ill children, neurologically impaired children, or those with gastroesophageal reflux. When administering cycled (or any EN) at night, it is prudent to elevate the head of the bed as a precaution against reflux. Table 21-7 provides cycled tube feeding rates.

Continuous to Bolus Tube Feeds

Bolus or intermittent EN is typically given several times a day over 15–45 minutes. When compared to continuous EN, the advantages of bolus feeds are the technical simplicity (no pump and minimal supplies are required) greater mobility of the patient, and a more natural hunger-satiety cycle; however, diarrhea, cramping, dumping syndrome, and delayed gastric emptying are more likely.[18] Slow, gradual, transition between continuous and bolus feeds will achieve

Table 21-7 Cycled tube feedings.

Add this rate to continuous TF rate:

Category/age	*Starting point*	*Incremental increases*	*Goal rate*	*Total volume/d*
ELBW	+ 1 mL/kg/hr	1 mL/kg/hr q 8 hr shift to goal	5 mL/hr × 22 hr	120mL/kg/d
VLBW	+ 2 mL/hr	2 mL/hr q 8 hr shift to goal	10 ml/hr × 22 hr	150 mL/kg/d
LBW	+ 2–5 mL/hr	2–5 mL/hr q 8 hr shift to goal	15 ml/hr × 20 hr	175 mL/kg/d
Neonate	+ 5 mL/hr	5–10 mL/hr q 2 hr to goal	25 ml/hr × 20 hr	500 mL/d
Up to 12 months	+ 10 mL/hr	10–15 mL/hr q 2 hr to goal	75 mL/hr × 16 hr	1,200 mL/d
1 to 3 years	+ 15 mL/hr	15–20 mL/hr q 2 hr to goal	90 mL/hr × 16 hr	1,440 mL/d
4 to 10 years	+ 20 mL/hr	20–25 mL/hr q 2 hr to goal	120 mL/hr × 14 hr	1,680 mL/d
11 to 18 years	+ 30 mL/hr	30 mL/hr q 2 hr to goal	150 mL/hr × 12 hr	1,800 mL/d

Infusion time less than 24 hours per day.

optimal tolerance. See Table 21-8 for suggested transitional increases.

Overnight Cyclic Tube Feeds with Daytime Bolus Tube Feeding

In conditions of extremely high energy requirements and lifestyle needs, continuous drip tube feeds are used overnight with addition intermittent or bolus feeds during the daytime.

TRANSITION FROM ENTERAL TO ORAL FEEDING

Changing from full EN to oral feeds is a psychological problem rather than a physiologic one. If EN has been successful, then gastrointestinal function is sufficient. In most cases where oral and esophageal function is intact, there is no physiologic impediment to oral feeding. Yet this transition can be difficult, prolonged, and frustrating. The difficulty in making this transition falls into twp of Chatoor's six categories of feeding problems: sensory food aversion and posttraumatic food aversion.[19] In sensory food aversion, the child's appetite is greatly influenced by external motivators. This type of feeding problem occurs during transition to solid foods with or without an underlying medical or motor delay condition. The child resists specific food tastes, textures, and odors. Posttraumatic food aversion is most com-

Table 21-8 Bolus tube feedings.

Age category	*Starting point*	*Incremental increases*	*Goal rate*	*Total volume/d*
ELBW	1 mL/kg q 2 hr	0.5 mL/kg every feed or every other feed to goal	12 mL q 3 hr 8 feeds/d	120 mL/kg/d
VLBW	2 mL/kg q 2 hr	1 mL/kg every feed or every other feed to goal	25 mL q 3 hr 8 feeds/d	150 mL/kg/d
LBW	5 mL/kg q 2 hr	2 mL/kg every feed or every other feed to goal	35 mL q 3 hr 8 feeds/d	175 mL/kg/d
Neonate	10–15 mL q 2 hr 10–12 feeds/d	10–20 mL every feed or every other feed to goal	90 mL q 3–4 hr 6–8 feeds/d	540–720 mL/d
Up to 12 months	30–60 mL q 2–3 8–10 feeds/d	15–60 mL every feed or every other feed to goal	150 mL q 4–5 hr 5–6 feeds/d	750–900 mL/d
1 to 3 years	60–90 mL q 2–3 8–10 feeds/d	60 mL every feed or every other feed to goal	180 mL q 4–5 hr 5–6 feeds/d	900–1,080 mL/d
4 to 10 years	75–90 mL q 3 hr 8 feeds/d	60 mL every feed or every other feed to goal	210 mL q 4–5 hr 5–6 feeds/d	1,050–1,260 mL/d
11 to 18 years	90–120 mL q 3 hr 8 feeds/d	60 mL every feed or every other feed to goal	240 mL q 5 hr 5–6 feeds/d	1,200–1,440 mL/d

mon when prolonged tube feeding and/or intubation were necessary. Frequently, simply the sight of food or the bottle, or even positioning the child for feeding causes stress and anxiety. Treatment for this type of feeding problem includes multidisciplinary oral motor therapy (by a feeding disorders team), supplementation, tube feeding, and appetite stimulants (see Chapters 11 and 12). Benoit and colleagues randomly assigned 64 tube fed children (ages 4 to 36 months) who had at least 1 month resistance to oral feeding to either a nutrition intervention or a behavior intervention for 7 consecutive weeks. The outcome of success, defined as infants no longer requiring tube feeding at the third visit (4.5 months after study start), was significantly higher in the behavioral group compared to the nutritional group. The success of the behavior therapy was attributed to the use of an extinction technique defined as removing the reinforcer to a response to decrease the occurrence of the response (for example, removing a spoon after food refusal reinforces food refusal, so not removing the spoon after food refusal is an extinction procedure).[20] Interventions that have proven helpful in both these types of food aversion are given in Table 21-9.

Table 21-9 Feeding problem interventions.

1. Reduce mealtime conflict;
2. Help the child develop an appetite, possibly with the use of appetite stimulants; and
3. Use supplemental feedings (30 calories/ounce) to reduce the conflict from attempting to get the child to consume adequate calories. Supplementation provides balanced and complete nutrition to prevent weight loss during the transitional period.
4. Consistent mealtime rules:
    i. Keep a limited meal time duration (30 minutes).
    ii. Do not become a short-order cook.
    iii. Minimize distractions during meals.
    iv. Provide a neutral attitude during meals. Do not give negative or positive support.
    v. Select age-appropriate foods.
    vi. Allow the child to make an age-appropriate mess.
    vii. Be a role model for eating.

MONITORING TRANSITIONAL AND COMBINATION FEEDING

Underhydration and overhydration are the most common complications of transitional NS and combination NS. It is accordingly important to routinely monitor intake, output, and body weight carefully. When using multiple modes of nutrition support concurrently or when changing from one to another, fluid balance must be maintained (Figure 21-1). During this time it could be difficult to assess a positive nutrition outcome based only on weight gain. Length velocity then has a higher assessment value.

Refeeding syndrome can occur during combination and transitional NS. Refeeding syndrome includes fluid balance abnormalities, abnormal glucose metabolism, hypophosphatemia, hypomagnesemia, and hypokalemia.[21] This complication is underreported in the literature. Observing a fall in phosphate levels after starting EN often makes the diagnosis of refeeding syndrome.[22]

CONCLUSION

Combined and transitional NS is essential for GI development and maintenance, prevention of NS related complications, and social and oral-motor development, as well as quality of life for the child and family. It is often an individualized and long process needing many resources, significant support, and much patience. Careful monitoring and intervention in the hospital and home determine its success and pace.

REFERENCES

1. Rogers EJ, Gilbertson HR, Heine RG, et al. Barriers to adequate nutrition in critically ill children. *Nutrition.* 2003;19:865–868.
2. Guedon C, Schmitz E, Lerebours E, et al. Decrease brushed border hydrolase activities without gross morphologic changes in human intestinal mucosa

after prolonged total parenteral nutrition of adults. *Gastroenterology.* 1986;90:373–378.

3. Castillo R, Feng J, Stevenson D, Kwong L. Altered maturation of small intestine function in the absence of intraluminal nutrients: rapid normalization with refeeding. *Am J Clin Nutr.* 1991;53:558–561.
4. Fang S, Kempley ST, and Gamsu HR. Prediction of early tolerance to enteral feeding in preterm infants by measurement of superior mesenteric artery blood flow velocity. *Arch Dis Child Fetal & Neonatal Ed.* 2001;85: F42–F45.
5. Faubion WC, Baker WL, Iott BA, et al. Cyclic TPN for hospitalized pediatric patients. *Nutr Supp Serv.* 1981;1(4):24.
6. Werlin SL, Wyatt D, Camitta B. Effect of abrupt discontinuation of high glucose infusion rates during parenteral nutrition. *J Pediatr.* 1994;124(3):441–444.
7. Bendorf K, Friesen CA, Roberts CC. Glucose response to discontinuation of parenteral nutrition in patients less than 3 years of age. *J Parenter Enter Nutr.* 1996;20(2):120–122.
8. Collier S, Crouch J, Hendricks K, Caballero B. Use of cycled parenteral nutrition in infants less than six months of age. *Nutr Clin Pract.* 1994;9:65–68.
9. Tyson JE, Kennedy KA. Trophic feedings for parenterally fed infants. *Cochrane Database of Systematic Reviews. 1, 2006.*
10. Simpson C, Schanler RJ, Lau C. Early introduction of oral feeding in preterm infants. *Pediatrics.* 2002;110:517–522.
11. McClure RJ, Newell SJ. Randomized controlled study of clinical outcome following trophic feeding. *Arch Dis Child Fetal Neonat Ed.* 2000;82:F29–F33.
12. Kliethermes PA, Cross ML, Lanese MG, et al. Transitioning preterm infants with nasogastric tube supplementation: increased likelihood of breastfeeding. *J Obstet, Gynecol, Neonatal Nurs.* 1999;28:264–273.
13. Lau C, Schanler RJ. Oral feeding in premature infants: advantage of a self-paced flow. *Acta Paediatr.* 2000;89:453–459.
14. Lau C, Sheena HR, Shulman RJ, Schanler RJ. Oral feeding in low birth weight infants. *J Pediatr.* 1997;130:561–569.
15. Hansen BW, SeSomery CH, Hagedom T, Kalnasy LW. Effect of enteral and parenteral nutrition on appetite in monkeys. *JPEN.* 1977;1:83–88.
16. Reifen R, Khoshoo V, Dinari G. Effect of parenteral nutrition on oral intake. *J Pediatr Endocrinol Metab.* 1999;12:203–205.
17. Campbell IT, Morton RP, Macdonald IA, Judd S, Shapiro L, Stell PM. Comparison of the metabolic effects of continuous postoperative enteral feeding and feeding at night only. *American J Clin Nutr.* 1990;52(6):1107–1112.
18. Lavine JE, Hattner RS, Heyman MB. Dumping in infancy diagnosed by radionuclide gastric emptying technique. *J Pediatr Gastroenterol Nutr.* 1988;7(4):614–618.
19. Chatoor I, Hirsch R, Ganiban J, Persinger M, Hamburger E. Diagnosing infantile anorexia nervosa: the observation of mother-infant interactions. *J Am Acad Child Adolesc Psychiatry.* 1998;37:959–967.
20. Benoit D, Wang EEL, Zlotkin SH. Discontinuation of enterostomy tube feeding by behavioral treatment in early childhood: a randomized controlled trial. *J Pediatr.* 2000;137:498–503.
21. Crook MA, Hally V, Panteli JV. The importance of the refeeding syndrome. *Nutrition.* 2001;17:632–637.
22. Afzal NA, Addai S, Fagbemi A, et al. Refeeding syndrome with enteral nutrition in children: a case report, literature review and clinical guidelines. *Clin Nutr.* 2002;21:515–520.

CHAPTER 22

Parenteral Nutrition Indications, Administration, and Monitoring

Robert J. Shulman and Sarah Phillips

INTRODUCTION

Parenteral nutrition (PN) can be lifesaving or life threatening, depending on when and how it is used. In infants and children who are unable to meet their nutritional requirements over extended periods, it can prevent death from malnutrition. On the other hand, if appropriate attention is not paid to the mechanical aspects of administration (e.g., catheter placement) or nutritional requirements (e.g., hypophosphatemia related to nutritional rehabilitation), death from iatrogenic causes can occur. Although PN often is thought of in terms of providing all nutritional support (i.e., total parenteral nutrition), it should be considered in situations where some nutritional needs can be met orally and/or enterally for extended periods of time. It is always important to maintain oral intake so that infants do not lose the desire or ability to feed. Oral and enteral intake also provide nutrients in direct contact with the gastrointestinal (GI) tract, which helps to maintain GI mucosal integrity and potentially decreases bacteria and bacterial product translocation across the GI mucosa.[1]

Indications for Parenteral Nutrition

Guidelines for the indications and use of PN are published.[2] Unfortunately, as pointed out in these recommendations, there are no prospective studies that clearly delineate at what ages and under what clinical situations PN should be initiated.[2] It is generally accepted that in preterm infants, adequate nutrition for growth should be provided within hours to a day of birth.[3] The same is likely true for term newborns. In older infants and children, indications for PN are less clear. For well nourished children, a week of suboptimal intake is probably not of major consequence. Beyond this time, it is generally accepted that adequate nutrition be provided.[2] There should be no delay for malnourished infants and children to receive adequate nutritional support because of the increased risk of infection and other complications.[2]

ADMINISTERING PARENTERAL NUTRITION

Prior to PN initiation, goals for this therapy must be established (Table 22-1). For example, deciding on the type of intravenous access (tunneled catheter, percutaneously implanted catheter) requires an assessment of the duration of intravenous nutrition to be provided. Similarly, the frequency of laboratory monitoring, use of supplemental enteral/oral nutrition, and educational needs of the family and patient are dependent on the overall goals that need to be achieved.[4]

Anthropometrics

The first steps in the administration of PN are dependent on accurate initial height and weight measurements. The basis for determining body

Table 22-1 Initiating and administering parenteral nutrition.

Step		*Notes and calculations*
1	Determine nutritional goals.	Does the patient require nutritional rehabilitation or maintenance of current status? Will duration of nutritional therapy be < 2 weeks or greater? Will full or partial calories be provided?
2	Determine weight to be used for calculations.	Use an admission weight or dry weight for initial calculations. Assess whether ideal body weight or an adjusted body weight is appropriate.
3	Assess venous access (Table 22-2 and Chapter 26).	Review/discuss IV access (patency, infiltrates, blood drawing, etc.) with nursing/medical staff. Review X-ray for line placement.
4	Assess fluid requirements (Chapter 23).	Check fluid status: intake/output balance, need for concentrated PN solution.
5	Assess protein requirements.	Check for protein loss via GI output, chest tube output, etc. Determine total grams protein in g/d, g/kg, and g/L.
6	Assess total energy requirements.	Percent of calories from protein (step 5); 40–60% of calories from carbohydrate; 20–50% of calories from fat. In general, 30% of calories will come from fat and 70% from the amino acids and dextrose solution.
7	Determine grams of dextrose.	Energy from carbohydrate ÷ 3.4 kcal/g dextrose = g dextrose.
8	Determine fat milliliters or grams (20% lipid).	Energy from fat (kcal/day) ÷ 2 kcal/mL = mL/day of lipid.
9	Determine energy density of solution (Table 22-3).	Check with pharmacist if the patient is fluid restricted and the solution must be concentrated.
10	Check glucose infusion rate = 6–14 mg/kg/min.	Glucose infusion rate (mg/kg/min) = grams dextrose/kg × 1,000 mg/g ÷ 1,440 minutes/d (the number of minutes will change depending on the duration of the infusion).
11	Determine electrolyte requirements (Chapter 23).	mEq/kg and total mEq/L. Determine K concentration (mEq/L) and infusion rate (mEq/kg /hour).
12	Check osmolality of solution (if peripheral).	mOsm/L = (g amino acids/L × 10) + (g dextrose/L × 5) + [(mEq Na +, K + Ca /L) × 2].

surface area, body mass index, fluid, energy, protein, and medication dosages are weight and length. Determine whether the dry weight, ideal body weight, or adjusted body weight is appropriate for calculations. It is important to keep in mind that daily changes in weight reflect changes in fluid status and measurement error more than actual fat and lean body mass gains or losses.[5]

Access

The next step in the administration of PN is the selection of appropriate access sites and the best delivery route (Table 22-2 and Chapter 26). Ideally, the selection of the access route should occur well in advance of PN order writing. Planning and foresight can save patients from

Table 22-2 Venous access for parenteral nutrition.

Type of access	*Duration of use*	*Comments*
Peripheral (solutions < 1,000 mOsm)		
Peripheral IV	< 7–10 days	• Tip of catheter generally in a small vein in the lower arm. • Change site on a routine basis. • Usual dwell time is 48–72 hours.
Midline	7–21 days	• Peripherally placed in the basilic, cephalic, or median antecubital vein. • Tip of catheter located in large vein of upper arm. • Cannot be used to draw blood.
Central (solutions > 1,000 mOsm)		
Peripherally inserted central venous catheter (PICC)	4–6 weeks	• Percutaneously placed, usually in the basilic vein. • Assess location of catheter for central placement. • Can migrate out of position if not sutured. • Single- or double-lumen catheters available.
Nontunneled (nonimplanted)	> 1 month	• Surgically placed central venous catheter. • Single-, double-, or triple-lumen catheters. • Not recommended for home use.
Tunneled (implanted)	> 1 month	• Surgically placed central venous catheter. • Single-, double- or triple-lumen catheters. • Good for long term home use.
Totally implanted venous access system (TIVAS) (port)	> 1 month	• Surgically placed central venous catheter. • Single- or double-lumen catheters. • Not indicated for continuous PN infusions.

needless discomfort and/or expense.[6] The selection of delivery route, peripheral or central, depends upon the duration of PN therapy, caloric needs, and the patient's nutritional status.

In general, with peripheral venous access, the catheter tip is in a vein other than the superior or inferior vena cava. Peripheral catheters are not appropriate for vesicant chemotherapy, PN solutions with osmolarity greater than 900–1,100 mOsm/L, medications with pH less than five or greater than nine, and solutions or medications with an osmolarity greater than 500 mOsm/L.[7]

A midline catheter is placed in one of the large veins of the upper arm (basilic, cephalic, or median antecubital). These lines allow for greater hemodilution than is possible in a standard peripheral vein infusion because they are advanced into the larger vessels of the arm. While midline catheters can withstand greater flow rates, the tip of the catheter is not advanced to the superior or inferior vena cava, and they are considered peripheral lines and are treated as such. Consequently, nursing assessment of peripheral vein and midline patency, evidence of phlebitis, or infiltration should be reviewed frequently by the practitioner to obviate complications and determine the potential need for central venous access. There is little advantage to a midline catheter over a standard peripheral vein catheter because of their tendency to fall out, clot, and contribute to thrombophlebitis.[8]

Patients who require PN solutions of an osmolarity greater than 1,000 mOsm/L and/or long term use (> 2 weeks) are candidates for central venous access. In general, there are 4 types of central venous catheters: peripherally inserted central catheter (PICC), nontunneled, tunneled, and totally implanted venous access devices (ports). A PICC line is inserted through the cephalic, basilic, or median cubital veins. Although inserted peripherally, the tip of the catheter resides in the superior or inferior vena cava, and therefore it is considered a central venous catheter. A PICC often can be used in place of a midline catheter with fewer complications and greater utility.[8] Nontunneled catheters offer the advantage of bedside placement. Tunneled catheters appear to be associated with somewhat fewer complications.[8] Totally implanted venous access devices carry the lowest risk of infection but are not appropriate for long term administration of PN because of the repeated need to pierce the skin to gain access to the catheter.[8,9]

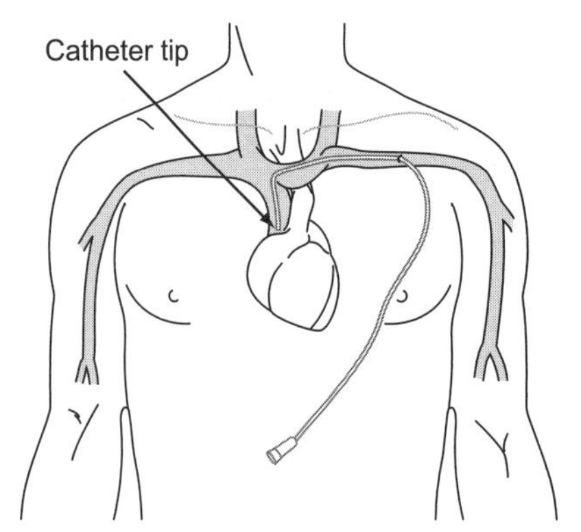

Figure 22-1 Desirable catheter position.

The assessment of catheter tip placement and patency of any catheter prior to administration of PN is essential for patient safety. The end of the catheter should be located at or near the top of the right atrium (Figure 22-1). Any child who has significant linear growth while a catheter is in place needs to have a chest radiograph to confirm that placement is still appropriate.[10]

Nutrition and Fluids

The patient's nutritional and medical status determines nutrient needs, nutrient mix, and rate of delivery. Minimum amounts of glucose, fat, and protein are required to replenish energy deficits and to prevent hypoglycemia, essential fatty acid deficiency, and hypoproteinemia. Feeding excess macronutrients can be associated with the development of hepatic steatosis, excessive CO_2 production, hyperglycemia and increased risk for infection, or prerenal azotemia.[11,13] Fluid restrictions might be required in renal failure, cardiac disease, or pulmonary disease. Volume restriction often requires PN solutions to be concentrated, and this could limit the delivery of adequate nutrients. In general, it is best to consider fluid (Chapter 23) and protein requirements first.[14] Patients with significant fluid restriction, for example, might need protein intake provided at the expense of energy intake. There are larger gains in protein accretion with increases in protein intake than with increases in energy intake.[14] Unless a patient has renal or liver impairment or disease, there is no reason to limit initial protein intake to less than calculated needs or to gradually advance over several days.[14]

There can be considerable intra- and interindividual variation as well as day-to-day variation in energy needs.[15] The dietary reference intakes (DRIs) (Chapter 8) give dietary allowances in age intervals from 0 to 0.5 years and from 0.5 to 1.0 years, and they reflect enteral requirements, making them difficult to use for PN.[16] Energy requirements for the hospitalized child can, therefore, be difficult to define with accuracy unless indirect calorimetry is used. Investigations and reviews have shown that increased energy needs in postsurgical patients are short lived, usually 12–24 hours.[17,18] In most cases, the provision of resting energy requirements is sufficient[19] for the critically ill child. Thus, a conservative approach to energy delivery initially minimizes the risk of overfeeding.[20] See Chapter 6 for further discussion of energy requirements.

Generally, 40–60% of calories from dextrose (glucose) and infusion rates of 6–14 mg/kg/day are appropriate for children. A gradual increase in glucose administration might be indicated in the preterm, severely malnourished, septic, or critically injured child. Table 22-3 lists the energy density of amino acid/dextrose solutions.

Intravenous fat provides energy and is required for essential fatty acids. The quantity of fat needed depends on several factors. Preterm, malnourished, diabetic, or septic patients, those who have impaired renal or hepatic function, and those who are critically ill are at increased risk for impaired fat clearance and are likely to develop hypertriglyceridemia and require cautious administration of intravenous fat emulsions.[21] Drugs such as steroids that are lipolytic could increase triglyceride levels. Generally, patients tolerate 20–40% of their total energy requirement supplied as fat emulsion. If more than 75–80% of energy is supplied by fat, ketosis could develop.

Intravenous fat emulsion may be started at the same time the amino acid/dextrose infusion is initiated. However, unlike the amino acid/dextrose solution, the rate of infusion of the fat emulsion is increased in a stepwise fashion. As noted previously, tolerance depends on a number of factors. Small, preterm infants might need to begin with 0.25 g/kg/day lipid and increase the rate by that amount every day, whereas an older child might tolerate a starting dose of 1 g/kg/day with increases in rate every 8–12 hours.

The rate of fat clearance is related to the amount infused per unit of time.[22] Thus, the longer the infusion duration, the less likely the patient will experience hypertriglyceridemia.

Table 22-3 Energy density of amino acid/dextrose solutions (kcal/mL).

	% Amino acids								
	1.0	*2.2*	*2.5*	*2.7*	*3.0*	*3.5*	*4.0*	*5.0*	*6.0*
% Dextrose									
7.5	0.30	0.35	0.36	0.37	0.38	0.40	0.42	0.46	0.50
10.0	0.38	0.43	0.44	0.45	0.46	0.48	0.50	0.54	0.58
12.5	0.47	0.52	0.53	0.54	0.55	0.57	0.59	0.63	0.67
15.0	0.55	0.60	0.61	0.62	0.63	0.65	0.67	0.71	0.75
20.0	0.72	0.77	0.78	0.79	0.80	0.82	0.84	0.88	0.92
25.0	0.89	0.94	0.95	0.96	0.97	0.99	1.01	1.05	1.09
30.0	1.04	1.09	1.10	1.11	1.12	1.14	1.16	1.20	1.24
35.0	1.23	1.28	1.29	1.30	1.31	1.33	1.35	1.39	1.43
40.0	1.40	1.45	1.46	1.47	1.48	1.50	1.52	1.56	1.60

Essential fatty acid deficiency is prevented by 0.5 g/kg/day for infants and 1.5 g/kg/day lipid infusion twice weekly for older children.[23] As with energy and protein, there can be significant interindividual variation in essential fatty acid requirements.[24,25] Depending on the patient's age, nutritional status, length of time on PN, and disease, the values cited above could be inadequate.

Vitamins and Minerals

The recommendations for vitamin and mineral administration are summarized in Tables 22-4 and 22-5. The delivery of vitamin and trace minerals is confounded by the fact that PN solutions contain trace minerals as contaminants,[26] and guidelines for pediatric vitamin and minerals were developed

Table 22-4 Infant and child parenteral multivitamin requirements and commercial preparations.

Vitamin (amount/d)	*Preterm infant**	*NAG-AMA Δ*	*Pediatric parenteral multivitamins† < 2.5 kg 40% of the vial (2 ml)*	*Pediatric parenteral multivitamins† > 2.5 yrs < 11 yrs > 2.5 yrs* < 11 yrs 100% of the vial (5 mL)*
A (μg)‡	500	700	280	700
C (mg)	25	80	32	80
D (IU)	160	400	160	400
E (mg)§	2.8	7	2.8	7
K (μg)	80	200	80	200
Thiamin (mg)	0.35	1.2	0.48	1.2
Riboflavin (mg)	0.15	1.4	0.56	1.4
Niacin (mg)	6.8	17	6.8	17
Pyridoxine (mg)	0.18	1	0.40	1
Folate (μg)	56	140	56	140
B_{12} (μg)	0.3	1	0.4	1
Pantothenic acid (mg)	2.0	5	2.0	5
Biotin (μg)	6	20	8	20

* Greene HL, Hambidge KM, Schanler R, Tsang RC. Guidelines for the use of vitamins, trace elements, calcium, magnesium, and phosphorus in infants and children receiving total parenteral nutrition: report of the Subcommittee on Pediatric Parenteral Nutrienet Requirements from the Committee on Cliniical Practice Issues of the American Society for Clinical Nutrition. *Am J Clin Nutr* 1988;48:1324–1342.

Δ Multivitamin preparations for parenteral use. A statement by the Nutrition Advisory Group. American Medical Association Department of Foods and Nutrition, 1975. *JPEN J Parenter Enteral Nutr.* 1979 Jul–Aug; 3(4):258–262.

† MVI-Pediatric (aaiPharma, Inc., Wilmington, NC).

‡ 500 μg = 1643 IU.

§ 1 mg = 1 IU.

NAG-AMA = Nutrition Advisory Group-American Medical Association in the late 1970s and 1980s. There is no recent reformulation of parenteral vitamin products.[27,28] PN vitamins available for children older than 11 years of age were recently reformulated. The use of this formula in younger children for long periods of time could put them at risk for excessive vitamin intakes. Additionally, nutrients are lost by adherence to the tubing or from photodegradation.[29] Both vitamin and mineral doses are based in part on patient weight, and so accurate weight measurements are critical, especially in the smaller or premature infant. Current vitamin and mineral formulations do not match well the requirements for malnourished patients, those with renal disease or liver disease, premature infants, and children with short bowel. These patients also will be more susceptible to vitamin and mineral excesses and deficiencies, thus, require close monitoring of vitamin and mineral status.

Because there is great variation in individual nutrient requirements, the point at which nutrient intakes are inadequate or excessive is not well defined. Nutrient delivery, therefore, should be tailored to the patient. Appropriate monitoring of the patient's response to treatment helps define adequate nutrient delivery.

Table 22-5 Adult parenteral multivitamin preparations.

Vitamin	*DRI/RDA 9–13 yr*	*Infuvite**	*M.V.I.-12 Δ*
A (IU)2	600 μg	3,300	3,300
D IU (μg)	200(5)	200 (5)	200 (5)
E (IU)	11	10	10
K (μg)	60	150	-
C (mg)	45	200	100
Thiamin (mg)	0.9	6	3
Riboflavin (mg)	0.9	3.6	3.6
Niacin (mg)	12	40	40
Pyridoxine (mg)	1	6	4
Folate (μg)	300	600	400
B_{12} (μg)	4	5	5
Pantothenic acid (mg)	1.8	15	15
Biotin (μg)	20	60	60

* Infuvite (Sabex, Inc., Boucherville, Canada).

Δ Multivitamin preparations for parenteral use. A statement by the Nutrition Advisory Group. American Medical Association Department of Foods and Nutrition, 1975. *JPEN J Parenter Enteral Nutr.* 1979 Jul–Aug; 3(4):258–262.

MVI-12 (aaiPharma, Inc., Wilmington, NC).

* Amended formula for adult multivitamin preparations.

† 500 μg = 1643 IU.

Source: Jeppesen PB, Hoy CE, Mortensen PB. Differences in essential fatty acid requirements by enteral and parenteral routes of administration in patients with fat malabsorption. *Am J Clin Nutr.* 1999;70:78–84.

MONITORING PEDIATRIC PARENTERAL NUTRITION

The goals of monitoring PN are to minimize complications and to assess the outcomes of treatment. The monitoring of PN includes assessment of metabolic factors, growth, and developmental and psychological parameters. Children with serious illnesses might be predisposed to vitamin and mineral deficiencies. Often the deficiencies are subtle and difficult to accurately assess and define.

Initial laboratory assessment is based on the patient's nutritional status, medical condition, and medications. Recommendations for monitoring electrolytes and minerals can be found in Table 22-6.[30,31]Serum electrolyte levels and blood sugars are measured daily until full PN is achieved and serum electrolytes are stable. Meticulous attention to blood drawing procedures (e.g., turning off fluids prior to blood draws, removing adequate amount of line contents before obtaining blood, obtaining appropriate blood volumes, and timing measurements with the middle or end of the PN infusion) minimizes error. An initial or baseline measurement of serum proteins, calcium, magnesium, phosphorous, and triglycerides can be helpful in some patients (e.g., malnutrition, liver, or renal disease or sepsis).

Patients with significant malnutrition, at risk for refeeding syndrome, liver or metabolic diseases, or who are PN dependent require more frequent monitoring of electrolytes and minerals. In addition, these patients require long term monitoring of vitamin and trace mineral status, growth, and developmental milestones. In patients at risk for refeeding syndrome, declines in potassium and phosphorous could last for 7–10 days.[32] It might be necessary during this period to monitor these minerals every day to every other day until serum levels are stable and in the normal range for age. If the amount of nutrition being provided is less than that required for catch-up weight gain or only enough to maintain weight, the refeeding syndrome will not develop. Consequently, the patient could be at risk for hypophosphatemia and hypokalemia weeks after the initiation of PN when energy intake is sufficient for tissue accretion and accelerated weight gain.

Glucose: Urine glucose, blood glucose levels, and the glucose infusion rate (mg glucose/kg/min) are used to monitor glucose delivery. The acute consequences of too much glucose include serum hyperosmolarity and osmotic diuresis. Hyperglycemia that requires insulin increases potassium, magnesium, and phosphorous uptake by cells. Therefore, these minerals need to be monitored more frequently when insulin is prescribed. Overfeeding in conjunction with excessive carbohydrate intake is associated with significant increases in CO_2 production and can affect liver function.[33,34]

Determining how much glucose is too much and when hyperglycemia is detrimental can be problematic. The exact intake at which a crossover occurs from beneficial to harmful is not known. Glucose tolerance and oxidative capacity are compromised by prematurity, sepsis, stress, hepatic and renal failure, malnutrition, steroid use, and diabetes.[35] These patients will need frequent urine glucose checks (every 8–12 hours or possibly more frequently). Premature infants, patients with liver disease, those at risk for cholestasis who are ventilated, hyperglycemic, or septic might benefit from limitations in glucose infusion rates.[32,33] Monitor glucose initially in patients on cyclic PN at the beginning, middle, and end of the discontinuation of the infusion to assess tolerance. Some patients, especially infants and patients prone to hypoglycemia (e.g., those with liver disease) might need prolonged ramping down times.

Fat: Lipoprotein lipase resides in the capillary bed, and patients who are malnourished have less capillary mass and slower rates of clearance than those who are not malnourished. In malnourished patients, tolerance of intravenous fat might need to be monitored more frequently than suggested in Table 22-6.

Hypertriglyceridemia is most likely to occur 4 hours after an infusion is initiated.[36,37] Triglyceride levels around 100 mg/dL–150 mg/dL are generally considered appropriate. Triglyceride levels

Table 22-6 Monitoring parenteral nutrition in pediatrics.

Parameter	*Initial*	*Follow-up*
Growth		
Weight	Daily	Daily to monthly
Length/stature	Weekly to monthly	Monthly
Head circumference	Weekly	Weekly to monthly
Body composition	Monthly	Monthly to annually
Metabolic (serum)		
Electrolytes	Daily to weekly	Weekly to monthly
BUN/creatinine	Weekly	Weekly to monthly
Ca, PO4, Mg	Twice weekly	Weekly to monthly
Acid/base	As indicated until stable	Weekly to monthly
Albumin/prealbumin	Weekly, every 2 weeks	Every 2 weeks to monthly
Glucose	Daily to weekly	Weekly to monthly
Triglyceride	Daily with changes	Weekly to monthly
Liver tests	At 2 weeks	Weekly to monthly
CBC	Weekly	Weekly to monthly
Platelets PT/PTT	Weekly	Weekly to monthly
Iron indices	As indicated	3–4 months
Trace elements	Monthly	Biannually to annually
Fat-soluble vitamins	As indicated	Biannually to annually
Carnitine	As indicated	Biannually to annually
Folate/B_{12}	As indicated	Biannually to annually
Ammonia	As indicated	As indicated
Metabolic (urine)		
Glucose/ketones	2 to 6 times per day	Daily to weekly
Specific gravity/urea n	As indicated	As indicated
Other		
Bone density	As indicated	As indicted
Verify line placement	Initially and as indicated with growth	Every 6–12 months
Developmental milestones	Monthly	Every 6–12 months
Occupational therapy	At 1 month, as indicated	Annually
Physical therapy		

vary depending on the analysis method. Some methods measure triglycerides by releasing free fatty acids from the molecule and measuring the free glycerol. Since fat emulsions contain free glycerol, the resulting serum triglyceride level might be overestimated. The American Gastroenterological Association Technical review on Parenteral Nutrition states that fat emulsions should not be administered to patients whose levels exceed 400 mg/dL.[38]

For individuals on long term PN, with little enteral intake and/or fat malabsorption, measurement of n-6 and n-3 fatty acids may be used to assess essential fatty acid status.[39]

Protein: In addition to albumin and prealbumin (transthyretin), patients with PN might need other parameters measured. In liver disease, the serum ammonia can be followed in patients when the direct bilirubin is elevated. In patients with short bowel syndrome, malabsorption, or protein-losing enteropathy enteric protein loss occurs, and fecal alpha-1-antitrypsin excretion is useful in detecting those losses and the need for additional protein intake. Blood urea nitrogen (BUN) can be used as a short term measure of protein intake, presuming that renal function and hydration are normal.

Liver Tests: PN therapy is associated with liver injury. The severity can vary from minimal with transient increases in liver-related blood tests to biliary cirrhosis and ultimately liver failure.[40] The younger the child or infant the greater the risk of developing disease. While the exact cause of liver disease is unknown, there are several factors that place children at risk. Small, preterm infants or patients who have undergone intestinal resection, had recurrent episodes of infection, lacked enteral feeds, or were overfed (carbohydrate, protein) are at greatest risk.[41]

Tests of liver status (ALT, GGT, bilirubin) should be performed in patients receiving PN for 2 weeks or greater. Some patients (preterm infants, those with liver disease or lack of enteral intake) will need more frequent assessments of liver status (e.g., weekly).

Vitamins: Preterm infants, children with liver or renal disease or short bowel syndrome, or those who are severely malnourished require close monitoring of vitamin status. Lipids and water soluble vitamins are lost during PN delivery.[25] Patients on long term PN with limited enteral intake and/or absorption should have vitamin levels checked (especially vitamin A and possibly riboflavin) because of potential losses in the administration set.

Carnitine: Patients who require long term PN should have carnitine (as pure L-carnitine) added to their PN solutions at a dose of 2–5 mg/kg/day. Plasma and red blood cell carnitine concentrations should be measured at baseline and at 4-month intervals until levels have stabilized, then yearly thereafter.[42]

Monitoring Trace Elements

Zinc: Patients at risk for zinc deficiency are those with gastrointestinal losses due to diarrhea, ileostomies, and nasogastric suction.[43] The assessment of zinc status, however, can be problematic. Serum zinc is a convenient but poor measure of marginal zinc status in individuals. Zinc is found primarily intracellularly, and a small portion is bound to plasma proteins. Diurnal rhythms, stress, infection, starvation, and plasma protein levels can affect plasma zinc levels. Currently, there is no single measure to accurately assess zinc status in humans. Zinc is important in many enzymes: lactic dehydrogenase, plasma ribonuclease, and plasma alkaline phosphatase, for example. However, a reliable zinc dependent enzyme to identify zinc status has not been identified. In the absence of a reliable zinc assessment, serial serum zinc levels may be used along with alkaline phosphatase to assess the effects of supplementation.

Manganese: Manganese is excreted in bile and can accumulate in patients with liver disease. Manganese is a frequent contaminant of PN solutions.[44] There is some evidence that manganese accumulation might be involved in the development of PN cholestasis.[45] Manganese levels should be monitored in patients receiving PN for greater than 30 days (see Copper section next). The best measure of manganese status is controversial. Whole blood levels appear to correlate (in adults) with MRI-documented cerebral manganese deposition. Most investigators use whole blood, red blood cell, or manganese superoxide dismutase.[46]

Copper: Copper, like manganese, is excreted in bile. Cholestatic conditions and liver disease could predispose patients to copper accumulation. Circulating copper levels are influenced by hormonal influences, malignancies, and inflammation. Copper and manganese supplementation is often decreased by one half to one fourth the standard dose in patients with cholestatic liver disease. However, there is no clear-cut evidence to support this practice. Some investigators argue that manganese should not be added to the PN of any patient with liver disease nor in those receiving PN for more than 30 days.[47,48] Whether the same holds true for copper is unknown. In the case of copper, there is a definite risk that too low a dose places the patient at risk for copper deficiency.[49]

Copper levels should be monitored every 3 to 6 months. Copper status is assessed with serum copper, ceruloplasmin levels or red cell superoxide dismutase, or hair copper.

Selenium: Knowledge regarding the adequacy of selenium intake is limited. Therefore, it is prudent to check serum selenium levels, particularly in preterm infants, and serum selenium levels and glutathione peroxidase activity in older infants and adolescents.

Chromium: Chromium status of patients on long term PN should be closely monitored. Chromium is a contaminant of PN solutions and the addition of chromium to PN at recommended levels can raise serum chromium levels above those that are desirable.[50] Patients at risk for chromium excess are preterm infants, those with renal disease, and those on long term PN. Chromium status can be assessed by measuring whole blood and urinary levels.

Iron: PN patients at risk for iron deficiency are preterm infants, long term PN patients, those with little or no enteral intake, and patients with significant malabsorption or fluid losses. Because iron is not routinely added to PN solutions, it must be administered orally, intramuscularly, or intravenously. Iron status should be monitored every 3 to 4 months by checking a complete blood count, reticulocyte count, and serum iron and transferrin levels.

Other: Frequent developmental, occupational, and physical therapy and psychological assessments are essential for maintaining developmental milestones in children on long term PN. Long term hospitalizations have been shown to disrupt normal feeding behaviors,[51] and developmental delays are a potential complication of prolonged hospitalization. Aversion to oral feeding could develop in children receiving long term PN or tube feedings.[52] Assessment and maintenance of oral motor function is essential in infants receiving PN and /or tube feedings.

Education: Assessment of learning and discharge planning needs should occur as soon as the patient begins PN therapy. PN education of families and patients decreases anxiety.[53] Frequent family meetings with the medical staff to review goals and planning help improve the families' ability to cope and their patient care skills.

CONCLUSION

PN can be life saving for infants and children who are unable to meet their nutritional requirements over extended periods of time. The administration of PN requires careful attention to the mechanical aspects of administration, nutritional requirements and monitoring. Frequent reassessment of the patient and therapy is necessary to safely provide this treatment.

REFERENCES

1. Sigalet DL, Mackenzie SL, Hameed SM. Enteral nutrition and mucosal immunity: implications for feeding strategies in surgery and trauma. *Can J Surg.* 2004;47(2):109–116.
2. ASPEN Board of Directors and the Clinical Guidelines Task Force. Guidelines for the use of parenteral and enteral nutrition in adult and pediatric patients. *J Parenter Enteral Nutr.* 2002;26:1SA–138SA.

3. Wilson DC, Cairns P, Halliday HL, Reid M, McClure G, Dodge JA. Randomised controlled trial of an aggressive nutritional regimen in sick very low birthweight infants. *Arch Dis Child Fetal Neonatal Ed.* 1997;77:F4–11.
4. Phillips SM. Pediatric parenteral nutrition clinical pathway. *Pediatric Nutrition: A Building Block for Life.* 2003;26:1–6.
5. Piug M. Body composition and growth. In: Walker WA and Watkins JB, eds. *Nutrition in Pediatrics.* Vol 2. Hamilton, Ontario, Canada: BC Decker; 1996:44–62.
6. Chung DH, Ziegler MM. Central venous catheter access. *Nutrition.* 1998;14(1):119–123.
7. Anonymous. Intravenous nursing. Standards of practice. Intravenous Nurses Society. *Intraven Nurs. 1998;21(1 suppl):S1–91.*
8. Moureau N, Poole S, Murdock MA, Gray SM, Semba CP. Central venous catheters in home infusion care: outcomes analysis in 50,470 patients. *J Vasc Interv Radiol.* 2002;13:1009–1016.
9. Shulman RJ, Rahman S, Mahoney D, Pokorny WJ, Bloss R. A totally implanted venous access system used in pediatric patients with cancer. *J Clin Oncol.* 1987;5:137–140.
10. Reed T, Phillips S. Management of central venous catheter occlusions and repairs. *J Intraven Nurs.* 1996;19(6):289–294.
11. Burke JF, Wolfe RR, Mullany CJ, Mathews DE, Bier DM. Glucose requirements following burn injury: parameters of optimal glucose infusion and possible hepatic and respiratory abnormalities following excessive glucose intake. *Ann Surg.* 1979;190(3):274–285.
12. Shikora SA, Benotti PN. Nutritional support of the mechanically ventilated patient. *Respir Care Clin N Am.* 1997;3(1):69–90.
13. Bistrian BR. Hyperglycemia and infection: which is the chicken and which is the egg? *JPEN.* 2001;25(4):180–181.
14. Shulman RJ, Phillips S. Parenteral nutrition in infants and children. *J Pediatr Gastroenterol Nutr.* 2003;36:587–607.
15. Jaksic T, Shew SB, Keshen TH, Dzakovic A, Jahoor F. Do critically ill surgical neonates have increased energy expenditure? *J Pediatr Surg.* 2001;36(1):63–67.
16. Barr SI, Murphy SP, Poos MI. Interpreting and using the dietary references intakes in dietary assessment of individuals and groups. *J Am Diet Assoc.* 2002;102(6):780–788.
17. Lloyd DA. Energy requirements of surgical newborn infants receiving parenteral nutrition. *Nutrition.* 1998;14(1):101–104.
18. Pierro A. Metabolism and nutritional support in the surgical neonate. *J Pediatr Surg.* 2002;37(6):811–822.
19. Schofield WN. Predicting basal metabolic rate, new standards and review of previous work. *Hum Nutr Clin Nutr.* 1985;39(suppl 1):5–41.
20. Chwals WJ. Overfeeding the critically ill child: fact or fantasy? *New Horiz.* 1994;2:147–155.
21. Dahn MS, Kirkpatrick JR, Blasier R. Alterations in the metabolism of exogenous lipid associated with sepsis. *JPEN.* 1984;8:169–173.
22. Kao LC, Cheng MH, Warburton D. Triglycerides, free fatty acids, free fatty acids/albumin molar ratio, and cholesterol levels in serum of neonates receiving long-term lipid infusions: controlled trial of continuous and intermittent regimens. *J Pediatr.* 1984;104:429–435.
23. Jeppesen PB, Hoy CE, Mortensen PB. Differences in essential fatty acid requirements by enteral and parenteral routes of administration in patients with fat malabsorption. *Am J Clin Nutr.* 1999;70:78–84.
24. Barr LH, Dunn GD, Brennan MF. Essential fatty acid deficiency during total parenteral nutrition. *Ann Surg.* 1981;193:304–311.
25. Wolfram G, Eckart J, Walther B, Zollner N. Factors influencing essential fatty acid requirement in total parenteral nutrition (TPN). *JPEN.* 1978;2:634–639.
26. Pluhator-Murton MM, Fedorak RN, Audette RJ, Marriage BJ, Yatscoff RW, Gramlich LM. Trace element contamination of total parenteral nutrition: 1. contribution of component solutions. *JPEN.* 1999;23(4):222–227.
27. American Medical Association Department of Foods and Nutrition. Multivitamin preparations for parenteral use: a statement by the Nutrition Advisory Group, 1975. *JPEN.* 1979;3:258–262.
28. Greene HL, Hambidge KM, Schanler R, Tsang RC. Guidelines for the use of vitamins, trace elements, calcium, magnesium, and phosphorus in infants and children receiving total parenteral nutrition: report of the Subcommittee on Pediatric Parenteral Nutrient Requirements from the Committee on Clinical Practice Issues of the American Society for Clinical Nutrition. *Am J Clin Nutr.* 1988;48:1324–1342.
29. Smith JL, Canham JE, Kirkland WD, Wells PA. Effect of Intralipid, amino acids, container, temperature, and duration of storage on vitamin stability in total parenteral nutrition admixtures. *JPEN.* 1988;12:478–483.
30. Davis AM. Initiation, monitoring, and complications of pediatric parenteral nutrition. In: Baker RD, Baker S, David A, eds. *Pediatric Parenteral Nutrition.* New York Chapman and Hall; 1977:212–237.
31. Conkin CA, Gilger MA, Jennings HC, et al. *Pediatric Residents' Nutrition Resource Handbook.* New York: Nestle; 2001.
32. Crook MA, Hally V, Panteli JV. The importance of the refeeding syndrome. *Nutrition.* 2001;17(7–8):632–637.
33. Nose O, Tipton JR, Ament ME, Yabuuchi H. Effect of the energy source on changes in energy expenditure, respiratory quotient, and nitrogen balance during total parenteral nutrition in children. *Pediatr Res.* 1987;21:538–541.

34. Burke JF, Wolfe RR, Mullany CJ, Mathews DE, Bier DM. Glucose requirements following burn injury: parameters of optimal glucose infusion and possible hepatic and respiratory abnormalities following excessive glucose intake. *Ann Surg.* 1979;190:274–285.
35. Kalhan SC. Kilic I. Carbohydrate as nutrient in the infant and child: range of acceptable intake. *Europ J Clin Nutr.* 1999;53:S94–S100.
36. Griffin EA, Bryan MH, Angel A. Variations in intralipid tolerance in newborn infants. *Pediatr Res.* 1983;17(6):478–481.
37. Zaidan H. Dhanireddy R. Hamosh M. Pramanik AK. Chowdhry P. Hamosh P Effect of continuous heparin administration on Intralipid clearing in very low-birth-weight infants. *J Pediatr.* 1982;101(4):599–602.
38. Koretz RL, Lipman TO, Klein S. AGA technical review on parenteral nutrition. *Gastroenterology.* 2001;121(4):970–1001.
39. Foote KD, MacKinnon MJ, Innis SM. Effect of early introduction of formula vs fat-free parenteral nutrition on essential fatty acid status of preterm infants. *Am J Clin Nutr.* 1991;54(1):93–97.
40. Meadows N. Monitoring and complications of parenteral nutrition. *Nutrition.* 1998;14(10):806–808.
41. Teitelbaum DH. Parenteral nutrition-associated cholestasis. *Curr Opin Pediatr.* 1997;9:270–275.
42. Borum PR. Should carnitine be added to parenteral nutrition solutions? *Nutr Clin Pract.* 2000;15:153–154.
43. Shulman RJ. Zinc and copper balance studies in infants receiving total parenteral nutrition. *Am J Clin Nutr.* 1989;49(5):879–883.
44. Hardy G. Reilly C. Technical aspects of trace element supplementation. *Curr Opin Clin Nutr Metab Care.* 1999;2:277–285.
45. Fok TF. Chui KK. Cheung R. Ng PC. Cheung KL. Hjelm M.. Manganese intake and cholestatic jaundice in neonates receiving parenteral nutrition: a randomized controlled study. *Acta Paediatr.* 2001;90:1009–1015.
46. Dickerson R. Manganese intoxication and parenteral nutrition. *Nutrition.* 2001;17:689–693.
47. Bertinet DB, Tinivella M, Balzola FA, et al. Brain manganese deposition and blood levels in patients undergoing home parenteral nutrition. *JPEN.* 2000;24:223–227.
48. Fitzgerald K, Mikalunas V, Rubin H, McCarthey R, Vanagunas A, Craig RM. Hypermanganesemia in patients receiving total parenteral nutrition. *JPEN.* 1999;23:333–336.
49. Fuhrman MP, Herrmann V, Masidonski P, Eby C. Pancytopenia after removal of copper from total parenteral nutrition. *JPEN.* 2000;24(6):361–366.
50. Hak EB. Storm MC. Helms RA Chromium and zinc contamination of parenteral nutrient solution components commonly used in infants and children. *Am J Health Syst Pharm.* 1998;55:150–154.
51. Geertsma MA, Hyams JS, Pelletier JM, Reiter S. Feeding resistance after parenteral hyperalimentation. *Am J Dis Child.* 1985;139(3):255–256.
52. Foy T, Czyzewski D, Phillips S, Baldwin J, Klish W. Treatment of severe feeding refusal in infants and toddlers. *Infants and Young Children.* 1997;3(Jan):26–35.
53. Laine L, Shulman RJ, Bartholomew K, Gardner P, Reed T, Cole S. An educational booklet diminishes anxiety in parents whose children receive total parenteral nutrition. *Am J Dis Child.* 1989;143(3):374–347.

Chapter 23

Parenteral Fluids and Electrolytes

Mathew P. Thomas and John N. Udall, Jr.

INTRODUCTION

Both water and electrolytes are essential for life. When disease or functional impairment of the gastrointestinal tract necessitates the use of parenteral nutrition (PN), it is water that constitutes the bulk weight of the PN solution. Water balance in infants and children receiving PN should be evaluated regularly. The administration of excess water with PN can result in edema and/or cardiac failure and insufficient water can lead to dehydration and shock.

Electrolytes are required in PN solutions to provide daily requirements and correct deficits. Standard formulas usually contain sodium, chloride, potassium, calcium, phosphorus, bicarbonate precursors, and magnesium.[1–5]

Both body water and electrolyte concentration can change dramatically in patients receiving PN, and they can fluctuate on a day-by-day basis in a variety of disease states. The decision to use a standard available formulation with maintenance water and electrolytes or an individualized formulation is based on a careful assessment of fluid and electrolyte balance.

FLUIDS

Fluid Requirements

As noted in Figure 23-1, water is the most abundant component of the human body, contributing 80% of the weight of the premature infant, 70% of the weight of the fullterm infant, and approximately 60% of the body weight of an adult.[6] Water is partitioned into two major compartments: intracellular water and extracellular water. The latter has been further subdivided into plasma space, interstitial lymph fluid space, and transcellular fluid space (cerebral spinal fluid, intestinal fluid, and renal fluid). Early in life, as the fetus matures *in utero*, body fat increases and body water decreases. This relationship of body fat and water continues after birth, with the amount of body water varying inversely with the fat content of the body. With increasing body fat, water compromises a smaller percentage of body weight. Individuals with excess body fat, therefore, have less body water as a percentage of total body weight. Because women tend to have more body fat than men, the percentage of their total body weight present as water is generally lower than that of men.

Three methods have been proposed to calculate maintenance fluids: (1) body surface area (1,500–1,700 mL/m^2), (2) body weight, and (3) calories expended (100 mL/100 kcal). Each method has its own pitfalls. Body surface area requires weight and height measurements and the use of a graph to calculate body surface area. This method does not address deviation from normal activity.[7] Requirements based on body weight or the Holliday-Segar formula (Table 23-1) are widely used because of the ease with which the formula can be remembered and applied. This formula also does not

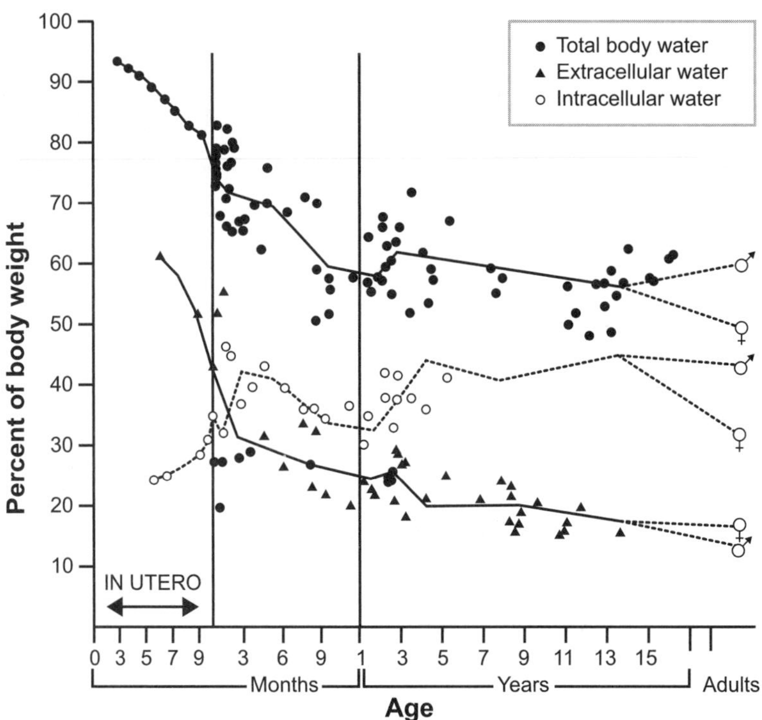

Figure 23-1 Body water compartments as percentages of body weight from early fetal life to adult life. ● total body water; ▲ extracellular water; ○ intracellular water. *Source:* Hill LL. Body composition, normal electrolyte concentrations, and the maintenance of normal volume, tonicity, and acid-base metabolism *Pediatr Clin North Am*, 1990;37:241–256. Reprinted with permission from Elsevier.

address variations in fluid requirements that arise from the variability in normal activity. The third method, estimation of daily fluid needs using the basal calorie method, requires a table, and it yields values slightly lower than the other methods.[7]

Fluid requirements vary with age and disease states.[8] The fluid requirements of hospitalized infants and children are also influenced by hydration status and whether there are gains or losses in body water from environmental factors.[9] Unappreciated gains in body water can occur with the use of incubators or mist tents saturated with water vapor. Other environmental factors, such as radiant warmers, ventilators, and phototherapy, could cause loss of body water. Prematurity or disease states associated with fever, vomiting, diarrhea, or polyuria might increase water requirements, and conditions such as congestive heart failure could limit the need for water. Approximately 40 mL of fluid per 100 calories metabolized is needed to replace insensible loss in 24 hours and 60 mL per 100 calories metabolized is necessary to replace urinary losses. Daily water loss in urine, stool, and insensible loss as a function of age is shown in Table 23-2. Patients who have fever or diarrhea might need adjustments in fluid calculations.[8] Fever increases insensible loss by 5 mL/kg /day for each degree of temperature above 38° C.

Some suggest that PN administered according to the accepted guidelines overhydrates children initially.[10] This premise is based on the observation that there is a rapid weight gain in the first few days of PN therapy and a disproportionate weight loss following the abrupt cessation of therapy. A number of years ago, Coran and his

Table 23-1 Calculation of daily fluid requirement using Holliday-Segar formula.

Body weight	*Amount of fluid per day*
1–10 kg	100 mL/kg
11–20 kg	1,000 mL + 50 mL/kg for each kg > 10 kg
> 20 kg	1,500 mL + 20 mL/kg for each kg > 20 kg

Source: From Boineau FG, Lewy JE. Estimation of parenteral fluid requirements. *Pediatr Clin North Am.* 1990;37:449–459. Reprinted with permission from Elsevier.

collaborators designed a study to explain this observation.[11] Eighteen infants receiving peripheral or central intravenous nutrition following major surgery were studied for periods ranging from 1 to 17 weeks. Total body water was measured using deuterium oxide, and extracellular fluid volume (EFV) was assayed using sodium bromide. Weight gain was noted in all infants. Mean body water as a percentage of total body weight was 82% prior to the initiation of intravenous nutrition in the 18 infants, decreased within the first week to 71%, and then stabilized for the remainder of the study at 75%. Mean extracellular fluid volume as a percentage of body weight was 56% prior to the start of intravenous nutrition, 47% during the first week of PN, and then stabilized at 40%. The authors concluded that during PN, total body water and EFV do not increase but remain unchanged or decrease in spite of weight gain. They suggest that weight gain during intravenous nutrition in infants is due to tissue accretion rather than fluid retention.[11]

Fluids in Special Disease States

On occasion, albumin may be added to PN solutions when the serum albumin concentration is less than 2.5g/dL, in an attempt to increase plasma oncotic pressure and improve fluid dynamics.[12,13] There is no agreement on the use of intravenous albumin in this manner.[14] Koretz reviewed randomized, controlled trials of IV albumin and evaluated clinical outcome in patients receiving PN.[15] He concluded that IV albumin is not effective in improving the clinical outcome of hypoalbuminemic patients who are receiving nutrition support. Expert panels question the efficacy and safety of albumin in critically ill patients with hypovolemia, burns, or hypoalbuminemia.[16] Additionally, the Food and Drug Administration distributed a letter in 1998, urging "... treating physicians to exercise discretion in the use of albumin and plasma protein fraction ..." until the results of further studies are available.[17] Other investigators suggest human albumin supplementation during PN results in significant increases in serum albumin concentration and colloid oncotic pressure. However,

Table 23-2 Maintenance water loss components based on age (mL/kg/d).

Component/age	*0–6 m*	*6 m–5 y*	*5 y–10 y*	*> 10 y*
Insensible	40	30	20	10
Urinary	60	60	50	40
Fecal	20	10	–	–
Total	120	100	70	50

Source: Adapted from Boineau FG, Lewy JE. Estimation of parenteral fluid requirements. *Pediatr Clin North Am.* 1990;37:257–264. Used with permission from Elsevier.

there is no apparent effect on free-water clearance, electrolyte-free water resorption, or sodium excretion.[18] Finally, the University Hospital Consortium published specific guidelines for the use of albumin in a variety of clinical situations.[19]

As noted earlier, some conditions dramatically increase a patient's need for fluid. Patients with jejunostomies or ileostomies could lose liters of fluid from ostomies, making fluid management difficult. Intravenous fluid requirements for these patients often exceed 3 liters per day. One group of investigators studied the effect of the somatostatin analogue, octreotide given subcutaneously on the fluid requirements of 10 patients with jejunostomies who were receiving home PN.[20] They noted that the administration of octreotide permitted an average reduction in intravenous fluid of 1.3 L/day. The authors concluded that octreotide has the potential to "improve the quality of life of jejunostomy patients with massive stomal losses, resistant to conventional medical treatment."[20]

Renal function, which is important in fluid balance, could be compromised in patients receiving long term PN. In one study of 13 children 9 $\pm$ 5 years (mean $\pm$ SD) who received PN for 8 $\pm$ 4 years all had decreased glomerular filtration rates (65.5 $\pm$ 11 mL/min per 1.73 m^2; range 49.5 to 83.7).[21] The children had normal blood pressure, urinary sediment, and serum creatinine concentrations. There was no relationship between the glomerular filtration rate and the diagnosis, number of episodes of infections, or antibiotics used, nor was the decrease in glomerular filtration rate related to underlying disease or the use of nephritic drugs. The duration of PN inversely correlated with the glomerular filtration rate ($r = 0.66$, $p < 0.001$). Long term PN is associated with a decreased glomerular filtration rate.[21] The mechanism is not known.

When calculating the rate at which fluids are given intravenously, the physician must not exceed the fluid rate that the patient can safely tolerate. Careful attention must be paid to the fluid rate when cardiac, pulmonary, renal, or neurologic diseases that might require restricted volumes are present. Serial weights, fluid intake (enteral and parenteral), and fluid output (urine, diarrhea, naso-gastric suction, etc.) need to be monitored closely along with serum electrolyte concentrations to maintain optimal hydration. The frequency of monitoring depends on the patient's health, stability of the disease process, and complicating factors. As a general rule, baseline laboratory tests must be performed within 24 hours of initiating PN. Changes in PN or changes in patient status might also warrant electrolyte monitoring.

ELECTROLYTES

There are at least 25 minerals present in the human body. Minerals, present in ionic form, are categorized as electrolytes. Electrolytes move from one body compartment to another in several ways.[6] One is by diffusion down a concentration gradient from a compartment of higher concentration to a compartment of lower concentration. Diffusion depends to an extent on the permeability of the membrane between the compartments and whether the molecule can diffuse freely across the membrane. Another mechanism by which fluid and electrolyte movement occurs is bulk flow. In this situation, water moves in bulk because of pressure differences across a porous membrane, creating a solvent drag. A third type of movement is by active transport of the electrolyte.[6]

As previously noted, total body water is divided into two compartments: intracellular fluid (ICF) and extracellular fluid (ECF). The fluid in these compartments has an ICF:ECF ratio of 2:1. The intracellular space contains potassium and magnesium as the major cationic components, with phosphates and sulfates as the anions. The plasma portion of the extracellular space has a significant concentration of sodium, chloride, and bicarbonate, with small amounts of potassium, calcium, magnesium, phosphate, sulfate, organic acid, and protein. Interstitial fluid is similar to plasma in electrolyte composition, but lacks significant amounts of protein.

The distribution of sodium and other electrolytes in the intracellular and extracellular spaces adheres to the law of electroneutrality. This law dictates that the total cations and total anions within a particular fluid space must be equal (Figure 23-2). Looking at the balance of cations and anions can be useful in the assessment of water and electrolyte problems and acid-base disturbances, i.e., anion gap metabolic acidosis versus nonion gap acidosis. These formulas are useful when correcting for free-water deficits in hypernatremic dehydration and symptomatic electrolyte disturbances.[22–24]

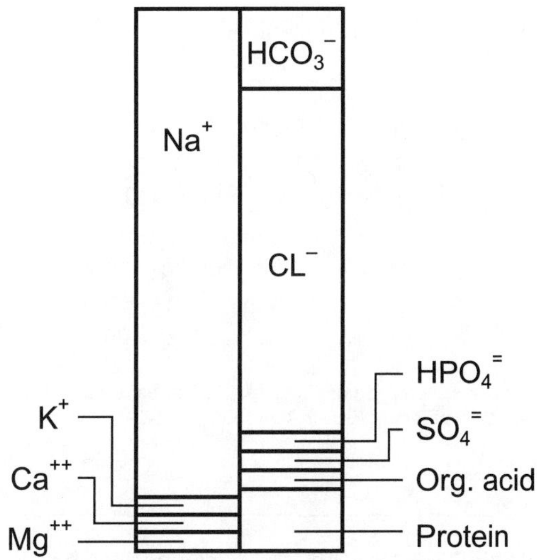

Figure 23-2 Electrolyte composition of plasma demonstrating electrochemical balance; cations equals anions. *Source:* Hill LL. Body composition, normal electrolyte concentrations, and the maintenance of normal volume, tonicity, and acid-base metabolism. *Pediatr Clin North Am.* 1990;37:241–256. Reprinted with permission from Elsevier.

Specific Requirements

The electrolytes important in PN that are discussed in this chapter are sodium, chloride, potassium, calcium, phosphorus, and bicarbonate. The daily intravenous requirements for these electrolytes are shown in Table 23-3. Watkins proposed formulas for the calculation of daily sodium (Table 23-4) and potassium (Table 23-5) based on weight.[25]

Table 23-3 Recommended daily intravenous intake of selected electrolytes.

Nutrient	*Preterm infants (mEq/kg/day)*	*Term infants (mEq/kg/day)*	*Children (mEq/kg/day)*	*Adults (mEq/day)*
Sodium	3–4.6	1.5–4.3	2	30.4
Potassium	2–3.1	1.4–3.1	2	20.5
Chloride	2–3	1.1–3.4	2	56.4
Calcium	1.41–2.35	1.41–1.88	0.47–0.94	0.235–0.47
Phosphates	1.8–2.7	1.8–2.7	1.8	0.9–1.8
Bicarbonate	NSR	NSR	NSR	NSR

NSR = no specific requirement.

Source: Adapted from American Medical Association. Parenteral and enteral nutrition. In: *AMA Drug Evaluations.* Chicago, Ill: American Medical Association; 1995:2307–2362.

Table 23-4 Daily sodium composition by weight.

Body weight	*Amount sodium per day*
1–10 kg	3 mEq/kg
11–20 kg	30 mEq + 1.5 mEq/kg for each kg > 10 kg
> 20 kg	45 mEq + 0.6m Eq/kg for each kg > 20 kg

Source: Adapted from Watkins SL. The basis of fluid and electrolyte therapy. *Pediatr Ann.* 1995;24:16–22.

Table 23-5 Daily potassium composition by weight.

Body weight	*Amount potassium per day*
1–10 kg	2 mEq/kg
11–20 kg	20 mEq + 1 mEq/kg for each kg > 10kg
> 20 kg	30 mEq + 0.4 mEq/kg for each kg > 20 kg

Source: Adapted from Watkins SL. The basis of fluid and electrolyte therapy. *Pediatr Ann.* 1995;24:16–22.

Sodium

Sodium is the major cation of ECF, and it functions principally in the control of water distribution and the osmotic pressure of body fluids. Sodium is provided in PN as a chloride, acetate, or phosphate salt. Chloride, acetate, and bicarbonate are important in acid-base balance.[26] The normal sodium requirement as shown in Table 23-3 is 1.5–4.6 mEq/kg/day.[27] The daily sodium intake ranges from 5% of the total body sodium stores in adults to 25% of total body sodium stores per day in extremely premature infants. Very-low-birth-weight (VLBW) infants require increased sodium because of poor renal sodium reabsorption. Infants with congestive heart failure, acute renal failure, or chronic diuretic therapy may need close monitoring of sodium intake. This cation is lost from the body primarily in urine, sweat, and stool.

Regulation of sodium balance and extracellular fluid is maintained by osmoreceptors in the supraoptic and paraventricular nuclei of the hypothalamus. As the concentration of plasma sodium increases, release of vasopressin or antidiuretic hormone (ADH) from the neurohypophysis occurs. In the kidney, ADH reduces excretion of solute-free water and increases water reabsorption, concentrating urine. When ADH is absent, urinary dilution occurs. Regulation of plasma osmolality is precise. The osmolality of a solution is the measure of the total number of particles in that solution. Under most conditions, the principal determinants of serum osmolaltiy are sodium (and its accompanying anions), glucose, and urea. An increase in osmolality of 1% leads to stimulation of thirst and ADH release. There are a number of clinically important stimuli of ADH release including physical injury, emotional stress, hypoxia, liver disease, adrenal insufficiency, cardiac failure, and most important, volume depletion.[28]

The problems of sodium imbalance that could occur in patients receiving PN are illustrated in the following report.[29] A 23-year-old man whose left leg was amputated following a motorcycle accident developed a postoperative ileus and sepsis. He was given antimicrobials administered in 5% dextrose (currently most hospitals use normal saline). This contributed 3 liters of free water to his fluid intake each day. With overhydration he developed rapid weight gain and edema of the lower extremity. He became hyponatremic, and the sodium content of the PN solution was increased to 140 mEq/L. Multiple doses of furosemide and albumin were administered, and fluids were restricted. Marked diuresis occurred; he lost 16 pounds and became hypernatremic. The furosemide was discontinued, and the content of sodium in the PN solution was decreased and finally eliminated. The authors conclude that several factors predisposed their patient to hyponatremia and then hypernatremia. First, the estimation of fluid and electrolyte requirement was complicated by the patient's loss of a significant amount of body weight when the left leg was amputated. Second, in the postsurgical period, the patient's hyponatremia was caused by the overzealous administration of large amounts of sodium-free fluid. The subsequent hypernatremia was explained by aggressive diuretic therapy and restriction of fluids. The report points out that the focus of the physician, in regard to PN fluid and electrolyte management, is often only on the volume and the electrolyte content of the PN solution. Free-water, sodium, and electrolytes can be administered by other means, including medication admixtures and supplemental intravenous fluids. These additional solutions and admixtures must be calculated as part of the total fluid and electrolyte therapy a patient receives.

The amount of sodium and other selected electrolytes found in standard PN solutions is shown in Table 23-6.[30,31] It is important to remember that excessive losses of sodium could occur in patients with vomiting, diarrhea, ostomies, glucosuria, or cystic fibrosis and in patients with renal or endocrine diseases. These losses should be replaced using separate intravenous lines.

Chloride

Chloride, the major extracellular anion, closely follows the physiologic disposition of sodium. Changes in acid-base balance are reflected by changes in serum chloride concentration. Chloride is essential to normal growth and development. This is underscored by the tragic story of infants who years ago developed metabolic alkalosis when fed a commercially available formula deficient in chloride.[32] When tested later, these children tended to weigh less than controls and scored lower on verbal, performance, and full-scale IQ tests.

Chloride excess can be detrimental. This situation was described in the early days of PN therapy. In one report, hyperchloremic metabolic acidosis was observed in 11 infants receiving PN containing mixtures of synthetic L-amino acids.[33] The observed acidosis was not caused by excessive gastrointestinal or renal loss of base, or the infusion of preformed excess hydrogen ion. Instead, it was secondary to PN mixtures that contained an excess of cationic amino acids (chloride salt of the amino acid) in relation to anionic amino acids. Metabolism of the cationic amino acids resulted in a net excess of hydrogen ion, explaining the observed acidosis.[33] Table 23-6 lists the recommendation for chloride in PN.

In another study, metabolic acidosis was noted in a large number of low birth weight infants receiving PN.[34] In this study, the newborns with higher chloride intakes had significantly increased serum chloride levels. PN fed infants received approximately 1–3 mEq/kg/day of chloride from intravenous and arterial lines flushed with normal saline. The total intravenous chloride load (flushes plus PN) was in excess of 6 mEq/kg/day. The authors concluded that if saline is used for intravenous and arterial line flushes, standard PN solutions should be reformatted with consideration of the total chloride load that would include the chloride in intravenous flushes.[34]

In an additional study, routine biochemical monitoring of parenterally fed newborn infants revealed plasma chloride levels higher than a widely quoted reference range.[35] The PN solutions were reformulated to reduce the chloride load using acetate salts instead of chloride salts. The authors then noted a decrease in plasma chloride and a decrease in acidosis during the

Table 23-6 Selected electrolyte concentrations used in parenteral nutrition.

Electrolyte	*Standard PN concentration (nonneonatal)*
Sodium	30–35 mEq/L
Chloride	30–35 mEq/L
Potassium	25–30 mEq/L
Acetate	10–67 mEq/L

Source: Zlotkin SH, Stallings, VA, Pencharz PB. Total parenteral nutrition in children. *Pediatr Clin North Am.* 1985;32:381–386. Reprinted with permission from Elsevier.

first 7 days of life.[35] These studies underscore the importance of accounting for not only the chloride provided in PN solutions but also the chloride present in intravenous flushes and medications.

Potassium

Potassium is the major cation of intracellular fluid and is essential in a variety of cell functions: control of cell volume and acid-base balance, isotonicity, DNA and protein synthesis, and maintenance of the electrical properties of cell membranes.[26] The intracellular concentration of potassium is 150–160 mEq/L and the extracellular concentration is 3–5 mEq/L. The large transcellular gradient is maintained by the Na-K adenosine triphosphate (ATPase) system, which pumps potassium into cells and sodium out of cells in a ratio of three sodium ions for every two potassium ions. There are approximately 50–60 mEq (2%) of potassium in ECF and 3,500 mEq (98%) in ICF.[36] Therefore, small shifts in cellular potassium can result in large changes in the measured intravascular potassium concentration. Muscle tissue is the major site of ICF potassium, and total body potassium and lean body mass are closely correlated. Hence, total body potassium is less in females compared to males since their lean body mass is less. If potassium is omitted from PN solutions used in the treatment of malnourished individuals, both negative potassium balance and negative nitrogen balance occurs.[37]

The concentration of potassium in standard PN solutions is shown in Table 23-6. The normal requirement of potassium is 2–3 mEq/kg/day. Potassium is available as chloride, phosphate, and acetate salts.[27] The amount of potassium might have to be altered if hypokalemia or hyperkalemia is present. During potassium deficiency, the decreased extracellular potassium results in an increase in the electronegativity across the cell membrane and hyperpolarization of the cell. This renders the attainment of threshold potential more difficult and explains the muscle weakness and paralytic ileus that accompany potassium deficiency. In potassium excess, there is an increase in extracellular potassium concentration, and this deceases the electronegativity across the membrane, thus rendering the cell hyperexcitable; the cell depolarizes more easily. If hyperkalemia is severe, the equilibrium potential might exceed the threshold potential and render the cell unable to return to its resting potential. This results in severe muscle weakness and diastolic arrest of the heart, a well-known consequence of hyperkalemia.

To avoid these serious complications of potassium imbalances, the potassium in PN solutions and in the vascular compartment should be monitored at appropriate intervals depending on the clinical state of the patient. The clinician should also keep in mind that serum potassium concentrations are influenced by shifts in acid-base balance. Changes in arterial pH affect the plasma potassium concentration.[38,39] In the acidotic state, hydrogen ion enters the cell and compels potassium to exit the cell to preserve electrical neutrality. For every decrease of 0.1U of pH, there is an estimated increase of serum potassium of 0.6 mEq/L. Hyperkalemia occurs in acidosis and hypokalemia in alkalosis.

Calcium and Phosphorus

Calcium and phosphorus are essential micronutrients for bone health. In PN, the concern is how to deliver adequate amounts of calcium and phosphorus without precipitation. See Chapters 25 and 27.

Calcium is predominantly an extracellular cation. In healthy adults, calcium comprises about 2% or 1,300 gm of body weight. At birth, calcium accounts for 0.9% of body weight. Most calcium is found in the skeleton (99%), the remainder is in the teeth, soft tissue, and extracellular fluid. Extracellular calcium exists in 3 forms: 40–45% protein bound (primarily albumin), 8–10% complexed as sulfate or phosphate salts, and about 45–50% in an unbound and physiologically active form.[40] During rapid growth, children need net calcium retention of 150–200 mg of calcium per day, whereas in adults, the net balance is zero.

Children have much higher requirements for calcium and phosphorus than adults when expressed as mg/kg/day (Table 23-7). The protein matrix of bone, referred to as osteoid, is mineralized with calcium and phosphorus. The mineralization process is regulated by many factors, including parathyroid hormone, vitamin D, calcium, magnesium, and phosphorus. Any disturbance in this process leads to the development of metabolic bone disease[41] (see Chapter 25). Evidence of metabolic bone disease includes hypercalciuria, hypercalcemia, hyperphosphatemia, and elevated serum alkaline phosphatase levels. Premature infants without adequate calcium supplementation develop rickets and fractures. In neonates, hypocalcemia could be due to hypercalciuria. The decreased plasma calcium could be associated with increased plasma phosphate. In patients with hypophosphatemia, supplementation of phosphate results in decreased calciuria and increased calcium retention.[42]

Phosphorus is a critically important element in every cell of the body. Approximately 85% of body phosphorus is in the skeleton and teeth, 14% is in soft tissue, and the remainder is in extracellular fluid. In infants and children, phosphorus balance, as with calcium, must be positive to meet the demands of skeletal growth. Phosphorus plays an important role in protein phosphorylation, nucleotide and phospholipid metabolism, and adenosine triphosphate (ATP) formation. Plasma membranes require phosphorus as a component of phospholipids. Phosphorus in the diet and in PN usually exists as potassium or sodium salt.

To meet the daily requirement of calcium and phosphorus in children, amounts of the minerals in PN could approach a critical concentration at which precipitation occurs. This PN complication can be minimized by keeping the product of these 2 ions (Ca × P) less than 300 in the PN solution. This is especially critical when patient fluid volume is restricted. Another rule of thumb is that precipitation could form in tubing if twice the calcium (mEq/L) plus the phosphate (mM/L) exceeds 50.

Many factors affect the solubility of calcium and phosphate in PN solutions, including concentration of calcium and phosphate, salt form of the calcium, concentration of amino acids, type of amino acid solution, concentration of dextrose, addition of cysteine (affects pH), temperature of solution, final pH, order of addition of calcium and phosphate to the PN solution, and agitation and time.[43,44]

Table 23-7 Adequate intake for calcium by age group.

Age group (years)	*Calcium intake (mg/day)*
0–0.5	210
0.5–1.0	270
1–3	500
4–8	800
9–13	1,300
14–18	1,300

Source: Institute of Medicine. *Dietary Reference Intakes for Calcium, Phosphorus, Magnesium, Vitamin D and Fluoride.* Washington, DC: National Academies Press; 1997.

Bicarbonate

There is no specific requirement for bicarbonate. The organic ions acetate, gluconate, lactate, and citrate are hydrogen ion acceptors and contribute bicarbonate equivalents during their metabolism. A decrease in plasma bicarbonate concentration results in metabolic acidosis. Acetate is most commonly used in PN solutions to prevent acidosis. When metabolized, acetate produces hydroxyl radicals, which increase the base excess if there is no disease that interferes with normal acetate metabolism.[26] The inherent acidity of PN solutions can be neutralized in part by the addition of acetate. As noted earlier, one group of investigators reformulated the anionic constituents of their PN solutions because the excess chloride load led to increased metabolic acidosis.[35] By reducing the chloride and increasing the acetate, phosphate, and gluconate concentration of PN solution, they were able to increase the plasma bicarbonate level from 21.7 to 25.3 mM/L, the pH from 7.31 to 7.35, and the base excess from –2.96 to 0.99.[35] Acetate may be added to PN solutions as sodium acetate or potassium acetate (Table 23-6).

An amino acid that has been shown to increase the need for acetate in the PN is cysteine. Cysteine, a conditionally essential amino acid for the neonate, is useful for enhancing calcium and phosphate solubility in PN solutions. Newborn infants receiving PN solutions to which cysteine HCL is added have lower carbon dioxide levels than newborns who received PN solutions without cysteine.[45] When cysteine is present in PN in appreciable amounts, an alkalizing agent such as acetate should be added to the PN.

Acetate does not precipitate with the calcium in PN solutions, whereas bicarbonate and chloride salts do precipitate. This is an added advantage of the use of sodium acetate and potassium acetate instead of the chloride salts.

STABILITY OF PN SOLUTIONS

Electrolytes and acetate influence pH, and, in turn, the stability of PN solution. Precipitation occurs when concentrations of calcium, phosphate, and minerals are not appropriate. In general, divalent ions (calcium, phosphate, and bicarbonate) form precipitates more readily than do monovalent ions. Monovalent ions, such as sodium, potassium, and chloride, rarely cause solubility problems. As noted previously, bicarbonate precursors can be given in the form of acetate to avoid precipitation. The acetate salts are both soluble and stable in PN solutions.

In order to minimize precipitation, PN solutions should be compounded as follows: patient-specific amounts of dextrose, amino acids, and sterile water for injection should be transferred into appropriate vinyl acetate bags, thereafter, additives should be introduced with electrolytes being added first, with the phosphate preceding the calcium. Vitamins should be added last.[46] Although total nutritional admixtures (TNAs: amino acids, carbohydrate, and lipids) have been used in pediatric patients, an FDA safety alert reported two deaths and at least two cases of respiratory distress that developed during peripheral infusion of TNAs.[47] The FDA notes that PN solutions "are made according to a variety of formulations and compounding protocols" and precipitation could occur, especially in TNAs. The FDA recommends visual inspection of PN solutions for turbidity before they leave the pharmacy and again at the bedside, immediately prior to infusion.[47]

CONCLUSION

Careful daily determination of fluid status using daily weights and accurate estimates of fluid intake and output are essential for good management of PN fed infants. Electrolyte monitoring is essential to avoid electrolyte imbalance. The requirements for fluid and electrolytes could vary with age and disease state. Thus, frequent monitoring of fluid and plasma electrolyte concentration and appropriate reformulation of the PN solution is necessary to maintain normal plasma electrolyte concentration in infants and children receiving PN.

REFERENCES

1. Bass DM, Udall JN Jr. Parenteral nutrition. In: Ichikawas I, ed. *Pediatric Textbook of Fluids and Electrolytes.* Baltimore, Md: Williams & Wilkins; 1990:469.
2. Arnold WC. Parenteral nutrition, and fluid and electrolyte therapy. *Pediatr Clin North Am.* 1990;37:449–459.
3. MacFarlane K, Bullock L, Fitzgerald JF. A usage evaluation of total parenteral nutrition in pediatric patients. *JPEN.* 1991;15:85–88.
4. Taylor L, O'Neill JA. Total parenteral nutrition in the pediatric patient. *Surg Clin North Am.* 1991;71:477–488.
5. Zlotkin SH, Stallings VA, Pencharz PB. Total parenteral nutrition in children. *Pediatr Clin North Am.* 1985;32:381–396.
6. Hill LL. Body composition, normal electrolyte concentrations, and the maintenance of normal volume, tonicity, and acid-base metabolism. *Pediatr Clin North Am.* 1990;37(2):241–256.
7. Roberts KB. Fluid and electrolytes: parenteral fluid therapy. *Pediatr Rev.* 2001;22(11):380–386.
8. Seigel NJ, Carpenter T, Gaudio KM. The pathophysiology of body fluids. In: Oski FA, ed. *Principles of practice of pediatrics.* 2nd ed. Philadelphia, Pa: J.B. Lippincott Company; 1994:64–79.

9. El-dahr SS, Chevalier RL. Special needs of the newborn infant in fluid therapy. *Pediatr Clin North Am.* 1990;37:323–332.
10. Heird WC, Driscoll JM Jr, Schullinger JN, Grebin B, Winters RW Intravenous alimentation in pediatric patients. *J Pediatr.* 1972;80(3):351–372.
11. Coran AG, Drongowski RA, Wesley JR. Changes in total body water and extracellular fluid volume in infants receiving total parenteral nutrition. *J Pediatr Surg.* 1984;19(6):771–776.
12. Mirtallo JM, Schneider PJ, Ruberg RL. Albumin in TPN solutions: potential savings from a prospective review. *JPEN.* 1980;4(3):300–302.
13. Brown RO, Bradley JE, Bekemeyer WB, Luther RW. Effect of albumin supplementation during parenteral nutrition on hospital morbidity. *Crit Care Med.* 1988;16:1177–1182.
14. DeGaudio AR. Therapeutic use of albumin. *Int J Artif Organs.* 1995;18:216–224.
15. Koretz RL. Intravenous albumin and nutrition support: going for the quick fix. *JPEN.* 1995;19:166–171.
16. Cochrane Injuries Group Albumin Reviewers. Human albumin administration in critically ill patients: systematic review of randomized controlled trials. *Br Med J.* 1998;317:235–240.
17. US Food and Drug Administration. Letter to Healthcare Providers, 1998. Available at: http://www.fda.gov/CBER/LTR/ALUBMIN.HTM. Accessed January 11, 2006.
18. Wojtysiak SL, Brown RO, Roberson D, Powers DA, Kudsk KA. Effect of hypoalbuminemia and parenteral nutrition on free water excretion and electrolyte-free water resorption. *Crit Care Med.* 1992;20:164–169.
19. Vermeulen LC, Ratko TA, Erstad BL, Brecher MF, Matuszewski KA. A paradigm for consensus: the University Hospital Consortium guidelines for the use of albumin, nonprotein colloid, and crystalloid solutions. *Arch Intern Med.* 1995;155:373–379.
20. O'Keefe SJ, Peterson ME, Flemning CR. Octreotide as an adjunct to home parenteral nutrition in management of permanent end-jejunostomy syndrome. *JPEN.* 1994;18(1):26–34.
21. Moukarzel AA, Ament ME, Buchman A, Dahlstrom KA, Vargas J. Renal function of children receiving long-term parenteral nutrition. *J Pediatr.* 1991;119:864–874.
22. Shils ME, Brown RO. Parenteral nutrition. In: Shils ME, Olson JA, Shike M, Ross AC, eds. *Modern Nutrition in Health and Disease.* 9th ed. Baltimore, Md: Williams and Wilkins; 1999:1657–1688.
23. Fluid and electrolytes. In: Foulkes D, ed. *The Harriet Lane Handbook.* 16th ed. St. Louis, Mo: Mosby; 2002:233.
24. American Medical Association. Parenteral and enteral nutrition. In: *AMA Drug Evaluations.* Chicago, Ill: American Medical Association; 1995:2307–2362.
25. Watkins SL. The basis of fluid and electrolyte therapy. *Pediatr Ann.* 1995;24:16–22.
26. Electrolyte solutions. In: Mary J. Reilly, Judith A. Kepler, eds. *American Hospital Formulary Service: Drug Information.* Bethesda, Md: American Society Of Hospital Pharmacists; 2003:pp 2467–2508.
27. Collier SB, Richardson DS, Gura KM, Duggan C. Parenteral nutrition. In: Hendricks KC, Duggan C, Walker WA, eds. *Manual of Pediatric Nutrition.* 3rd ed. Hamilton, Ontario; BC Decker; 2000:82.
28. Avner ED. Clinical disorders of water metabolism: hyponatremia and hypertnatremia. *Pediatr Ann.* 1995;24(1):23–30.
29. Sunyecz L, Mirtallo JM. Sodium imbalance in a patient receiving total parenteral nutrition. *Clin Pharm.* 1993;12(2):138–149.
30. Mourkarzel AA, Ament ME. Home parenteral nutrition in infants and children. In: Rombeau J, ed. *Clinical Nutrition: Parenteral Nutrition.* Philadelphia, Pa: W.B. Saunders; 1993:791–813.
31. Heird WC, Hay W, Helms RA, Storm MC, Kaskyap S, Dell RB. Pediatric parenteral amino acid mixture in low birth weight infants. *Pediatrics.* 1988;81:41–50.
32. Malloy MH. The follow-up of infants exposed to chloride-deficient formulas. *Adv Pediatr.* 1993;40:141–158.
33. Heird WC, Dell RB, Driscoll JM, Grebin B, Winters RW. Metabolic acidosis resulting from alimentation mixtures containing synthetic amino acids. *N Engl J Med.* 1972;287:843–948.
34. Groh-Wargo S, Ciasccia A, Moore J. Neonatal metabolic acidosis: effect of chloride from normal saline flushes. *JPEN.* 1988;12(2):159–161.
35. Richards CE, Drayton A, Jenkins H, Peters TJ. Effect of different chloride infusion rates on plasma base excess during neonatal parenteral nutrition. *Acta Paediatr.* 1993;82(8):678–682.
36. Aizman R, Granquist L, Celsi G. Potassium homeostasis: ontogenic aspects. *Acta Paediatr.* 1998;87:609–617.
37. Rudman D, Millikan WJ, Richardson TJ, Bixter TJ, Stackhouse WJ, McGarrity WC. Elemental balances during intravenous hyperalimentation of underweight adult subjects. *J Clin Invest.* 1975;55(1):94–104.
38. Mandal AK. Hypokalemia and hyperkalemia. *Med Clin North Am.* 1997;81:611–639.
39. Cohn JN, Kowey PR, Whelton PK, Prisant LM. New guidelines for potassium replacement in clinical practice: a contemporary review by the National Council on Potassium in Clinical Practice. *Arch Intern Med.* 2000;160:2429–2436.
40. Weaver CM, Heaney RP. Calcium. In: Shils ME, Olson JA, Shike M, Ross AC, eds. *Modern Nutrition in Health and Disease.* 9th ed. Baltimore, Md: Williams and Wilkins; 1999:141–155.

41. Seidner DL, Licata A. Parenteral nutrition associated metabolic bone disease: pathophysiology evaluation and treatment. *Nutr Clin Pract.* 2000;15:163–170.
42. ASPEN Board of Directors. Guidelines for the use of parenteral and enteral nutrition in adult and pediatric patients. *JPEN.* 2002;26:1SA–138SA.
43. Mascarenhas MR, Kerner JA, Stallings VA. Parenteral and enteral nutrition. In: Walker WA, Durries PR, Hamilton JR, Walker-Smith JA, Watkins JB, eds. *Pediatric Gastrointestinal Disease.* 3rd ed. Hamilton, Ontario: B.C. Decker, Inc; 2000:1705–1752.
44. Sacks SG, Canada T. New strategies in specialized nutrition support. *Hosp Pharm Rep.* June 1997;42–51.
45. Line L, Schulman RJ, Pitter D, Leftists CH, Adams J. Cysteine usage increases the need for acetate in neonates who receive total parenteral nutrition. *Am J Clin Nutr.* 1991;54(3):565–567.
46. Rollins CJ, Elsberry VA, Pollack KA, Pollack PF, Udall JN Jr. Three-in-one parenteral nutrition: a safe and economical method of nutritional support for infants. *JPEN.* 1990;14(3):290–294.
47. US Food and Drug Administration. *FDA Safety Alert: Hazards of Precipitation Associated with Parenteral Nutrition.* Washington, DC: Department of Health & Human Services; April 18, 1994.

CHAPTER 24

Macronutrients

Susan S. Baker and Robert D. Baker

INTRODUCTION

The macronutrients, proteins, fats, and carbohydrates are essential under all conditions. This chapter provides a general review of the functions, requirements, special uses, and monitoring tools for each of the macronutrients.

PROTEIN

Proteins are essential for all metabolic functions and serve as the main structural elements of the body, as biochemical catalysts, and as regulators of gene expression. Proteins are complex, and their function is influenced by the availability of energy and nutrients such as minerals, vitamins, and trace elements. The average content of nitrogen in dietary protein is 16% by weight, and nitrogen metabolism is often considered synonymous with protein metabolism. Proteins consist of amino acids that have been categorized as essential (or indispensable) and nonessential (or dispensable). The nine essential amino acids, histidine, isoleucine, leucine, lysine, methionine, phenylalanine, threonine, tryptophan, and valine, are those that cannot be synthesized from precursors and hence must be provided in the diet. However, as more information on protein and intermediary metabolism becomes available, the definition of essential becomes blurred. Laidlaw and Kopple propose adding a third category of amino acid, conditionally indispensable, or conditionally essential.[1] Conditionally essential amino acids are those amino acids that are synthesized from other amino acids; however, their synthesis is limited and under special physiological conditions, might not meet requirements.[1] These amino acids can be especially important in the neonate, for whom it is likely that alanine, aspartate, glutamate, serine, and perhaps asparagine are conditionally indispensable.[2]

Unlike energy and other nutrients, the body has little in the way of protein reserves that can be mobilized during times of insufficient intake. In a 70 kg adult, the reservoir of labile protein is estimated at about 1% of total body protein. More than half of the body protein is present as skeletal muscle, skin, and blood. The liver and kidneys are metabolically active tissues that contain about 10% of total body protein. Brain, heart, lung, and bone account for about 15% of whole body protein. The distribution of protein among these organs varies with age; the newborn has proportionately more brain and visceral tissue and less muscle than at any other time of life. When exogenous protein is inadequate, functional body proteins are used. The body can adapt to a wide range of protein intakes; however, pathologic conditions such as infection or trauma can cause substantial protein loss as demand for amino acids increases or as amino acid carbon skeletons are used to meet energy demands. If these extra needs are not met, a serious depletion of body protein mass occurs. Skeletal muscle is the largest single contributor to protein loss.

The establishing of protein requirements is based on the assumptions that adequate energy is provided so the carbon skeletons of amino acids are not needed as an energy source and the protein quality is high. Table 24-1 lists estimates of protein requirements by age. Protein quality is determined by digestibility, not a factor in parenteral nutrition (PN), and the indispensable amino acid composition of the protein. If the content of a single indispensable amino acid is less than the requirement, that amino acid limits the utilization of other amino acids, preventing normal rates of protein synthesis even when the total nitrogen is adequate. Proposed amino acid requirements of the nine indispensable amino acids for infants, based on the amino acid composition of human milk, children, and adults have been reviewed.[3] Data exists, however, to suggest that histidine is conditionally essential for infants to 6 months of age[4] and cysteine is conditionally essential in low birth weight infants.[5] Table 24-2 lists examples of the amino acid composition of some parenteral solutions. Enteral products contain complete proteins so that requirements are met if a specified volume is consumed.

The most reliable method to assess the adequacy of dietary protein, enteral or parenteral, is nitrogen balance—the difference between nitrogen intake and the amount excreted in urine, feces, skin, and sweat (see Chapter 7 and Table 29-3). This measurement is not practical clinically, especially for children. There is no reliable clinical measure of protein status. In infants and children, failure to gain weight or length can be used to assess the overall nutritional adequacy of a diet, and failure to gain length occurs with

Table 24-1 Estimates of protein requirements by age.

Age	*IOM recommendations (g/kg/day)**	*RDA (g/kg/day)†*	*Estimate for healthy patients (g/kg/day)‡*
Low birth weight	None	None	3–4
Fullterm–6 mo	1.52 (AI)§	1.52	2–3
7–12 mo	1.1 (EAR)**	1.5	2–3
1–3 years	0.88	1.1	1–1.2
4–8 years	0.76	0.95	1–1.2
Adolescence			
Boys	0.76	0.76	0.9
Girls	0.76	0.76	0.8
Critically ill	None	None	1.5

* Adapted from Institute of Medicine. *Dietary Reference Intakes for Energy, Carbohydrates, Fiber, Fat, Fatty Acids, Cholesterol, Protein, and Amino Acids.* Washington, DC: National Academies Press; 2002/2005.

† Adapted from Shulman RJ, Phillips S. Parenteral nutrition in infants and children. *J Pediatr Gastroenterol Nutr.* 2003;36:587–607.

‡ Adapted from ASPEN Board of Directors and the Clinical Guidelines Task Force. Guidelines for the use of parenteral and enteral nutrition in adult and pediatric patients. *JPEN.* 2002;26(suppl 1):1SA-138SA.

§ AI = adequate intake, a recommended average daily nutrient intake level based on observed or experimentally determined approximations or estimates of nutrient intake by a group (or groups) of apparently healthy people that are assumed to be adequate—used when an RDA cannot be determined.

**EAR = estimated average requirement, the average daily nutrient intake level estimated to meet the requirement of half the healthy individuals in a particular life stage and gender group.

Source for § and **: Subcommittee on the Tenth Edition of the RDAs, Food and Nutrition Board. *Recommended Dietary Allowances.* Washington, DC: National Academy Press; 1989.

Table 24-2 Amino acid composition of commonly available parenteral solutions.

	Product (vendor)					
	For infants less than 1 year		*For children older than 1 year through adulthood*			
	TrophAmine (B. Braun)	*Aminosyn-PF (Abbott)*	*Aminosyn-HBC (Abbott)*	*Aminosyn-II (Abbott)*	*Travasol (Baxter)*	*Novamine (Baxter)*
Total nitrogen (g/L of a 10% solution)	15.5	15.2	16	15.3	16.5	23.9
Protein equivalent (approximate g/L of a 10% solution)	97	100	100	100	100	100
PH (range)	5.5 (5.0–6.0)	5.0 (5.0–6.5)	5.2 (4.5–6.0)	5.8 (5.0–6.5)	6.0 (5.0–7.0)	5.6 (5.2–6.0)
Essential amino acids, mg/100 mL of a 10% solution						
Isoleucine	820	760	1,127	660	600	500
Leucine	1,400	1,200	2,251	1,000	730	693
Lysine	820	677	378	1,050	580	787
Methionine	340	180	294	172	400	500
Phenylalanine	480	427	325	298	580	693
Threonine	420	512	388	400	420	500
Tryptophan	200	180	126	200	180	167
Valine	780	673	1127	500	580	640
Nonessential amino acids, mg/100 mL of a 10% solution						
Alanine	540	698	943	993	2,070	1,447
Arginine	1,200	1,227	717	1,018	1,150	980
Aspartic acid	320	527	–	700	–	289
Glutamic acid	500	820	–	738	–	500
Glycine	360	385	943	500	1,030	693
Histidine	480	312	220	300	560	596
Proline	680	812	640	722	680	596
Serine	380	495	316	530	500	667
Taurine	25	70	–	–	–	–
Tyrosine	240	44	47	270	40	26

Source: Manufacturers' product information, February 2005.

borderline inadequate protein intake.[6] Other anthropometrics are less sensitive. The most commonly used clinical tools to assess protein status are albumin and prealbumin.

Most individuals can tolerate a wide range of protein intakes. Fomon reviewed adverse outcomes with increased protein intakes in healthy formula and breastfed infants.[7] Diets high in protein were associated with an increase in renal solute load, a potential safety concern for water balance in the infant. Transient tyrosinemia as a consequence of delay in maturation of p-hydroxyphenylpyruvic acid oxidase can occur. The elevated levels can last as long as 6 weeks, raising a concern for long term sequelae.

High protein diets can alter the serum amino acid profile. The significance of this in infants and children who are already ill and could have an abnormal profile secondary to the primary disease is not known. The tolerable upper limit in healthy populations for individual amino acids is estimated in a report by the Institute of Medicine.[3] The report cautions, however, that the studies might not have carefully monitored for adverse outcomes.

Specialized dietary amino acids, enteral or parenteral, have been proposed for a variety of clinical situations, including trauma, liver failure, metabolic stress, improvement of immune function, and others. Branched-chain enriched preparations, glutamine enhanced solutions, and a solution specially designed for infants are most commonly used.

The term immunonutrition refers to the use of specific nutrients, arginine, glutamine, nucleotides and omega-3 fatty acids alone or in combination to influence nutritional, immunologic, and inflammatory parameters in the laboratory and in clinical studies. The use of immunonutrition was systematically reviewed.[8] The primary outcomes of interest were mortality and number of patients with new infectious complications. In the 22 papers that met the inclusion criteria, the reviewers found no consistently used standard definition of what constitutes immunonutrition. Pneumonia, intra-abdominal abscess, sepsis, line sepsis, wound infection and urinary tract infections were identified as primary adverse outcomes. Secondary outcomes included length of hospital and intensive care unit stays and duration of mechanical ventilation. From this review, the authors concluded that immunonutrition might decrease infectious complication rates, but the treatment effect varies depending on the patient population, the intervention, and the quality of the study. In surgical patients, immunonutrition was associated with a reduction in infectious complication rates and shorter length of hospital stay without adverse effects on mortality. In critically ill patients, immunonutrition was not associated with any apparent clinical benefit and could be harmful in some subgroups of patients. Thus, immunonutrition is not recommended for all critically ill patients.

Protein energy malnutrition is common in patients with liver disease. As the liver disease progresses and encephalopathy ensues, branched-chain enriched parenteral solutions could offer benefits.[9] However, strong clinical studies have not been performed to support the use of branched-chain enriched parenteral solutions in all patients with liver disease.[10] Branched-chain enriched amino acid solutions can offer benefits for patients who have hepatic encephalopathy, and these solutions are recommended for such patients.[11–13]

The use of glutamine was systematically reviewed.[14] Fourteen randomized trials compared the use of glutamine supplementation in surgical and critically ill patients. The review concluded that in surgical patients, glutamine supplementation (doses > 0.20 g/kg/day) could be associated with a reduction in infectious complication rates and shorter hospital stay. In critically ill patients, glutamine supplementation could be associated with a reduction in complications and mortality rates. The authors caution, however, that further, separate studies of the surgical and critically ill groups need to be performed, and they must be powered large enough to detect clinically important differences using parenterally delivered glutamine. There was no evidence of harm with glutamine supplementation.

Two amino acid solutions are specifically designed for infants less than 1 year of age. Use of these solutions results in plasma amino acid concentrations that approximate the profile seen in breastfed infants. The difference between these two solutions and others is that they contain taurine, glutamate, and aspartate; reduced amounts of methionine, glycine, and alanine; and increased arginine and leucine. Although there are differences between the two solutions, both have shown benefits in term and preterm infants.[15–17] There appears to be no difference in occurrence or magnitude of cholestasis between children who receive either of the two solutions.[18] Use of these solutions is recommended for infants less than 1 year of age. In addition to the differing amino acid composition, these solutions are more acidic and permit the solubilization of a higher concentration of calcium and phosphorus than the amino acid mixtures prepared for adults.

Enteral formulas are fed to infants less than a year of age if a mother chooses not to breastfeed, if a medical contraindication to breastfeeding exists, or an infant fails to thrive on human milk. For infants born prematurely, human milk is inadequate as a sole food but has a role in promoting the health and development of these infants. The protein sources in enteral formulas include cow milk, soy proteins, hydrolyzed cow milk proteins, and mixtures of single amino acids.

CARBOHYDRATES

Carbohydrates are polyhydroxy aldehydes or ketones or their derivatives, and they serve as an energy source. Monosaccharides or simple sugars such as glucose, fructose, mannose, galactose, ribulose, or xylose cannot be hydrolyzed into simpler compounds. Reducing sugars are alcohol forms of glucose and fructose such as sorbitol and mannitol, respectively. Disaccharidases such as sucrose, lactose, isomaltose, maltose, and trehalose, are two monosaccharides in glycosidic linkage, and require disaccharidases of the surface membrane of the small intestines to cleave the linkage so absorption can take place. Carbohydrates are stored as starch in plants and as glycogen in animals. Starch is a plant polysaccharide that consists of linear chains of glucose molecules linked by α-1,4 glucosidic bonds (amylose) and of branched chains with branch points made up of α-1,6 linkages (amylopectin). Glycogen is similar to amylopectin in structure. Oligosaccharides are carbohydrates containing 3 to 10 monosaccharide units, and polysaccharides are those polymers with more than 10 monosaccharide units.

In a recent review of carbohydrates,[3] the lower limit of dietary carbohydrate compatible with life was noted to be zero, provided adequate amounts of fat and protein are consumed. The amount of carbohydrate needed for optimum health in humans is unknown. Only the central nervous system and cells dependent on anaerobic glycolysis, such as red blood cells, white blood cells, and the medulla of the kidney have an absolute requirement for glucose. The central nervous system can adapt to a fat-derived fuel. The carbohydrate requirement for infants and children is listed in Table 24-3.

Glucose is the major energy source in PN because it is safe, economical, and readily available. Other sugars, fructose, sorbitol, glycerol, and xylitol have been suggested as useful energy sources for specific conditions such as diabetes or after a trauma, but they are not readily available or used. Glucose in PN solutions is in the monohydrous form containing 3.4 kcal/g, and it is available commercially in concentrations of 2.5–70%. The glucose concentration of parenteral solutions that can be safely administered is limited by osmolality. Concentrations higher than about 12.5% sclerose peripheral veins, increasing the incidence of phlebitis and shortening the time that a vein could be used for infusion. Glucose solutions higher than 12.5% must be administered in a central vein. Glucose is calculated to provide 60–75% of nonprotein calories. Estimated parenteral energy requirements are provided in Table 24-4.

Initiation of glucose infusion should occur in an incremental fashion to prevent hyperosmolarity and hyperinsulinemia. See Table 24-5 for glucose concentration guidelines and Table 24-6

Table 24-3 Requirements for carbohydrates by age and gender.

Age	*Requirement (g/day)*
0–6 months*	60
7–12 months*	95
1–3 years†	130
4–8 years†	130
Boys†	
9–13 years	130
14–18 years	130
Girls†	
9–13 years	130
14–18 years	130
Men†	
19–30 years	100
Women†	
19–30 years	100

* AI.
† RDA.

Source: Constructed from Institute of Medicine. *Dietary Reference Intakes for Energy, Carbohydrates, Fiber, Fat, Fatty Acids, Cholesterol, Protein, and Amino Acids.* Washington, DC: National Academies Press; 2002/2005.

Table 24-4 Estimates of parenteral energy requirements.

Age (years)	*Energy (kcal/kg/day)*	*Carbohydrate (mg/kg/min)**
Premature infant	80–120	10–18
Term infant	90–120	11–18
1–3	75–90	9–14
4–6	65–75	8–11
7–10	55–75	7–11
11–18	40–55	7–8.5

* Estimate based on 60-75% of nonprotein calories as glucose.

Source: Lee PC, Werlin SL. Carbohydrates. In: Baker RD, Baker SS, Davis AM, eds. *Pediatric Parenteral Nutrition.* New York, NY: Chapman and Hall; 1997:99–107. Reproduced with permission.

for information on complications of glucose infusion. Glucose infusion rate (GIR) can be calculated using the following equation:

$$\text{GIR} = \frac{\text{g/kg/day glucose} \times 1{,}000}{1{,}440 \text{ min/day}}$$

A GIR of 12–14 mg/kg/min is tolerated in a healthy child, and infants can safely be given a GIR of 8–12 mg/kg/min. In adult patients, there is no apparent correlation between glucose clearance and the rate of oxidation of glucose.[19] Increases in the rate of glucose infusion from 4–7 mg/kg/min are associated with an increase in the rate of glucose oxidation. At higher rates, fat is synthesized without further increase in oxidation. High glucose loads, i.e., those containing more than 25% glucose and delivered at > 26 mg/kg/min, might not be beneficial to infants and could contribute to hepatosteatosis. In critically ill children, it is unlikely that overfeeding glucose will enhance energy balance or reduce protein catabolism (see Chapter 6). Complications associated with glucose infusions are listed in Table 24-6. Estimates of glucose utilization by the brain vary with age.[20]

The American Academy of Pediatrics recommends that insulin not be routinely added to PN solutions because responses to the addition of this hormone by infants are unpredictable.[21] For persistently hyperglycemic infants, insulin could improve tolerance of glucose.[22] However, there are a limited number of studies assessing clinical outcomes of infants treated with insulin.[23–25] Concerns about the use of insulin in the neonate include the possibility that suppression of muscle proteolysis could be undesirable, the composition of the resultant weight gain is not clearly understood, that serum glucose is driven to tissues other than the brain, and the possibility that glucose is converted to fat rather than being oxidized.[21]

Glucose intolerance can develop in critically ill patients, such as those who have experienced trauma, burns, sepsis, or cancer. For these patients, the infusion rate is limited to 5–7 mg/kg/min.[26] Infusion of excess glucose causes

Table 24-5 Glucose concentration in parenteral solutions.

	Premature infant (< 1,000 g or 28 weeks gestation)	*Infant*	*Child (1–10 years)*	*Adolescent (11–18)*
Begin infusion	5–7.5% or glucose concentration in current IV	5–7.5% or glucose concentration in current IV	10% or percent higher than concentration in current IV	10% or percent higher than concentration in current IV
Advance	2.5% each day as tolerated	2.5% each day as tolerated	5% each day as tolerated	5% each day as tolerated
Usual GIR upper limit (mg/kg/min)	8–12	12–14	8–10	5–6
Peripheral maximum concentration (%)	12	12.5	12.5	12.5
Central glucose concentration (%)	20–25	25	25	25
Monitor at initiation and with every increase	Urine glucose	Urine glucose	Urine glucose	Urine glucose

Source: Lee PC, Werlin SL. Carbohydrates. In: Baker RD, Baker SS, Davis AM, eds. *Pediatric Parenteral Nutrition*. New York, NY: Chapman and Hall; 1997:99–107. Reproduced with permission.

Table 24-6 Commonly reported complications of glucose infusions.

Complication	*Usual cause*	*Prevention or treatment*
Phelibitis	High osmolarity	Limit glucose concentration to 12.5% for peripheral administration
Refeeding syndrome	Rapid refeeding of a malnourished patient	Refeed slowly, monitor serum phosphorus, potassium, calcium, and magnesium
Hepatosteatosis	All nonprotein calories provided as carbohydrate or excessive calories	Provide 30% of calories as lipid; reassess energy
Cholestasis	Infant fed exclusively by PN	Enteral feeding
CO_2 retention	High GIR in a patient with respiratory failure	Decrease GIR
Hypoglycemia	Abrupt discontinuation of PN or decrease in GIR	Taper PN
Hyperglycemia	High GIR, stress, burns, sepsis, incorrect glucose concentration	Decrease GIR, add insulin

GIR = glucose infusion rate.
PN = parenteral nutrition.

Source: Lee PC, Werlin SL. Carbohydrates. In: Baker RD, Baker SS, Davis AM, eds. *Pediatric Parenteral Nutrition.* New York, NY: Chapman and Hall; 1997:99–107. Reproduced with permission.

hyperglycemia, glucosuria, dehydration, and the conversion of glucose to fat. When hyperglycemia occurs, the infusion rate can be decreased, or insulin can be added to the therapy. Exogenous insulin enhances the movement of substrate from the periphery to the liver and increases fat synthesis and storage. This can lead to hepatosteatosis; hence insulin is not commonly used in critically ill patients outside the neonatal age group.

Enteral feeding products contain a variety of carbohydrates including simple sugars, glucose and fructose, disaccharides, sucrose and lactose, and more complex carbohydrates such as corn syrup solids and maltodextrins. The source of maltodextrins can be corn or other vegetables such as soy or tapioca. Some formulas contain nondigestable carbohydrates such as fructooligosaccharides or soy fibers.

Most enteral formulas for infants contain lactose as the major carbohydrate to mimic human milk. Lactose free cow milk based or soy infant formulas use corn syrup solids with or without sucrose as the carbohydrate source. Enteral foods designed for children older than 1 year are generally lactose free.

The dextrose equivalent (DE) is a measure of reducing power compared to a dextrose standard of 100. The higher the DE, the greater the extent of starch depolymerization and the smaller the average polymer size.

The US Food and Drug Administration (FDA) defines maltodextrins as nonsweet nutritive saccharide polymers that consists of D-glucose units linked primarily by α-1,4 bonds and have a DE less than 20. Maltodextrins are prepared as a white powder or concentrated solution by partial hydrolysis of a starch such as corn, potato, tapioca, or rice.[27]

The FDA defines corn syrup solids as dried glucose syrup with a DE of 20 or higher. They are considered a generally regarded as safe (GRAS) food ingredient (see Chapter 15). Corn syrup solids are sweet, viscous, and used by the food industry to improve texture, especially in low fat foods. They serve as an energy source in some enteral foods.

Fructooligosaccharides and fiber are nondigestible carbohydrates that add bulk and serve as prebiotics (see Chapter 3 for a discussion of prebiotics).

FAT

Fat is an important fuel source. It aids in the absorption of certain vitamins; serves to maintain membrane structure and function; is a precursor for prostaglandins, thromboxanes, and leukotrienes; and because of its influence on the phospholipid composition of membranes, it affects enzyme activities and regulatory functions. Fats could modulate immune response and influence gene expression.[28] Adequate intakes for fat by age and gender are listed in Table 24-7.

Dietary fat consists of triacyl glycerol, phospholipids, and cholesterol. Humans use both animal and plant as fat sources. Dietary fat supply governs the fatty acid (FA) composition of the body. Except for lenoleic and lenolenic acid, tissue metabolic processes modify dietary FAs and synthesize FAs de novo.

Triacylglycerol accounts for 98% of dietary fat and is a glycerol molecule with esterified FAs that are saturated or unsaturated. Glycerol compounds with one or two esterified FAs occur in small amounts, mostly as intermediates in the synthesis or degradation of glycerol-containing lipids. The chain length of FAs and the number, position, and form of double bonds determines the melting point, water solubility, energy content, digestibility, and metabolic properties of the triacylglycerol. FAs are classified as short chain, less than 8 carbons, medium chain, 8–10 carbons, and long chain, ≥ 16 carbons. FAs are further described as saturated (having no double bonds), monosaturated (1 double bond), or polyunsaturated (containing 2 or more double bonds). FAs can exist in the cis or trans position with respect to double bonds. Almost all plant and animal FAs that are used for metabolic processes and in

Table 24-7 Adequate intake (AI) for fat intake by age and gender.

Age	*Total fat*	*n-6 PPUFA >12 months; lenoleic acid > 12 months (g/day)*	*n-3 PUFA > 12 months; lenolenic acid > 12 months (g/day)*
0–6 months	31	4.4	0.5
7–12 months	30	4.6	0.5
1–3 years	None	7	0.7
4–8 years	None	10	0.9
Boys 9–13 years	None	12	102
Boys 14–18 years	None	16	1.6
Girls 9–13 years	None	10	1.0
Girls 14–18 years	None	11	1.1

Source: Adapted from Standing Committee on the Scientific Evaluation of Dietary Reference Intakes Food and Nutrition Board Institute of Medicine. *Dietary Reference Intakes for Energy, Carbohydrate, Fiber, Fat, Fatty Acids, Cholesterol, Protein and Amino Acids (Macronutrients)*. Washington, DC: National Academy Press; 2002.

tissue structure are in the cis position. Trans FAs are formed by rumen bacteria and by chemical hydrogenation of FAs. Trans FAs are not essential and provide no known benefit.

Structured lipids are triglycerides chemically synthesized using acidolysis, enzyme catalysis and transesterification.[28–31] Structured lipids are medium chain FAs and select long chain FAs attached to a glycerol backbone. The functional properties of these tailor-made fats can improve nutritional or physical properties and depend on the type of FAs and the position of their attachment to glycerol. Long chain FAs are chosen for the functional properties they impart to the final product or for their biological function after ingestion. They might provide a means of delivering desired FAs for nutrition or therapeutic purposes or for targeting specific diseases and metabolic conditions.[32] Medium chain FAs are chosen as a readily available source of energy that, in general, does not contribute to fat storage.

Considerable emphasis has been placed on n-6 and n-3 FAs. FAs in which the first double bond occurs 3 carbons from the methyl end are termed omega-3 FAs, also noted as ω-3 or n-3 FAs. The major sources of n-3 FAs in the diet are soybean and canola oils and fatty fish oil. N-3 polyunsaturated fatty acids (PUFA) are important as structural membrane lipids, especially in nervous tissue and the retina. The n-3 PUFA, linolenic acid, is an essential FA. FAs in which the first double bond occurs six carbons from the methyl end are termed omega-6 FAs, also noted as ω-6 or n-6 FAs. Dietary sources include corn, safflower, soybean, and sunflower oils. Linoleic acid, an essential fatty acid, is an n-6 PUFA and serves as a precursor to the eicosanoids. There is evidence that dietary n-3 and n-6 could influence the inflammatory and immune response.[33] N-3 fatty acids might have a beneficial effect on chronic inflammatory diseases such as rheumatoid arthritis, inflammatory bowel disease, lupus, multiple sclerosis, and others.[34]

Human milk is the preferred nutrient source for infants. Infant formulas attempt to replicate human milk both in content and performance. Human milk contains about 55% of the calories as fat and most of the fat is saturated or monounsaturated FAs. It contains linolenic acid, eicosapentaenoic acid, and docosahexaenoic acid (DHA). Human milk also has a relatively high cholesterol content. The FA content of human milk varies with maternal diet. Infant formulas contain a mixture of vegetable oils, mostly soybean, safflower, sunflower, coconut, and palm; have lower cholesterol content; and until recently did not contain arachadonic acid (AA) or DHA. Infant formulas contain linoleic and linolenic acid as precursors for the long chain polyunsaturated fatty acids (LCPUFA). Because of concern over whether LCPUFA are essential nutrients in infancy, AA and DHA were recently added to formula designed for term infants. A recent Cochrane review found little evidence from randomized trials to support the hypothesis that LCPUFA supplementation confers a benefit for visual or general development of term infants.[35] There seems to be a general consensus that AA and DHA are beneficial for preterm infants. However, another recent Cochrane review failed to find long term benefits for preterm infants whose diet was supplemented with these LCPUFA. The infants in the reports were relatively mature, healthy preterm infants. There was no evidence that supplementation of formula with n-3 and n-6 LCPUFA impaired the growth of preterm infants.[36] Similarly, supplementation of infant formula with LCPUFA does not influence the growth of term infants.[37]

Infant formulas and enteral feeding products mostly contain the vegetable oils palm, olein, sunflower, safflower, soy, coconut, corn, canola, and lecithin in various concentrations to meet energy and FA requirements. Some formulas contain medium chain triglyceride (MCT) oils and a few have beef or deodorized fish oils.

MCTs are often used in enteral formulas and offer several advantages. They are more water soluble than long chain triglycerides, intraluminal hydrolysis occurs more rapidly and more completely than the hydrolysis of long chain triglycerides, and they require little or no lipase or bile salts for substantial absorption to occur.

MCTs are transported directly into the blood via the portal system, bypassing the lymphatic system. MCT enriched formulas are often used to overcome malabsorption caused by pancreatic insufficiency, chronic liver disease, or bowel resections, for chyluria, chylous fistulas and protein-losing enteropathy. MCTs do not contain essential FAs, and when MCT oil enriched formulas are used, especially in the first year of life, care must be taken that adequate essential FAs are provided. MCT oils provide 8.2 to 8.4 kcal/g compared to 9 kcal/g for long chain triglycerides.

Lipids are administered to virtually all patients who receive PN. Initially, intravenous fats were given to patients who had no oral intake to overcome essential fatty acid deficiency (EFAD); however, since intravenous lipids are the most calorically dense component of PN, intravenous fats are considered an important source of calories, especially for patients who are fluid restricted. Thus intravenous lipids have at least two roles, avoiding or treating EFAD and as a source of energy.

There are a number of reasons to choose fat predominant PN solutions over glucose predominant ones. Glucose results in a higher specific dynamic action and thus, higher resting energy expenditures and higher metabolic rates. Glucose predominant PN can result in a respiratory quotient of greater than 1.0, indicating the use of energy for lipogenesis (see Chapter 6). Finally, glucose metabolism results in an increased CO_2 elimination by the lungs when compared to fat metabolism. This fact can be of importance to mechanically ventilated patients and those with marginal lung function. In general, the ratio of calories derived from glucose to the calories derived from fats in the range of 3:1 to 2:1 minimizes CO_2 stress.[38,39]

Intravenous fats consist of three components: an aqueous phase, a lipid phase, and an emulsifier. The lipid phase supplies most of the calories and the essential FA. Glycerin is present in the aqueous phase and raises the tonicity as well as incidentally supplying calories. The emulsifier is usually egg phospholipid. Soybean oil, safflower oil, and mixtures of the two have been used as sources of lipid. The caloric density of 10% lipid emulsions is 1.1 kcal/mL, 20% emulsion is 2.0 kcal/mL and 30% is 3.0 kcal/mL (available for 3-in-1 solutions only). Intravenous fat emulsions with higher concentrations of phospholipids (10% versus 20 or 30%) should be avoided since the higher phospholipids produce high levels of triglycerides, cholesterol, and phospholipids.

Preventing EFAD is 1 of the 2 major reasons for administering intravenous fats. The essential fats for humans are lenoleic acid (C18:2ω6), arachidonic acid (C20:4ω6), and lenolenic acid (C18:3ω3). EFAD has been described in children and adults who have no exogenous source of fats for 3 weeks or more. In the preterm infant, EFAD is seen after only 1 week without essential FAs. Symptoms of EFAD include scaly skin rash, sparse hair, susceptibility to infection, failure to thrive, hypotonia, increased red cell fragility, and electroencephalographic and electrocardiographic changes. In EFAD, the ratio of trienoic to tetraenoic acids increases to greater than 0.2.[40] In older children and adults, EFAD can be prevented by supplying 0.5–1.0 g/kg/day as intravenous lipid, and for premature infants, 0.6–0.8 g/kg/day prevents EFAD. Others suggest measuring n-6 and n-3 long chain polyunsaturated fatty acids for EFAD status.[41]

For the most part, intravenous fats are handled in the circulation in much the same fashion as very low density lipoprotein (VLDL) particles. Lipoprotein lipase, present in the capillary endothelium, reduces the triglycerides at the core of the particle, while the polar lipids, at the surface of the VLDL, are removed to form nascent high density lipoprotein (HDL). Lecithin-cholesterol acyl transferase (LCAT), released into the circulation from the liver, works to convert the nascent HDL into mature HDL.[42] Lipoprotein lipase at the endothelial surface and LCAT in circulation are key in clearing the infused lipid from the circulation. Lipids can be cleared by other mechanisms such as endothelial cell endocytosis via cell surface heparin sulphate proteoglycans in a receptor-independent manner.[43]

Other factors negatively affect the clearance rate of intravenous fat emulsions. Low levels of lipoprotein lipase found in severely malnourished states slow the rate of fat clearance. Hypertriglyceridemia might develop in hypermetabolic states such as sepsis, trauma, or organ dysfunction during intravenous fat infusion. Concurrent administration of medications such as steroids alters tolerance to intravenous fat because steroids have a lipolytic effect.[43] Continuous intravenous propofol infusions and amphotericin B are sources of fat and calories and must be included when planning and monitoring PN.

The amount of lipid that can be given safely by the intravenous route is limited by the rate of clearance of lipids from circulation. Two to three g/kg/day lipid can be safely administered to premature infants, term babies, and older children. Serum triglycerides must be monitored to assure that the clearing mechanism has not been overwhelmed. It has been suggested that heparin might enhance clearance. In a randomized trial of 2 heparin doses, the drug caused increase in circulating free fatty acids, presumably because of release of the lipoprotein lipase into circulation. There was no increase in lipid utilization.[44] It was concluded that heparin was of no benefit for fat metabolism. Administering IV lipid over 20 hours while allowing 4 hours for lipid clearing has been proposed as another method of facilitating lipid clearance. Evidence does not support this practice.[45]

Tolerance to intravenous fat infusion can be evaluated by measuring serum triglyceride levels 4 hours after starting a fat infusion or increasing the fat infusion rate since this is the time that hypertriglyceridemia is most likely to occur.[46] The American Gastroenterological Association Technical Review on Parenteral Nutrition reports that intravenous fat emulsion should not be given to patients with serum triglyceride levels above 400 mg/dL; however, there is no data to support this statement.[12] There is general agreement to decrease fat infusion rates when serum levels approach 400 mg/dL.

Lipid emulsions used for parenteral administration contain phytosterols. These are plant-derived isoflavones that possess estrogenic properties. Their importance, either beneficial or detrimental, as a part of PN is not known. Phytoestrogens, present in soy based formulas, have been implicated as a cause of decreased bone mineral content in premature infants. Whether these compounds figure in PN bone disease is speculation. Early menarche and thelarche in females fed soy formulas has been found in some studies[47] and disputed by other studies.[48] The importance of phytosterols in infused lipid emulsions as feminizing compounds has not been studied. To date there is no proof that phytosterols play a role in PN-associated cholestasis, although this relationship has been suggested.[49] Neither liver nor pancreatic disease are contraindications to the use of intravenous fat emulsions.

Several new intravenous fat solutions are available. An olive and soybean-based emulsion (ratio 4:1) with fewer polyunsaturated fatty acids and more alpha-tocopherol than standard soybean oil emulsion was found to enhance linoleic acid conversion and improve vitamin E status in premature infants.[50] MCT (50% MCT/50% LCT) fat infusion can increase net fat oxidation in infants after surgery as long as the carbohydrate calories do not exceed resting energy expenditures.[51] It is important to note that MCTs do not provide essential fatty acids and do not require carnitine for oxidation.[52]

ENERGY SOURCES IN PN

A controversy surrounds the issue of whether protein should be considered a calorie source and whether it should be included in the calculation of total energy. Some basic principles agreed upon are: a minimum amount of glucose must be provided to prevent hypoglycemia, and too much causes excessive CO_2 production and/or hepatic steatosis.[53] A minimum amount of intravenous fat prevents EFAD, and an extreme amount leads to hypertriglyceridemia and pulmonary vascular lipid deposition. Adequate amounts of amino acids must be provided to prevent hypoproteinemia; however, excessive amounts result in metabolic acidosis and hyperammonemia. In order to determine the appropriate types and amounts of carbohydrate, fat, and protein in PN, size, age, and clinical condition must be considered for each pediatric patient.

CONCLUSION

Macronutrients, protein, carbohydrates, and fats are important nutrients. But as knowledge about macronutrients increases, it becomes clear that they are active in directing metabolic pathways. This opens the possibility of using them as "nutriceuticals" to influence specific disease states.

REFERENCES

1. Laidlaw SA, Kopple JD. Newer concepts of the indispensable amino acids. *Am J Clin Nutr.* 1987;46:593–605.
2. Pencharz BP, House JD, Wykes LJ, Ball RO. What are the essential amino acids for the preterm and term infant? In: Bindels JG, Goedhart A, Visser HKA, eds. *Recent Developments in Infant Nutrition: Nutricia Symposia.* Vol 9. Dordrech, the Netherlands: Kluwer Academic Publishers; 1996:278–296.
3. Institute of Medicine. *Dietary Reference Intakes for Energy, Carbohydrates, Fiber, Fat, Fatty Acids, Cholesterol, Protein, and Amino Acids.* Washington, DC: National Academies Press; 2002/2005.
4. Snyderman SE. The protein and amino acid requirements of the premature infant. In: Visser HKA, Toreistra JA, eds. *Nutrica Symposium: Metabolic Processes in the Fetus and Newborn Infant.* Leiden, the Netherlands: Stenfert Kroese; 1971:128–143.
5. Sturman JA, Gaull GE, Raiha NCR. Absence of cystathionase in human fetal liver. Is cysteine essential? *Science.* 1970;169:74–76.
6. Jelliffe DB. The assessment of the nutritional status of the community. *WHO Monograph Series No. 53.* Geneva, Switzerland: World Health Organization; 1966.
7. Fomon SJ. *Nutrition of Normal Infants.* St. Louis, Mo: Mosby-Year Book, Inc; 1993.
8. Heyland DK, Novak F, Drover JW, Minot J, Xiangyao S, Suchner U. Should immunonutrition become routine in critically ill patients? A systematic review of the evidence. *JAMA.* 2001;286:944–953.
9. Naylor CD, O'Rourke K, Detsky A, Baker JP. PN with branched-chain amino acids in hepatic encephalopathy. *Gastroenterology.* 1989;97:1033–1042.
10. Nompleggi DJ, Bonkovsky HL. Nutritional supplementation in chronic liver disease: an analytical review. *Hepatology.* 1994;19(2):518–533.
11. ASPEN Board of Directors and the Clinical Guidelines Task Force. Guidelines for the use of parenteral and enteral nutrition in adult and pediatric patients. *JPEN.* 2002;26(suppl 1):1SA–138SA.
12. Korletz RL, Lipman TO, Klein S. AGA technical review on PN. *Gastroenterology.* 2001;121:970–1001.
13. Klein S, Kinney J, Jeejeebhoy K, et al. Nutrition support in clinical practice: review of published data and recommendations for future research directions. *JPEN.* 1997;21:133–156.
14. Novak F, Heyland D, Alison A, Drover JW, Xiangyao S. Glutamine supplementation in serious illness: a systematic review of the evidence. *Crit Care Med.* 2002;30:2022–2029.
15. Heird WC, Dell RB, Helms RA, et al. Amino acid mixture designed to maintain normal plasma amino acid patterns in infants and children requiring PN. *Pediatrics.* 1987;80:401–408.
16. Heird WC, Hay W, Helms RA, Storm MC, Kashyap S, Dell RB. Pediatric parenteral amino acid mixture in low birth weight infants. *Pediatrics.* 1988;81:41–50.
17. Helms RA, Christensen ML, Mauer EC, Storm MC. Comparison of a pediatric versus standard amino acid formulation in preterm neonates requiring PN. *J Pediatr.* 1987;110:466–470.
18. Gura KM, Sandler R, Lo C. Aminosyn PF or trophamine: which provides more protection from cholestasis associated with total PN? *J Pediatr Gastroenterol Nutr.* 1995;21:374–382.
19. Wolfe RR, Allsop JR, Burke JF. Glucose metabolism in man: responses to intravenous glucose infusion. *Metabolism.* 1979;28:210–220.
20. Kalhan SC, Kilic I. Carbohydrate as nutrient in the infant and child: range of acceptable intake. *Eur J Clin Nutr.* 1999;53:S94–S100.
21. American Academy of Pediatrics Committee on Nutrition. *Pediatric Nutrition Handbook.* 5th ed. Elk Grove Village, Ill: American Academy of Pediatrics; 1998:375.
22. Vaucher YE, Walson PD, Morrow G III. Continuous insulin infusion in hyperglycemic, very low birth weight infants. *J Pediatr Gastroenterol Nutr.* 1982;1:211–215.
23. Binder ND, Raschko PK, Benda GI, Reynolds JW. Insulin infusion with PN in extremely low birth weight infants with hyperglycemia. *J Pediatr.* 1989;114:273.
24. Collins JW, Hoppe M, Brown K, et al. A controlled trial of insulin infusion with glucose intolerance. *J Pediatr.* 1991;118:921.
25. Poindexter BB, Karn CA, Denne SC. Exogenous insulin reduces proteolysis and protein synthesis in extremely low birth weight infants. *J Pediatr.* 1998;132:948.

26. Jeevanandam M, Mamias L, Schiller WR. Elevated urinary C-peptide excretion in multiple trauma patients. *J Trauma.* 1991;31:334–338.
27. US Department of Agriculture. Commercial item description, January 26, 2001. Available at: http://www.ams.usda.gov/fqa/aa20124c.htm. Accessed July 10, 2005.
28. Gonzalez Moreno PA, Robles Medina A, Camacho Rubio F, Camacho Paez B, Molina Grima E. Production of structured lipids by acidolysis of an EPA-enriched fish oil and caprylic acid in a packed bed reactor: analysis of three different operation modes. *Biotechnol Prog.* 2004;20(4):1044–1052.
29. Iwasaki Y, Yamane T. Enzymatic synthesis of structured lipids. *Adv Biochem Eng-Biotechnol.* 2004;90:151–171.
30. Hamam F, Shahidi F. Synthesis of structured lipids via acidolysis of docosahexaenoic acid single cell oil (DHASCO) with capric acid. *J Agricultural Food Chem.* 2004;52(10):2900–2906.
31. Sellappan S, Akoh CC. Synthesis of structured lipids by transesterification of trilinolein catalyzed by lipozyme IM60. *J Agricultural Food Chem.* 2001;49(4):2071–2076.
32. Lee KT, Akoh CC. Structured lipids; synthesis and applications. *Food Rev Int.* 1998;14:17–34.
33. Grimble RF. Symposium on 'evidence-based nutrition:' nutritional modulation of immune function. *Proc Nutr Soc.* 2001;60:389–397.
34. Calder PC. N-3 polyunsaturated fatty acids and inflammation: from molecular biology to the clinic. *Lipids.* 2003;38:343–352.
35. Simmer K. Long chain polyunsaturated fatty acid supplementation in infants born at term (review). The Cochrane Database of Systematic Reviews; 2005:1.
36. Simmer K, Patole S. Long chain polyunsaturated fatty acid supplementation in preterm infants. The Cochrane Database of Systematic Reviews; 2005:1.
37. Makrides M, Gibson RA, Udell T, Ried K. International LCPUFA investigators: supplementation of infant formula with long-chain polyunsaturated fatty acids does not influence the growth of term infants. *Am J Clin Nutr.* 2005;81:1094–1101.
38. Nose O, Tipton JR, Ament ME. Administration of lipid improves nitrogen retention in children receiving isocaloric TPN. *Pediatr Res.* 1985;19:228A.
39. Sauer P, Van Aerde J, Smith J, et al. Substrate utilization in newborn infants fed intravenously with or without a fat emulsion. *Pediatr Res.* 1984;18:804A.
40. Uauy R, Treen M, Hoffman D. Essential fatty acid metabolism and requirements during development. *Semin Perinatol.* 1989;13:118.
41. Foote KD, MacKinnon MJ, Innis SM. Effect of early introduction of formula vs fat-free parenteral nutrition on essential fatty acid status of preterm infants. *Am J Clin Nutr.* 1991;54:93–97.
42. Eisenberg S. Very low density lipoprotein metabolism. *Prog Biochem Pharmacol.* 1979;15:139.
43. Olivecrona G, Olivecrona T. Clearance of artificial triacylglycerol particles. *Curr Opin Clin Nutr Metabol Care.* 1998;1(2):143–151.
44. Spear ML, Stahl GE, Hamossh M, et al. Effect of heparin dose and infusion rate on lipid clearance and bilirubin binding in premature infants receiving intravenous fat emulsions. *J Pediatr.* 1988;112:94.
45. Kao LC, Cheng MH, Warburton D. Triglycerides, free fatty acids, free fatty acids/albumin molar ratio, and cholesterol levels in serum of neonates receiving long-term lipid infusions: controlled trial of continuous and intermittent regimens. *J Pediatr.* 1984;104(3):429–435.
46. Griffin EA, Bryan HM, Angel A. Variations in intralipid tolerance in newborn infants. *Pediatr Res.* 1983;17:478–481.
47. Freni-Titulaer LW, Cordero JF, Haddock L, et al. Premature telarche in Puerto Rico: a search for environmental factors. *Am J Dis Child.* 1986;140:1263–1277.
48. Strom BL, Schinnar R, Ziegler EE, et al. Exposure to soy-based formula in infancy and endocrinological and reproductive outcomes in young adulthood. *JAMA.* 2001;286(7):807–814.
49. Clayton PT, Bowron A, Mills KA, Massoud A, Milla PJ. Phytosterolemia in children with parenteral nutrition-associated liver disease. *Gastroenterology.* 1993;105:1808.
50. Gobel Y, Koletzko B, Bohles HJ, et al. Parenteral fat emulsions based on olive and soybean oils: a randomized clinical trial in preterm infants. *J Pediatr Gastroenterol Nutr.* 2003;37(2):161–167.
51. Donnell SC, Lloyd DA, Eaton S, Pierro A. The metabolic response to intravenous medium-chain triglycerides in infants after surgery. *J Pediatr.* 2002;141:689–694.
52. Heine RG, Bines JE. New approaches to parenteral nutrition in infants and children. *J Pediatr Child Health.* 2002;38:433–437.
53. Shulman RJ, Phillips S. Parenteral nutrition in infants and children. *J Pediatr Gastroenterol Nutr.* 2002;36:587–607.

CHAPTER 25

Minerals, Trace Elements, and Vitamins, Enteral and Parenteral

Jatinder Bhatia, Amy Gates, and Robert D. Baker

INTRODUCTION

This chapter reviews the role of minerals, trace elements, and vitamins in enteral (EN) and parenteral nutrition (PN). PN requirements for calcium, phosphorus, and magnesium are not defined. Since there is an overall inability to provide enough calcium and phosphorus to meet the needs of an infant, child, or an adult, careful attention to mineral homeostasis is warranted. For the infant or child receiving PN, there are trace element preparations containing chromium, copper, iodide, manganese, selenium, zinc, and molybdenum (Table 25-1). Vitamins are essential nutrients (see Chapter 8). Health depends on an adequate supply of vitamins. Infants and children requiring either EN or PN could have special vitamin requirements. Monitoring vitamin levels for adequacy and toxicity is important.

CALCIUM, PHOSPHORUS, AND MAGNESIUM

The minerals calcium, phosphorus, and magnesium are vital to intermediary metabolism serving in energy transfer. Calcium and phosphorus also serve a structural function, and calcium is a regulator for a variety of intracellular processes. Presumably, calcium and phosphorus are actively transported across the placenta against a concentration gradient.[1] Between the time a fetus weighs 1,000 g and 4,400 g at term, whole body calcium content increases by 86%, phosphorus by 82%, and magnesium by 78%.[2]

Premature Infants

The fetus accumulates between 13 and 33 g of calcium[3] during the third trimester, a period of rapid skeletal mineralization. Maternal adaptation to this calcium requirement includes a twofold increase in the intestinal absorption of calcium, mediated by a doubling of free and bound maternal 1,25-dihydroxyvitamin D. Fetal phosphorus levels are higher than maternal levels, suggesting active transport;[4] however, the regulation of this active transport is not clear.[5]

Magnesium is the fourth most abundant mineral and the most abundant intracellular divalent cation in the body. Term newborn infants have about 0.8g of magnesium, with 80% being accreted in the last trimester of pregnancy.[6] Magnesium is distributed in bone (~ 65%), intracellular space (~ 34%), and in the extracellular fluid. In plasma, magnesium exists either as a protein-bound fraction, free ionic form, or is bound to anions such as phosphate and oxalate.[7] Magnesium is ultrafiltrable and freely filtered at the renal glomerulus. The protein-bound fraction reacts to alterations in pH in a manner similar to calcium and the ionized fraction of magnesium is physiologically important. Prolonged maternal therapy with Mg for tocolysis has been associated with metabolic bone disease in the infant.[8]

Table 25-1 Parenteral trace element combinations.

	Trace element dose							
	Chromium Cl (mcg/mL)	*Copper SO4 (mg/mL)*	*Iodide (mcg/mL)*	*Manganese SO4 (mg/mL)*	*Selenious acid (mcg/mL)*	*Zinc SO4 (mg/mL)*	*Molybdenum (mcg/mL)*	*How supplied*
Neotrace-4	0.85	0.1	0	0.03	0	1.5	0	2-mL vials
PTE-4	1	0.1	0	0.025	0	1	0	3-mL vials
PTE-5	1	0.1	0	0.025	15	1	0	3-mL vials
MTE-5	4	0.4	0	0.1	20	1	0	10-mL vials
MTE-6	4	0.4	25	0.1	20	1	0	10-mL vials
MTE-7	4	0.4	25	0.1	20	1	25	10-mL vials

Source: From product information, July 2005.
PTE = pediatric trace element
MTE = multiple trace elements

Parenteral Nutrition

Prolonged total PN cannot supply adequate minerals because of the insolubility of calcium and phosphorus (Chapter 27). Therefore, the infant born early in the third trimester and dependent on PN is born in a state of osteopenia aggravated by inadequate calcium intake. In premature infants, it might not be possible to deliver these minerals in quantities that simulate intrauterine mineral accretion, but severe bone disease can be reduced. Since the amount of calcium that can be delivered is limited, maneuvers that decrease urinary calcium losses have been explored. Factors that promote hypercalciuria are increased calcium intake,[9] decreased phosphate intake,[9] increased amino acid infusion,[10] metabolic acidosis,[11] and cycling PN infusions.[12]

Enteral Nutrition

High calcium, cow's milk based formulas appear to result in more bone mineral accretion in premature infants.[13,14] However, in one study, premature breastfed individuals had higher bone mineral content at 5 years when compared to premature individuals fed a high calcium formula.[15] Despite this study, it is generally accepted that premature infants, breastfed or formula fed, require more calcium than is present in human milk and thus need supplementation.[16,17]

Phosphorus metabolism and requirements of the premature infant are largely extrapolated from studies performed on fullterm breastfed babies. The extrapolation might not be justified, because premature infants do not experience the maturation of kidney function and the drop in phosphorus intake until later than the term infant does (see Term Infants and Children section).

The net retention of magnesium in premature infants consuming human milk has been determined to be 10–15 mg/day; that represents 45% absorption.[18,19] Formulas based on either cow milk or soy protein have a higher magnesium content than human milk.[20–22] The fraction absorbed from formulas is the same or higher than from human milk resulting in formula fed babies absorbing the same or more magnesium compared to babies fed breast milk.

Term Infants and Children

Many chronic diseases are associated with trace element depletion. Approximately 99% of total body calcium is found in bone, while 85% of phosphorus is in bone, and 50–60% of magnesium is in bone. Bone acts as a reservoir for calcium, phosphorus, and magnesium, so serum levels often do not reflect total body content. This makes it difficult to identify deficiency states. Less than 1% of the total body Ca, P, and Mg are in the circulation. Because serum calcium is tightly controlled at the expense of bone, calcium deficiency is a state of chronic bone loss. Calcium circulates in 3 forms: 45% is in the biologically active ionized form; 45% is bound to protein, mainly albumin; and 10% is complexed with phosphate, lactate, and citrate.[23] Measurement of ionized calcium, because it is the active form, better reflects calcium homeostasis than does measuring total serum calcium (Chapter 7). Fifty percent of phosphorus exists in circulation as free ions, 10% is protein bound, and 40% is in a complex with Ca, Mg, and Na as salts. Phosphorus deficiency can be a serious acute problem when malnourished patients are refed and sufficient phosphorus is not provided.[24] Magnesium is mainly an intracellular anion, so serum Mg levels might not accurately reflect total body magnesium status.

Parenteral Nutrition

Peak bone mass is attained in late adolescence and is determined by nutritional factors, genetics, mechanical factors, and the environment.[25] PN should supply adequate minerals to attain optimal peak bone mass. Metabolic bone disease is common in premature infants and in children receiving long term PN.[26,27] The hypocalcemia associated with metabolic bone disease results from not supplying adequate calcium and from urinary calcium losses. Because calcium and phosphorus will complex with each other and form a precipitate, there are limitations to the amounts of calcium and phosphorus that can be supplied in PN solutions[28] (Chapter 27). These limitations spurred nutritionists to seek creative ways of providing the minerals, such as alternating intravenous solutions of high calcium concentration with high phosphorus content. These strategies have no proven benefit. Amino acid solutions designed for children under 1 year have added cysteine. Cysteine lowers the pH enough to permit the addition of calcium and phosphorus in significant amounts.[29]

Children on long term PN do not experience bone pain or fractures since metabolic disease associated with PN is mostly asymptomatic.[30] Aluminum present as a contaminant in PN solutions and in additives can lead to decreased bone mineralization.[31] Parenteral amino acid solutions prepared from casein hydrolysates were contaminated with aluminum. Aluminum contamination is associated with osteopenia, growth arrest, fractures, and pain.[32–34] Since the discontinuation of these solutions, metabolic bone disease has become less of a problem. However, osteopenia remains a problem for children.[35,36] A study of children who had bowel resections of varying length necessitating PN support for 1 to 67 months showed appropriate bone mineralization for their weight and height after the PN solutions were discontinued.[37] The bone mineralization was less than that of healthy children of the same age. Although this observation is encouraging, the study must be viewed with caution since more than half of the children had relatively small amounts of bowel removed and required PN for less than 8 months.

Enteral Nutrition

Calcium recommendations during the first 6 months of life are based on the amount of calcium present in human milk. Human milk calcium content is remarkably constant, averaging 264 mg/L for the first 6 months and 210 mg/L during the second 6 months of lactation.[38] Based on an absorption coefficient of about 60% and an average intake of 780 mL/day, the adequate intake (AI) was set at 210 mg/day.[39] Using similar methodological calculations, the AI for infants 7–12 months was set at 270 mg/day.[39] The coefficient of calcium absorption from formula (38%) is much less than from human milk; however, the calcium content of formula (520 mg/L) is almost twice as high as the calcium content of human milk. Soy based and special formulas are even higher in calcium; they are around 700 mg/L. Because of the higher calcium content, formula fed infants absorb at least as much calcium as breastfed infants. Breastfed babies are at risk of developing vitamin D deficient rickets, and the American Academy of Pediatrics advises supplementation.[40] Table 25-2 gives enteral recommendations for calcium intake.

In the United States, nutritional deficiency of calcium and phosphorus during childhood years is relatively rare because milk is fortified with vitamin D. Pediatric formulas intended for enteral tube feeding contain 800 mg to 1.5 gm/L of calcium.

Adolescents undergo a growth spurt, dramatically increasing the demand for bone minerals. At the same time that the adolescent growth spurt requires additional calcium and phosphorus, teenagers might be decreasing the amount of calcium and phosphorus-containing products in their diets, replacing milk with soft drinks, tea, or coffee. National surveys show that adolescents are not getting enough calcium.[41]

Inorganic phosphorus (P_i) in the breastfed term infant falls dramatically from birth to about 6 weeks. This decline is probably due to a decrease in the P_i in human milk and to an increase in the glomerular filtration rate of the infant.[42] The renal phosphate excretion mechanism reaches full functional capacity at about 6 weeks of age.[43] At this point, the human infant should be able to adapt to a wide range of phosphorus intake.

Magnesium recommendations for term infants were set using human milk as a standard. Human milk contains 43 mg/L and remains relatively constant for the first year of lactation.[20,44] The AI for 0–6 months is 30 mg/day and for 7–12 months is 75 mg/day. The goal of these intakes is to allow accretion of 10 mg/day (DRI). The recommendation for growing children and adolescents is based on achieving a positive magnesium balance of approximately 8–10 mg/day.

Development of Bone Mass

Skeletal Ca accumulation remains the critical factor for increments in bone mass; however, other nutrients are required as demonstrated in chronically undernourished infants and children who have depressed rates of bone turnover compared to recovery periods.[45] Estimated amounts of adequate calcium intake during the first 2 decades of life are depicted in Table 25-2. It is only in the second decade of life that differences in males and females become apparent. Males gain and accumulate more calcium than females. Skeletal development during infancy depends on a balanced nutrient intake provided by either human milk or formula for the first 6 months. The addition of complementary feeds at 4 to 6 months of age and the type of food added could change the balance of total nutrient intake and affect skeletal development.

Table 25-2 Adequate intake of calcium.

Age	*AI*
0 through 6 months	210 mg/day
7 through 12 months	270 mg/day
1 through 3 years	500 mg/day
4 through 8 years	800 mg/day
9 through 18 years	1,300 mg/day

Source: Adapted from Institute of Medicine. *Dietary Reference Intakes for Vitamin A, Vitamin K, Arsenic, Boron, Chromium, Copper, Iodine, Iron, Manganese, Molybdenum, Nickel, Silicon, Vanadium, and Zinc.* Washington, DC: National Academy Press; 2001:197–223.

Refeeding Syndrome

The refeeding syndrome frequently accompanies the nutritional rehabilitation of malnourished individuals. The refeeding syndrome is a set of metabolic and functional complications that occurs as a result of intracellular shifts of elements. During rapid nutritional rehabilitation, profound hypophospatemia, hypomagnesemia, and hypokalemia can precipitate acute respiratory and circulatory collapse. Neurologic manifestations of the refeeding syndrome include weakness, lethargy, paralysis, and confusion. Deaths have been documented.[24] Phosphorus, magnesium, and potassium must be carefully monitored in malnourished patients. Aggressive supplementation and correction of low values prevents the adverse outcomes of refeeding syndrome.

ZINC

Zinc is essential for growth. It is involved in chromosome replication; regulation of the translation of genetic information; provides structure for zinc-finger proteins; stabilizes ribosomes and membranes; and is a component of a number of enzymes.[46] Zinc deficiency in humans impairs cell-mediated immunity.[47] Signs of zinc deficiency include dermatitis, alopecia, diarrhea, and immune deficiency (see Table 25-3 for biomarkers of zinc and other micronutrients). Zinc status is difficult to monitor. Stress, infections, and trauma all alter circulating zinc levels. Merely administering PN diminishes plasma zinc by about 30%.[48] Despite these shortcomings, serum zinc is commonly used to monitor zinc nutriture. Zinc is lost from the body through urine, sweat, and stool. High zinc losses occur in diarrhea and excessive ostomy output. Zinc status should be assessed, and zinc should be supplemented if deficiency exists.

Premature Infants, Term Infants, and Children

Parenteral Nutrition

Severe, PN associated zinc deficiency mimics acrodermatitis enteropathethica.[49] With zinc deficiency, relatively more fat accrues than lean tissue.[48] The composition of the tissue acquired during nutritional rehabilitation could be affected by zinc status. Zinc is excreted

Table 25-3 Suggested biomarkers from selected micronutrients.

Micronutrient	*Preferred biomarker*	*Functional biomarker*
Vitamin A	Plasma retinol	Dark adaptation, impression cytology
Iodine	Urinary iodine, serum thyroid-stimulating hormone	Goiter prevalence, severity
Iron	Serum ferritin; iron; % saturation; transferrin receptors, free erythrocyte porphyrin	Hemoglobin concentration; microcytic anemia
Vitamin D	Plasma 25-hydroxyvitamin D	Parathyroid hormone
Vitamin C	Plasma vitamin C	None available
Vitamin B_1	Erythrocyte transketolase activation coefficient	None in common use
Vitamin B_2	Erythrocyte glutathione reductase activation coefficient	None in common use
Folate	Serum or red blood cell folate	Plasma homocysteine; leukocyte nucleus lob count
Vitamin B_{12}	Serum vitamin B12; holotranscobalamin	Methylmalonic acid
Calcium	Serum calcium (corrected for bound serum protein)	Alkaline phosphatase activity
Selenium	Plasma or red cell selenium; glutathione peroxides activity	None in common use
Copper	Cu-Zn superoxide dismutase	None in common use
Zinc	Serum Zn (might be affected by acute phase reaction)	Growth rate, severity of diarrheal episodes

Source: Adapted from Bates CJ. Assessment of micronutrient status in mothers and young infants. In: Delange FM, West KP, eds. *Micronutrient Deficiencies in the First Months of Life.* Vevey, Switzerland: Nestle, Ltd; 2003:3.

via the biliary tract; therefore, in the face of cholestatic disease, the parenteral administration of zinc should be closely monitored and reduced or discontinued if zinc accumulation is suspected. The same is true for copper. Acute zinc toxicity can cause pancreatitis.[50] Chronic toxicity has not been described in pediatric patients receiving PN.

Enteral Nutrition

The amount of zinc in human milk is initially high at 4 mg/L, but drops rapidly to 1.2 mg/L at 6 months postpartum.[51] The measured zinc intake by breastfed babies at 3 months of age was 1 mg/day.[52] Thus, with an AI of 2 mg/day, a 6-month-old infant who is exclusively breastfed is at risk of becoming zinc deficient. Infants starting on complementary feeds should be introduced to foods high in zinc at an early stage.

A number of nutrients are known to interfere with zinc absorption. Key among these are iron[53] and phytates.[54] Fiber foods tend to contain large amounts of phytates. Recent recommendations to increase the fiber intake of children might adversely affect their zinc status.

COPPER

Copper is important in many enzyme systems, especially those that involve oxygen, hydrogen peroxide, and superoxide. Copper is necessary for the formation of melanin, for catecholamine synthesis, and for cross-linking of elastin and collagen.[55] Copper circulates bound to ceruloplasmin, which could have antioxidant properties of its own. Unlike serum zinc as an indicator of zinc, serum copper is a good indicator of copper status.

Premature Infants, Term Infants, and Children

Premature infants are at special risk of becoming copper deficient because copper accumulates in the fetus during the third trimester. Signs of copper deficiency include: hypochromic, microcystic anemia; depigmentation of skin and hair; hypothermia; and hypotonia.

Parenteral Nutrition

Copper deficiency has been described in long term PN patients frequently.[56,57] As for zinc, parenteral copper administration should be done cautiously in the face of cholestatic disease, since the biliary tract is the major route of excretion. Because of concern that copper overload could occur in cholestasis, a number of regimens have been used to limit or omit copper from PN solutions. None are supported by evidence-based medicine.

Enteral Nutrition

Zinc interferes with copper absorption, but it is unclear whether this is clinically relevant as the amount of zinc needed to decrease copper absorption is far more than that contained in an ordinary diet. This interaction becomes relevant when large amounts of zinc are ingested as part of a complementary medicine treatment. Zinc can be used to inhibit the absorption of copper in Wilson's disease.[58] Iron could interfere with copper absorption. It has been postulated that copper absorption is decreased in infants consuming high iron formulas.[59]

MANGANESE

Manganese has 2 known functions, as cofactor for the enzyme pyruvate carboxylase and as a part of the mitochondrial form of superoxide dismutase.

Premature Infants, Term Infants, and Children

Parenteral Nutrition

Manganese deficiency in long term PN has not been described, however, toxicity has. High levels of manganese have been implicated as a causative factor in the cholestatic effect of PN and also in basal ganglia damage resulting in Parkinson's disease in adults on long term PN. Fell et al. have monitored basal ganglia damage associated with manganese accumulation in children on long term PN using MRI. This group also followed the cholestatic effects of manganese in children. Their study supports a causative role for manganese in both of these complications of PN.[60]

Enteral Nutrition

Only a small fraction of ingested manganese is absorbed (1.35–5%).[61] It is taken up by the blood, delivered to the liver, and rapidly excreted through the biliary system into the gastrointestinal tract. Almost all of the manganese leaves the body in the feces. There could be a gender factor important in manganese absorption, as there is apparently a longer half-life in men than in women.[61]

CHROMIUM

The metabolic role of chromium is poorly understood. Proof that chromium plays a part in a glucose tolerance factor, thought to activate insulin, is lacking. Two cases of chromium deficiency have been described in adults receiving PN. The symptoms of the described cases include glucose intolerance, hyperosmolarity, dehydration, and glucosuria. Symptoms responded poorly to insulin, but insulin responsiveness was restored with administration of chromium.[62]

Premature Infants, Term Infants, and Children

Parenteral Nutrition

Chromium deficiency in children receiving PN has not been described; however, chromium excess has been reported.[63] Chromium toxicity results in skin irritation and carcinogenesis in animals.[64] The trivalent chromic ions present in PN solutions are not highly toxic, so excessive chromium from PN is not likely to be harmful.

Enteral Nutrition

The Daily Reference Intakes (DRIs) set the adequate intake of chromium for infants 0–12 months by determining the amount in human milk. Adequate Intake (AI) for older children and adolescents were determined by extrapolation from adult data.[65]

IODINE

Iodine is essential, and its deficiency has been described in children.[66] The major role of iodine is its function in thyroid hormones. Because of the importance of the thyroid hormones, iodine is essential for the developing brain, muscle, heart, pituitary gland, and kidneys. Iodine is also important in nonthyroid-dependent functions such as bacterial killing through the action of myeloperoxidase and in the prevention of fibrocystic disease of the breast.

Premature Infants

Parenteral Nutrition

Ibrahim et al. studied a group of extremely premature infants on PN who were in negative iodine balance.[67] Since the absorption of iodine is good, the parenteral dose should be similar to the enteral recommendation. One μg/kg/day administered parenterally is recommended for the very low birth-weight infant.

Enteral Nutrition

The enteral recommendation is 30 μg/kg/day.[68,69] An AI of 110 μg/day from 0–6 months and 130 μg/day from 7–12 months of age is recommended. Estimated Average Requirement (EAR) for 1- through 8-year-olds is 65 μg/day; for 9- through 13-year-olds, it is 73 μg/day; and for 14 through 18-year-olds, it is 95 μg/day.

Term Infants and Children

Parenteral Nutrition

Iodine is a minor contaminating component of many PN solutions and is present in antiseptics used to cleanse the skin at the catheter insertion site. PN patients receive measurable iodine from both of these sources.[70] No toxicity has been found in subjects receiving 20 times the RDA for iodine. Any pediatric patient receiving long term PN requires supplemental iodine.

Enteral Nutrition

The consequences of iodine deficiency are mental retardation, hypothyroidism, goiter, cretinism, and abnormalities in growth and development. After table salt producers began fortifying it with potassium iodide, iodine deficiency all but disappeared. Recently, there has been an increased use of sea salt that is not fortified. It remains to be seen whether iodine deficiency will reappear.

SELENIUM

Selenium is at the catalytic site of glutathione peroxidase, an enzyme that catalyzes the reduction of H_2O_2 to H_2O. Selenium is also at the active site of types one and three iodothyronine deiodinase, which is important in the synthesis and degradation of triiodothyronine.[71]

Premature Infants, Term Infants, and Children

Parenteral Nutrition

One study did not show a correlation between selenium supplementation and thyroid function in very low-birth-weight infants receiving long term PN,[72] but selenium deficiency has been reported in children receiving PN.[73–75] The ASCN guidelines list the parenteral selenium requirements at 2.0 µg/kg/day for preterm infants, term infants and children.[76] Selenium toxicity is described.[77]

Enteral Nutrition

Rarely has selenium deficiency been described outside of the context of PN. Plants take up selenium, present in the soil, and humans ingest the plants. There are areas of the world where the soil is very low in selenium; however, in the developed world, food distribution is so broad that selenium deficiency is unlikely even in geographic areas low in selenium.

IRON

Iron deficiency is the most common cause of anemia in children.[78] However, anemia is a manifestation of the severe end of the iron deficiency spectrum, as iron is used for erythropoesis at the expense of other tissues including brain. Iron deficiency adversely affects behavior and neurodevelopment.[79] Iron deficiency is common among children receiving long term PN. It occurs as a result of the underlying condition necessitating PN rather than a result of PN itself. Long term PN without iron supplementation results in iron deficiency and iron deficiency anemia. Causes of anemia other than iron deficiency could be present and should be searched for before assuming that anemia is due to iron deficiency. Other causes of anemia include the anemia of chronic disease, zinc deficiency, vitamin E deficiency, and hemolysis. Chronic blood loss from stool, urine, or vomitus can lead to iron deficiency. These sources of loss should be corrected when possible. A number of tests are useful in assessing iron nutrition, including assessments of ferritin, free erythrocyte protoporphyrin, zinc protoporphyrin, transferrin saturation, transferrin receptors, mean corpuscular volume, and finally hemoglobin and hematocrit (Chapter 7). Hemoglobin and hematocrit are readily accessible but represent severe, end-stage iron deficiency. Ferritin is an early marker of iron deficiency, reflecting liver stores of iron; however, ferritin is also an acute phase reactant, making interpretation of ferritin test results problematic. Changes in protoporphyrin levels reflect early alteration of erythropoesis. In the context of a child suspected to be iron deficient, a combination of these tests is recommended.[80]

Premature Infants

Parenteral Nutrition

Prematurely born infants are at particular risk for deficiency as iron is transferred to the fetus via the placenta during the last trimester. Iron precipitates as iron phosphate from lipid emulsions and 3-in-1 solutions. Iron dextrans are compatible with PN solutions that do not contain lipid.[81]

Enteral Nutrition

Because of the increased risk of iron deficiency, all prematurely born infants, breastfed or formula fed, should receive iron supplementation. Breastfed premature infants should receive 2 mg/kg/day elemental iron starting at 1 month of age and continuing through the first year. Formula fed premature infants should get 1 mg/kg/day elemental iron in addition to the iron contained in the formula.[82]

Term Infants and Children

Parenteral Nutrition

Iron can be given either intravenously or intramuscularly as iron dextran.[83] Iron sucrose can be given intravenously.[84] Inorganic salts of iron are used in PN solution in Europe.[85] Some report increased infection rates in children receiving iron supplementation.[86] Other reports have not found this association.[87] A meta-analysis found no association between iron therapy and infection.[88] Iron homeostasis is regulated at the level of gastrointestinal absorption. Parenterally administered iron bypasses this control mechanism, making iron overload possible. Iron administration should be reduced or eliminated if overload is present.[89]

Enteral Nutrition

The term infant experiences an interval of about 4 months when erythropoesis is low. Therefore the demand for iron is low. Between 4 and 6 months of age, erythropoesis accelerates, and the demand for iron increases. The term infant is born with iron stores adequate for about 4–6 months. Human milk has very little iron (about 1 mg Fe/L); however, the term breastfed infant is unlikely to become iron deficient despite low iron intake, if iron-containing complementary foods are introduced in a timely fashion. If iron stores were low to begin with, or if iron-containing complementary foods are not introduced, the term breastfed infant might become iron deficient. If there is no clear source of iron other than human milk by 6 months of age, supplementation with 1 mg/kg/day elemental iron must be given.[82] Most formulas available in the United States contain 12 mg/L iron, an amount that will supply iron requirements through the first year of life. Even low iron formula contains 4 mg/L iron, enough iron to prevent depletion of iron stores in most infants.

The risk of iron deficiency continues into the toddler years. Growth of the erythron, while slower, is still substantial. Toddlers' diets are typically not high in iron-containing foods. Various reports place the prevalence of iron deficiency among toddlers at 2–9%.[90,91] Adolescent girls are also at risk because of the onset of menstrual blood loss and demands of increased growth. In the context of pediatric nutrition support, iron status should be evaluated and supplemental iron given in the face of either depleted stores or anemia. It is important to investigate the underlying reason for abnormal iron status.

MOLYBDENUM

In the human, molybdenum is known to be a cofactor in only 3 enzymes, sulfite oxidase, xanthine oxidase, and aldehyde oxidase. These enzymes function in the metabolism of sulfur amino acids and heterocyclic compounds. A true molybdenum deficiency state has not been described in humans. That molybdenum is essential is inferred from two lines of reasoning: (1) in an inborn error of metabolism that results in complete absence of the molybdenum-dependent enzyme, sulfite oxidase neurologic damage and death occurs in the neonatal period,[92] and (2) in long term PN without molybdenum, an amino acid imbalance that is correctible by intravenous administration of molybdenate occurs.[93]

Premature Infants, Term Infants, and Children

The absorption of molybdenum appears to be nearly complete via a passive, nonmediated process. The implication of the almost complete absorption is that enteral and parenteral requirements should be similar. Regulation of molybdenum homeostasis is at the level of the kidney.[94,95]

An AI of 3 μg/kg/day is established for infants from 0–12 months. For older children, the EAR was extrapolated from adult data using the metabolic weight ($kg^{0.75}$). The EAR for children 1–3 years old is 13 μg/day; for 4 through 8-year-olds, it is 17 μg/day; for 9 to 13-year-old children, it is 26 μg/day; and for those 13–18, it is 33 μg/day.[96]

VITAMINS

Vitamins are essential nutrients (Chapter 8). Health depends on an adequate supply of vitamins. Long term high intakes of fat-soluble vitamins A, D, E, and K can cause toxicity. For infants and children with chronic fat malabsorption (cystic fibrosis, other reasons for exocrine pancreatic deficiency, or liver disease) higher intakes of fat-soluble vitamins might be indicated, but vitamin levels should be monitored. For patients who have nonfunctional gastrointestinal tracts dependent on PN, there is little flexibility to individualize vitamin administration since only two intravenous vitamin preparations are available (see Chapter 22 for a discussion of parenteral vitamins; also see Table 25-4). Patients who have at least a partially functioning gastrointestinal tract can take vitamin supplements as

Table 25-4 Parenteral multivitamin combinations.

Vitamin Dose	A (IU)	D (IU)	E (IU)	K (mcg)	C (mg)	B_1 (mg)	B_2 (mg)	B_3 (mg)	B_5 (mg)	B_6 (mg)	B_{12} (mcg)	Biotin (mcg)	Folic acid mcg
MVI-Pediatric 5 mL	2,300	400	7	200	80	1.2	1.4	17	5	1	1	20	140
MVI-12 5 mL	1,650	100	5	0	50	1.5	1.8	20	7.5	2	2.5	30	200
MVI-concentrate 1 mL	2,000	200	1	0	100	10	2	20	5	3	0	0	0
Cernevit 2.5 mL	1,750	110	5.6	0	62.5	1.2	1.4	17	5	1	1	20	140

Source: From product information, July 2005.

individual vitamins or as a multivitamin. Vitamin supplements come in liquid, chewable, and pill (capsule or tablet) forms (see Table 25-5). All enteral nutrition products that are medical foods (Chapter 15) contain adequate vitamins to meet the daily requirement, provided a minimum volume, usually 1 liter, is consumed.

Human milk is deficient in vitamin D. All infant formulas sold in the United States must have a minimum vitamin D concentration of 40 IU/100 kcal and a maximum vitamin D concentration of 100 IU/100 kcal. If an infant is receiving at least 500 mL/day of an infant formula, that infant is receiving the recommended amount of vitamin D. Infants who are fed solely on human milk or receive less than 500 mL/day of an infant formula must have their diet supplemented with vitamin D.[97]

CHOLINE AND CARNITINE

Intravenous vitamin preparations for PN do not contain choline or carnitine. Choline is an essential nutrient (see Chapter 8 for a discussion of essential nutrients) for health. Choline functions as a precursor for acetylcholine, phospholipids, and betaine. Endogenous synthesis of choline via the sequential methylation of phosphatidylethanolamine occurs, but choline is an essential nutrient because the *de novo* synthesis rate is not adequate to meet the demand for the nutrient when other nutrients are available in amounts sufficient to sustain normal growth and function. Choline is abundant in foods, so deficiency is unlikely except in the most extreme cases, such as patients on long term PN. Insufficient choline intake is associated with hepatocellular damage such as that caused by fatty liver,[98] and it might cause or contribute to liver abnormalities sometimes seen in patients on PN. There is no guidance on when choline should be added to PN solutions or the dose that should be prescribed except in the case of hepatic steatosis.[99] A multicenter clinical trial is in progress to assess the effect of choline chloride on the reversal of hepatic steatosis.[100] Parenteral choline chloride is manufactured in China.

Carnitine might be an essential nutrient in neonates, especially for those infants born prematurely.[101] It is a quaternary amine synthesized from the amino acid lysine. Carnitine, as acyltransferases and translocases, is required for the transfer of activated fatty acyl groups within subcellular compartments and across intracellular membranes. Thus, fatty acid oxidation is dependent on carnitine. Carnitine is required for long chain polyunsaturated fatty acids to enter the mitochondria of cells. Carnitine deficiency is associated with cardiomyopathy, encephalopathy, nonketotic hypoglycemia, hypotonia, poor growth, and frequent infections.[102] Human milk, the diet, and infant formulas are rich sources of carnitine. For infants on PN who are at risk of developing carnitine deficiency, especially premature infants, an intravenous preparation, Carnitor (Sigma-Tau, Gaithersburg, MD)[103] is available. An initial dose of 8–10mg/kg/day (50.0–62.5 μmol/kg/day) is reported as a safe starting dose. Blood levels should be closely monitored.

Carnitine benefits the respiratory status of ventilator dependent adults[104] and increases stabilization and physical performance of adults with chronic respiratory insufficiency.[105] Iafolla noted a decrease in infant apnea episodes 48 hours after treatment with oral carnitine.[106] Subsequently, Iafolla supplemented healthy, preterm 34-week-gestation infants with carnitine and found a significant decrease in apnea episodes and early weaning from ventilators.[107] However, a recent Cochrane review of carnitine treatment trials in preterm infants with apnea found that none of the existing trials met the review criteria of randomized or quasirandomized treatment trials with a placebo group.[108] The reviewers concluded that there is insufficient evidence at this time to support the use of carnitine for the treatment of apnea of prematurity, and further studies are needed.

CONCLUSION

The essence of pediatric nutrition support is attention to detail. Evaluating, administering, and reevaluating each of the vitamins and trace elements might appear to be tedious details; however, a good outcome can be directly related to how much effort is put into each of these details.

Table 25-5 Vitamin/mineral/trace element combinations.

Product	Dose	A (IU)	D (IU)	E (IU)	C (mg)	K (mcg)	Folic acid (mg)	B_1 (mg)	B_2 (mg)	B_3 (mg)	B_6 (mg)
Drops											
Vi-Daylin or Poly-Vi-Sol (carbohydrate-free)	1 mL	1,500	400	5	35	0	0	0.5	0.6	8	0.4
Poly-Vi-Flor 0.25											
Vi-Daylin w/fluoride	1 mL	1,500	400	5	35	0	0	0.5	0.6	8	0.4
Poly-Vi-Flor 0.5	1 mL	1,500	400	5	35	0	0	0.5	0.6	8	0.4
Tri-Vit (Tri-Vi-Sol)	1 mL	1,500	400	0	35	0	0	0	0	0	0
Tri-Vit w/fluoride 0.25 (Tri-Vi-Flor 0.25)	1 mL	1,500	400	0	35	0	0	0	0	0	0
Tri-Vit w/Fluoride 0.5 (Tri-Vi-Flor 0.5)	1 mL	1,500	400	0	35	0	0	0	0	0	0
Vi-Dalyin w/iron	1 mL	1,500	400	5	35	0	0	0.5	0.6	8	0.4
Vi-Daylin/F w/iron	1 mL	1,500	400	4.2	35	0	0	0.5	0.6	8	0.4
ADEKs	1 mL	1,500	400	40	45	100	0	0.5	0.6	6	0.6
Liquid											
Vi-Daylin	5 mL	2,500	400	11	60	0	0	1.05	1.2	13.5	1.05
Vi-Daylin w/iron	5 mL	2,500	400	11	60	0	0	1.05	1.2	13.5	1.05
Theragran	5 mL	5,000	400	0	200	0	0	10	10	100	4.1
Chewable tablets (pediatrics)											
Poly-Vi-Sol	1 tablet	2,500	400	15	60	0	0.3	1.05	1.2	13.5	1.05
Poly-Vi-Flor 0.5	1 tablet	2,500	400	15	60	0	0.3	1.05	1.2	13.5	1.05
Poly-Vi-Flor 1.0	1 tablet	2,500	400	15	60	0	0.3	1.05	1.2	13.5	1.05
Vitamax	1 tablet	5,000	400	200	60	150	0.2	1.5	1.7	20	2
Flintstones Complete Bugs Bunny	1	5,000	400	30	60	0	0.4	1.5	1.7	20	2
ADEKs	1	4,000	400	150	60	150	0.2	1.2	1.3	10	1.5
Tablets (adult)											
Nephro-Vite	1	0	0	0	60	0	0.8	1.5	1.7	20	10
Theragran	1	5,500	400	30	120	0	0.4	3	3.4	30	3
Theragran-M	1	5,500	400	30	120	0	0.4	3	3.4	30	3

Source: From product information, July 2005.

Table 25-5 Vitamin/mineral/trace element combinations (continued).

Product	*Dose*	*Pantothenic acid (mg)*	*Biotin (mcg)*	*B_{12} (mcg)*	*Fluoride (mg)*	*Calcium (mg)*	*PO4 (mg)*	*Mg (mg)*	*Iron (mg)*	*Zinc (mg)*
Drops										
Vi-Daylin or Poly-Vi-Sol (carbohydrate-free)	1 mL	0	0	0.4	0	0	0	0	0	0
Poly-Vi-Flor 0.25										
Vi-Daylin w/fluoride	1 mL	0	0	0.4	0.25	0	0	0	0	0
Poly-Vi-Flor 0.5	1 mL	0	0	0.4	0.5	0	0	0	0	0
Tri-Vit (Tri-Vi-Sol)	1 mL	0	0	0	0	0	0	0	0	0
Tri-Vit w/fluoride 0.25 (Tri-Vi-Flor 0.25)	1 mL	0	0	0	0.25	0	0	0	0	0
Tri-Vit w/Fluoride 0.5 (Tri-Vi-Flor 0.5)	1 mL	0	0	0	0.5	0	0	0	0	0
Vi-Dalyin w/iron	1 mL	0	0	0	0	0	0	0	10	0
Vi-Daylin/F w/iron	1 mL	0	0	0	0.25	0	0	0	10	0
ADEKs	1 mL	3	15	4	0	0	0	0	0	5 (ZnSO4)
Liquid										
Vi-Daylin	5 mL	0	0	4.5	0	0	0	0	0	0
Vi-Daylin w/iron	5 mL	0	0	4.5	0	0	0	0	10	0
Theragran	5 mL	21.4	0	5	0	0	0	0	0	0
Chewable tablets (pediatrics)										
Poly-Vi-Sol	1 tablet	0	0	4.5	0	0	0	0	0	0
Poly-Vi-Flor 0.5	1 tablet	0	0	4.5	0	0	0	0	0	0
Poly-Vi-Flor 1.0	1 tablet	0	0	4.5	0	0	0	0	0	0
Vitamax	1 tablet	10	200	6	0	0	0	0	0	0
Flintstones Complete Bugs Bunny	1	10	40	6	0	100	100	20	18	15
ADEKs	1	10	50	12	0	0	0	0	0	7.5 glucon
Tablets (adult)										
Nephro-Vite	1	10	300	6	0	0	0	0	0	0
Theragran	1	10	15	9	0	0	0	0	0	0
Theragran-M	1	10	15	9	0	40	0	100	27	15

Source: From product information, July 2005.

REFERENCES

1. Husain SM, Mughal MZ. Mineral transport across the placenta. *Arch Dis Child.* 1992;67:874–878.
2. Widdowson EM, Spray CM. Chemical development in utero. *Arch Dis Child.* 1951;26:205–214.
3. Givens MH, Macy IC. The chemical composition of the human fetus. *J Biol Chem.* 1933;102:7–17.
4. Lanske B, Karaplis AC, Lee K, et al. PTH/PThrP receptor in early development and Indian hedgehog-regulated bone growth. *Science.* 1996;273:663–666.
5. Stulic J, Stulcova B. Placental transfer of phosphate in anesthetized rats. *Placenta.* 1996;17:487–493.
6. Key LL, Carpenter TO. Metabolism of calcium, phosphorus, and other divalent ions. In: Ichikawa I, ed. *Pediatric Textbook of Fluids and Electrolytes.* Baltimore, Md: Williams and Wilkins; 1990:98–106.
7. Widdowson EM, McCance RA. The metabolism of calcium, phosphorus, magnesium and strontium. *Pediatr Clin North Am.* 1965;12:595.
8. Aikawa JK. *Magnesium: Its Biologic Significance.* Boca Raton, Fla: CRC Press; 1981: 43–56.
9. Larchet M, Garabedian M, Bourdeau A, Gorski AM, Goulet O, Ricour C. Calcium metabolism in children during long term total parenteral nutrition: the influence of calcium, phosphorus, and vitamin D intakes. *J Pediatr Gastroenterol Nutr.* 1991;13(4):367–375.
10. Lipkin EW, Ott SM, Chesnut CH III, Chait A. Mineral loss in the parenteral nutrition patient. *Am J Clin Nutr.* 1988;47(3):515–523.
11. Karton MA, Rettmer R, Lipkin EW, Ott SM, Chait A. D-lactate and metabolic bone disease in patients receiving long-term parenteral nutrition. *JPEN.* 1999;13(2):132–135.
12. Wood RJ, Bengoa JM, Sitrin MD, Rosenberg IH. Calciuretic effect of cyclic versus continuous total parenteral nutrition. *Am J Clin Nutr.* 1985;41(3):614–619.
13. Greer FR, Steichen JJ, Tsang RC. Effect of increased calcium, phosphorus, and vitamin D intake on bone mineralization in very low birth weight infants fed formulas with polycose and medium change triglycerides. *J Pediatr.* 1982;100:951–955.
14. Pittard WB III, Geddes KM, Sutherland SE, Miller MC, Hollis BW. Longitudinal changes in the bone mineral content of term and premature infants. *Am J Dis Child.* 1990;144:36–40.
15. Bishop NJ, Dahlenburg SL, Fewtrell MS, Morley R, Lucas A. Early diet of preterm infants and bone mineralization at age five years. *Acta Paediatrica.* 1996;85:230–236.
16. Bishop NJ, King FJ, Lucas A. Increased bone mineral content in preterm infants fed with a nutrient enriched formula after discharge from hospital. *Arch Dis Child.* 1993;68:573–578.
17. Chan GM. Growth and bone mineral status of discharged very low birth weight infants fed different formulas or human milk. *J Pediatr.* 1993;123:439–443.
18. Atkinson SA, Chappell JE, Clandinin MT. Calcium supplementation of mothers' milk for low birthweight infants: problems related to absorption and excretion. *Nutr Res.* 1987;7:813–823.
19. Schanler RJ, Garza C, Smith EO. Fortified mothers' milk for very low birth weight infants: results of macromineral balance studies. *J Pediatr.* 1985;107:767–774.
20. Allen JC, Keller RP, Archer P, Neville MC. Studies in human lactation: milk composition and daily secretion rates of macronutrients in the first year of lactation. *Am J Clin Nutr.* 1991;54:69–80.
21. Fomon SJ, Nelson SE. Calcium, phosphorus, magnesium and sulfur. In: Fomon SJ, ed. *Nutrition of Normal Infants.* St. Louis, Mo: Mosby-Year Book, Inc; 1993:192–216.
22. Greer FR. Calcium, phosphorus and magnesium: how much is too much for infant formulas? *J Nutr.* 1989;119:1846–1851.
23. Koo W, Tsang RC. Calcium, magnesium and phosphorus and Vitamin D. In: Tsang R, Lucas A, Uauy R, and Zlotkin S, eds. *Nutritional Needs of the Premature Infant.* Philadelphia, Pa: Williams and Wilkins, Inc; 1993:134–141.
24. Weinsier RL, Krumdieck CL. Death resulting from overzealous total PN: the refeeding syndrome revisited. *Am J Clin Nutr.* 1980;34:393–399.
25. Matkovic V. Calcium intake and peak bone mass. *New Engl J Med.* 1992;327(2):119–120.
26. Kien CL, Browning C, Jona J, Starshak RJ. Rickets in premature infants receiving parenteral nutrition: a case report and review of the literature. *JPEN.* 1982;6(2):152–156.
27. Shike M, Shils ME, Heller A, et al. Bone disease in prolonged parenteral nutrition: osteopenia without mineralization defect. *Am J Clin Nut.* 1986;44(1):89–98.
28. Dunham B, Marcuard S, Khazanie PG, Meade G, Craft T, Nichols K. The solubility of calcium and phosphorus in neonatal total PN solutions. *JPEN.* 1991;15:608–611.
29. Heird WC, Hay W, Helms RA, et al. Pediatric parenteral amino acid mixture in low birth weight infants. *Pediatrics.* 1988;81:41–50.
30. Ament ME. Bone mineral content in patients with short bowel syndrome: the impact of PN. *J Pediatr.* 1998;132:386–388.
31. Klein GL. Metabolic bone disease of total parenteral nutrition. *Nutrition.* 1998;14(1):149–152.

32. Ott SM, Maloney NA, Kleein GL, et al. Aluminum is associated with low bone formation in patients receiving chronic PN. *Ann Intern Med.* 1983;98:910–914.

33. Klein GL, Ott SM, Alfrey AC, et al. Aluminum as a factor in the bone disease of long term PN. *Trans Assoc Am Physicians.* 1982;15:155–164.

34. Klein GL, Alfrey AC, Miller NL, et al. Aluminum loading during total PN. *Am J Clin Nutr.* 1982;35:1425–1429.

35. Vargas JH, Klein GL, Ament ME, et al. Metabolic bone disease of total PN: course after changing from casein to amino acids in parenteral solutions with reduced aluminum content. *Am J Clin Nutr.* 1988;48:1070–1078.

36. Dellert SF, Farrell MK, Specker BL, Heubi JE. Bone mineral content in children with short bowel syndrome after discontinuation of PN. *J Pediatr.* 1998;132:516–519.

37. Schmidt-Sommerfeld E, Snyder G, Rotti TM, et al. Catheter-related complications in 35 children and adolescents with gastrointestinal disease on home PN. *JPEN.* 1990;14:148–151.

38. Atkinson SA, Alston-Mills BP, Lonnerdal B, Neville MC, Thompson MP. Major minerals and ionic constituents of human and bovine milk. In: Jensen RJ, ed. *Handbook of Milk Composition*. San Diego,Calif: Academic Press; 1995:593–619.

39. Institute of Medicine. *Dietary Reference Intakes for Calcium, Phosphorus, Magnesium, Vitamin D, and Fluoride*. Washington, DC: National Academy Press; 1997:91–106.

40. Gartner LM, Greer FR. Section on Breastfeeding and Committee on Nutrition, American Academy of Pediatrics. Prevention of rickets and vitamin D deficiency: new guidelines for vitamin D intake. *Pediatrics*. 2003;111:908–910.

41. Suitor CW, Gleason PM. Using dietary reference intake-based methods to estimate the prevalence of inadequate nutrient intake among school-aged children. *J Am Diet Assoc.* 2002;102:530–536.

42. Greer FR, Tsang RC, Levin RS, Searcy JE, Wu R, Steichen JJ. Increasing serum calcium and magnesium concentrations in breast-fed infants: longitudinal studies of minerals in human milk and in sera of nursing mothers and their infants. *J Pediatr.* 1982;100:59–64.

43. Brodehl J, Gellissen K, Weber H-P. Postnatal development of tubular phosphate reabsorption. *Clin Nephrol.* 1982;17:163–171.

44. Dewey KG, Finley DA, Lonnerdal B. Breastmilk volume and composition during late lactation (7–20 months). *J Pediatr Gastroenterol Nutr*. 1984;3:713–720.

45. Branca F, Robins SP, Ferro-Luzzi A. Golden MH. Bone turnover in malnourished children. *Lancet.* 1992;340:1493.

46. Prasad AS. Zinc: an overview. *Nutrition.* 1995;11(1 Suppl):93–99.

47. Beck FW, Prasad AS, Kaplan J, Fitzgerald JT, Brewer GJ. Changes in cytokine production and T cell subpopulations in experimentally induced zinc-deficient humans. *Am J Physiol.* 1997;272(6 Pt 1):E1002–1007.

48. Golden BE, Golden MH. Plasma zinc, rate of weight gain, and the energy cost of tissue deposition in children recovering from severe malnutrition on a cow's milk or soya protein based diet. *Am J Clin Nutr*. 1981;34(5):892–899.

49. Anonymous. Acrodermatitis enteropathica—hereditary zinc deficiency. *Nutrition Reviews*. 1975;33:327–9.

50. Main AN, Hall MJ, Russell RI, Fell GS, Mills PR, Shenkin A. Clinical experience of zinc supplementation during intravenous nutrition in Crohn's disease: value of serum and urine zinc measurements. *Gut.* 1982;23(11):984–991.

51. Krebs NF, Reidinger CJ, Hartley S, Robertson AD, Hambridge KM. Zinc supplementation during lactation: effects on maternal status and milk zinc concentration. *Am J Clin Nutr.* 1995;1:1030–1036.

52. Krebs NF, Reidinger CJ, Robertson AD, Hambridge KM. Growth and intakes of energy and zinc in infants fed human milk. *J Pediatr.* 1994;124:32–39.

53. O'Brien KO, Zavaleta N, Caulfield LE, Wen J, Abrams SA. Prenatal iron supplements impair zinc absorption in pregnant Peruvian women. *J Nutr*. 2000;130:2251–2255.

54. Oberleas D, Muhrer ME, O'Dell BL. Dietary metal-complexing agents and zinc availability in the rat. *J Nutr*. 1966;90:56–62.

55. Solomon NW. Zinc and copper. In: Shils ME, Young VR, eds. *Modern Nutrition in Health and Disease.* Philadelphia, Pa: Lea and Febiger; 1988:238–262.

56. Karpel JT, Peden VH. Copper deficiency in long-term parenteral nutrition. *J Pediatr*. 1972;80(1):32–36.

57. Koo WW. Parenteral nutrition-related bone disease. *JPEN.* 1992;16(4):386–394.

58. Brewer GJ, Hill GM, Prasad AS, Cossack ZT, Rabbani P. Oral zinc therapy for Wilson's disease. *Ann Intern Med.* 1983;99:314–319.

59. Lonnerdal B, Hernell O. Iron, zinc, copper and selenium status in breast-fed infants and infants fed trace element fortified milk-based infant formula. *Acta Paediatr.* 1994;83:367–373.

60. Fell JM, Reynolds AP, Meadows N, et al. Manganese toxicity in children receiving long-term parenteral nutrition. *Lancet.* 1996;347(9010):1218–1221.

61. Finley JW, Johnson PE, Johnson LK. Sex affects manganese absorption and retention by humans from a diet adequate in manganese. *Am J Clin Nutr.* 1994;60:949–955.

62. Freund H, Atamian S, Fischer JE. Chromium deficiency during total parenteral nutrition. *JAMA.* 1979;241(5):496–498.
63. Moukarzel AA, Song MK, Buchman AL, et al. Excessive chromium intake in children receiving total parenteral nutrition. *Lancet.* 1992;339(8790):385–388.
64. Katz SA, Salem H. The toxicology of chromium with respect to its chemical speciation: a review. *J Appl Toxicol.* 1993;13(3):217–224.
65. Institute of Medicine. *Dietary Reference Intakes for Vitamin A, Vitamin K, Arsenic, Boron, Chromium, Copper, Iodine, Iron, Manganese, Molybdenum, Nickel, Silicon, Vanadium, and Zinc.* Washington, DC: National Academy Press; 2001:197–223.
66. Mirmira, P. Kimiagar M, Azizi F. Three-year survey of effects of iodized oil injection in schoolchildren with iodine deficiency disorders. *Exp Clin Endocrinol Diabetes.* 2002;110(8):393–397.
67. Ibrahim M, de Escobar GM, Visser TJ, et al. Iodine deficiency associated with parenteral nutrition in extreme preterm infants. *Arch Dis Child Fetal Neonatal Edition.* 2003;88(1):F56–57.
68. Ares S, Escobar-Morreale HF, Quero J, et al. Neonatal hypothyroxinemia: effects of iodine intake and premature birth. *J Clin Endocrinol Metabol.* 1997;82(6):1704–1712.
69. Delange F, Bourdoux P, Chanoine JP, et al. Physiology of iodine nutrition during pregnancy, lactation and early postnatal life. In: Berger H, ed. *Vitamins and Minerals in Pregnancy and Lactation: Nestle's Nutrition Workshop Series.* Vol 16, New York, NY: Vevey/Raven Press; 1988:205–214.
70. Moukarzel AA, Buchman AL, Salas JS, et al. Iodine supplementation in children receiving long-term parenteral nutrition. *J Pediatr.* 1992;121(2):252–254.
71. Larsen PR, Berry MJ. Nutritional and hormonal regulation of thyroid hormone deiodinases. *Ann Rev Nutr.* 1995;15:323–352.
72. Klinger G, Shamir R, Singer P, Diamond EM, Josefsberg Z, Sirota L. Parenteral selenium supplementation in extremely low birth weight infants: inadequate dosage but no correlation with hypothyroidism. *J Perinatol.* 1999;19(8 Pt 1):568–572.
73. Kien C, Ganther HE. Manifestations of chronic selenium deficiency in a child receiving total parenteral nutrition. *Am J Clin Nutr.* 1983;37(2):319–328.
74. Van Caillie-Bertrand M, Degenhart HJ, Fernandes J. Selenium status of infants on nutritional support. *Acta Paediatr Scand.* 1984;73(6):816–819.
75. Hatanaka N, Nakaden H, Yamamoto Y, Matsuo S, Fujikawa T, Matsusue S. Selenium kinetics and changes in glutathione peroxidase activities in patients receiving long-term parenteral nutrition and effects of supplementation with selenite. *Nutrition.* 2000;16(1):22–26.
76. Greene HL, Hambidge KM, Schanler R, Tsang RC. From the Committee on Clinical Practice Issues of the American Society for Clinical Nutrition. Guidelines for the use of vitamins, trace elements, calcium, magnesium, and phosphorus in infants and children receiving total parenteral nutrition: report of the Subcommittee on Pediatric Parenteral Nutrient Requirements. *Am J Clin Nutr.* 1988;48(5):1324–1342.
77. Levander OA. A global view of human selenium nutrition. *Ann Rev Nutr.* 1987;7:227–250.
78. Looker AC, Dallman PR, Carroll MD, Gunter EW, Johnson CL. Prevalence of iron deficiency in the United States. *JAMA.* 1997;277(12):973–976.
79. Nokes C, van den Bosch C, Bundy DAP. *The Effects of Iron Deficiency and Anemia on Mental and Motor Performance, Educational Achievement and Behavior in Children: A Report of the International Nutrition Anemia Consultative Group.* Washington, DC; International Nutritional Anemia Consultative Group, 1998.
80. Glader BE. Screening for anemia and erythrocyte disorders in children. *Pediatrics.* 1986;78(2):368–369.
81. Mayhew SL, Quick MW. Compatibility of iron dextran with neonatal parenteral nutrient solutions. *Am J Health-System Pharm.* 1997;54(5):570–571.
82. Committee on Nutrition. Iron Deficiency *American Academy of Pediatrics, Committee on Nutrition Pediatric Nutrition Handbook.* 5th ed. Elk Grove Village, Ill: American Academy of Pediatrics; 2004:299–312.
83. Reed MD, Bertino JS Jr, Halpin TC Jr. Use of intravenous iron dextran injection in children receiving total parenteral nutrition. *Am J Dis Child.* 1981;135(9):829–831.
84. Van Wyck DB, Cavallo G, Spinowitz BS, et al. Safety and efficacy of iron sucrose in patients sensitive to iron dextran: North American clinical trial. *Am J Kidney Dis.* 2000;36(1):88–97.
85. Michaud L, Guimber D, Mention K, et al. Tolerance and efficacy of intravenous iron saccharate for iron deficiency anemia in children and adolescents receiving long-term parenteral nutrition. *Clin Nutr.* 2002;21(5):403–407.
86. Murray MJ, Murray AB, Murray MB, Murray CJ. The adverse effect of iron repletion on the course of certain infections. *BMJ.* 1978;2(6145):1113–1115.
87. Baltimore RS, Shedd DG, Pearson HA. Effect of iron saturation on the bacteriostasis of human serum: in vivo does not correlate with in vitro saturation. *J Pediatr.* 1982;101(4):519–523.
88. Gera T, Sachdev HP. Effect of iron supplementation on incidence of infectious illness in children: systematic review. *BMJ.* 2002;325(7373):1142.

89. Ben Hariz M, Goulet O, De Potter S, et al. Iron overload in children receiving prolonged parenteral nutrition. *J Pediatr*. 1993;123(2):238–241.

90. Sherry B, Mei Z, Yip R. Continuation of the decline in prevalence of anemia in low-income infants and children in five states. *Pediatrics*. 2001;107:677–682.

91. Hay G, Sandstad B, Whitelaw A, Borch-Iohnsen B. Iron status in a group of Norwegian children aged 6–24 months. *Acta Paediatr*. 2004;93:592–598.

92. Johnson JL. Molybdenum. In: O'Dell BL, Sunde RA, eds. *Handbook of Nutritionally Essential Mineral Elements. Clinical Nutrition in Health and Disease*. New York, NY: Marcel Dekker; 1997:413–438.

93. Abumrad NN, Schneider AJ, Steel D, Rogers LS. Amino acid intolerance during prolonged total parenteral nutrition reversed by molybdate therapy. *Am J Clin Nutr*. 1981;34:2551–2559.

94. Turnlund JR, Keyes WR, Peiffer GL. Molybdenem absorption, excretion and retention studied with stable isotopes in young men at five intakes of molybdenum. *Am J Clin Nutr*. 1995;62:790–796.

95. Turnlund JR, Keyes WR, Peiffer GL. Molybdenem absorption, excretion and retention studied with stable isotopes in young men during depletion and repletion. *Am J Clin Nutr*. 1995;61:1102–1109.

96. Institute of Medicine. *Dietary Reference Intakes for Vitamin A, Vitamin K, Arsenic, Boron, Chromium, Copper, Iodine, Iron, Manganese, Molybdenum, Nickel, Silicon, Vanadium, and Zinc*. Washington, DC: National Academy Press; 2001:424–441.

97. Lawrence M, Gartner MD, Frank R, Greer MD. Prevention of rickets and vitamin D deficiency: new guidelines for vitamin D intake. *Pediatrics*. 2003;111:908–910.

98. Zeisel SH. Choline deficiency. *J Nutr Biochem*. 1990;1:332–349.

99. Buchman AL, Dubin MD, Moukarzel AA, et al. Choline deficiency: a cause of hepatic steatosis during parenteral nutrition that can be reversed with intravenous choline supplementation. *Hepatology*. 1995;22(5):1399–1403.

100. Total parenteral nutrition-associated liver disease. ClinicalTrials.gov identifier NCT00031135; Illinois Northwestern University. Available at: http://www.clinicaltrials.gov/ct/gui/show/nct00031135. Accessed March 6, 2006.

101. Borum PR. Carnitine in neonatal nutrition. *J Child Neurol*. 1995;10:S8–24.

102. Winter SC. Szabo-Aczel S. Curry CJ. Hutchinson HT. Hogue R. Shug A. Plasma carnitine deficiency: clinical observations in 51 pediatric patients. *Am J Dis Child*. 1987;141:660.

103. Sapsfore AL. Parenteral nutrition: energy, carbohydrate, protein and fat. In: Groh-Wargo S, Thompson M, Cox JH, Hartline JV, eds. *Nutritional Care for High-Risk Newborns*. Chicago, Ill: Precept Press, Inc; 2000:137.

104. DalNegro R, Pomari G, Zoccatelli O, Turoo P. L-carnitine rehabilitative respiratory physiokinesitherapy: metabolic and ventilatory response in chronic respiratory insufficiency. *Int J Clin Pharmacol Ther Toxicol*. 1986;27:14–20.

105. DalNegro R, Turoo P, Pomari G, DeConti F. Effects of L-carnitines on physical performance in chronic respiratory insufficiency. *Int J Clin Pharmacol Ther Toxicol*. 1988;26:269–272.

106. Iafolla AK, Browning IB, Roe CR. Familial infantile apnea and immature beta oxidation. *Pediatr Pulmonol*. 1995;20:167–171.

107. Iafolla AK, Roe CR. Carnitine deficiency in apnea of prematurity. *Pediatr Res*. 1995;37:309A.

108. Kumar M, Kabra NS, Paes B. Carnitine supplementation for preterm infants with recurrent apnea (review). The Cochrane Collaboration 2005. http://www.thecochranelibrary.com. Accessed June 26, 2005.

CHAPTER 26

Central Venous Catheters in Parenteral Nutrition

H. Biemann Othersen, Jr., Joshua B. Glenn, Katherine Hammond Chessman, and Edward P. Tagge

INTRODUCTION

For children with difficult venous access, the ability to keep a line in a high-flow vein, such as the superior vena cava near the atrium, has allowed the infusion of concentrated solutions for parenteral nutrition (PN). Additionally, the administration of chemotherapeutic agents, toxic and sclerotic to peripheral veins, has been possible without the concomitant pain and obliteration of peripheral veins. This technique allows physicians to salvage many small infants who otherwise would die.

The modern era of PN began approximately 40 years ago when Wilmore and Dudrick, in a landmark paper, reported the successful treatment with PN of a newborn infant with intestinal atresia suffering progressive malnutrition from short gut syndrome.[1] Since that time, technical refinements in catheter materials and design have increased catheter longevity, permitting the infusion of drugs, nutritional fluids, and the withdrawal of blood without attendant needle punctures. In this area, technical changes occur constantly.

At the Medical University of South Carolina (MUSC), staff began using central lines for total PN in 1968 when the pharmacists, who were working with Dudrick and Wilmore, came from the University of Pennsylvania to Charleston to help in constituting the new intravenous solutions. Thus, in 2006, the surgical staff at MUSC has 38 years of experience in this technique, then known as "hyperalimentation" and now termed PN.

INDICATIONS

The indications for the placement of a central line catheter (CVC) include:

1. The need for PN that will be required for longer than 5 days.
2. The administration of concentrated chemotherapeutic agents over a period exceeding 3 to 4 weeks.
3. Venous access in a chronically ill child, requiring multiple venous punctures for blood sampling and for administration of intravenous drugs.
4. Absence of peripheral IV access for any reason.
5. The administration of antibiotics over a period of 3 to 6 weeks for treatment of resistant cardiac, osseous, or other infections.
6. Critical care monitoring of central venous pressure or pulmonary capillary pressure.

OPERATIVE TECHNIQUE

Percutaneous Cannulation

There are three basic systems for percutaneous cannulation: through the needle, over the needle, and the Seldinger technique using a guide wire.

A typical example of a through-the-needle technique is the intracath type of device that uses a large, thin walled needle and a special guard to protect the catheter. The catheter is advanced into the vessel through the needle. This technique is no longer used for central venous access in children because it requires fairly large needles and stiff catheters.

The over-the-needle technique is usually applied for peripheral arterial and venous access. The over-the-needle position protects the catheter from the needle point. Small needles, such as a 24-gauge, can be used. A wire guide facilitates this procedure. Once the vessel is punctured, the wire is advanced through the needle, the catheter is passed over the needle and over the wire into the vessel. A new device uses this technique for placement of central catheters through a peripheral vein (PCVC or peripheral CVC). Another name for these lines is peripherally inserted central catheter (PICC). This technique does not require the use of guide wires or introducers and can be done at the bedside by trained nursing staff or in radiology by interventional radiologists. It allows placement of a long soft line into a central vein through which PN can be delivered.

The Seldinger guide-wire technique is used when large vessels, such as the internal jugular vein, subclavian, or femoral veins, are needed. The vein is punctured by a thin-walled needle, a guide wire is inserted and passed into the appropriate location, which is verified by fluoroscopy or plain radiographs. The needle is withdrawn and the puncture site is then enlarged. Since most catheters used for PN are soft, it is necessary to insert a peel-away introducer sheath to allow the placement of the catheter in its desired central position.

Commonly used sites with the Seldinger technique include the subclavian vein and the internal jugular vein. The subclavian vein is one of the most common sites used for older children, but it can also be employed for small infants.[2] The success rate of central passage varies from 70 to 98%. Coagulopathy, if uncorrected, is a contraindication for placement of a line in the subclavian vein using the Seldinger guidewire technique. The incidence of pneumothorax varies between 1 and 5% but is increased when high ventilatory pressures are used in children with respiratory distress syndrome. Figure 26-1 illustrates the landmarks used for

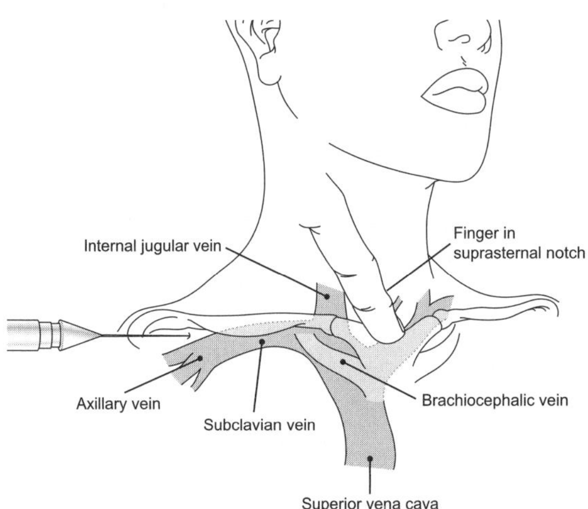

Figure 26-1 Landmarks and technique used for catheterization of the subclavian vein. *Source:* Rowe MI. Vascular access. In: Rowe MI, O'Neil JA, Grosfeld JL, ed. *Essentials of Pediatric Surgery*. Chicago, Ill: Mosby Year Book; 1995:146. Reproduced with permission.

percutaneous catheterization of the subclavian vein. In general, the right subclavian vein is preferred for cannulation because the thoracic duct is vulnerable to injury as it joins the left subclavian vein at the internal jugular junction. The infraclavicular approach is preferable but supraclavicular access can also be used. The Trendelenburg position is helpful in promoting distention of these veins. It is best to stop mechanical ventilation during puncture of the vein in order to avoid the occurrence of pneumothorax. Catheters are advanced over a guide wire and peelaway sheaths are introduced with fluoroscopic control. Final placement of the catheter is checked with C-arm fluoroscopy, but it is important to obtain a chest radiograph to confirm final placement of the line and the absence of complications such as pneumothorax or hemothorax.

However, a recent retrospective study of 1,039 CVCs placed in 824 patients showed that when central lines were placed under fluoroscopic control, a postoperative chest X-ray is not necessary unless there is clinical suspicion of a complication of the procedure.[3]

The internal jugular vein also has a high success rate for cannulation and a low incidence of pneumothorax (less than 0.1%). Since bleeding can be more easily controlled by compression in this location, the jugular vein can be used even if uncorrected coagulopathy is present. Again, the right vein is the preferred site. Internal jugular cannulation should not be performed if a tracheostomy is present, extracorporeal membrane oxygenation is contemplated, or in the face of increased intracranial pressure. Figure 26-2 illustrates the course and the technique employed for cannulation of the internal jugular vein. When using the percutaneous technique, as with subclavian vein puncture, it is helpful to have the patient in the Trendelenburg position and to stop mechanical ventilation during puncture. It is important to note that this vein can also be accessed by cutdown technique. This approach is usually only required in small, premature infants. In such cases, distal jugular ligation is often necessary.

All these techniques require that the patient remain very still, and for that reason, significant sedation or general anesthesia is almost always necessary in infants and small children.

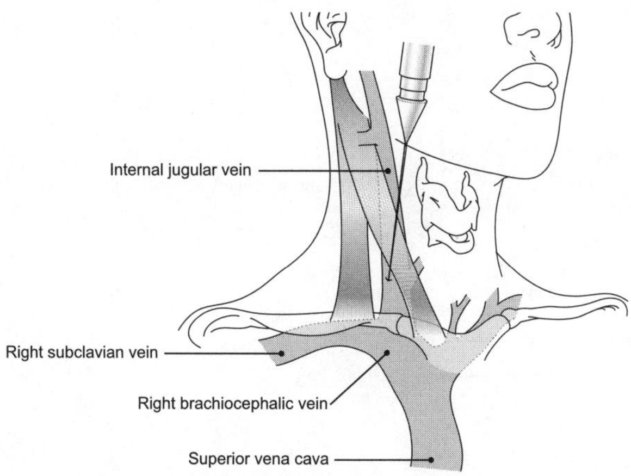

Figure 26-2 Technique employed for catheterization of the internal jugular vein. Note that the needle is inserted between the 2 muscular heads of the sternocleidomastoid muscle, just above the clavicle. *Source:* Rowe MI. Vascular access. In: Rowe MI, O'Neil JA, Grosfeld JL, ed. *Essentials of Pediatric Surgery*. Chicago, Ill: Mosby Year Book; 1995:145. Reproduced with permission.

Venesection

There are several different sites for venous cutdown for catheter placement. The most commonly used sites are the antecubital, external jugular, facial, intercostal, cephalic, saphenofemoral, and umbilical sites.

The external jugular vein is superficial, usually visible, and of sufficient size to accommodate a relatively large catheter. A 4.2 French catheter can be passed through the external jugular vein in an infant as small as 3 kg. The smallest catheter, a 2.7 French, can be used for tiny, premature infants. Figure 26-3 illustrates the course of the external jugular vein as it runs across the sternocleidomastoid muscle from the angle of the mandible and perforates the deep cervical fascia, just under the middle of the clavicle, to join the subclavian vein. The best way to advance the catheter into a central position using the cutdown technique is to incise 50% of the lumen of the external jugular vein and advance the catheter under both direct vision and fluoroscopic control.

The facial vein is a reliable route for central venous catheterization, particularly in infants, since the vein tends to be large in children less than 1 year of age, and it enters the internal jugular vein directly. It is important to avoid damage to the mandibular branch of the facial nerve during dissection. The pulsations of the facial artery provide a helpful landmark to identify this nerve. Either the anterior facial or the common facial veins can be used for catheterization. Again, fluoroscopic control is necessary to determine final position. Figure 26-4 illustrates the anatomy of the facial vein.

Central venous catheterization can be consistently accomplished using the upper cephalic vein even in children with occlusion of the jugular venous system. The upper cephalic vein has a constant location. Figure 26-5 illustrates the landmarks used to identify the cephalic vein as it enters the subclavian vein. The triangle formed by the anterior head of the deltoid muscle, the uppermost pectoralis major muscle, and the clavicle indicates the site of venesection. The

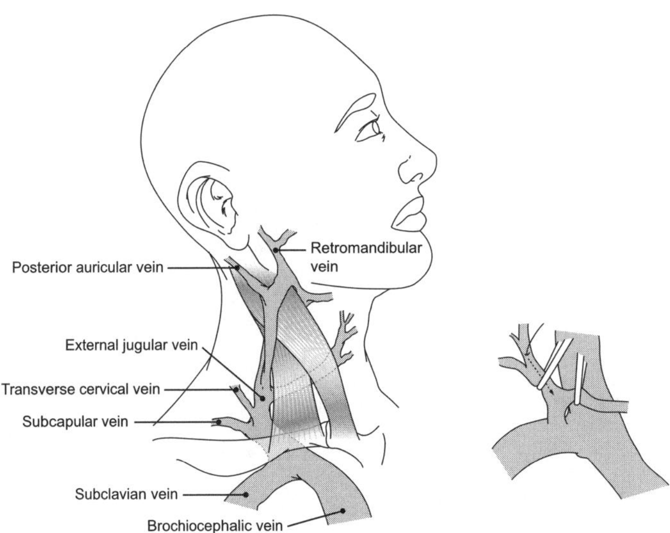

Figure 26-3 The course of the external jugular vein as it joins the subclavian vein in the lower neck. *Source:* Rowe MI. Vascular access. In: Rowe MI, O'Neil JA, Grosfeld JL, ed. *Essentials of Pediatric Surgery*. Chicago, Ill: Mosby Year Book; 1995:140. Reproduced with permission.

cephalic vein is found lying deep in the groove between those muscles. Under direct vision, a catheter can be passed into the subclavian vein and then centrally into the superior vena cava with fluoroscopic control.

The saphenofemoral venous cutdown is a simple, rapid technique with a high success rate. The complication rate is low and the technique can be used in small, preterm infants. This technique allows access to the iliac veins and the inferior vena cava for placement of a central line. The incision is made just below the inguinal ligament at the level of the junction between the greater saphenous and femoral veins. The femoral vein does not have to be manipulated or exposed as the incision is made in the saphenous vein. This vein is usually large enough to allow passage of at least a 4.2 French catheter. The catheter tip is advanced to a position high above the hepatic veins. Placement at the level of the renal veins is not desirable since renal vein thrombosis could result.

Umbilical vein catheterization is a simple procedure that allows rapid placement of a large bore catheter into the central venous system of newborn infants. The main disadvantages include a high incidence of catheter sepsis, tip malposition, risk of liver abscess, portal vein thrombosis, and perforation into the peritoneal cavity. Cannulation is usually possible up to 7 days after birth. Most authors agree that the catheter should not remain in place for prolonged periods of time. Thus, it is not a desirable route for long term PN. The catheter is advanced so that the tip is located close to the right atrium. In 60% of cases, the catheter passes from the umbilical vein, through the ductus venosus, into the inferior vena cava. Once the cava is entered, the catheter might go down into the legs, but generally goes up toward the heart. As it is advanced, it passes into the right atrium and, since the foramen ovale is immediately adjacent to the entrance of the inferior vena cava, it might pass into the left atrium and enter a pulmonary vein. Although measurement of the catheter length can be a guide in detecting the location of its tip, the tip's position must be checked by a radiograph of the chest or abdomen prior to use.

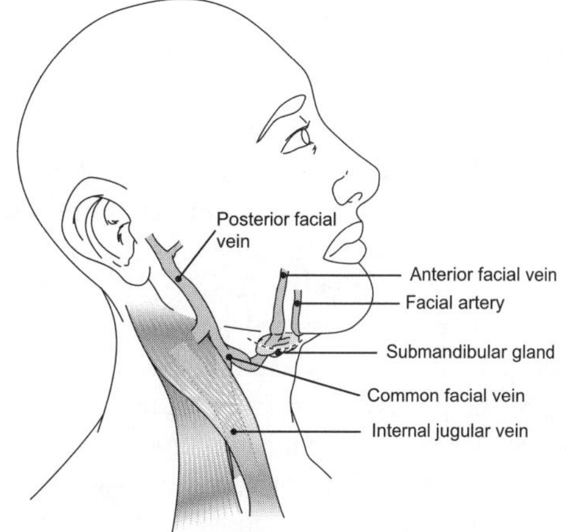

Figure 26-4 Anatomy of the facial vein. The pulsations of the facial artery are a useful landmark. Note that the facial vein joins the internal jugular vein. *Source:* Rowe MI. Vascular access. In: Rowe MI, O'Neil JA, Grosfeld JL, ed. *Essentials of Pediatric Surgery*. Chicago, Ill: Mosby Year Book; 1995:141. Reproduced with permission.

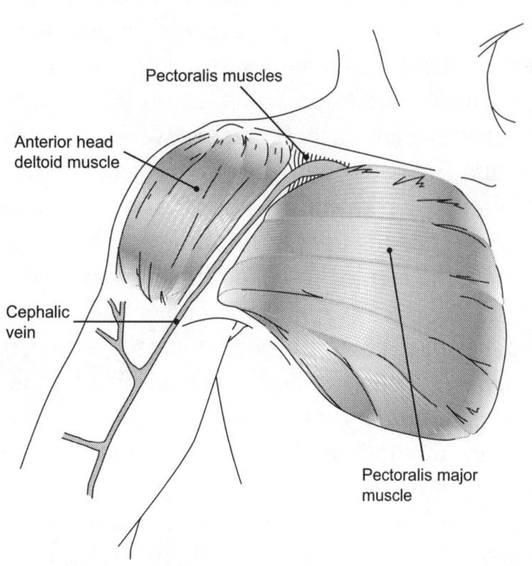

Figure 26-5 Landmarks used to identify the cephalic vein as it enters the subclavian vein in the chest. *Source:* Rowe MI. Vascular access. In: Rowe MI, O'Neil JA, Grosfeld JL, ed. *Essentials of Pediatric Surgery*. Chicago, Ill: Mosby Year Book; 1995:143. Reproduced with permission.

Patients on long term PN who no longer have adequate peripheral or central veins for placement of new catheters and have thrombosis of the innominate, subclavian, or even vena cava can have a central line placed via the azygos vein through one of the right posterior intercostal veins. The lower 8 right intercostal veins directly join the azygos vein, which enters the chest through the aortic hiatus. The intercostal vein can be exposed through a short, transverse incision in the right side of the posterior chest and a catheter can be advanced into the central circulation.

An additional alternative is the use of percutaneous transhepatic venous catheterization with the aid of interventional radiology. Central venous catheters can be advanced into hepatic vein branches, reaching the vena cava and right atrium.

In complicated cases, venographic or Doppler ultrasound studies of the upper and lower extremity veins, as well as central veins, are useful to determine the patency of the venous circulation prior to attempting catheter placement. Once the exact anatomy is identified, skilled interventional radiologists and surgeons can obtain access to certain occult veins with passage of central venous lines under fluoroscopic control.

Central venous access can be a very challenging and frustrating problem in the management of children dependent on long term PN. The careful and judicious use of central lines is essential to avoid the elimination of peripheral and central veins. The clinician must remember that once a vein has been accessed by cutdown technique, it is unlikely that it can be used again. In addition, thrombosis of any major vein (i.e., jugular, subclavian, femoral, or iliac) will preclude its use in the future. Such conditions could make children with limited venous access a challenging problem, with significant morbidity and mortality related to the lack of venous access sites and associated comorbid conditions.

NEW TECHNIQUES OF INSERTION

In a series of 452 children undergoing operation for congenital heart disease, the distance from the skin insertion site to the radiographic junction of the superior vena cava and the right atrium was measured. The following formulae were developed: correct length of insertion (cm) = (height in cm/10) – 1 for patients 100 cm or less in height and (height in cm/10) – 2 for patients greater than 100 cm in height.[4] Tunneling of noncuffed femoral central venous lines was found to decrease colonization of the lines in critically ill children.[5] In a study of the size of the subclavian vein in children, it was found that using a posterior shoulder roll and turning the head to the right (the classical position) significantly decreased the cross-sectional area of the subclavian vein. Maintaining the head with the chin midline and without a shoulder roll optimized the size of the subclavian vein.[6] The fluoroscopic landmark for the junction of the superior vena cava and the right atrium in children was found to lie at the sixth thoracic vertebral level or the interspace above or below.[7] In a child with most venous access sites thrombosed, the ovarian vein was cannulated with a catheter for an implantable port.[8,9]

MAINTENANCE OF CENTRAL VENOUS CATHETERS

Meticulous care of CVCs is required to decrease catheter related complications. An appropriate catheter care regimen starts with good hand hygiene and aseptic technique during insertion. After placement, routine dressing changes with skin antisepsis, careful management of catheter connections and tubing during solution administration, and maintenance of catheter patency are all important in minimizing complications.[9] Each institution should develop standardized protocols for CVC use and care. Prepackaged CVC dressing kits are recommended as a convenient, cost-effective method of standardizing CVC dressing changes for both hospitalized and home patients.

A variety of antiseptics have been used for skin antisepsis of catheter insertion sites, including 70% isopropyl alcohol, 3% hydrogen peroxide, 1–2% povidone-iodine, 10–100% acetone, and 0.5%, 1%, and 2% chlorhexidine solutions. Alcohol, hydrogen peroxide, and chlorhexidine have a high level of antiseptic activity while povidone-iodine and acetone have less antiseptic activity. Alcohol is associated with the most rapid antisepsis but its effect is short lived compared to that of chlorhexidine. Alcohol is also associated with significant drying of the skin. Jakobsen et al. demonstrated a 67% decrease in infection rates with the use of povidone-iodine ($p < 0.01$) that contradicted an earlier study showing no decrease in infection with povidone-iodine.[10,11] Most regimens include the combination of either alcohol or acetone with either povidone-iodine or chlorhexidine. In July 2000, the Food and Drug Administration (FDA) approved a 2% chlorhexidine gluconate/70% isopropyl alcohol antiseptic that has become widely used for hospital and home catheter care. A chlorhexidine-impregnated sponge (Biopatch™) has been used in adult patients under the CVC dressing. Data with the use of the patch are limited in children. One randomized, controlled study evaluated the use of the patch in 705 neonates. There was a substantial decrease in colonized catheter tips in infants using the patch compared with the group that had standard dressings (15% versus 24%; relative risk = 0.6; 85% confidence interval = 0.5=0.9), but no difference in the rates of catheter related bloodstream infection (CRBSI) were noted. A localized contact dermatitis developed in 15% of infants weighing less than 1,000 g and in 1.5% in those weighing more than 1,000 g ($p < 0.0001$).[12]

Semipermeable, transparent polyurethane dressings such as Op-siter or Tegaderm® are most commonly used for CVC dressings. Transparent dressings permit continuous visual inspection of the CVC site while reliably securing the catheter. Several investigators have shown a higher rate of infection with the use of transparent dressings when compared to gauze.[13,14] The difference is likely due to a lower rate of colonization of the gauze dressing because it allows less moisture accumulation.[15] Kellam et al. found that for premature infants receiving PN, a transparent dressing changed every 7 days preserved skin integrity and prevented accidental catheter dislodgment but did not change infection rates when compared to a silk tape and gauze dressing changed every 48 hours.[16] A meta-analysis assessed studies that compared the risk for CRBSI for groups using transparent dressings compared to groups using gauze dressing.[17] Risk of CRBSI did not differ between the groups. Dressing type, therefore, is a matter of preference. Gauze is preferred when blood is oozing from the insertion site, especially immediately after insertion. It is generally recommended that tape and gauze dressings be changed at least every 48 hours and transparent dressings every 2–7 days. The dressing must be changed if the occlusive seal is broken or if the dressing becomes wet or soiled. More frequent dressing changes combined with the use of a topical antibiotic such as triple antibiotic ointment or mupirocin might be warranted if the exit site becomes inflamed or purulent.

Aseptic technique must be followed during PN solution preparation and administration because PN solutions can support bacterial and fungal growth. However, contamination of catheter hub and tubing connections is a more common cause of infection than contamination of PN solutions.[18,19] Care must be taken to avoid contamination during tubing or solution changes. Some clinicians recommend swabbing all connections with povidone-iodine during manipulations. Routine care of both temporary and permanent CVCs usually includes the use of heparin flushes to prevent clot formation, although saline flushes have been shown to be equally effective for maintenance of patency.[20,21] Some catheters (e.g., Groshong) require only a saline flush after use. Because thrombi and fibrin deposits on CVCs might serve as a nidus for microbial colonization, the use of anticoagulants like heparin might have a role in the prevention of CRBSI.

Flushing is not required during continuous infusions but is necessary at the beginning and end of intermittent infusions (e.g., cyclic PN, intermittent antibiotics, chemotherapy). Unused CVCs must be flushed routinely—at least once daily for external catheters, monthly for implantable ports, and usually once every 8 to 12 hours for peripherally inserted CVCs (e.g., PICCs). The appropriate heparin volume depends on the type and size of the catheter. Most pediatric CVCs can be flushed adequately with 1–5 mL of a 10-unit/mL heparin solution. Implantable ports require larger volumes and are usually flushed with 5 mL of 100-unit/mL heparin for monthly flushes and 10-unit/mL heparin for daily or more frequent flushes.

In an attempt to prevent CRBSI, various antibiotic lock solutions have been proposed. The antibiotic lock technique flushes the catheter but then fills the lumen with an antibiotic solution and leaves the solution to dwell in the lumen for various lengths of time depending on the frequency of CVC use. The results of the use of several catheter lock solutions have been published. One lock solution containing heparin 10 units/mL, plus vancomycin 25 mcg/mL, and another solution containing heparin 9.75 units/mL, vancomycin 25 mcg/mL and ciprofloxacin 2 mcg/mL have been shown to be more effective than heparin alone in increasing time to the first episode of CRBSI in children.[22–24]

Routine use of thrombolytic agents has also been investigated as a method of decreasing CRBSI. In a prospective, randomized, double-blind trial of catheter flushes of central lines in children with cancer, a combination of urokinase and heparin was compared to heparin alone. The catheters were flushed monthly. No significant difference could be demonstrated in the number of documented bacteremic events.[25] Because the use of vancomycin is an independent risk factor for the acquisition of vancomycin-resistant enterococci, vancomycin-containing antibiotic lock solutions should not be used routinely, but they can be used in selected cases. Anecdotally, a number of other antibiotic lock solutions have been used in clinical practice, the content of which is dictated by blood or CVC culture results.

COMPLICATIONS OF CENTRAL VENOUS CATHETERS

CVC use is associated with many complications, the most common being infection and thrombosis. These complications necessitate catheter removal and reinsertion in 20–40% of cases, at additional costs and risks to the patient.[26–28] In addition, venous access could be limited in children requiring long term PN, thus mandating that every CVC be used for as long as possible before removal.

Infection

Catheter related infection can occur either systemically or locally, and can include local site infection, CRBSI, septic thrombophlebitis, endocarditis, and other metastatic infections such as osteomyelitis, endophthalmitis, and lung and brain abscesses. The incidence of CRBSI depends on the type and site of catheter, frequency of catheter manipulation, and patient related factors including underlying disease and acuity. The estimated cost of CRBSI is substantial, both in terms of morbidity and the financial resources expended.[29–31] The Centers for Disease Control has published clinical and surveillance definitions for catheter related infections (Table 26-1). The National Nosocomial Infection Surveillance System (NNIS) collects data on the incidence and etiologies of hospital acquired infections in a group of nearly 300 hospitals in the United States. Data issued in August 2001 revealed that the pooled mean for catheter associated bloodstream infection rates in high risk nurseries ranged from 3.8/1,000 catheter days in term infants weighing more than 2,500 g to 11.3/1,000 catheter days in premature neonates weighing less than 1,000 g. In the pediatric population, rates ranged from 3.4/1,000 catheter days in patients with a primary respiratory diagnosis to 9.7/1,000 catheter days in burned patients. From 1995 to 2000, the pooled mean CRBSI rate for all pediatric intensive care units reporting to NNIS was 7.7/1,000 catheter days.[32] Infection is the complication that most frequently leads to CVC removal (20–30%).[23,28,33–35] Catheter related infections could be caused by the introduction of microorganisms into the blood or catheter site at the time of CVC insertion, colonization of the catheter insertion site, hematogenous seeding of

Table 26-1 CDC clinical definitions for CVC-related infections.

Localized catheter colonization: Significant microorganism growth (> 15 CFU) from the CVC tip, SC segment, or hub.
Exit site infection: Erythema or induration within 2 cm of the CVC exit site, without BSI or purulence.
Clinical exit site infection (tunnel infection): Tenderness, erythema, or site induration > 2 cm from the CVC site along the SC tract of a tunneled catheter, without BSI.
Pocket infection: Purulent fluid in the SC pocket of a totally implanted CVC that might or might not be associated with spontaneous rupture and drainage or necrosis of the overlaying skin, without BSI.
Infusate-related BSI: Growth of the same organism from the infusate and blood cultures (preferably percutaneously drawn) with no other source of infection.
CVC-related BSI: Bacteremia/fungemia in a patient with a CVC with at least 1 positive peripheral blood culture, clinical signs of infection (e.g., fever, chills, hypotension), and no apparent source for the BSI except the CVC with 1 of the following:

- Positive semiquantitative (> 15 CFU/CVC segment) or quantitative (> 103 CFU/CVC segment) culture with the same organism isolated from the CVC segment and peripheral blood.
- Simultaneous quantitative blood cultures with a 5:1 ratio CVC versus peripheral blood.
- Differential time of CVC culture versus peripheral blood culture positivity of > 2 hr.

Abbreviations: BSI = bloodstream infection; CFU = colony forming units; CVC = central venous catheter; SC = subcutaneous.

the catheter tip during periods of bacteremia or fungemia, or contamination of nutrient solutions during preparation or administration. The fibrin sheath surrounding the catheter provides a nidus for infection. Additionally, in children with short bowel syndrome, the gastrointestinal tract could be the source of infection through bacterial or fungal translocation into the blood.[36] Children who require PN from early infancy appear to have a higher frequency of sepsis than those who begin PN after 1 year of age. Patients with short bowel syndrome have the highest frequency of infection.[37]

The most important route of catheter related bacterial contamination is thought to be migration of organisms from the skin along the subcutaneous tract into the vein. Another important source of infection is catheter hub contamination during catheter tubing manipulations. In fact, in 6 of 10 cases, the isolated bacteria was found on the skin of nurses who changed the PN bag.[38] Meticulous catheter care is extremely important to decrease infectious complications. Schwartz et al. found a vancomycin-heparin lock solution to be effective in preventing bacteremia with vancomycin susceptible organisms in a small number of children with channeled CVCs.[22] However, a recent study found this technique to be ineffective.[39] In children and adults, most CRBSIs are caused by coagulase negative staphylococci. Other organisms associated with CRBSIs are *Staphylococcus aureus*, gram-negative bacteria (e.g., *Escherichia coli, Pseudomonas aeruginosa, Klebsiella pneumoniae)*, *Enterococcus*, and *Candida* species. Antimicrobial or antiseptic impregnated catheters and cuffs are approved by the FDA for use in children weighing more than 3 kg. However, all of the studies that have evaluated the use of these catheters have been conducted in adults with triple lumen, noncuffed catheters. Materials used to coat catheters and cuffs include chlorhexidine/silver sulfadiazine, minocycline/rifampin, platinum/silver, and silver.

In a study involving 397 patients in a pediatric ICU, no association was found between the duration of catheterization and the daily probability of infection ($r = -0.21$; $p > 0.1$).[40] With the limited vascular access sites in children and the lack of evidence to support it, the practice of routine catheter changes is discouraged.

Initial treatment of CVC related sepsis requires administration of appropriate empiric antibiotics with modifications based on the results of culture and sensitivity data. Emergency catheter removal is generally recommended when the patient has a severe clinical course or when antibiotics fail to sterilize the blood cultures after 48–72 hours. Catheter salvage has been reported in 50–75% of cases when a bacterial pathogen was isolated.[37,41] Candida infections are more difficult to treat even with maximal antifungal therapy and in most cases the CVC must be removed.[37, 41–43] Some clinicians use thrombolytic agents such as urokinase or alteplase (recombinant tissue plasminogen activator [rt-PA]) concomitantly with antibiotics to salvage infected catheters, but a randomized trial evaluating bolus urokinase in catheter related sepsis showed no benefit from its use. Recombinant tissue plasminogen activator has not been studied for this application.[44]

Thrombosis

Thrombotic occlusion occurs with an estimated frequency of 25%, develops over time, and is heralded by progressive difficulty in flushing the catheter or aspirating blood through the catheter. Two forms of clot could occur. The first is the formation of a fibrin sheath at the catheter tip. The fibrin sheath is a consistent finding on all indwelling catheters regardless of the type of material used. The amount of sheath varies, however, depending on the catheter material's thrombogenicity; polyurethane > polyvinyl chloride > silicone > hydromer-coated polyurethane.[45] The fibrin sheath can be an embolic hazard during CVC removal if it is stripped off as the catheter is withdrawn. A second type of thrombus forms on the outside wall of the catheter and/or on the wall of the vessel adjacent to the catheter (mural thrombus). Mural thrombi occur within 48 hours of catheter insertion.

Attempts to prevent the development of catheter related thrombosis have included the administration of salicylates, dextran, or heparin. Catheters have also been coated with salicylates, heparin, and antibiotics. These techniques have not been successful for the prevention of thrombosis or infection during long term use. Routine addition of heparin to infused solutions (500–2,000 units/liter) might decrease thrombotic complications during long term catheter use and is recommended by the manufacturers of most peripherally inserted CVCs.[46]

Children experience higher CVC occlusion rates than adults; 10% of children receiving home PN with gastrointestinal disease, 13–16% of pediatric oncology patients, 31% of infants,[36] and 40% of children with cystic fibrosis experience occlusion.[28,37,43,47,48] Occlusion occurs because of formation of a fibrin sheath at the catheter tip, drug or mineral precipitation, lipid deposition within the CVC lumen, abutment of the catheter tip against the vessel wall, kinks in the CVC, and tight sutures at the venous insertion site. Risk factors for catheter occlusion include inadequate flushing and retrograde blood flow resulting in blood in the CVC lumen. Restoration of catheter patency is preferable to CVC replacement because it is generally quicker, less expensive, and preserves central access sites.

Traditional methods of restoring CVC patency include instillation of heparinized saline flushes, aspiration, and positional maneuvers. These techniques should be instituted immediately upon discovery of occlusion; however, they are often unsuccessful and might result in catheter rupture or forceful dislodgement of the thrombus and pulmonary embolization. Streptokinase, urokinase, rt-PA, and reteplase have been used successfully to restore patency to CVCs occluded by a fibrin sheath or thrombus formation.[48–60]

Although both streptokinase and urokinase have been used to restore patency, rt-PA is preferred because it is readily available and lacks antigenicity. Urokinase (Open-Cath™ Abbott Laboratories) was previously preferred because of its availability in a 5,000 units/mL concentration in 1 mL and 1.8-mL vials. However, the product was removed from the US market in 1999 because of FDA concerns with the manufacturing process.

Since the removal of urokinase from the market, rt-PA has become the preferred thrombolytic agent for catheter clearance. In addition to availability, the advantages of rt-PA include greater affinity for fibrin than urokinase and a very low incidence of allergic reaction compared to streptokinase where the development of antistreptococcal antibodies limits its use. The instilled volume of rt-PA used in clinical trials ranges from 0.1 to 2 mL. Others used a volume equal to the priming volume of the catheter plus 10%, to a maximum of 2 mL. The volume injected should always approximate the internal volume of the CVC. In general, 0.5–1 mL for most catheters and 1.8 mL for implantable ports provides an adequate volume without increasing risk. The FDA labeled manufacturer's package insert states that the appropriate dose for those weighing more than 30 kg is 2 mg/2 mL and for those weighing from 10 to 30 kg, 110% of the internal volume of the catheter, not to exceed 2 mg/2 mL. No information is given for those weighing less than 10 kg, but rt-PA has been used safely in premature infants. If the CVC has multiple lumens, then rt-PA should be instilled into each lumen. Concentrations of rt-PA used in clinical trials varied from 0.25 mg/mL to 2 mg/2 mL. One common approach is to use 0.5 mg/mL for children weighing less than 10 kg and 1–2 mg/1–2 mL for those patients weighing more than 10 kg. Efficacy rates are similar. The lowest dose decreases risk and cost. Cumulative success rates in clinical trials with rt-PA are 55–89% with 1 instillation, 86.8% with 2 instillations, and 90.6% with 3 instillations.[56–58,60] More than 3 instillations are not recommended. Recommended dwell times are variable based on clinical trials and range from 20 minutes to 24 hours. Most clinicians recommend a 20- to 30-minute dwell time prior to the first attempt at aspiration. If this is unsuccessful, allowing the rt-PA to dwell for an additional 30–60 minutes prior to repeating the dose is often helpful. For some resistant catheters, allowing the rt-PA to remain in the catheter overnight has been successful.

The rt-PA is generally instilled into the CVC using a 10-mL syringe. Care should be taken to avoid generating excess pressure. Due to the nature of the material, some ballooning will occur with gentle pressure, allowing the solution to enter the catheter. However, excessive force can result in dislodgement of the clot into the systemic circulation or catheter rupture. One technique developed to address this issue is the use of a stopcock to create a vacuum to pull the rt-PA into the catheter. In this method, a 3-way stopcock is attached directly to the hub of the catheter with the off valve facing the catheter. An empty 10-mL syringe is attached to the side port of the stopcock, and the rt-PA dose in a 10-mL syringe is attached to the straight port of the stopcock. With the stopcock open, the empty syringe is aspirated back to the 1 mL mark. The stopcock is then turned open to the rt-PA syringe. The negative pressure created will pull the rt-PA into the catheter without force being exerted into the internal lumen of the catheter.[61] This method has been challenged. After patency has been restored, gently aspirating back 3–5 mL is recommended to remove any residual rt-PA or clot.

Occasionally, traditional methods of rt-PA instillation fail to resolve the occlusion. Continuous infusions of urokinase were successfully used in the past.[48,51] Continuous infusion rt-PA (2 mg infused over 4–6 hours) has been used by some clinicians, but there are no published studies evaluating this method. The use of rt-PA and other thrombolytics for catheter occlusion is rarely associated with adverse effects. Jacobs et al. reported no adverse effects when rt-PA was used to treat 320 CVC occlusions in 228 children.[57] Bleeding is rarely reported and is unlikely when the smaller doses of rt-PA are used. For most patients, if recommended rt-PA guidelines are used, the delivered dose is 0.02–0.03 mg/kg, which is well below therapeutic thrombolytic doses. In some instances, rt-PA cannot be instilled into the catheter. Early in the use of rt-PA for catheter occlusions, there was no specific packaging for this indication. Most facilities used a 50-mg vial and diluted the contents with sterile water for injection to a final concentration of 1 mg/1 mL. This was then divided into 1 mL or 2 mL aliquots in 5 mL sterile vials and frozen for up to 6 months.[62] The rt-PA was then thawed for 20 minutes prior to administration. Cathflo Activase® (Genentech) is 2 mg rt-PA in 2 mL specifically for catheter occlusions. Wholesale price is $82.33 from Genentech (March, 2006). This makes treatment of catheter occlusions more cost effective compared to replacement of the CVC. The solutions should be reconstituted immediately before use; swirled, not shaken, to avoid denaturing the protein; and administered within 8 hours of reconstitution. As of January 2006, information regarding catheter occlusions was available at http://www.cathflo.com.

Nonthrombotic Occlusion

Drug and mineral precipitation can be prevented by flushing before and after drug administration, attention to calcium and phosphate concentrations in infused solutions, and avoidance of simultaneous administration of incompatible drugs or solutions. Commonly implicated drugs in CVC occlusions include phenytoin, diazepam, and etoposide. Lipid deposition has been reported to occur more frequently with the use of total nutrient admixtures (TNA). TNA are solutions in which the lipid, carbohydrate, protein, and all minerals are mixed together in a single bag, also called 3-in-1 solutions. Lipid deposition can be prevented by the avoidance of TNA or by using dual chamber bags, which prevent mixing of the lipid with the other components until just prior to administration.

Conventional methods to restore patency or thrombolytics are ineffective for nonthrombotic occlusions. Because most drug and mineral precipitation is pH dependent, patency can be restored with the instillation of 0.2–1 mL of 0.1 N hydrochloric acid (HCl) for 30–120 minutes.[63,64] Two to three instillations might be required. This weak acid solution lowers the pH at the site of the precipitate, increasing solubility. Weak HCl can also be used to restore patency to implantable ports that have been occluded for up to 4 days.[65] Some drug precipitates, due to their chemical nature, will require an alkaline solution such as sodium bicarbonate (1 mEq/mL) to restore patency. The pharmacist is an excellent resource for determining the need for either HCl or sodium bicarbonate.

Catheter occlusion with a waxy lipid substance occurs more commonly with the use of TNA.[66,67] Thrombolytics and HCl are ineffective in such occlusions; however, a solution of 70% ethanol has been used to restore patency in lipid occluded catheters.[68] In this study, one 3 mL instillation was sufficient to restore patency. However, if 1 instillation is ineffective, careful, repeated instillations over several days might dissolve the lipid layer and restore patency. Small volumes (e.g., 1 mL) might be advisable in infants and children to avoid the side effects of ethanol administration, particularly when repeated instillations are necessary.

OTHER COMPLICATIONS

In addition to infection and thrombosis, there are numerous reports of complications resulting from misplaced catheter tips.[68-,70] Regardless of the site or technique of insertion, the catheter might not traverse the anticipated path and the tip can be positioned to deliver the concentrated solutions into heart muscle, pericardium, retroperitoneum, or spinal cord. Cardiac perforation or tamponade, paraplegia, or retroperitoneal infusion could be the result. The position of the catheter tip *must* be absolutely verified either by fluoroscopy or X-ray prior to infusion of fluids.

PICCs share similar complications as other central lines. The long dwell time of PICC lines predisposes them to additional complications. PICC lines are prone to fracture and migration during placement and throughout their life span. Catheter thrombosis and infection are common.[70,71]

CENTRAL VENOUS CATHETERS

The catheters employed can be Teflon, polyethylene, polyurethane, or silicone. Table 26-2 describes characteristics of each material. The silicone elastomer is the most commonly used

Table 26-2 Characteristics of catheter materials.

Material	*Thrombogenicity and tip characteristics*	*Stiffness*	*Pressure monitor*
Teflon	Moderate firm tip irritates endothelium; smooth catheter surface	Stiff	Yes
Polyethylene	High, firm tip; rough catheter surface	Stiff	Yes
Polyurethane	Low; soft	Softness in vessel	Yes
Silicone elastomer	Low; smooth and soft tip	Very soft	No, too soft

catheter today for PN via a central line.[72] In addition to fluid administration, central lines allow venous access for blood sampling. In general, if a child requires continuous or continual PN or if multiple drug administrations or blood sampling are required, a Broviac-type catheter with a Dacron cuff is appropriate. On the other hand, for a patient who will receive only intermittent chemotherapeutic drugs or antibiotics, the implantation of a subcutaneous reservoir allows the child to function without a line that exits from the skin. The disadvantage of the reservoir is that each time it is accessed, a needle must penetrate the skin.

As the techniques for PICC have improved, their number now greatly exceeds those inserted at operation. Some details have changed. During operative insertion we previously confirmed catheter location by chest radiograph. We now use portable fluoroscopy. We have used catheters of Teflon and polyurethane, but now almost all are of silicone rubber. In bone marrow transplantations, our pediatric hematologists request a double-lumen subcutaneous reservoir with double-lumen central line.

CONCLUSION

One of the truly outstanding medical advancements in the past 50 years has been the development of techniques and materials that allow the use of CVCs for administration of PN. This method of central administration of concentrated solutions has been especially valuable in small, premature infants, neonates, and children who, prior to 1965, could not have been sustained by the peripheral route. Central venous lines have allowed children with limited venous access to undergo prolonged therapy with antibiotics and chemotherapeutic agents without the attendant pain of peripheral venous spasm, thrombosis, and multiple needle punctures. Thus, central lines have been life-saving for many children and continue to enhance the quality of life.

In spite of many advances in techniques and the development of catheters with special qualities to prevent thrombosis or infection, maintenance of long term catheters in small children requires attention to detail from a team of dedicated health care professionals.

REFERENCES

1. Dudrick WD. Growth and development of an infant receiving all nutrients exclusively by vein. *JAMA*. 1968;203:140.
2. McGovern TM, Brandt B. Percutaneous infraclavicular subclavian venous access in infants and children. *Contemp Surg*. 1994;45:335.
3. Janik JE, Cothren CC, Janik JS, et al. Is a routine chest x-ray necessary for children after fluoroscopically assisted central venous access? *J Pediatr Surg*. 2003;38(8):1199–1202.
4. Andropoulos DB, Bent ST, Skjonsby B, Stayer SA. The optimal length of insertion of central venous catheters for pediatric patients. *Anesth Analg*. 2001;93(4):883–886.
5. Nahum E, Levy I, Katz J, et al. Efficacy of subcutaneous tunneling for prevention of bacterial colonization of

femoral central venous catheters in critically ill children. *Pediatr Infect Dis J.* 2002;21(11):1000–1004.

6. Lukish J, Valladares E, Rodriguez C, et al. Classical positioning decreases subclavian vein cross-sectional area in children. *J Trauma.* 2002;53(2):272–275.
7. Connolly B, Mawson JB, MacDonald CE, Chait P, Mikailian H. Fluoroscopic landmark for SVC-RA junction for central venous catheter placement in children. *Pediatr Radiol.* 2000;30(10):692–695.
8. Shankar KR, Anbu AT, Losty PD. Use of the gonadal vein in children with difficult central venous access: a novel technique. *J Pediatr Surg.* 2001;36(6):E3.
9. Evans NJ, Bamba M, Rombeau JL. Care of central venous catheters. In: Rombeau JL and Caldwell CM, ed. *Clinical Nutrition: Parenteral Nutrition.* Philadelphia, Pa: W. B. Saunders; 1993:353–366.
10. Jakobsen CJ, Grabe N, Damm MD. A trial of povidone-iodine for prevention of contamination of intravenous cannulae. *Acta Anaesthesiol Scand Suppl.* 1986;30(6):447.
11. Prager RL, Silva J Jr. Colonization of central venous catheters. *South Med J.* 1984;77(4):458–461.
12. Garland JS, Alex CP, Mueller CD, et al. A randomized trial comparing povidone-iodine to a chlorhexidine gluconate-impregnated dressing for prevention of central venous catheter infections in neonates. *Pediatrics.* 2001;107(6):1431–1436.
13. Conly JM, Grieves K, Peters B. A prospective, randomized study comparing transparent and dry gauze dressings for central venous catheters. *J Infect Dis.* 1989;159(2):310–319.
14. Maki DG, Ringer M. Evaluation of dressing regimens for prevention of infection with peripheral intravenous catheters: gauze, a transparent polyurethane dressing, and an iodophor-transparent dressing. *JAMA.* 1987;258(17):2396–2403.
15. Toltzis P, Goldmann DA. Current issues in central venous catheter infection. *Annu Rev Med.* 1990;41:169–176.
16. Kellam B, Fraze DE, Kanarek KS. Central line dressing material and neonatal skin integrity. *Nutr Clin Pract.* 1988;3(2):65–68.
17. Hoffmann KK, Weber DJ, Samsa GP, Rutala WA. Transparent polyurethane film as an intravenous catheter dressing. A meta-analysis of the infection risks. *JAMA.* 1992;267(15):2072–2076.
18. Stotter AT, Ward H, Waterfield AH, Hilton J, Sim AJ. Junctional care: the key to prevention of catheter sepsis in intravenous feeding. *JPEN.* 1987;11(2):159–162.
19. Linares J, Sitges-Serra A, Garau J, Perez JL, Martin R. Pathogenesis of catheter sepsis: a prospective study with quantitative and semiquantitative cultures of catheter hub and segments. *J Clin Microbiol.* 1985;21(3):357–360.
20. Murphy LM, Lipman TO. Central venous catheter care in parenteral nutrition: a review. *JPEN.* 1987;11(2):190–201.
21. Smith S, Dawson S, Hennessey R, Andrew M. Maintenance of the patency of indwelling central venous catheters: is heparin necessary? *Am J Pediatr Hematol Oncol.* 1991;13(2):141–143.
22. Schwartz C, Henrickson KJ, Roghmann K, Powell K. Prevention of bacteremia attributed to luminal colonization of tunneled central venous catheters with vancomycin-susceptible organisms. *J Clin Oncol.* 1990;8(9):1591–1597.
23. Henrickson KJ, Axtell RA, Hoover SM, et al. Prevention of central venous catheter-related infections and thrombotic events in immunocompromised children by the use of vancomycin/ciprofloxacin/heparin flush solution: A randomized, multicenter, double-blind trial. *J Clin Oncol.* 2000;18(6):1269–1278.
24. Carratala J, Niubo J, Fernandez-Sevilla A, et al. Randomized, double-blind trial of an antibiotic-lock technique for prevention of gram-positive central venous catheter-related infection in neutropenic patients with cancer. *Antimicrob Agents Chemother.* 1999;43(9):2200–2204.
25. Aquino VM, Sandler ES, Mustafa MM, Steele JW, Buchanan GR. A prospective double-blind randomized trial of urokinase flushes to prevent bacteremia resulting from luminal colonization of subcutaneous central venous catheters. *J Pediatr Hematol Oncol.* 2002;24(9):710–713.
26. Mirro J Jr, Rao BN, Kumar M, et al. A comparison of placement techniques and complications of externalized catheters and implantable port use in children with cancer. *J Pediatr Surg.* 1990;25(1):120–124.
27. Stanislav GV, Fitzgibbons RJ Jr, Bailey RT Jr, Mailliard JA, Johnson PS, Feole JB. Reliability of implantable central venous access devices in patients with cancer. *Arch Surg.* 1987;122(11):1280–1283.
28. Wiener ES, McGuire P, Stolar CJ, et al. The CCSG prospective study of venous access devices: an analysis of insertions and causes for removal. *J Pediatr Surg.* 1992;27(2):155–163; discussion 163–164.
29. Anonymous. National Nosocomial Infections Surveillance (NNIS) system report, data summary from January 1992–April 2000, issued June 2000. *Am J Infect Control.* 2000:28(6):429–448.
30. Anonymous. National Nosocomial Infections Surveillance (NNIS) System Report, Data Summary from January 1992–June 2001, issued August 2001. *Am J Infect Control.* 2001;29(6):404–421.
31. Prevention CfDCa. National Nosocomial Infections Surveillance System report, data summary from January 1992–June 2001, issued August 2001. *Am J Infect Control.* 2001;6:404–421.
32. http://www.cdc.gov/mmwr/PDF/rr/rr5110.pdf (Accessed March 8, 2006).
33. Richards MJ, Edwards JR, Culver DH. Gaynes. Nosocomial infections in pediatric intensive care units

in the United States: National Nosocomial Infections Surveillance System. *Pediatrics.* 1999;103:103–109.

34. Johnson PR, Decker MD, Edwards KM, Schaffner W, Wright PF. Frequency of broviac catheter infections in pediatric oncology patients. *J Infect Dis.* 1986;154(4):570–578.
35. Keohane PP, Jones BJ, Attrill H, et al. Effect of catheter tunnelling and a nutrition nurse on catheter sepsis during parenteral nutrition: a controlled trial. *Lancet.* 1983;2(8364):1388–1390.
36. Sitges-Serra A, Linares J, Perez JL, Jaurrieta E, Lorente L. A randomized trial on the effect of tubing changes on hub contamination and catheter sepsis during parenteral nutrition. *JPEN.* 1985;9(3):322–325.
37. Kurkchubasche AG, Smith SD, Rowe MI. Catheter sepsis in short-bowel syndrome. *Arch Surg.* 1992;127(1):21–24; discussion 24–25.
38. Schmidt-Sommerfeld E, Snyder G, Rossi TM, Lebenthal E. Catheter-related complications in 35 children and adolescents with gastrointestinal disease on home parenteral nutrition. *JPEN.* 1990;14(2):148–151.
39. de Cicco M, Panarello G, Chiaradia V, et al. Source and route of microbial colonisation of parenteral nutrition catheters. *Lancet.* 1989;2(8674):1258–1261.
40. Rackoff WR, Weiman M, Jakobowski D, et al. A randomized, controlled trial of the efficacy of a heparin and vancomycin solution in preventing central venous catheter infections in children. *J Pediatr.* 1995;127(1):147–151.
41. Stenzel JP, Green TP, Fuhrman BP, Carlson PE, Marchessault RP. Percutaneous central venous catheterization in a pediatric intensive care unit: a survival analysis of complications. *Crit Care Med.* 1989;17(10):984–988.
42. King DR, Komer M, Hoffman J, et al. Broviac catheter sepsis: the natural history of an iatrogenic infection. *J Pediatr Surg.* 1985;20(6):728–733.
43. Dato VM, Dajani AS. Candidemia in children with central venous catheters: role of catheter removal and amphotericin B therapy. *Pediatr Infect Dis J.* 1990;9(5):309–314.
44. Eppes SC, Troutman JL, Gutman LT. Outcome of treatment of candidemia in children whose central catheters were removed or retained. *Pediatr Infect Dis J.* 1989;8(2):99–104.
45. La Quaglia MP, Caldwell C, Lucas A, et al. A prospective randomized double-blind trial of bolus urokinase in the treatment of established Hickman catheter sepsis in children. *J Pediatr Surg.* 1994;29(6):742–745.
46. Borow M, Crowley JG. Evaluation of central venous catheter thrombogenicity. *Acta Anaesthesiol Scand Suppl.* 1985;81:59–64.
47. Fabri PJ, Mirtallo JM, Ruberg RL, et al. Incidence and prevention of thrombosis of the subclavian vein during total parenteral nutrition. *Surg Gynecol Obstet.* 1982;155(2):238–240.
48. Hartman GE, Shochat SJ. Management of septic complications associated with Silastic catheters in childhood malignancy. *Pediatr Infect Dis J.* 1987;6(11):1042–1047.
49. Bagnall HA, Gomperts E, Atkinson JB. Continuous infusion of low-dose urokinase in the treatment of central venous catheter thrombosis in infants and children. *Pediatrics.* 1989;83(6):963–966.
50. Cassidy FP Jr, Zajko AB, Bron KM, Reilly JJ Jr, Peitzman AB, Steed DL. Noninfectious complications of long-term central venous catheters: radiologic evaluation and management. *AJR Am J Roentgenol.* 1987;149(4):671–675.
51. Haire WD, Lieberman RP, Lund GB, Edney J, Wieczorek BM. Obstructed central venous catheters. Restoring function with a 12-hour infusion of low-dose urokinase. *Cancer.* 1990;66(11):2279–2285.
52. Curnow A, Idowu J, Behrens E, Toomey F, Georgeson K. Urokinase therapy for Silastic catheter-induced intravascular thrombi in infants and children. *Arch Surg.* 1985;120(11):1237–1240.
53. Tschirhart JM, Rao MK. Mechanism and management of persistent withdrawal occlusion. *Am Surg.* 1988;54(6):326–328.
54. Wachs T. Urokinase administration in pediatric patients with occluded central venous catheters. *J Intraven Nurs.* 1990;13(2):100–102.
55. Zajko AB, Reilly JJ Jr, Bron KM, Desai R, Steed DL. Low-dose streptokinase for occluded Hickman catheters. *AJR Am J Roentgenol.* 1983;141(6):1311–1312.
56. Winthrop AL, Wesson DE. Urokinase in the treatment of occluded central venous catheters in children. *J Pediatr Surg.* 1984;19(5):536–538.
57. Maloney K, Nelson T, Gill J. The use of aliquoted and frozen TPA in central venous line occlusions. *Blood.* 1999;94:29a.
58. Jacobs BR, Haygood M, Hingl J. Recombinant tissue plasminogen activator in the treatment of central venous catheter occlusion in children. *J Pediatr.* 2001;139(4):593–596.
59. Choi M, Marizinotto V, Chan A, Andrew M. Use of tissue plasminogen activator to clear blocked central venous lines in pediatric patients: a prospective cohort study. *Blood.* 1999;94:25a.
60. Terrill KR, Lemons RS, Goldsby RE. Safety, dose, and timing of reteplase in treating occluded central venous catheters in children with cancer. *J Pediatr Hematol Oncol.* 2003;25(11):864–867.
61. Haire WD, Atkinson JB, Stephens LC, Kotulak GD. Urokinase versus recombinant tissue plasminogen activator in thrombosed central venous catheters: a double-blinded, randomized trial. *Thromb Haemost.* 1994;72(4):543–547.

62. Hooke C. Recombinant tissue plasminogen activator for central venous access device occlusion. *J Pediatr Oncol Nurs.* 2000;17(3):174–178.

63. Calis KA, Cullinane AM, Horne MK III. Bioactivity of cryopreserved alteplase solutions. *Am J Health Syst Pharm.* 1999;56(20):2056–2057.

64. Duffy LF, Kerzner B, Gebus V, Dice J. Treatment of central venous catheter occlusions with hydrochloric acid. *J Pediatr.* 1989;114(6):1002–1004.

65. Shulman RJ, Reed T, Pitre D, Laine L. Use of hydrochloric acid to clear obstructed central venous catheters. *JPEN.* 1988;12(5):509–510.

66. Kupensky DT. Use of hydrochloric acid to restore patency in an occluded implantable port: a case report. *J Intraven Nurs.* 1995;18(4):198–201.

67. Messing B, Beliah M, Girard-Pipau F, Leleve D, Bernier JJ. Technical hazards of using nutritive mixtures in bags for cyclical intravenous nutrition: comparison with standard intravenous nutrition in 48 gastroenterological patients. *Gut.* 1982;23(4):297–303.

68. Main J, Pennington CR. Catheter blockage with lipid during long term parenteral nutrition. *Br Med J.* 1984;289:734.

69. Pennington CR, Pithie AD. Ethanol lock in the management of catheter occlusion. *JPEN.* 1987;11(5):507–508.

70. Sztajnbok J, Troster EJ. Acute abdomen due to late retroperitoneal extravasation from a femoral venous catheter in a newborn. *Sao Paulo Med J.* 2002;120(2):59–61.

71. Pettit J. Assessment of infants with peripherally inserted central catheters: Part 1. Detecting the most frequently occurring complications. *Adv Neonatal Care.* 2002;2(6):304–315.

72. Chow LM, Friedman JN, Macarthur C, et al. Peripherally inserted central catheter (PICC) fracture and embolization in the pediatric population. *J Pediatr.* 2003;142(2):141–144.

73. Rowe MI. Vascular access. In: Rowe MI, O'Neil JA, Grosfeld JL, ed. *Essentials of Pediatric Surgery.* Chicago, Ill: Mosby Year Book; 1995:138–151.

74. Caldwell MD, Jonsson HT, Othersen HB Jr. Essential fatty acid deficiency in an infant receiving prolonged parenteral alimentation. *J Pediatr.* 1972;81(5):894–898.

CHAPTER 27

Pharmacy Considerations in Pediatric Parenteral Nutrition

I-Fen Chang, Thuy Anh Sorof, and Ngoc Yen Thi Nguyen

INTRODUCTION

More than a quarter of a century has elapsed since the first report of normal growth and development using intravenous nutrition in animals.[1] In 1968, Wilmore and Dudrick introduced the first long term experience using parenteral nutrition (PN) in humans,[2] and by the early 1970s, intravenous nutrition was shown to sustain growth and development in premature infants.[3] Over the last few decades, PN evolved to play a pivotal role in improving the quality of care of patients unable to use the gastrointestinal (GI) tract. Clinical advances and research underpin evidence-based protocols that improve patient care and minimize complications.

The expansion of indications, creation of disease-specific solutions, and development of automation in the preparation and delivery of PN opened new opportunities and challenges. This is particularly true for pediatric patients. This chapter addresses issues that a pharmacist might encounter in the preparation and delivery of PN, with a focus on routes of administration, compatibility of medications with PN, and the evaluation of the effects of medications on nutrients and electrolytes.

The therapeutic goal of PN in children is to maintain proper nutrition status and achieve normal growth and development. A balanced PN solution should provide the optimal combination of macronutrients and micronutrients to meet the patient's nutritional needs. Macronutrients are the bulk of the solution and are composed of water, dextrose, protein, and lipid emulsions. Micronutrients support the metabolic activities necessary for cellular homeostasis and include vitamins, trace elements, and electrolytes. Monitoring and adjustments must be individualized and are dictated by fluid and electrolyte balance, changes in organ function, metabolic stress, and coadministration of medications.[4]

FLUIDS

The first step in initiating PN is to determine the amount of fluid (see Chapter 23) to be used in the PN solution. Fluid requirements are dependent on patient size, hydration status, surgical procedures, coadministered medications, and the underlying disease state. Fluid restriction might be necessary, particularly if the patient has cardiac, renal, or hepatic insufficiency. In this situation, the administration of fluids other than PN (e.g., blood products, replacement fluids, saline or heparin flushes, and medications) must be included in determining fluid needs. Medications should be diluted in the minimum amount of fluid possible that is considered safe for administration. The PN solution should be prepared using the most concentrated solution, especially if large amounts of proteins are needed. For example, 70% dextrose, 15% amino acid, and 20 or 30% lipid emulsion should be used as the base in compounding the PN solution.

ACCESS SITE FOR PN

The administration of PN requires the placement of an appropriate venous access device (see Chapter 26) to safely deliver the hypertonic solution. Catheter selection is highly dependent on patient factors and the duration of therapy. Central venous access is achieved by advancing the catheter tip into the right atrium or superior or inferior vena cava via cannulation of the subclavian, internal jugular, or femoral vein. Catheter tip placement anywhere else is considered peripheral access. The Intravenous Nursing Society recognizes midline, midclavicular, and short peripheral as peripheral access.[5]

PERIPHERAL PARENTERAL ROUTE

Peripheral parenteral nutrition (PPN) should be used when central venous access is not possible, not warranted, or when a short length of therapy is expected. PPN is an option for supplementation in patients as enteral feeds are advanced or as a bridge until central access can be obtained. On occasion, the medical condition of the patient might preclude placement of a central line. For example, patients with radical head/neck surgery, low platelet counts, or recurrent episodes of sepsis might benefit from peripheral nutrition support.

PPN is usually composed of a dilute solution of amino acids, dextrose, and micronutrients. It is difficult to provide adequate nutrition via PPN for children. To do so requires large volumes. For this reason, PPN might be contraindicated in patients who are fluid restricted.

Several factors can influence the successful provision of PPN. Maintaining peripheral access for an appropriate amount of time without infusion site complications such as phlebitis, thrombosis, or infiltration is essential. Some of the tactics employed to reduce the risk of infusion site complications include limiting osmolarity of the formulation, inclusion of lipid emulsion in PPN solution, and the addition of heparin or hydrocortisone to the PPN formulation.

OSMOLARITY OF PPN FORMULATION

The incidence of thrombophlebitis in PPN is directly related to the osmotic content of the solution and the delivery rate.[6–7] The maximum osmolarity of PPN preparations should not exceed 900 mOsm/L;[8] dextrose concentration should be less than 12.5% (625 mOsm/L) and amino acid concentration less than 4% (40gm/L).[4] Higher concentrations in a peripheral line increase the risk of thrombophlebitis. Because dextrose, amino acids, and electrolytes are the major contributors to osmolarity, the following equation is one of the methods by which osmolarity can be calculated:

$$\text{Osmolarity (mOsm/L)} = (\text{total grams dextrose/liter}) \times 5 + (\text{total grams amino acid/liter}) \times 10 + (\text{total mEq cations/liter}) \times 2$$

LIPID EMULSION

Because the amount of carbohydrates that can be provided is limited by osmolarity, lipids are a major calorie source. Lipid emulsions appear to protect peripheral veins while providing an increase in caloric intake without drastically increasing osmolarity. The osmolarity of lipid emulsions is approximately 300 mOsm/L; it is relatively isotonic. Animal studies show that lipid emulsions reduce endothelial damage from amino acid solutions.[9] Peripheral vein patency time is increased in neonates given a high fat PN formulation compared to a low fat formulation of the same osmolarity.[10] Similarly, Williams et al. demonstrated no significant difference in the incidence of thrombophlebitis between patients receiving lipid-based formulations with an osmolarity of 650 mOsm/kg and those receiving an osmolarity of 860 mOsm/kg.[11] Tolerance to osmolarities of approximately 1,300 mOsm/L lipid admixtures have been reported in adults.[12] Lipid-based formulations improve venous patency time, but close monitoring is essential for patients receiving peripheral hyperosmolar solutions.

HEPARIN AND HYDROCORTISONE

Addition of heparin and hydrocortisone to PPN increases tolerance to hyperosmolar solutions. Several randomized studies show that heparin and hydrocortisone have a synergistic effect in reducing thrombophlebitis.[13–15] For example, Alpan et al. showed that in premature infants, 1 unit of heparin per mL of PPN was associated with a 30% reduction in the incidence of thrombophlebitis (5.7% versus 17.2%) and a doubling in duration of catheter patency.[16] Fonkalsrud et al. found the addition of 1 unit/mL of heparin and 10 mg/L of hydrocortisone to solutions of 5% dextrose or to a solution containing 5% dextrose with 0.45% sodium chloride produce nearly the same results in phlebitis as buffering the solution to a pH of 7.2 to 7.5.[17] Heparinization and addition of hydrocortisone to PPN solutions reduce the incidence of complications associated with peripheral lines. Although heparin has been used for many years, some caution is necessary. Heparin can cause a transient fall in platelet count 1–3 days after initiation of treatment. In most patients, this is of no clinical significance; the platelet levels return to normal within a few days of the discontinuation of heparin. In some patients, heparin-induced thrombocytopenia (HIT), a life and limb threatening complication of heparin therapy, can occur. HIT is likely an immune-mediated syndrome that can be precipitated even by minute quantities of heparin given to flush catheters.[18] In addition, heparin must be used with caution in patients who are at increased risk of bleeding. Caution is also needed when using heparin flushes as heparinization can result.

CENTRAL PARENTERAL ROUTE

Central parenteral nutrition (CPN) solutions are usually hypertonic solutions that must be administration via a central vein. Central veins have a high blood flow, which can quickly dilute the hypertonic solution. Central venous catheters vary in composition, lumen size, and number of injection ports (see Chapter 26). They can be placed for short or long term access. Radiographic verification of correct placement is necessary prior to initiating CPN.

CPN is used for patients who require PN for more than 7–10 days or those who have high nutritional requirements, poor peripheral venous access, or fluctuating fluid requirements. Disadvantages associated with CPN include the risks associated with catheter insertion and catheter related infections. In addition, the risk of more serious catheter related trauma and technical problems is higher than with peripheral venous access.

COMPATIBILITY OF ADDITIVES WITH PN

Considerable effort has focused on the compatibilities of PN formulations, especially calcium and phosphate solubility. These studies provide compatibility information for the specific amino acid products and concentrations tested under the specific conditions of the study models (for example, duration, temperature, and solution constituents). PN formulations are patient specific and often differ from the studies in compositions, concentrations, product brands, and clinical settings. Therefore, clinicians must appreciate the limitations of the studies when interpreting compatibility information in the clinical setting.

Unique to pediatric PN solutions are 3 challenges: IV access, fluid restriction, and requirement for high levels of calcium and phosphate. For fluid restricted, PN dependent patients, PN formulations are optimized by maximizing the concentrations of individual components, such as amino acid, dextrose, calcium, and phosphate. For these patients, the PN solution can also be used as a delivery vehicle for medications such as H-2 antagonists and iron dextran. The ability to deliver multiple agents in 1 solution is attributed to the titratable acid property of amino acids. Amino acids and electrolytes are buffers that render PN solutions resistant to pH changes. A standard PN solution contains on the average 10 components, including dextrose, amino acids, electrolytes, trace minerals, and vitamins. When medications are added, the risk for incompatibilities increases. The following sections outline some common compatibility issues that clinicians might encounter.

Calcium and Phosphorus

Calcium and phosphate solubility in PN solutions is highly sensitive to pH. Calcium can react with phosphate to form either monobasic or dibasic calcium phosphate. As the pH of the PN solution increases, more dibasic phosphate is available to bind to free calcium, forming the insoluble dibasic calcium phosphate salt. As the pH decreases, monobasic phosphate is available to bind with calcium to form monobasic calcium phosphate, which is relatively soluble.[19] The buffering capacity of amino acids improves the compatibility of calcium and phosphate salts, allowing a higher concentration of each in the solution. The buffering capacity varies greatly among commercially available crystalline amino acid products and depends in part on the amount of acetic acid and the inherent buffering properties of the amino acids.[20] When amino acids solutions are diluted with dextrose and water, the overall titratable acidity is decreased.[19,21] In addition, at midrange, pH amino acid solutions form soluble complexes with calcium and phosphate, decreasing free concentrations of the salts that would be available for interaction.[22] High dextrose concentrations decrease pH, but this does not seem to be a major factor affecting calcium and phosphate solubility.[23] Lipid emulsions can increase solution pH. Thus, a PN solution with low amino acid concentration and high molar concentrations of calcium and phosphate is highly likely to precipitate.[19]

Calcium and phosphate compatibility is also dependent on temperature, the calcium salt used, the order in which the salts are added to the solution, and shelf time. Temperature contributes to catheter occlusion in preterm infants placed in incubators and in septic patients with indwelling catheters.[24] As the temperature of the solution rises, the degree of calcium and phosphate complex dissociation increases, creating an environment for calcium and phosphate ions to form calcium phosphate salts.[19,22,24,25] Because calcium gluconate dissociates to a lesser degree than calcium chloride, the gluconate salt is preferred in PN solutions.[22] To further minimize interaction of calcium and phosphate, phosphate should be added early in the mixing process, and calcium should be added last. Despite precautions, precipitation can occur at times other than formula preparation. For example, the risk for precipitation increases with standing time and slow infusion rates.[19,23,26] Incompatibilities of borderline concentrations of salts could become apparent 12 or more hours after mixing.[27]

Measures that avoid precipitation include: (1) consulting compatibility curves for the specific amino acid brand and final amino acid concentration, (2) avoiding solutions with borderline compatibilities whenever possible, and (3) adding cysteine hydrochloride 40 mg per gram of protein to decrease the pH of the solution.[26,28]

Insulin

Insulin is chemically stable in PN. However, determining an appropriate dose can be complicated. Insulin adsorbs to the solution container, delivery system, and in-line filter. Losses of insulin to the delivery system varying from 3 to 60% are reported. Adsorption occurs within 15 seconds of contact and could take up to 5 hours before binding sites are saturated.[29,30] The time necessary to achieve uniform delivery of insulin appears to depend largely on the infusion flow rate and extent of administration set binding. The extent of adsorption is dependent on insulin concentration, type and length of administration set, type of container, and temperature.[31–33] Addition of extra insulin to compensate for the losses has been suggested, as has the addition of albumin to minimize insulin adsorption.[34,35] Neither is recommended, since the benefits of these practices are negligible.[29,36]

Albumin

Albumin is visually compatible in PN formulations for up to 24 hours. However, PN solutions containing albumin promote bacterial and fungal growth.[37] Consideration must be given to cost and the indication for its use. Albumin should not exceed 25 g/liter, since occlusion of in-line filters has been noted at higher concentrations.

Vitamin A

The availability of vitamin A from PN solutions is poor because of the chemical properties of the lipid-soluble vitamin. Vitamin A adsorbs onto the plastic matrix of intravenous administration sets. Increases in exposure time and temperature enhance diffusion and decrease availability of vitamin A. Studies show vitamin A losses up to 75% after 24 hours in PVC bags. Photodegradation or oxidation is responsible for 16% of the loss.[38–41] The clinical significance of this loss has important implications for patients receiving long term PN therapy, especially neonates and patients who must heal wounds. Because vitamin A availability from PN formulations is unpredictable, supplementation via the intramuscular or oral route for patients at risk for vitamin A deficiency should be considered.

Iron Dextran

Iron dextran, 100 mg/liter in nonlipid-containing PN, is chemically stable for up to 18 hours.[42] Iron dextran at 10 mg/liter PN containing TrophAmine < 1.5% results in the formation of rust-colored precipitants within 12 to 24 hours of preparation at room temperature.[43] At amino acid concentrations of 2 and 2.5%, PN appears to be stable for up to 48 hours at room temperature. It is not recommended to use iron dextran in PN formulations containing lipid. When added to lipid-containing solutions, iron dextran can destabilize lipid particles, causing the formation of large droplets. These droplets could be dangerous if infused.[44]

An iron manufacturer issued a black box warning regarding the risk of severe anaphylactic reactions associated with the use of iron dextran. Therefore, it is advisable to administer a test dose prior to initiation of iron therapy via PN. Still, allergic reactions can occur with subsequent doses.[45–46]

Thiamine

Thiamine degradation occurs rapidly in PN solutions containing > 160 mg/liter of bisulfite at pH values > 6.[47] Under these conditions, thiamine undergoes hydrolysis, rendering it inactive. One study tested thiamine at the dose of 3 mg per 500 mL of undiluted FreAmine III 8.5% (pH = 6.5) and Travasol 5.5% (pH = 5.5). After 24 hours at room temperature, only 3–8% and 29% of added thiamine remained in the FreAmine and Travasol solutions, respectively. Under refrigerated conditions for 24 hours, thiamine availability improved to 37% and 67%, respectively. The higher availability observed with Travasol was attributed to the solution's lower pH.[47] Thiamine degradation apparently does not have clinical significance since the study condition did not reflect the conditions of PN formulations commonly prescribed. A later study demonstrated negligible thiamine loss simply by diluting Travasol to 4.25% in dextrose 25% solution. The final bisulfite concentration produced was approximately 0.05%.[48]

H-2 Antagonists

Cimetidine is stable over a wide range of conditions and mixtures. Concentrations ranging from 80 mg/liter to 1,000 mg/liter are stable at room temperature up to 72 hours with negligible drug loss.[49–51] Ranitidine is less stable. At concentrations ranging from 50 to 100 mg/liter, up to 20% loss was observed after 24 hours at room temperature.[52] If PN solutions are refrigerated, ranitidine losses are 6–10% after 48 hours.[53,54] The stability of famotidine at concentrations of 20–50% is comparable to cimetidine.[55,56]

Y-Site Compatibility

Critically ill patients often receive multiple intravenous medications but have a limited number of injection ports or access. Table 27-1 provides

Table 27-1 Y-site compatibility of medications with PN and lipids.

Drug	*PN*	*Lipids*
Acetazolamide	I	NI
Acyclovir	I	NI
Albumin	Y	NI
Alprostadil	NI	NI
Amikacin	Y	I
Amiodarone	NI	NI
Ampho-B	I	I
Ampicillin	I	Y
Atracurium	Y	NI
Caffeine citrate	Y	Y
Calcium chloride	Concentration dependent	NI
Calcium gluconate	Concentration dependent	Y
Cefazolin	Y	Y
Cefotaxime	Y	Y
Ceftazidime	Y	Y
Ceftriaxone	Y	Y
Cefuroxime	Y	Y
Cimetidine	Y	Y
Clindamycin	Y	Y
Dexamethasone	Y	Y
Diazepam	Y	NI
Digoxin	Y	Y
Dobutamine	Y	NI
Dopamine	Y	Y
Epinephrine	Y	NI
Esmolol	NI	NI
Famotidine	Y	Y
Fentanyl	Y	Y
Fluconazole	Y	NI
Fosphenytoin	Y	NI
Furosemide	Y	Y
Ganciclovir	Y	NI
Gentamicin	Y	Y
Heparin	Y	Y
Hydrocortisone	Y	Y

Table 27-1 Y-site compatibility of medications with PN and lipids (continued).

Drug	*PN*	*Lipids*
Immune globulin	Y	I
Indomethacin	I	NI
Insulin	Y	Y
Isoproterenol	Y	Y
Levothyroxine	NI	NI
Lidocaine	Y	Y
Lorazepam	Y	I
Magnesium sulfate	Y	I
Methylprednisolone	Y	Y
Metoclopramide	Y	Y
Midazolam	I	I
Morphine	Y	Y
Nafcillin	Y	Y
Nitroglycerin	Y	NI
Nitroprusside	Y	NI
Norepinephrine	Y	Y
Octreotide	Y	Y
Pancuronium	NI	NI
Penicillin G potassium	Y	Y
Phenobarbital	Y	I
Phytonadione	Y	NI
Ranitidine	Y	Y
Rifampin	NI	Y
Sodium bicarbonate	I	I
Terbutaline	NI	NI
Ticarcillin	Y	Y
Ticarcillin/clavulanate	Y	Y
Tobramycin	Y	Y
Vancomycin	Y	Y
Vasopressin	NI	NI
Vecuronium	Y	NI

Y = compatible at the Y-site; N = not compatible; NI = no information. Information applies to PN solutions with 10–20% dextrose, amino acid 2–4%.

Sources: Information compiled from Trissel LA. *Handbook on Injectable Drugs*. 12th ed. Bethesda, Md: American Society of Health-System Pharmacists; 2003: and Zenk KE, Sills JH, Koeppel RM. *Neonatal Medications and Nutrition: A Comprehensive Guide*. Santa Rosa, Calif: NICU INK Book Publishers; 1999.

compatibility information on PN solutions and commonly used intravenous medications that may be added at a Y-site.

EVALUATION OF DRUG LABORATORY AND DRUG NUTRIENT INTERACTIONS

Patients receiving PN frequently receive medications that can cause electrolyte imbalances (Table 27-2). The imbalances occur through a number of mechanisms, including enhanced or diminished renal excretion, centrally mediated alterations in total body fluid balance, and transcellular shifting. In addition to creating metabolic disturbances, medications could affect a patient's electrolyte load simply by containing sodium or potassium as a part of their formulation (Table 27-3). When drugs are initiated or discontinued, frequent monitoring of electrolytes

Table 27-2 Medications that can affect electrolytes and nutrients.

	Effects on electrolyte					
Drug	*Sodium*	*Potassium*	*Magnesium*	*Phosphorus*	*Acid/base imbalance*	*Glucose*
ACE inhibitors		↑				
ARBs (angiotension receptor blockers)		↑				
Amphotericin		↓	↓	↓	√	
β2 receptor agonists		↓				↑
Biphosphonates		↓	↓	↓		
Calcineurin inhibitors		↑	↓			↑
Cidofovir		↓			√	↑
Cisplatinol	↓	↓	↓	↓		
Cyclophosphamide	↓					
Corticosteroids		↓				↑
Diuretics (loop, thiazide, carbonic anhydrase inhibitors)	↓↑	↑			√	
Diuretics (potassium sparing)		↑				
Foscarnet		↓	↓	↓↑		
Insulin		↓				↓
Sodium polystyrene sulfonate		↓				
Vincristine	↓					

↓↑ = increase or decrease, ↓ = decrease, ↑ = increase, √ affects acid/base balance.

Sources: Information compiled from package inserts.

Table 27-3 Sodium content of common injectable medications.

Drug	*Dosage unit*	*Sodium content (mEq)*
Albumin 5 and 25%	1 L	130–160
Ampicillin sodium	1 gm	3
Cefazolin sodium	1 gm	2
Cefotaxime sodium	1 gm	2.2
Cefoxitin sodium	1 gm	2.3
Ceftriaxone sodium	1 gm	3.6
Cefuroxime	1 gm	2.4
Metronidazole	500 mg	14
Nafcillin sodium	1 gm	2.9
Penicillin G sodium	1,000,000 units	2
Phenobarbital sodium	65 mg	0.3
Phenytoin sodium	1 gm	3.8
Ticarcillin disodium	1 gm	5.2
Thiopental sodium	1 gm	3.8

Sources: Information compiled from package inserts.

is recommended. Preemptive modification of the electrolyte content of the PN is not advisable because the time course and extent of the changes are not predictable. PN should not be used to correct electrolyte abnormalities. Electrolyte corrections are made via a separate line, and if that is not possible, the PN is discontinued until electrolyte stability is assured.

Medications can cause electrolyte imbalance and affect acid-base homeostasis. Amphotericin B, loop diuretics, and cidofovir are examples of drugs that create acid-base disturbances through renal mediated mechanisms. When a patient receiving PN is on multiple medications, collaboration among pharmacists, dieticians, and physicians is critical to assure a comprehensive approach to management (see Chapter 14 for a discussion of drug nutrient interactions).

Propofol can contribute to caloric intake. Propofol is formulated in a 10% lipid emulsion and when administered in high doses for prolonged periods, can provide up to one third to one fourth of a patient's total daily lipid requirements.

Finally, when transitioning from PN to enteral feeds, electrolyte requirements could change. Variations in salt solubility and individual absorption kinetics can dramatically impact the effect of oral electrolyte supplementation. Increased frequency of monitoring is again recommended during this period of transition.

CONCLUSION

The provision of PN is considered the standard of care for many patients. Appropriate patient selection, assessment, and monitoring are keys in achieving successful nutritional therapy and preventing unnecessary complications. PN formulations should be individualized based on the patient's diagnosis and nutritional requirements. In addition, the impact of medications on calories, electrolytes, and acid/base balance should be taken into consideration. A multidisciplinary team of clinicians composed of physicians, dieticians, and pharmacists should be highly involved in all levels of the nutritional support.

REFERENCES

1. Dudrick SJ, Wilmore DW, Vars HM, Rhoads JE. Long-term parenteral nutrition with growth and development and positive nitrogen balance. *Surgery.* 1968;64:134.
2. Wilmore DW, Dudrick SJ. Growth and development of an infant receiving all nutrients exclusively by vein. *JAMA.* 1968;203:860–864.
3. Driscoll JM, Heird WC, Schullinger JN, Gongaware RD, Winters RW. Total intravenous alimentation in low birth weight infants: a preliminary report. *J Pediatr.* 1972;81:145–153.
4. Acra SA, Rollins C. Principles and guidelines for parenteral nutrition in children. *Pediatric Ann.* 1999;28(2):113–120.
5. Intravenous Nurses Society. Intravenous nursing: standards of practice, revised. *J Intraven Nurs.* 1998;21(Jan–Feb; 1 suppl):S1–91.
6. Timmer JG, Schipper HG. Peripheral venous nutrition: the equal relevance of volume load and osmolarity in relation to phlebitis. *Clin Nutr.* 1993;12:261–265.
7. Kuwahara T, Asanami S, Tanura T, Keneda S. Effects of pH and osmolarity on phlebitic potential of infusion solutions for peripheral parenteral nutrition. *J Toxicol Sci.* 1998;23:77–85.
8. Maki DG, Ringer M. Risk factors for infusion-related phlebitis with small peripheral venous catheters: a randomized controlled trial. *Ann Int Med.* 1991;114:845–853.
9. Fujuwara T, Kawaeasaki H, Fonkalsrud EW. Reduction of post-infusion venous endothelial injury with intralipid. *Surg Gynecol Obstet.* 1984;158:57–65.
10. Pineault M, Chessex P, Piedboeuf B, Bisaillon S. Beneficial effect of infusing a lipid emulsion on venous patency. *JPEN.* 1989;13:637–640.
11. William N, Wales S, Irving MH. Prolonged peripheral parenteral nutrition with an ultrafine cannula and low-osmolarity feed. *Br J Surg.* 1996;83:114–116.
12. Hoheim DF, O'Callaghan TA, Joswiak BJ, Boysen DA, Bommarito AA. Clinical experience with three-in-one admixtures administered peripherally. *Nut Clin Pract.* 1990;5:118–122.
13. Messing B, Levere X, Rigaud D, et al. Peripheral venous complications of hyperosmolar (960 mOsm) nutritive mixture: the effect of heparin and hydrocortisone. A multicenter double-blinded random study in 98 patients. *Clin Nutr.* 1986;5:57–61.
14. Reid I, Keane FB, Monson JR, Tanner WA. Thrombophlebitis following peripherally administered parenteral nutrition: a randomized clinical study of the effect of infusion additives. *Surg Res Comm.* 1990;9:69–77.
15. Madan M, Alexander DJ, Mellor E, Cooke J, McMahon MJ. A randomized study of the effects of osmolarity and heparin with hydrocortisone on thrombophlebitis on peripheral intravenous nutrition. *Clin Nutr.* 1991;10:309–314.
16. Alpan G, Eyal F, Springer C, Glick B, Goder K, Armon J. Heparinization of alimentation solutions administered through peripheral veins in premature infants: a controlled study. *Pediatrics.* 1984;74(3):375–378.
17. Fonkalsrud EW, Carpenter K, Masuda JY, Beckerman JH. Prophylaxis against postinfusion phlebitis. *Surg Gynecol Obstet.* 1971;133(2):253–256.
18. Heeger PS, Backstrom JT. Heparin flushes and thrombocytopenia. *Ann Intern Med.* 1986;105:143.
19. Eggert LD, Rusho WJ, MacKay MW, Chan GM. Calcium and phosphate compatibility in parenteral nutrition for neonates. *Am J Hosp Pharm.* 1982;39:49–53.
20. Sturgeon RJ, Athanikar NK, Henry RS, Jurgens RW Jr, Welco AD. Titratable acidities of crystalline amino acid admixtures. *Am J Hosp Pharm.* 1980;37:388–390.
21. Knight PH, Cuchanan S, Clathworthy HW. Calcium and phosphate requirements of preterm infants who require prolonged hyperalimentation. *JAMA.* 1980;243:1244–1246.
22. Henry RS, Harbison H, Sturgeon RJ, Athanikar N, Welco A, Van Leuven M. Compatibility of calcium chloride and calcium gluconate with sodium phosphate in mixed TPN solution. *Am J Hosp Pharm.* 1980;37:673–674.
23. Poole RL. Problems with preparation of parenteral nutrition solutions. In: Kerner JA, ed. *Manual of Pediatric Parenteral Nutrition.* New York, NY: John Wiley & Sons, Inc; 1983:129–136.
24. Robinson LA, Wright BT. Central venous catheter occlusion caused by body-heat-mediated calcium phosphate precipitation. *Am J Hosp Pharm.* 1982;39:120–121.
25. Dunham B, Marcuard S, Khazaine PG, Meade G, Craft T, Nichols K. The solubility of calcium and phosphorus in neonatal total parenteral nutrition solutions. *JPEN.* 1991;15:608.
26. Fitzgerald KA, MacKay MW. Calcium and phosphate solubility in neonatal parenteral nutrient solutions containing Aminosyn PF. *Am J Hosp Pharm.* 1987;44:1396–1400.

27. Schuetz DH, King JC. Compatibility and stability of electrolytes, vitamins, and antibiotics in combination with 8% amino acid solution. *Am J Hosp Pharm.* 1978;35:33–44.
28. Lenz GT, Mikrut BA. Calcium and phosphate solubility in neonatal parenteral nutrient solutions containing Aminosyn-PF or TrophAmine. *Am J Hosp Pharm.* 1988;45:2367–2371.
29. Weber SS, Wood WA, Jackson EA. Availability of insulin from parenteral nutrient solutions. *Am J Hosp Pharm.* 1977;34:353–357.
30. Petty C, Cunningham NL. Insulin adsorption by glass infusion bottles, polyvinlychloride infusion containers, and intravenous tubing. *Anesthesiology.* 1974;40:400–404.
31. Goldberg NJ, Levin SR. Insulin adsorption to an in-line membrane filter. *N Engl J Med.* 1978;298:1480.
32. Hirsch JI, Wood JH, Thomas RB. Insulin adsorption to polyolefin infusion bottles and polyvinyl chloride administration sets. *Am J Hosp Pharm.* 1981;38:995–997.
33. Twardowski ZJ, Nolph KD, McGary TJ, Moore HL. Influence of temperature and time on insulin adsorption to plastic bags. *Am J Hosp Pharm.* 1983;40:583–586.
34. Peterson L, Caldwell J, Hoffman J. Insulin adsorbance to polyvinyl chloride surfaces with implications for constant-infusion therapy. *Diabetes.* 1976;25:72–74.
35. Genuth SM. Constant intravenous insulin infusion in diabetic ketoacidosis. *JAMA.* 1973;223:1348–1351.
36. Tate J, Cowan GS. Insulin kinetics in hyperalimentation solution and routine intravenous therapy. *Am Surg.* 1977;43:811–816.
37. Mirtallo JM, Schneider PJ, Ruberg RL. Albumin in TPN solutions: potential savings from a prospective review. *JPEN.* 1980;4:300–302.
38. Hartline JV, Zachman RD. Vitamin A delivery in total parenteral nutrition solution. *Pediatrics.* 1976;58:448–451.
39. Shenai JP, Stahlman MT, Chytil F. Vitamin A delivery in total parenteral alimentation solution. *J Pediatr.* 1981;99:661–663.
40. Howard L, Chu R, Feman S, Mintz H, Oversen L, Wolf B. Vitamin A deficiency from long-term parenteral nutrition. *Ann Intern Med.* 1980;93:576–577.
41. Niemiec PW, Walker JZ. Vitamin A availability from parenteral nutrition delivery systems. *Nutr Support Serv.* 1983;3:53–56.
42. Wan KK, Tsallas G. Dilute iron dextran formulation for addition to parenteral nutrient solutions. *Am J Hosp Pharm.* 1980;37:206–210.
43. Mayhew SL, Quick MW. Compatibility of iron dextran with neonatal parenteral nutrient solutions. *Am J Health Syst Pharm.* 1997;54:570–571.
44. National Advisory Group on Standards and Practice Guidelines for Parenteral Nutrition. Safe practices for parenteral nutrition formulations. *JPEN.* 1998;22:49–66.
45. InFeD product information. Watson Pharma, Inc, Corona, Calif; 2001.
46. DexFerrum product information. American Regent Laboratories, Inc, Shirley, NY; 2001.
47. Scheiner JM, Araujo MM, DeRiter E. Thiamine destruction by sodium bisulfite in infusion solutions. *Am J Hosp Pharm.* 1981;38:1911–1913.
48. Bowman BB, Nguyen P. Stability of thiamine in parenteral nutrition solutions. *JPEN.* 1983;7:462–464.
49. Tsallas G, Allen LC. Stability of cimetidine hydrochloride in parenteral nutrition solutions. *Am J Hosp Pharm.* 1982;39:484–485.
50. Cano SM, Montoro JB, Pastor C, et al. Stability of cimetidine in total parenteral nutrition. *J Clin Nutr Gastroenterol.* 1987;2:40–43.
51. Mitrano FP, Baptista RJ. Stability of cimetidine HCL and copper sulfate in a TPN solution, DICP. *Ann Pharmacother.* 1989;23:429–430.
52. Cano SM, Montoro JB, Pastor C, Pou L, Sabin P. Stability of ranitidine hydrochloride in total nutrient admixtures. *Am J Hosp Pharm.* 1988;45:1100–1102.
53. Williams MF, Hak LJ, Dukes G. In vitro evaluation of the stability of ranitidine hydrochloride in total parenteral nutrient mixtures. *Am J Hosp Pharm.* 1990;47:1574–1579.
54. Walker SE, Bayliff CD. Stability of ranitidine hydrochloride in total parenteral nutrient solution. *Am J Hosp Pharm.* 1985;42:590–592.
55. Distefano JE, Mitrano FP, Baptista RJ, Der MM, Silvetri AP, Palombo JD. Stability of famotidine 20 mg/mL in total parenteral nutrient solution. *Am J Hosp Pharm.* 1989;46:2333–2335.
56. DiStefano JE, Mitrano FP, Baptista RJ, Der MM, Silvestri AP, Palombo JD, Bistrian BR. Long-term stability of famotidine 20 mg/L in a total parenteral nutrient solution. *Am J of Hosp Pharm.* 1989;46(11):2333–5. 57

CHAPTER 28

Nutrition Support for Children with Developmental Disabilities

Shirley Ekvall and Valli Ekvall

INTRODUCTION

It is a challenge to provide appropriate nutrition safely for children with developmental disabilities. Malnutrition, overnutrition, and undernutrition are common.[1–4] Often malnutrition is not recognized and not treated, or is inadequately treated. The most common reasons for inappropriate treatment include the difficulty of performing an assessment, the difficulty of supplying the nutrients because of problems with oral intake, and the reluctance of caregivers to encourage normal growth which might cause them to be unable to lift or move larger children and adolescents. This chapter discusses the assessment of children with developmental disabilities, nutritional problems that might occur, and special cases, such as a ketogenic diet and specific developmental abnormalities.

Developmental disabilities (DDs) describe a diverse group of severe, chronic conditions that are due to mental and/or physical impairments. DDs are associated with problems in all major life activities such as language, mobility, learning, self-help, and independent living. DDs begin any time during development up to 22 years of age and usually last throughout a person's lifetime.[5] Malnutrition and gastrointestinal problems that adversely affect nutrition, such as feeding difficulties, nutritional deficiencies, aspiration, gastritis, gastroesophageal reflux, constipation, and hepatitis are common in children with DDs.[6–8] For example, feeding problems occur in about 25% of the general population and in 80% of children with a DD.[9] Children with DDs might require more or less nutrients than nonimpaired children because of their activity level.

Cerebral palsy (CP) is an umbrella-like term used to describe a group of chronic, developmental disorders impairing control of movement that appear in the first few years of life and generally do not worsen over time. The disorders are caused by faulty development of or damage to motor areas in the brain that disrupt the brain's ability to control movement and posture. Symptoms of CP include difficulty with fine motor tasks, maintaining balance, or walking, as well as involuntary movements. The symptoms differ from person to person and might change over time. CP can be associated with other medical disorders, including seizures or mental impairment, but CP does not always cause profound handicap. CP can be congenital or acquired. Some causes include head injury, jaundice, Rh incompatibility, prematurity, and rubella. Symptoms of CP could change over time, but by definition CP is not progressive.[10]

HISTORY AND PHYSICAL EXAMINATION

Before beginning nutrition support (NS), a complete medical history, including review of systems, family history, and social history must be obtained. In addition, a careful dietary history consisting of food recall, 4-day food records, or food tables is important. The history should include information on feedings such as how often feeds are offered, who feeds the child, how long each feeding takes, the child's activity level, muscle tone, and the types of physical activity the child performs and how often they are performed. Important items that should be discussed in the feeding history are listed in Table 28-1.

A physical examination with an accurate weight/height ratio and careful anthropometrics including triceps, subscapular, and calf skinfold thickness[11–12] should be performed. A standard stadiometer can be used in the absence of scoliosis, spasticity, or joint contractures. When these findings are present, then upper arm and lower leg length provide an accurate and reproducible measure of linear growth.[13,14] Physical findings of concern include orofacial anomalies, dental caries, sensitive gag reflex, decreased or increased muscle tone, the presence of an abdominal mass suggesting an impaction, and indicators of malnutrition. Observation of a feed provides a wealth of information that can assist in the assessment of the child's feeding and the challenges the child and caretaker(s) might need to overcome.

Table 28-1 Feeding history and skills for children with neurological impairment or developmental delays.

- Developmental status
- Neurologic status
- Physical activity
- Mobility
- Feeding history
  - Diet history
  - 4-day diet diary, include fluids
  - 4-day physical activity diary
  - Supplemental feedings, including oral feedings, tube feedings, vitamins, and minerals
  - Herbal supplements
  - Feeding difficulties in the past
  - Length of time to complete a meal
- Swallowing difficulties
- Choking
- Recurrent pneumonia
- Pain when eating
- Vomiting
- Difficulty with textures or thickness of solids or liquids
- Current use of occupational therapy/physical therapy/speech therapy
- Developmental stimulation activities
- School programs
- Nutritional status
- Caregiver's willingness to consider tube feedings
- Stooling history
- Surgery history

FOCUSED LABORATORY TESTS

In addition to the usual nutritional laboratory assessment (Chapter 7), specialized studies could be helpful. Swallowing studies using video fluoroscopy that are evaluated by a radiologist and a trained speech therapist assess how the patient handles liquids, solids, and various textures, as well as how body postures affect oromotor function (see Chapter 12). The speech therapist also assesses muscle tone, head control, whether the suck is weak or absent, hand-to-mouth coordination, quality of lip closure, tongue thrust, the gag reflex, and coordination of swallowing. Swallowing function studies also provide an assessment of the risk for aspiration.[15] Fiberoptic endoscopic swallowing evaluation allows the observation of secretions and the swallowing of foods in the pharyngeal phase.[16]

Further assessment depends on the symptoms and findings. For example, an upper gastrointestinal series confirms normal anatomy; a gastric emptying study identifies delayed emptying; a flat plate assesses for stool impaction; a pH probe provides information on acid reflux; and an endoscopy with biopsies can diagnose allergy, infection, or inflammation. Stool studies help identify if infection or malabsorption are present.

Medications could interfere with nutrients (see Chapter 14 for a discussion of drug nutrient interactions), and assessment of specific nutrient levels, metabolites, or functions might be necessary. Deficiencies of micronutrients often occur with anticonvulsant therapy. Long term use of some anticonvulsants can alter folate and vitamin D metabolism. It might be necessary to supplement both.

QUALITY OF LIFE ISSUES

The quality of life of the child and family must be assessed, especially with respect to feedings. Families often find a trade-off exists between the child's enjoyment of the eating experience and the amount of time spent feeding the child. Many times, supplements provide this balance. One study involving approximately 340 children with neurological impairment found that 8% received caloric supplements and 8% received tube feeds.[17]

GASTROINTESTINAL PROBLEMS THAT AFFECT NUTRITION

Reflux

The prevalence of gastroesophageal reflux, the involuntary passage of gastric contents into the esophagus, is higher in children with DDs and can be manifested by vomiting, gagging, grimacing in pain after or during swallowing, food aversion, irritability, hematemesis, failure to thrive, or occult blood loss in stools, or it can be silent. The most common cause of reflux is inappropriate relaxation of the lower esophageal sphincter, but delayed gastric emptying and perhaps low esophageal sphincter tone might predispose to reflux. Prolonged supine positioning, reliance on liquid feeds, and increased abdominal pressure caused by spasticity, seizures, or cough contribute to reflux. It is important to consider reflux, since undiagnosed reflux can cause esophagitis that is painful and could be associated with blood loss, which, in turn, can cause iron deficiency anemia. Esophagitis can lead to strictures or Barrett's esophagus. Not all vomiting is caused by reflux, however, and increased intracranial pressure, metabolic abnormalities, anatomic abnormalities, infections, and food or medication allergy must be considered. A pediatric gastroenterologist should be consulted to assess and provide treatment guidance.

Constipation

The prevalence of constipation in children with DDs is unknown, but most care providers believe it is common. Constipation is associated with diminished muscle tone and activity, low fiber intake, low fluid intake, and some medications. Constipation is thought to be associated with gassiness, abdominal pain, vomiting, decreased food intake, early satiety, and poor feeding. If an impaction is present, diagnosed by physical examination or abdominal radiographs, disimpaction must be performed before stool softeners can be effective.[18] Polyethylene glycol 3350 (PEG) is often used for both disimpaction and maintenance therapy. Other osmotic agents such as sorbitol, lactulose, or milk of magnesia may also be used. Mineral oil should be avoided if there is any risk of aspiration.

Oral Health

Dental hygiene, the prevention of cavities and gingival disease, and aggressive treatment when oral disease develops are important for all children with DDs, even those receiving enteral feedings. Good dental care prevents the development of more serious problems such as abscesses, and it reduces the risk of aspiration from oral secretions. Good care also prevents chronic pain from carious teeth.

NUTRITION ALTERATIONS WITH NEUROLOGICAL DELAYS

Failure to thrive is common in children with DDs; 20–30% of children with DDs are underweight for age and 8–14% are obese.[19] Children with DDs are at risk for malnutrition for many reasons, the most common being insufficient food intake, not the underlying neurological, muscular, or mental abnormality. About 33% of children with CP have oromotor dysfunction, and 25% have moderately or severely impaired self-feeding skills.[20] Increased nutrient losses can also occur because of vomiting, diarrhea, or simply food wastage during feedings. In a retrospective chart review, Duncan et al.[21] showed that less than 75% of the Recommended Daily Allowance (RDA) for calories was administered to 95% of children, 58% for calcium, 68% for phosphorus, and 74% for vitamin D.

For children with CP intrauterine events, prematurity or intrauterine growth retardation might contribute to their nutritional problems.

A serious problem in providing nutrition for children with DDs is the lack of information on their nutrient requirements, especially energy requirements. It is likely that nonambulatory children and adolescents with CP have reduced energy requirements when compared to the normal population.[2,19,21–25] This lack of critical information necessary in setting nutritional goals makes it easy to under or over estimate caloric needs.

Bone Health

Children with DDs, especially CP, are at risk for diminished bone mineral density (BMD). Many factors contribute to the development of low BMD. Some of these factors are impaired weight bearing ambulation, immobilization after orthopedic procedures, poor growth, poor nutrition, low vitamin and mineral intake, anticonvulsant use and little or no sun exposure.[21,25] In addition, CP is often associated with prematurity and prematurity is a risk for the development of metabolic bone disease.[26] Children with low BMD and CP are at risk for fractures, and it is reported that roughly 26% of children with CP develop fractures.[21] Many children have multiple fractures.[27–29] The femur is most commonly involved. Fractures are painful, they increase the work load of care providers, and they might require hospitalization and surgical treatment. A report of children with CP treated for 12 months with pamidronate showed an improvement in age-normalized BMD z-scores.[30] The drug had no side effects that required treatment. While this is promising, others recommend caution in the use of biphosphonates in children and the need for larger trials.[31]

NS is associated with improved rates of linear growth, weight gain, bone mineralization, attitude and behavior of the child, and family lifestyle. Improved nutrition promotes healing of pressure sores and could reduce or prevent aspiration pneumonia, especially if gastrostomy feedings are used.

Indications for Nutrition Support

The indications for nutritional intervention are listed in Table 28-2, and those for enteral intervention are listed in Table 28-3. Nutrition therapy alone usually does not improve oromotor function. Nutrition therapy should be considered for children whose neurologic status is complicated by moderate or severe malnutrition and linear growth failure, especially when the bone age delay is more than two standard deviations from the mean for chronologic age.[32] In contrast, dietary restriction might be needed for any child whose BMI is greater than the 80th percentile.

There is little indication for parenteral nutrition in children with DDs who have a functioning gastrointestinal tract. But parenteral nutrition can be used if the gastrointestinal tract cannot fully support the child. There are important ethical issues, risks, and benefits associated with parenteral nutrition involving children and adolescents with DDs that require honest discussion between the physicians and the child's care providers.

Approach to Nutrition Support

There are no intrinsic intestinal abnormalities in most neurologic disorders. Malnutrition itself could impose changes in intestinal morphology and function, but these are transient. Enteral tube feedings are mandatory in any child with neurologic handicaps who cannot meet his or her fluid or nutrient requirements by oral feeding alone (Table 28-4 outlines nutrition support for chil-

Table 28-2 Indications for nutrition intervention.

Primary therapy for oromotor feeding difficulties
Supportive therapy
Preoperative nutritional rehabilitation
Drug nutrient interactions
- Vitamin D
- Folic acid

Abnormalities of specific laboratory tests
- Anemia
- Hypoalbuminemia
- Serum mineral deficiencies
- Serum vitamin deficiencies
- Prolonged prothrombin time
- Depressed alkaline phosphatase
- Lactose intolerance

Complications of neurologic disorders
- Malnutrition
- Growth failure
- Obesity

Table 28-3 Indications for enteral tube placement.

Nutritional
- Inability to meet daily fluid requirement
- Inability to meet daily nutrient requirements by the oral route
- Moderate/severe wasting (< 80% weight-for-height)
- Moderate/severe linear stunting (< 90% height-for-age)

Neurologic
- Orofacial abnormalities associated with swallowing difficulties
- Gastroesophageal reflux unresponsive to medications
- Recurrent complications of swallowing difficulties (aspiration, pneumonia, esophagitis)

dren with developmental disabilities). Evidence of moderate wasting (< 80% weight-for-height) or linear stunting (< 90% height-for-age) indicates the need for aggressive nutritional rehabilitation. Orofacial abnormalities associated with persistent swallowing difficulties, gastroesophageal reflux unresponsive to medical management, and recurrent complications from these warrant the use of tube feedings.

Use of supplemental nasogastric or gastrostomy feedings in children with cerebral palsy has a significant, positive effect on nutritional status. Weight gain and body fat stores are improved.[33] The greatest positive effect occurs when supplemental nutrition is initiated in the first year of life.[34]

Several issues must be considered: the route of enteral refeeding, the method of formula administration, the amount of nutrients required, and the source of the nutritional supplement (Table 28-4). In general, a percutaneous endoscopic gastrostomy (PEG) tube is the feeding route of choice. The advantages of PEG include the possibility of placement under sedation, avoidance of laparotomy, minimal postoperative discomfort, minimal likelihood of postoperative ileus, and the ability to use the tube within hours of placement. Tube feedings are discussed in Chapter 20.

The targeted amount of nutritional therapy administered via the enteral route varies, depending on the energy requirements and tolerance level of the child. The precise energy requirements for nutritional rehabilitation and restoration with a positive therapeutic outcome are not known. In practice, the amount of enteral feedings associated with a positive therapeutic outcome is highly variable. Children with CP demonstrate short term weight gains of 33% at a rate of 24–29 g/day, or 1.5–3.3 g/kg body weight while receiving dietary energy intakes that range from 40 to 150 kcal/kg/day body weight.[34–36] One study showed that approximately 85% of the weight gain was fat, and 15% was lean body mass.[33] Over 6 months, weight-for-age and weight-for-height measurements increased 20%, and length-for-age measurements increased 4%. Although no further increases in length occurred, body weight increased another 10% over the next 18 months. Not all children, however, achieved such positive outcomes. In one series, 75% of children with CP remained below the fifth percentile for

Table 28-4 Approach to nutrition support in children with developmental disabilities.

Route of tube feeding
- Nasogastric
- Gastrostomy
- Jejunostomy

Method of formula administration
- Continuous drip
- Intermittent bolus
- Combined continuous nighttime and intermittent daytime bolus

Amount of nutrients
- Individualize energy based on ideal body weight for chronologic age (10th–25th percentile) in the malnourished child
- Individualize energy based on multiples (1.0–1.2) of the resting metabolic rate in obese children

Source of nutrition supplement
- Polymeric formula specific for children
- Whey based formula for children with emesis

height, 33% remained underweight for height, and 21% became overweight for height after gastrostomy feedings.[33] The relationship between dietary energy intakes and weight gain could not be predicted on the basis of activity level, muscle tone, seizure control, or the presence of infection.[33] The earlier the nutritional intervention, however, the more favorable the outcome.

Complications Associated with Nutrition Support

Complications of nutrition support in general are discussed in Chapter 20. Complications specific for children with DDs are the continuation of undernutrition and the development of obesity.

Undernutrition can persist because of inappropriate prescription of enteral feedings, because caretakers are unconvinced of its value and hence limit feedings, and because caretakers fear that with normal growth the child with DDs will become too large for them to physically move.

Overfeeding causes obesity. This happens because of overly aggressive nutrient prescriptions or caretakers providing more than prescribed. One cause of obesity is the lack of enteral feeds designed for children with DDs. All enteral formulas for children older than 1 year of age contain 1 kcal or more/mL. To provide adequate minerals, vitamins, and trace elements, children must consume 1 liter of these formulas. In many instances this is simply too many calories. Providing less than 1 liter or diluting the formulas compromises the delivery of essential nutrients. The availability of a reduced calorie formula that contains the same density of other nutrients would be very useful.

Follow-up is essential to observe for overfeeding that can lead to serious obesity problems and reduced mobility. Nutrition support can be discontinued if 75% of the RDA/DRI and 90% of the fluid requirement can be met by mouth.[16]

Monitoring

Depending on the nutritional status and the nutrition therapy that is required, children with DDs should be monitored every 1–4 months. At that time, an interval feeding history and physical examination should be performed. Laboratory tests are performed on an as needed basis. Attention should be paid to fluid balance, and urine specific gravity might be useful. Adjustments in the nutrition therapy can be made so that undernutrition does not continue or so that overnutrition does not develop.

KETOGENIC DIET

Sometimes the ketogenic diet is prescribed for refractory seizures.[37] This is a high fat diet that is used to induce ketosis.[38]

A vitamin and mineral supplement must be prescribed for all children on ketogenic diets. Parents also must monitor urine ketones and specific gravity daily by urine chemstick. Serum beta-hydroxy-butyrate levels are a measure of serum ketones and can be used to monitor for ketosis. Some commercially available products permit easier administration of the ketogenic diet by gastrostomy tube feedings. A dietitian is necessary to design, monitor, and teach the diet. Vitamin D and folate must be carefully monitored.

NEUROMUSCULAR DISEASES

Children with neuromuscular disease might be underweight or obese. Feeding difficulty is often encountered in neuromuscular diseases. In Duchenne type muscular dystrophy, self-feeding becomes a challenge because of poor strength in the body's trunk and limbs. Swallowing dysfunction usually occurs late in the disease. In spinal muscular atrophy, oromotor dysfunction occurs as the disease progresses. In congenital myotonic dystrophy, supplemental feeding is often required from birth because of inadequate suck and swallow.[39] In Guillain-Barré syndrome, nasogastric feeding might be necessary because of poor swallowing, especially when severe neuropathy is present.[40]

MYELOMENINGOCELE

Obesity is a common problem for children with myelomeningocele, especially for those who have higher spinal lesion levels, because mobility is limited. Children with myelomeningocele have low lean body mass and high body fat content, particularly in the lower extremities.[41] In one study, when estimation of caloric needs was based on lean body mass, about a 50% reduction in lean body mass was found after age 8 years.[41] Using current growth charts, it is recommended that the child remain between the 25th and 50th percentile for weight on the Centers for Disease Control growth curves. Segmental and special growth charts are also useful.[11–13] Low calorie, nutrient rich foods and physical activity should be encouraged.

DOWN SYNDROME

Children with Down syndrome exhibit abnormal feeding patterns caused by impaired jaw and tongue functions, and a continuous "smooth sequence of feeding actions."[42] Parents of children with Down syndrome typically do not volunteer information on the extent of the child's feeding difficulty, partly due to the tendency of these parents to be controlling in their interactions with the children. For this reason, information on feeding should be solicited by the dietitian along with an observation of the child feeding. Children with Down syndrome typically have difficulty gaining weight during infancy, followed by a tendency to gain too much weight later in life. The growth of children with Down syndrome should be plotted on growth curves specifically validated for this syndrome and available on the web site of the National Down Syndrome Society.[43] Children with Down syndrome are at increased risk for celiac disease, and they should be monitored using a quantitative serum IgA level and a serum transglutaminase antibody test.[44]

Rett Syndrome

Rett syndrome, a progressive syndrome affecting young girls, is characterized by psychomotor retardation, ataxia, seizures, autistic behavior, and death. Oromotor dysfunction occurs frequently and nutrition support is required early in treatment. Severe scoliosis is common, progressive, and could further hamper the ability to eat.[45] Growth failure is a common feature in Rett syndrome. Children with Rett syndrome might be 2 standard deviations below the norm for height and weight-for-height.

Caregiver Education

An interdisciplinary feeding team consisting of a gastroenterologist, nutritionist, occupational therapist/speech therapist, and behavioral psychologist is recommended to provide optimal evaluation and care for the child with a complex feeding disorder. Intervention should include treatment of the medical condition, behavioral modification, and parent/caregiver education and training in care giving and feeding skills. The use of home health nurses and nutritionists for follow-up visits in the home ensures that feeding tubes/pumps are used correctly and monitors for potential complications with the nutrition/therapy. These in-home professionals can give providers needed support.[46–47]

For the caregiver, there are some helpful keys to feeding behavior. Reinforce appropriate feeding behavior[46,47] and avoid negative oral stimulation if possible at feeding time. Examples of negative stimulation include the insertion of a nasogastric tube or giving medicine that has an unpleasant taste. Appropriate positioning should be ensured and might require holding or placing the child in an infant seat or wheelchair for feedings. Structure such as consistent mealtimes is important.[48] Positive oral motor stimulation can be promoted using a soft toothbrush just prior to or during the feeding.

Medical Home

The concept of consistent, family centered care in the child's own community, a "medical home," has become the standard for treatment for children with DDs or special health care needs.[44] The medical home should provide preventative services, immunizations, developmental and growth assessments, screening, health care, supervision, and family counseling in health/psychosocial issues. Surveys show that 70–90% of children with special health care needs have nutrition related problems.[10,47–52] The professionals treating this population need to be aware of the community services and organizations that are available to these families.[47,49,51,53]

CONCLUSIONS

Children with developmental disabilities are at high risk for overnutrition and undernutrition and require careful periodic nutrition assessments. The gastrointestinal tracts of DD children are usually normal. The problems commonly encountered are poor feeding skills and environmental deterrents to good nutrition. Neither of these problems should result in suboptimal nutritional status, if treated properly.

REFERENCES

1. Samson-Fang L, Fung E, Stallings VA, et al. Relationship of nutritional status to health and societal participation in children with cerebral palsy. *J Pediatr.* 2002;141:637–643.
2. Stallings VA, Zemel BS, Davies JC, Cronk CE, Charney EB. Energy expenditure of children and adolescents with severe disabilities: a cerebral palsy model. *Am J Clin Nutr.* 1996;64:627–634.
3. Stallings VA, Cronk CE, Zemel BS, Charney EB. Body composition in children with spastic quadriplegic cerebral palsy. *J Pediatr.* 1995;126:833–839.
4. Jones M, Campbell KA, Duggan C, et al. Multiple micronutrient deficiencies in a child fed an elemental formula. *JPGN.* 2001;33:602–605.
5. Centers for Disease Control, National Center on Birth Defects and Developmental Disabilities. Developmental disabilities: what are developmental disabilities? Available at: http://www.cdc.gov/ncbddd/dd/default.htm. Accessed May 19, 2005.
6. Reilly S, Skuse D, Problete X. Prevalence of feeding problems and oral motor dysfunction in children with cerebral palsy: a community survey. *J Pediatr.* 1996;129:877–882.
7. Dahl M, Thommessen M, Rasmussen M, Selberg T. Feeding and nutritional characteristics in children with moderate or severe cerebral palsy. *Acta Paediatr.* 1996;85:697–701.
8. Thomas AG, Akobeng AK. Technical aspects of feeding the disabled child. *Curr Opin Clin Nutr Metab Care.* 2000;3(3):215–221.
9. Manikam R, Perman JA. Pediatric feeding disorders. *J Clin Gastroenterol.* 2000;30(1):34–46.
10. National Institute of Neurological Disorders and Stroke. NINDS cerebral palsy information page. Available at: http://www.ninds.nih.gov/disorders/cerebral_palsy/cerebral_palsy.htm. Accessed May 19, 2005.
11. Ekvall S, Cerniglia F. Myelomeningocele. In: Ekvall S, Ekvall V, eds. *Pediatric Nutrition in Chronic Diseases and Developmental Disorders.* 2nd Ed. New York, NY: Oxford University Press; 2005:97–104.
12. LaFollette Atencio P, Ekvall S, Oppenheimer S, Grace E. Effect of level of lesion and quality of ambulation on growth chart measurements in children with myelomeningocele: a pilot study. *J Am Diet Assoc.* 1992;92(7):858–861.
13. Belt-Niedbala B, Ekvall S, Cook CM, Oppenheimer S, Wessel, J. Linear growth measurement: a comparison of single arm length and arm span. *Dev Med Child Neurol.* 1986;28:319–334.

14. Spender QW, Cronk CE, Charney EB, Stallings VA. Assessment of linear growth of children with cerebral palsy: use of alternative measures to height or length. *Devel Med and Child Neurol.* 1998;31:206–214.
15. Morton RE, Bonas R, Fourie B, Minford J. Videofluoroscopy in the assessment of feeding disorders of children with neurological problems. *Dev Med Child Neurol.* 1993;35(3):388–395.
16. Lewis G, Ekvall S, Ekvall V. Nutrition in the neurological child. In: *American Society for Parenteral and Enteral Nutrition Support Practice Manual.* Silver Spring, MD ;1998:1–8.
17. Strauss DJ, Shavelle RM, Anderson TW. Life expectancy of children with cerebral palsy. *Pediatr Neurol.* 1998;18:143–149.
18. Baker SS, Liptak GS, Colletti, RB, et al. Constipation in infants and children: evaluation and treatment. *JPGN.* 1999;29:612–626.
19. Stallings VA, Charney EB, Davies JC, Cronk CE. Nutritional status and growth of children with diplegic or hemiplegic cerebral palsy. *Dev Med Child Neurol.* 1993;35:997–1006.
20. Thommessen M, Heiberg A, Kase BF, et al. Feeding problems, height and weight in different groups of disabled children. *Acta Paediatr Scand.* 1991;80:527–533.
21. Duncan B, Barton LL, Lloyd J, Marks-Katz M. Dietary considerations in osteopenia in tube-fed nonambulatory children with cerebral palsy. *Clin Pediatr.* 1999;38:133–137.
22. Dickerson RN, Brown RO, Hanna DL, Williams JE. Energy requirements of non-ambulatory, tube-fed adult patients with cerebral palsy and chronic hypothermia. *Nutrition.* 2003;19:741–746.
23. Taylor SB, Shelton JE. Caloric requirements of a spastic immobile cerebral patient: a case report. *Arch Phys Med Rehabil.* 1995;76:281–283.
24. Hogan SE. Energy requirements of children. *Can J Diet Prac Res.* 2004;65:124–130.
25. Krick J, Murphy PE, Markham JFB, Shapiro BK. A proposed formula for calculating energy needs of children with cerebral palsy. *Devel Med Child Neurol.* 1992;34:481–487.
26. Miller ME. The bone disease of preterm birth: a biomechanical perspective. *Pediatr Res.* 2003;53:10–15.
27. Henderson RC. Bone density and other possible predictors of fracture risk in children and adolescents with spastic quadriplegia. *Dev Med Child Neurol.* 1997;39:224–227.
28. Lee JJK, Lyne ED. Pathologic fractures in severely handicapped children and young adults. *J Pediatr Orthop.* 1990;10:497–500.
29. Mc Ivor WC, Samilson RL. Fractures in patients with cerebral palsy. *J Bone Joint Burg Am.* 1966;48:858–866.
30. Henderson RC, Lark RK, Kecskemethy H, Miller F, Harche HT, Bachrach SJ. Biphosphonates to treat osteopenia in children with quadriplegic cerebral palsy: a randomized placebo-controlled clinical trial. *J Pediatr.* 2002;141:644–651.
31. Whyte MP, Wenkert D, Clements KL, McAlister WH, Mumm S. Bisphosphonate-induced osteopetrosis. *N Eng J Med.* 2003;349(5):457–463.
32. Motil, KJ. Enteral nutrition in the neurologically impaired child. In: Baker SS, Baker RD, Davis A, eds. *Pediatric Enteral Nutrition.* New York, NY: Chapman and Hall;1994:217–237.
33. Fung EB, Samson-Fang L, Stallings VA, et al. Feeding dysfunction is associated with poor growth and health status in children with cerebral palsy. *J Am Diet Assoc.* 2002;102:361–373.
34. Rempel GR, Colwel SO, Nelson RP: Growth in children with cerebral palsy fed via gastrostomy. *Pediatrics.* 1988;82(6):957–967.
35. Sanders KD, Cox K, Cannon R, et al. Growth response to enteral feeding by children with cerebral palsy. *JPEN.* 1990;14:23–26.
36. Patrick J, Boland M, Stoski D, et al. Rapid correction of wasting in children with cerebral palsy. *Dev Med Child Neurol.* 1986;28:743–746.
37. Vining EP. The ketogenic diet. *Adv Exp Med Biol.* 2002;497:225–229.
38. Sinha Sr, Kossoff EH. The ketogenic diet. *The Neurologist.* 2005;11:161–170.
39. Hageman AT, Gabreels FJ, Liem KD, Renkawek K, Boon JM. Congenital myotonic dystrophy: a report on thirteen cases and a review of the literature. *J Neurol Sci.* 1993;115(1):95–101.
40. Iannaccone S. Muscular dystrophy. In: Ekvall S, ed. *Pediatric Nutrition in Chronic Diseases and Developmental Disorders*, 1st Ed. New York, NY: Oxford University Press; 1993:103–105.
41. Grogan C, Ekvall S. Body composition of children with myelomeningocele determined by K, urinary creatinine and anthropometric measures. *J Am Coll Nutr.* 1999;18:316–325.
42. Spender Q, Stein A, Dennis J, Reilly S, Percy E, Cave D. An exploration of feeding difficulties in children with Down syndrome. *Dev Med Child Neurol.* 1996;38(8):681–689.
43. National Down Syndrome Society. Growth charts. Available at: http://www.ndss.org/content.cfm?fuseaction=InfoRes.HlthArticle&article=603. Accessed January 23, 2006.
44. Children's Digestive Health and Nutrition Foundation/North American Society of Pediatric Gastroenterology, Hepatology and Nutrition. Diagnosis and treatment of celiac disease in children: clinical practice guideline

summary. Available at: http://www.celiachealth.org/pdf/celiac8.pdf. Accessed January 23, 2006.

45. Bassett GS, Tolo VT. The incidence and natural history of scoliosis in Rett syndrome. *Dev Med Child Neurol.* 1990;32(11):963–966.
46. Bayerl CT, Ries JD, Bettencourt MF, Fisher P. Nutrition issues of children in early intervention programs: primary care team approach. *Semin Pediatr Gastroenterol Nutr.* 1993;(4):11–13.
47. Ekvall S, Ekvall V. Early intervention and nutrition. In: Stevens F, Ekvall S, eds. *Empowering Children Through Early Intervention with Good Nutrition—Focusing on Culturally Diverse Children with Special Health Care Needs.* Manual IV, MCHB. Rockville, Md: HRSA; 2002:7–20.
48. US Dept of Health and Human Services. *Healthy People 2010: Understanding and Improving Health.* Washington, DC: US Government Printing Office; November 2000. Stock No. 017-001-001-00-550-9.
49. Position of the American Dietetic Association: providing nutrition services for infants, children, and adults with developmental disabilities and special health care needs. *J Am Diet Assoc.* 2004;104(1):97–107.
50. Sullivan PB, Lambert B, Rose M, Ford-Adams M, Johnson A, Griffiths P. Prevalence and severity of feeding and nutritional problems in children with neurological impairment: Oxford feeding study. *Dev Med Child Neurol.* 2000;42(10):674–684.
51. Morris SE, Klein MD. Pre-feeding skills: *Pre-Feeding Skills: A Comprehensive Resource for Mealtime Development.* 2nd ed. Tuscon, Ariz: Communication Skills Builders; 2001.
52. Wadie GM, Lobe TE. Gastroesophageal reflux disease in neurologically impaired children: the role of the gastrostomy tube. *Semin Laparosc Surg.* 2002;9(3):180–189.
53. Cloud H, Ekvall S, Hicks L. Feeding in children with developmental delays. In: Ekvall S, Ekvall V, eds. *Pediatric Nutrition in Chronic Diseases and Developmental Disorders.* 2nd ed. New York, NY: Oxford University Press; 2005:172–182.

ACKNOWLEDGMENTS

We wish to acknowledge L. Glen Lewis, MD, gastroenterologist, for his earlier input and Valeria Cohran, MD, gastroenterologist, for her recent input to this chapter.

CHAPTER 29

Nutrition Support for Pediatric Burns and Critical Care

Theresa Mayes and Michele M. Gottschlich

INTRODUCTION

In the past 20 years, advances in wound and surgical care, pharmacokinetics, pulmonary treatment, fluid resuscitation, and nutritional therapy improved the survival of critically ill and burned patients. However, children remain at high risk of morbidity because their immune, gastrointestinal, and renal systems are immature, they have small total body reserves and fluid resuscitation requirements may acutely be misinterpreted. Furthermore, children require additional nutritional consideration for growth and development. The catabolic state produced by burns and critical illness presents a challenge to ensure that the nutrient requirements for the stress of illness, as well as growth and development, are achieved. This chapter discusses the pathophysiological alterations of critical illness and their nutritional implications. Particular attention is given to the evaluation of energy and protein needs, the method of nutrient delivery, formula selection, early and perioperative feeding, and nutrition assessment techniques.

METABOLIC RESPONSE TO INJURY

Cuthbertson and Tilstone describe the metabolic response to trauma as two phases, the ebb and flow.[1] During the initial ebb, or shock phase, which usually lasts 3 to 5 days following injury, cardiac output, temperature, blood pressure, and oxygen consumption decrease, resulting in catabolism. With transition to the flow state, elevated circulatory and catabolic hormone responses drive nutrient requirements up. In addition, the rise in glucagon to insulin ratio supports gluconeogenesis, lipolysis, and protein degradation. Derangements in counterregulatory hormones and cytokines affect both the humoral and cell-mediated components of the immune system, which increases the susceptibility of the organism to infection. Burns evoke the most pronounced manifestation of the postinjury metabolic response. Despite the etiology of injury, however, alterations in metabolism occur to some degree, making it necessary to determine the energy and protein demands as a foremost nutrition goal.

ENERGY

An increase in energy requirements accompanies critical illness. For burns, the degree of hypermetabolism is related to the extent of injury, although an energy ceiling is reached when approximately 50% total body surface area is involved.[2] The causes of hypermetabolism are many. Aside from the elevations noted with general trauma and infection, the stress of illness releases catecholamines that drive metabolism up.[3–7] Pain and anxiety control reduce metabolism. For burns, raising room temperature and applying an impermeable dressing lessens the metabolic response. Gottschlich et al. suggest that sleep deprivation could be an additional cause of postburn hypermetabolism.[8] This is a fascinating concept that requires further consideration, not only in burns, but also in all critically ill pediatric patients.

Caloric reserves in children are low, but caloric requirements are higher per meter squared of body surface area than that of adults, so deficiencies develop readily. For this reason, the determination of energy needs and provision of calories to meet these needs are critical.[1]

Calorie needs may be estimated or measured. Formulas used to estimate calorie requirements begin with recommendations from standard reference tables such as those of the World Health Organization[9] and the Dietary Reference Intake (DRI),[10] or they can be derived from an equation such as the Harris Benedict equation.[11] Factors are added for the stress of injury. Equations that estimate energy requirements for critically ill infants and children have been proposed;[12–15] however, Briassoulis and colleagues caution that a number of equations grossly overestimate energy expenditure.[16] Equations to calculate energy requirements for burned children also exist[17–22] (Table 29-1), but recent studies show that the energy demands of burned children are lower than previously estimated.[20–22] These observations and other reports suggest that during stress, a shift in energy expenditure from growth to functions associated with the acute illness occurs.[22–24] Energy needed for activity is decreased in acutely injured individuals.

Indirect calorimetry is an option for spontaneously breathing patients who weigh 4 kg or more. Indirect calorimetry in stable, ventilator-dependent children, primarily less than 3 years of age, is limited because uncuffed endotracheal tubes are often used. Recent data, however, shows that cuffed endotracheal tubes can be used with no increased risk of postextubation stridor or significant long term sequelae.[25] Thus, Joosten et al. recommend the use of cuffed endotracheal tubes in small children. They also show that indirect calorimetry with uncuffed endotracheal tubes can be successfully achieved if the difference in inspiratory and expiratory tidal volume measurements is less than 10%.[26] Older children tolerate cuffed endotracheal tubes, and accurate indirect calorimetry measurements can be achieved. The figure for resting energy expenditure (REE) measured by indirect calorimetry is modified by a multiplication factor that accounts for environmental factors. Environmental factors include repositioning, suctioning, pain, anxiety, physical therapy, and dressing changes.

Table 29-1 Formulas for calculating energy requirements of pediatric burned patients.

Reference	*Age (yr)*	*% BSAB*	*Calories per day*
Curreri[17]	0–1	< 50	Basal + (15 × % BSAB)
	1–3	< 50	Basal + (25 × % BSAB)
	4–15	< 50	Basal + (40 × % BSAB)
Davies and Lilijedahl[18]	Child	Any	60 W + (35 × % BSAB)
Hildreth[19–21]	< 15	> 30	(1,800/m² BSA) + (2,200/m² BSAB)
	< 12		(1,800/m² BSA) + (1,300/m² BSAB)
Mayes[22]	< 3	10–50	108 + 68 W + (3.9 × % BSAB)
	5–10	10–50	818 + 37.4 W + (9.3 × % BSAB)

W = weight in kilograms BSA= body surface area BSAB = body surface area burned

The estimation of appropriate calories is a dynamic process that changes with the status of the patient. For example, surgical procedures, sepsis, organ failure, and even wound closure are associated with transient variations in metabolic demand. Therefore, it is imperative that patient assessment is an ongoing process and that energy needs are adjusted as necessary.

PROTEIN

Protein requirements of critically ill children depend on the type of illness or injury and the preexisting protein state. Whether a child is malnourished and requires repletion or not must be determined during the initial and ongoing assessment. For most injured or ill children, the protein requirement is based on the DRI, to which stress factors are added. For sick or injured children, assuming energy needs are met and positive nitrogen balance is achieved, the nonprotein calorie to nitrogen ratio is 150:1 to 200:1[27] or 2.8 grams protein per kg.[28] In contrast, studies in burned patients show that the provision of 20–23% of calories as protein decreases infection and improves survival.[29] This level of protein is about 2.5–4.0 grams per kg or a nonprotein calorie to nitrogen ratio of 80:1. This amount of protein supports resistance to infection, replenishes preexisting or injury-driven depletion, maintains muscle mass, and in the case of burn or other wound type, supports replacement of exudative losses to permit healing.

When a high protein diet is prescribed, close monitoring is essential to avoid amino acid imbalance, azotemia, hyperammonemia, or metabolic acidosis. High protein diets have historically been avoided in children less than 1 year of age. However, if fluid intake is not restricted, renal and hepatic function are not compromised, and if metabolic pathways are sufficiently mature, a diet with 4f g protein per kg body weight per day is tolerated by infants 6 months or older.[30]

An ongoing study at the Shriners Hospital for Children in Cincinnati, Ohio, supports the safe provision of this level of protein in children with burns in excess of 30% total body surface area. Whether high protein intakes are beneficial in burned children less than 3 years of age is not known, but preliminary evidence suggests high protein intakes are associated with improved outcomes.

ROUTE OF NUTRIENT DELIVERY

The anticipated duration of feeding, aspiration risk, and function of the gastrointestinal tract determine the route of feeding. Enteral nutrition (EN) support is recognized as the preferred method of nutrient delivery for patients with an intact gastrointestinal system.[31–43] The enteral route offers immune advantages over the parenteral route. Intestinal blood flow is increased, gastrointestinal function preserved, mucosal atrophy lessened, and bacterial translocation and postoperative sepsis are reduced.[34,35,37,39,44–54] EN is less expensive than intravenous feeds, and risks associated with parenteral nutrition (PN) such as pneumothorax, bleeding, infection, air embolism, pulmonary or hepatic dysfunction, and decreased utilization of nutrients are not issues with EN. Chapter 20 discusses the advantages and disadvantages of various enteral feeding routes.

Concurrent use of enteral feeds and inotrope agents might be associated with bowel necrosis;[55–60] other evidence suggests that enteral feeding is protective against necrosis.[61–65] Until the relationship between inotropic agents and enteral feedings is better understood, it might be prudent to provide minimal gastrointestinal stimulation during vasopressor therapy.[65] Peripheral PN, where the dextrose concentration is limited to 10–12.5%, is a feeding option for well nourished patients who require supplemental nutrition for a period of less than 2 weeks.[31] Peripheral PN cannot meet the high calorie requirements of critically ill or injured children and so in this setting its use is limited.[66]

FORMULA SELECTION

Enteral Support

The choice of enteral formula depends on the age of the patient, the condition of the gastrointestinal tract, and the disease state. Ideally, nutrition intervention should prevent loss of lean body mass, support immunocompetence, maximize organ function, and facilitate wound healing. Special formulas are considered whenever fluid and electrolyte restriction, organ failure, septicemia, burns, or other presenting conditions alter specific nutrient requirements.

Term infants less than 6 months of age should be fed human milk with human milk fortifiers added as needed. When infants are not breastfed, an infant formula is appropriate. Additional carbohydrate, protein, or vitamins and minerals can be added as needed.

Enteral formulas for children are designed to meet the DRI for healthy children, not critically ill or injured children. Enteral products that might augment immunity, promote wound healing, prevent and reverse respiratory failure, and enhance weight gain are available for adults. In many instances, with appropriate clinical monitoring, these products may be safely used in children.

The type and content of fat in the formula is important because fats affect immune function.[67–71] Omega-6 fatty acids, most notably, linoleic acid, have a negative impact on immunocompetence[71–74] and facilitate proteolysis.[70,75,76] Omega-3 fatty acids are precursors of biologic metabolites that are anti-inflammatory, immune enhancing, and vasodilating agents.[77–87] In addition, omega-3 fatty acids have competitive and inhibitory effects on the conversion of linoleic acid to its immune compromising metabolites, 1 and 2 series prostaglandins.[88–93] Formulas supplemented with omega-3 fatty acids have superior immune effects over the standard omega-6 fatty acid containing formulas.[67,71,72] Several omega-3 fatty acid supplemented formulas are available; however, none are made specifically for infants and children, and none provide the lower fat ratio required by burn patients.

The optimal enteral product for burned patients is not available, but many formulas approximate the composition recommended by the latest research. One study[94] found that formula osmolality, drugs used to prevent stress ulcers, and hypoalbuminemia did not have an adverse effect on intestinal nutrient absorption. It might be prudent to limit the high linoleic acid (omega-6 fatty acids) in the diet of critically ill patients because low fat, omega-3 fatty acid supplemented diets seem to be beneficial for burned patients.[67]

Parenteral Support

PN support might become necessary for patients with abdominal trauma, persistent intestinal ileus, severe diarrhea, superior mesenteric artery syndrome, and other conditions that interfere with digestion and absorption or when sufficient calories and protein cannot be delivered enterally. When PN is used, simultaneous provision of trophic enteral feeds whenever feasible is recommended to promote gut function and maintain the mucosal barrier. As the rate of enteral feeding is increased, the rate of PN is decreased.

Daily intravenous fat is immunosuppressive, and its administration is discouraged in burned patients. If the amount of fat in the trophic enteral feed provides 1–2% of the calorie requirement as linoleic acid and 1–2% of calories are derived from a marine source or α-linolenate, then intravenous fat is not necessary. If PN is the sole nutrient source, then a fat emulsion bolus should be given 3 times a week to meet the essential fatty acid requirements.

This conservative approach to the provision of intravenous fat in critically ill patients is a source of disagreement among caregivers because some studies show fat is the preferred substrate in the critically ill.[28,95–98] Many studies show that excessive energy in the form of carbohydrate drives the respiratory quotient (RQ) to a value in excess of 1.0, indicative of net fat synthesis. At least 1 study included subjects in negative nitrogen balance.[28] It is possible that the RQ was greater than 1.0 because insufficient protein was provided; i.e., the substrate was not sufficiently mixed to meet requirements. Studies are needed to discern whether high carbohydrate intake combined with increased protein and decreased fat consumption sufficiently modifies substrate to lower RQ. Parenteral lipid emulsions are associated with physiologic derangements such as decreased pulmonary diffusion, decreased peripheral oxygenation, altered leukocyte function, hyperphospholipidemia, hypercholesterolemia, and changes in prostaglandin metabolism.[99–101] In addition, high fat diets, enteral or parenteral, result in decreased cell-mediated immunity.[102–112] Furthermore, Hart et al. suggest that carbohydrate is more effective than fat at improving skeletal muscle protein balance because carbohydrate reduces muscle catabolism in association with higher insulin levels.[113] Despite these conflicting observations, 0.5 g lipid emulsion/kg/d is generally given intravenously.

EARLY FEEDING

Some authors apply the term early to a feeding time within a few hours of surgery or injury, while for others, early means initiation of feeds within days of surgery or injury. The term early feeding can refer to PN, EN, or a combination of both.

Early PN is used for patients with compromised gastrointestinal function. Combination enteral and parenteral feeds are provided to patients whose gastrointestinal tracts cannot tolerate the necessary volume of feeds. In most instances, early EN without PN is safe, well tolerated, and less costly. Even when gastroparesis is present postburn or with head trauma, the small bowel is intact, functional, and serves as a viable option for nutrient delivery via the naso-duodenal or naso-jejunal route.

A correlation might exist between early EN and a reduction of hypermetabolism postinjury.[48,102–108,112–121] Reduced catabolic hormones, decreased weight loss, improved nitrogen retention, enhanced wound healing, and shorter hospital stays are associated with early feeding. Early, aggressive EN has risks. Empirical evidence suggests an association between early feeding and hypotension, splanchic hypoperfusion, and intestinal necrosis.[122–130]

Postpyloric tube feeding is ideal in the critically ill because it allows for early initiation of nutrition support, within hours of injury or surgery. Once the feeding is started, it is not necessary to decrease the rate or withhold feedings for therapies such as dressing changes, rehabilitative therapy, surgery, intravenous line changes, and supine or prone positioning. Transpyloric EN should be given a high priority in the care of these patients.

Burned patients who received adequate fluids during resuscitation safely tolerate postpyloric feeding initiation and advancement within hours of injury. Patients with inadequate fluid resuscitation could be at increased risk for intestinal necrosis. Therefore, under-resuscitated patients are provided trophic enteral feels until the resuscitation period is completed.

The early provision of fluids is crucial for survival after burns. Inappropriate or miscalculated fluid resuscitation can result in death. One of the most frequently used pediatric fluid replacement calculations is the modified Parkland formula[131]

Table 29-2 Pediatric fluid calculations for resuscitation and maintenance postburn.

Modified Parkland Formula	
Total resuscitation fluids = (mL/24 hr)	[4 mL × % burn × weight (kg)] + [basal fluid requirements (1,500 × m^2)]
	½ of calculated fluid volume given in the first 8 hours
	½ of calculated fluid volume given in the next 16 hours
Maintenance Fluid Calculation	
Total maintenance fluids = (mL/hr)	Basal fluids + evaporative losses
=	$\frac{1500 \text{ mL} \times m^2 + (35 + \% \text{ burn}) \times m^2}{24 \text{ hr}}$

Source: Warden GD. Burn shock resuscitation. *World J Surg.* 1992;16:16–23.

(Table 29-2). This formula should serve only as a guide and should not replace the evaluation of vital signs, blood pressure, and urinary output. During resuscitation and throughout the acute postburn phase, children must be given enough fluid to maintain urine output at 1 to 2 mL/kg/hour. The goal for urine output for older children, roughly greater than 15 years of age, is 30 to 50 mL/hour.

Perioperative Feeding

The objective of perioperative feeding is to maintain or replete nutrition stores at the time of operation in an effort to minimize malnutrition related complications. Studies supporting the use of perioperative nutrition are reported in adult patients; consequently, a similar approach to nutrition support is used in pediatrics. Enteral provision of nutrients is preferred in the perioperative feeding period. PN is reserved for patients who have compromised gastrointestinal function.

Preoperative Feeding

Preoperative nutrition support is reserved for surgery patients whose condition is weakened by a malnourished state or for those whose surgical procedure must be delayed and in whom malnutrition develops. Nutrition support repletes and maintains nutrition stores. PN should be used only for severely malnourished patients for at least 1 week before surgery.[132,133] EN should be used for at least 10 days prior to surgery.[134]

Intraoperative Feeding

Intraoperative enteral feeding is a concept that might alarm some caregivers; however, this concept deserves attention. Successful intraoperative enteral feeding is possible in pediatric burn patients and contributes to a reduction in morbidity.[135] Strict safety guidelines, including diligent monitoring of duodenal tube placement and rigorous attention to nasogastric output in the operating room, are necessary.

Often tube feeds are stopped for unnecessarily long periods of time. Sometimes feedings are withheld for 12 or more hours before surgery. This practice compromises nutritional status and possibly the immune response at a time when efforts to replete and maintain nutritional stores are critical. For this reason, an interdisciplinary effort is needed to implement a protocol that reduces the amount of time feeds are withheld. An example protocol could include withholding duodenal tube feeds 2 hours before the scheduled surgery time. Feeds would then be resumed as a priority in the immediate postoperative period. Ongoing education of physicians and nurses as to the relevance of this feeding practice in reducing morbidity is essential to its success.

Postoperative Feeding

Depending on the age of the child (the younger child has lower reserves), if the period of absent or decreased nutrition support is expected to extend for more than 3–5 days after surgery, then early postoperative nutrition support could be beneficial. Postoperative nutrition support is necessary for all severely malnourished children.

VENTILATED POPULATION

Critically ill patients who require prolonged ventilator support are at nutritional risk because they cannot eat. Patients who require more than 3 to 5 days of ventilator support should be considered for supplemental nutrition support. If mechanical dependency is expected to be long term, feeding should begin immediately. If the gut is viable, it should be used. Tube placement beyond the ligament of Treitz is standard to avoid aspiration. Overfeeding calories increases CO_2 retention and the work of breathing and prolongs ventilator dependency (see Chapter 6 for a discussion of overfeeding). For this reason, indirect calorimetry, with appropriate interpretation of respiratory quotient, should be performed at regular intervals.

Orally intubated infants and toddlers undergo multiple, repeated, traumatic oral/facial experiences such as suctioning, application of tape to the face, repeated intubations, etc. Oral intubation deprives infants of the pleasure of food, soothing hand-to-mouth behaviors, and pacifiers. Furthermore, in thermally injured infants and children, burned areas of the face are painfully cleansed multiple times each day. After they are extubated, these experiences can cause the child to react negatively to food. The infant might cry, grimace, clamp its mouth shut, or refuse to suck. This is learned defensive behavior caused by negative oral/facial experiences. Patients presenting with these symptoms should be referred to an occupational therapist and speech pathologist to coordinate a care plan. To prevent oral aversion, critically ill infants should be nasally intubated. Patients who need long term mechanical ventilation should have a tracheosotomy tube placed. Nasoendotracheal and tracheostomy tube placements permit positive oral stimulation that offsets the negative stimulus of medical treatments. A pacifier, lollipop licks, oral discovery of hands, playing with age appropriate toys, or biting a teething ring can serve as positive stimuli. Infants who exhibit signs of opposition to feeds should not be forced to consume food via syringe or other means. This simply worsens the aversion.

OBSTACLES PREVENTING ADEQUATE NUTRITION

Complications related to EN such as ileus, diarrhea, constipation, abdominal distention, and regurgitation most often cause providers to reduce or stop enteral feeds. If the gastrointestinal problem prevents delivery of adequate nutrition for a period greater than 3–5 days, PN should be instituted.

Fluid restriction and the need for frequent procedures and diagnostic tests that require a fasted state are the most common barriers to delivery of adequate nutrition in critically ill children.[136] For fluid restricted patients, concentrating of enteral feeds can be beneficial. Strict monitoring of gastrointestinal and metabolic tolerance is necessary. Ongoing reevaluation of energy needs is vital. Because calorie goals are often overestimated by energy equations a patient may already be receiving nutrition that approximates their caloric requirements. After a period of fasting, the tube feeding rate can be temporarily increased as tolerated so the estimated 24-hour volume is delivered.

NUTRITIONAL ASSESSMENT

Assessment of the critically ill child is an integral component of the nutrition care plan. Thorough guidelines of assessment of pediatric patients receiving supplemental nuttrition are listed in Table 29-3. The initial evaluation should occur within 24 hours of admission. Patient acuity determines the frequency of further nutritional evaluations.

Nitrogen balance is used to verify the adequacy of protein intake. The standard equation accounts for nonurinary insensible losses. The factor for insensible losses is age dependent in children[137] (Table 29-4). Chapters 7 and 24 discuss nitrogen balance. Experience at the burn center of the Shriners Hospital for Children in Cincinnati, Ohio, shows that a nutritional regimen that maintains nitrogen balance (using the standard equation adjusted for age) at + 2 to + 3 in children less than 5 years of age and between + 5 and + 10 in older children is sufficient for wound healing.

Daily calculation of nitrogen balance is encouraged in burned children with a weekly review of the trend. This practice is applicable to other critical illnesses as well; however, lower nitrogen balance values are acceptable for the general critical care population given that there are no additional nitrogen losses via open wound.

CONCLUSION

Critical illness elicits pathophysiologic aberrations that have an impact on nutritional status. Appropriate nutrition support prevents malnutrition and positively affects outcomes. The type of injury determines which nutrients are needed and in what quantities. In general, the provision of a high calorie, high protein, low fat, low omega-6 fatty acid diet is desirable. Early and continuous feeding promotes optimal conditions for wound

Table 29-3 Nutrition Assessment Guidelines for Pediatric Parenteral and Enteral Nutrition

Initial	*Daily*	*Weekly*
COLLECT INFORMATION		
Demographics	Calorie and Protein Intake	Weight (daily for some populations)
• Age		
• Percent TBSA burned	Fluid Intake Output	
• Percent full thickness burn		
• Inhalation injury	Labs:	Visceral Protein Labs
	• BUN/creatinine	
Ventilatory Status	• Glucose	
• FIO_2	• Electrolytes	Nitrogen Balance Trend
• Cuffed vs uncuffed ETT	• Nitrogen balance	
	• Urine specific gravity, glucose/acetone	
Gastric Decompression (Y/N)		Triglycerides (biweekly PN only)
	• Complete blood cell count	
Anthropometrics	Tolerance:	
• Weight for age (correct for prematurity at least 1 year)	• Intra-abdominal pressure	
	• Abdominal girth	Bile Acids (PN only)
• Height for age (length for infants)	• Nausea	
	• Vomiting	
• Weight for height	• Distention	Liver Function
• Head circumference (< 3 years)	• Stool frequency and consistency	
		Minerals (Ca, P, Mg–daily for burns)
OBTAIN APPROPRIATE HISTORIES	• Gastric residuals	
Past Medical History	• Clinical course	
Social History	• Sepsis	
Concomitant Injuries	• Infection	Vitamins, Trace Elements (as needed)
Routine Medications	• Surgeries	
Referring Hospital Course (as applicable)	• Fluid status	
	• Medications	
	• Respiratory status	Wound Healing (% open wound, as applicable)
CALCULATE		
Calorie and Protein Needs	Appropriateness of diet/enteral or PN order	
Growth Percentiles (NCHS statistics)		
		Indirect Calorimetry:
DETERMINE FEEDING ROUTE		
Oral		• REE
Orogastric		• RQ
Nasoenteral		
Parenteral		
INITIATE ASSESSMENT TOOLS		
Indirect Calorimetry		
24-Hr. Urinary Urea Nitrogen (daily)		
Obtain Baseline Visceral Protein Labs		
Initiate Calorie/Protein Intake Monitoring		

TBSA, total body surface area; ETT, endotracheal tube; PN, parenteral nutrition; REE, resting energy expenditure; RQ, respiratory quotient

Table 29-4 Calculation of nitrogen balance.

Nitrogen balance	=	Nitrogen intake – Nitrogen output
Nitrogen intake	=	grams of protein in ÷ 6.25
Nitrogen output	=	UUN + 2 (for children 0–4 years old)
		UUN + 3 (for children > 4–10 years old)
		UUN + 4 (for children > 10 years old)

UUN = urine urea nitrogen

Source: O'Neil CE, Hustler D, Hildreth MA. Basic nutritional guidelines for pediatric burn patients. *J Burn Care Rehabil.* 1989;10:278–284.

healing and immune competence. The requirements for normal growth and development of children in addition to that imposed by the injury present a challenge for the clinician. This challenge is fueled by the lack of a diet therapy research base for children.

REFERENCES

1. Cuthbertson D, Tilstone WJ. Metabolism during the postinjury period. *Adv Clin Chem.* 1969;12:1–55.
2. Wilmore DW. Nutrition and metabolism following thermal injury. *Clin Plast Surg.* 1974;1:603–619.
3. Clowes GHA. Metabolic responses to injury. Part I. The production of energy. *J Trauma.* 1963;3:149–195.
4. Bessey PQ, Walters JM, Aoki TT, Wilmore DW. Combined hormonal infusion simulates the metabolic response to injury. *Ann Surg.* 1984;200:264–281.
5. Matthews DE, Pesola G, Campbell G. Effect of epinephrine upon amino acid and energy metabolism in humans. *Am J Physiol.* 1990;258:E948–E956.
6. Stalen MF, Matthews DE, Cryer PE, Bier PM. Physiologic increments in epinephrine stimulate metabolic rate in humans. *Am J Physiol.* 1987;253:E322–E330.
7. Wilmore DW, Long JM, Mason AD, Skreen RW, Pruitt BA. Catecholamines: mediator of the hypermetabolic response to thermal injury. *Ann Surg.* 1974;180:653–669.
8. Gottschlich MM, Jenkins ME, Mayes T, et al. A prospective clinical study of the polysomnographic stages of sleep following burn injury. *J Burn Care Rehabil.* 1994;15:486–492.
9. World Health Organization. *Energy and Protein Requirements. Report of a Joint FAO/WHO/UNU Expert Consultation.* Technical Report Series 724. Geneva, Switzerland: WHO; 1985:206.
10. Institute of Medicine. *Dietary Reference Intakes,* Washington, DC: National Academy Press; 2002.
11. Harris JA, Benedict FS. *Biometric Studies of Basal Metabolism in Man.* Washington, DC: Carnegie Institute of Washington; 1919. Publication 279.
12. White MS, Shepherd RW, McEniery JA. Energy expenditure in 100 ventilated, critically ill children: improving the accuracy of predictive equations. *Crit Care Med.* 2000;28:2307–2312.
13. Talbot FB. Basal metabolism standards for children. *Am J Dis Child.* 1938;55:455–459.
14. Schofield WN. Predicting basal metabolic rate, new standards and review of previous work. *Hum Nutr Clin Nutr.* 1985;39(suppl 1):5–41.
15. Swinamer DL, Phang PT, Jones RL, Grace M, King EG. Twenty-four hour energy expenditure in critically ill patients. *Crit Care Med.* 1987;15:637–643.
16. Briassoulis G, Venkataraman S, Thompson AE. Energy expenditure in critically ill children. *Crit Care Med.* 2000;28:1166–1172.
17. Day T, Dean P, Adams MC, Luterman A, Ramenofsky ML, Curreri PW. Nutritional requirements of the burned child: the Curreri junior formula. *Proc Am Burn Assoc.* 1986;18:86. Abstract.
18. Davies JWL, Lilijedahl SL. Metabolic consequences of an extensive burn. In: Polk HC, Stone HH, eds. *Contemporary Burn Management.* Boston, Mass: Little, Brown & Co; 1971:151–169.
19. Hildreth MA, Herndon DN, Parks DH, Desai MH, Rutan T. Evaluation of a caloric requirement formula in burned children treated with early excision. *Trauma.* 1987;27:188–189.
20. Hildreth MA, Herndon DN, Desai MH, Duke MA. Reassessing caloric requirements in pediatric burn patients. *J Burn Care Rehabil.* 1988;9:616–618.
21. Hildreth MA, Herndon DN, Desai MH, Broemeling LD. Current treatment reduces calories required to

maintain weight in pediatric patients with burns. *J Burn Care Rehabil.* 1990;11:405–409.

22. Mayes T, Gottschlich MM, Khoury J, Warden GD. Evaluation of predicted and measured energy requirements in burned children. *JADA.* 1996;96:24–29.
23. Ford E. Nutrition support of pediatric patients. *NCP.* 1996;11:183–191.
24. Turi RA, Petros AJ, Eaton S, et al. Energy metabolism of infants and children with systemic inflammatory response syndrome and sepsis. *Ann Surg.* 2001;233:581–587.
25. Deakers TW, Reynolds G, Stretton M, Newth CJ. Cuffed endotracheal tubes in pediatric intensive care. *J Pediatr.* 1994;125:57–62.
26. Joosten KF. Verhoeven JJ. Hop WC. Hazelzet JA Hazelzet JA. Indirect calorimetry in mechanically ventilated infants and children: accuracy of total daily energy expenditure with 2 hour measurements. *Clin Nutr.* 1999;18:149–152.
27. Hovasi-Cox J, Cooning SW. Parenteral nutrition. In: Queen P, Lang C, eds. *Handbook of Pediatric Nutrition.* Gaithersburg, Md: ASPEN Publishers; 1993:279–314.
28. Coss-Bu JA, Klish WJ, Walding D, Stein F, Smith O, Jefferson LS. Energy metabolism, nitrogen balance, and substrate utilization in critically ill children. *Am J Clin Nutr.* 2001;74:664–669.
29. Alexander JW, MacMillen BG, Stinnett JD, et al. Beneficial effects of aggressive protein feeding in severely burned children. *Ann Surg.* 1980;192:505–517.
30. Gottschlich MM. Nutrition in the burned pediatric patient. In: Samour PQ, Helm KK, Lang CF, eds. *Handbook of Pediatric Nutrition.* 2nd ed. Sudbury, MA: Jones and Bartlett;1999:495–511.
31. ASPEN Board of Directors. Guidelines for the use of parenteral and enteral nutrition in adult and pediatric patients. *JPEN.* 1993;17:55A–95A.
32. American Burn Association. Practice guidelines for burn care. *J Burn Care Rehabil.* 2001;22:59S–66S.
33. ASPEN Board of Directors. American Society for Parenteral and Enteral Nutrition. Standards for hospitalized pediatric patients *Nutr Clin Pract.* 1996;11:217–28.
34. Kudsk KA, Croce MA, Fabian TC, et al. Enteral versus parenteral feeding: Effects on septic morbidity after blunt and penetrating abdominal trauma. *Ann Surg.* 1992;215:503–513.
35. Moore FA, Moore EE, Jones TN, McCroskey BL, Peterson VM. TEN vs TPN following major abdominal trauma—reduced septic morbidity. *J Trauma.* 1989;29:916–923.
36. Bower RH, Talamini MA, Sax HC, Hamilton F, Fischer JE. Postoperative enteral vs. parenteral nutrition: a randomized controlled trial. *Arch Surg.* 1986;121:1040–1045.
37. Moore FA, Feliciano DV, Andrassy RJ, et al. Early enteral feeding, compared with parenteral, reduces postoperative septic complications. The results of a meta-analysis. *Ann Surg.* 1992;216:172–183.
38. Kudsk KA. Gut mucosal nutritional support—enteral nutrition as primary therapy after multiple system trauma. *Gut.* 1994;35:S52–S54.
39. Herndon DN, Barrow RE, Stein M, et al. Increased mortality with intravenous supplemental feeding in severely burned patients. *J Burn Care Rehabil.* 1989;10:309–313.
40. Suchner V, Senftleben U, Eckart T, et al. Enteral versus parenteral nutrition: effects on gastrointestinal function and metabolism. *Nutrition.* 1996;12:13–22.
41. Kudsk KA, Minard G, Wojtysiak SL, Croce M, Fabian T, Brown RO. Visceral protein response to enteral versus parenteral nutrition and sepsis in patients with trauma. *Surgery.* 1994;116:516–523.
42. Peterson VM, Moore EE, Jones TN, et al. Total enteral nutrition vs. total parenteral nutrition after major torso injury: attenuation of hepatic protein reprioritization. *Surgery.* 1988;104:199–207.
43. Moore EE, Jones TN. Benefits of immediate jejunostomy feeding after major abdominal trauma: a prospective, randomized trial. *J Trauma.* 1986;26:874–881.
44. Suchner V, Senftleben U, Eckart T, et al. Enteral versus parenteral nutrition: effects on gastrointestinal function and metabolism. *Nutrition.* 1996;12:13–22.
45. Alverdy JC, Chi HS, Sheldon G. The effect of parenteral nutrition on gastrointestinal immunity: the importance of enteral stimulation. *Ann Surg.* 1985;202:681–684.
46. Levine GM, Deren JJ, Steiger E, et al. Role of oral intake in maintenance of gut mass and disaccharide activity. *Gastroenterology.* 1994;67:975–982.
47. Kotani J, Usami M, Nomura H, et al. Enteral nutrition prevents bacterial translocation but does not improve survival during acute pancreatitis. *Arch Surg.* 1999;134:287–292.
48. Gianotti O, Nelson JL, Alexander JW, Chalk CL, Pyles T. Post injury hypermetabolic response and magnitude of translocation: prevention by early enteral nutrition. *Nutrition.* 1994;3:225–231.
49. Braga M, Gianotti L, Constantini E, et al. Impact of enteral nutrition of intestinal bacterial translocation and mortality in burned mice. *Clin Nutr.* 1994;13:256–261.
50. Inoue S, Epstein MD, Alexander JW, Trocki O, Jacobs P, Gura P. Prevention of yeast translocation across the gut by a single enteral feeding after burn injury. *JPEN.* 1989;13:565–571.
51. Alverdy JC, Aoys E, Moss GS. Total parenteral nutrition promotes bacterial translocation from the gut. *Surgery.* 1988;104:185–190.

52. Lowry SF. The route of feeding influences injury responses. *J Trauma.* 1990;30:S10–S15.
53. Waters B, Kudsk KA, Jarvi EJ, Brown RO, Fabian TC, Wood GC. Effect of route of nutrition on recovery of hepatic organic anion clearance after fasting. *Surgery.* 1994;115:370–374.
54. Braga M, Gianotti L, Gentilini O, Parisi V, Salis C, DiCarlo V. Early postoperative enteral nutrition improves gut oxygenation and reduces costs compared with total parenteral nutrition. *Crit Care Med.* 2001;29:242–248.
55. Scaife CL, Saffle JR, Morris SE. Intestinal obstruction secondary to enteral feedings in burn trauma patients. *J Trauma.* 1999;47:859–863.
56. Munshi IA, Steingrub JS, Wolpert I. Small bowel necrosis associated with early postoperative jejunal tube feeding in a trauma patient. *J Trauma.* 2000;49:163–165.
57. Riegel T, Allgeier C, Gottschlich M, Warden G, Kagan R. Fluid resuscitation, inotropic agents, and early feeding: is there a relation to bowel necrosis? *J Burn Care Rehabil.* 2003;25:S61.
58. Lawlor DK, Inculet RI, Malthaner RA. Small bowel necrosis associated with jejunal tube feeding. *Can J Surg.* 1998;41:459–462.
59. Myers JG, Page CP, Steward RM, Schwesinger WH, Sirinek KR, Aust JB. Complications of needle catheter jejunostomy in 2,022 consecutive applications. *Am J Surg.* 1995;170:547–550.
60. Wilson MD, Dziewulski P. Severe gastrointestinal haemorrhage and ischemic necrosis of the small bowel in a child with 70% full-thickness burns: a case report. *Burns.* 2001;27:763–766.
61. Inoue S, Lukes S, Alexander JW, Trocki O, Silberstein EB. Increased gut blood flow with early enteral feeding in burned guinea pigs. *J Burn Care Rehabil.* 1989;10:300–308.
62. Roberts PR, Black KW, Zaloga GP. Enteral nutrition blunts decrease in mesenteric blood flow (MBS) during high dose phenylephrine administration. *Crit Care Med.* 1999;27:135S.
63. Gosche JR, Garrison RN, Harris PD, Cryer HG. Absorptive hyperemia restores intestinal blood flow during *Escherichia coli* sepsis in the rat. *Arch Surg.* 1990;125:1573–1576.
64. Purcell PN, Davis K, Branson RD, et al. Continuous duodenal feeding restores gut blood flow and increases gut oxygen utilization during PEEP ventilation for lung injury. *Am J Surg.* 1993;165:188–194.
65. Gottschlich MM, Jenkins ME, Mayes T, Khoury J, Kagan RJ, Warden GD. An evaluation of the safety of early vs delayed enteral support and effects on clinical nutritional and endocrine outcomes after severe burns. *J Burn Care Rehabil.* 2002;23:401–415.
66. Klotz KA, Wessel J, Hennies G. Goals of pediatric nutrition support and nutrition assessment. In: Merritt JF, ed. *A.S.P.E.N. Nutrition Support Practice Manual.* Gaithersberg, MD: ASPEN Publishers;1998:1–14.
67. Gottschlich MM, Jenkins M, Warden GD, et al. Differential effects of three enteral dietary regimens on selected outcome variables in burn patients. *JPEN.* 1990;14(3):225–226.
68. Beisel WR, Edelman R, Nauss K, Suskind R. Single-nutrient effects on immunologic functions. *JAMA.* 1981;245(1):53–58.
69. Fiser RH, Rollins JB, Beisel WR. Decreased resistance against infectious canine hepatitis in dogs fed high-fat ration. *Am J Vet Res.* 1972;33(4):713–719.
70. Mochizuki H, Trocki O, Dominioni L, Alexander JW. Optimal lipid content for enteral diets following thermal injury. *JPEN.* 1984;8(6):638–646.
71. Alexander JW, Saito H, Trocki O, Ogle CK. The importance of lipid type in the diet after burn injury. *Ann Surg.* 1986;204(1):1–8.
72. Trocki O, Heyd TJ, Waymack JP, Alexander JW. Effects of fish oil on postburn metabolism and immunity. *JPEN.* 1987;11(6):521–528.
73. Arturson MG. Arachidonic acid metabolism and prostaglandin activity following burn injury. In: Ninnermann J, ed. *Traumatic injury: infection and other immunologic sequelae.* Baltimore, Md: University Press; 1983:57–78.
74. Eliner JJ. Suppressor cells of man. *Clin Imunol Rev.* 1981;1(1):119–123.
75. Baracos V, Rodemann HP, Dinarello CA, Goldberg AL. Stimulation of muscle protein degradation and prostaglandin E_2 release by leukocyte pyrogen (interleukin 1): a mechanism for the increased degradation of muscle proteins during fever. *N Engl J Med.* 1983;308(10):553–558.
76. Rodeman HP, Goldberg AL. Arachidonic acid, prostaglandin E, and F, alpha influence rates of protein turnover in skeletal and cardiac muscle. *J Biol Chem.* 1982;257(4):1632–1638.
77. Foitzik T, Eibl G, Schneider P, Wenger FA, Jacobi CA, Buhr HJ. Omega-3 fatty acid supplementation increases anti-inflammatory cytokines and attenuates systemic disease sequelae in experimental pancreatitis. *JPEN.* 2002;26:351–356.
78. Grimm H, Mayer K, Mayer P, Eigenbrodt E. Regulatory potential of n-3 fatty acids in immunological and inflammatory processes. *Br J Nutr.* 2002;87(suppl 1): S59–S67.
79. Tashiro T, Yamamori H, Takagi K, et al. N-3 versus n-6 polyunsaturated fatty acids in critical illness. *Nutrition.* 1998;14:551–553.
80. Mascioli E, Leader L, Flores E, Trimbo S, Bistrian B, Blackburn G. Enhanced survival endotoxin in guinea

pigs fed IV fish oil emulsion. *Lipids.* 1988;23:623–625.

81. Koch T, Heller A, Breil I, et al. Alterations of pulmonary capillary filtration and leukotriene synthesis due to infusion of a lipid emulsion enriched with n-3 fatty acids. *Clin Intensive Care.* 1995;6:112–120.
82. Breil I, Koch T, Heller A, et al. Alteration of n-3 fatty acid composition in lung tissue after short-term infusion of fish oil emulsion attenuates inflammatory vascular reaction. *Crit Care Med.*1996;24:1893–1902.
83. Garcia-Garmendia JL, Garnaco-Montero J, Ortiz-Leyba C, et al. Cytokine levels in critically ill septic patients fed with an enteral diet supplemented with fish oil and vitamin E. *Clin Nutr.* 1998;17(suppl 1):6.
84. Endres S, Ghorbani R, Kelley VE, et al. The effect of dietary supplementation with n-3 polyunsaturated fatty acids on the synthesis of interleukin-1 and tumor necrosis factor by mononuclear cells. *N Engl J Med.* 1989;320:265–271.
85. Meydani SN, Lichtenstein AH, Cornwall S, et al. Immunologic effects of National Cholesterol Education Panel Step-2b diets with and without fish-derived n-3 fatty acid enrichment. *J Clin Invest.* 1993;92:105–113.
86. Calder PC. N-3 polyunsaturated fatty acids and cytokine production in health and disease. *Ann Nutr Metab.* 1997;41:203–234.
87. Calder PC. Dietary fatty acids and lymphocyte functions. *Proc Nutr Soc.* 1998;57:487–502.
88. Steinberg G, Slayton WH, Howton DR, Mead JF. Metabolism of essential fatty acids. IV. Incorporation of lineolate into arachidonic acid. *J Biol Chem.* 1956;220(1):257–264.
89. Holman RT. Nutritional and metabolic interrelationships between fatty acids. *Proc FASEB.* 1964;23:1062–1067.
90. Holman RT. Essential fatty acid deficiency. *Prog Chem Fats Lipids.* 1970;9:275–348.
91. Hwang DH, Carroll AE. Decreased formation of prostaglandins derived from arachidonic acid by dietary linolenate in rats. *Am J Clin Nutr.* 1980;33(3):590–597.
92. Marshall LA, Szezesnwski A, Johnston PV. Dietary alpha-linolenic acid and prostaglandins synthesis: a time course study. *Am J Clin Nutr.* 1983;38(6):895–900.
93. Meng HC. Fat emulsions in parenteral nutrition. In: Fischer JE, ed. *Total Parenteral Nutrition.* Boston, Mass: Little, Brown; 1976:305–334.
94. Gottschlich MM, Warden GD, Michel MA, et al. Diarrhea in tube-fed burn patients: incidence, etiology, nutritional impact and prevention. *JPEN.* 1988;12:338–345.
95. Sheridan RL, Yu YM, Prelack K, Young VR, Burke JF, Tompkins RG. Maximal parenteral glucose oxidation in hypermetabolic young children: a stable isotope study. *JPEN.* 1998:22;212–216.
96. Tappy L, Schwarz JM, Schneiter P, et al. Effects of isoenergetic glucose-based or lipid-based parenteral nutrition on glucose metabolism, de novo lipogenesis, and respiratory gas exchanges in critically ill patients. *Crit Care Med.* 1998;26:860–867.
97. Askanazi J, Rosenbaum SH, Hyman AI, Silverberg PA, Eilic-Emili J, Kinney JM. Respiratory changes induced by the large glucose loads of total parenteral nutrition. *JAMA.* 1980;243:1444–1447.
98. Giovannini I, Boldrini G, Castagneto M, et al. Respiratory quotient and patterns of substrate utilization in human sepsis and trauma. *JPEN.* 1983;7:226–230.
99. Heird WC. Lipid metabolism in parenteral nutrition. In: Fomon SJed. *Energy and Protein Needs During Iinfancy* San Diego, Calif: Academic Press. 1986:215–229.
100. Periera GR, Fox WW, Stanley CA, Baker L, Schwartz JG. Decreased oxygenation and hyperlipemia during intravenous fat infusions in premature infants. *Pediatrics.* 1980;66:26–30.
101. Levene MI, Wigglesworth JS, Desai R. Pulmonary fat accumulation after Intralipid infusion in the preterm infant. *Lancet.* 1980;2:815–818.
102. Strunk RC, Kunke KS, Kolski GB, et al. Intralipid alters macrophage membrane fatty acid composition and inhibits complement (C2) synthesis. *Lipids.* 1983;18:493–500.
103. Fischer GW, Hunter KW, Wilson SR, et al. Diminished bacterial defenses with Intralipid. *Lancet.* 1980;2:819–820.
104. Sorbrado J, Moldawer LL, Pomposelli J, et al. Lipid emulsions and reticuloendothelial system function in healthy and burned guinea pigs. *Am J Clin Nutr.* 1985;42:855–863.
105. Hamawy KJ, Modawer LL, Georgieff M, et al. The effect of lipid emulsions on reticuloendothelial system function in the injured animal. *JPEN.* 1985;9:559–565.
106. Jarstrand C, Berghem L, Lahnborg G. Human granulocyte and reticuloendothelial system function during Intralipid infusion. *JPEN.* 1978;2:663–670.
107. Hessor I, Flemming M, Haug A. Postmortem findings in three patients treated with intravenous fat emulsions. *Arch Surg.* 1979;114:66–68.
108. Seidner DL, Mascioli EA, Istfan NW, et al. Effects of long-chain triglyceride emulsions on reticuloendothelial system function in humans. *JPEN.* 1989;13:614–619.
109. Robin AP, Arain I, Phuangsab A, Holian O, Roccaforte P, Barrett JA. Intravenous fat emulsion acutely suppresses neutrophil chemiluminescence. *JPEN.* 1989;13:608–613.

110. Kohelet D, Peller S, Arbel E, Goldberg M. Preincubation with intravenous lipid emulsion reduces chemotactic motility of neutrophils in cord blood. *JPEN.* 1990;14:472–473.

111. Salo M. Inhibition of immunoglobulin synthesis in vitro by intravenous lipid emulsion (Intralipid). *JPEN.* 1990;14:459–462.

112. McArdle AH, Palmason C, Brown RA, et al. Protection from catabolism in major burns: a new formula for the immediate enteral feeding of burn patients. *J Burn Care Rehabil.* 1983;4:245–250.

113. Hart DW, Wolf SE, Zhang X-J, et al. Efficacy of a high-carbohydrate diet in catabolic illness. *Crit Care Med.* 2001;29:1318–1324.

114. Jenkins M, Gottschlich M, Alexander JW, Warden GD. Effect of immediate enteral feeding on the hypermetabolic response following severe burn injury. *JPEN.* 1989;13:12S.

115. McArdle AH, Palmason C, Brown RA, Brown HC, Williams HB. Early enteral feeding of patients with major burns: prevention of catabolism. *Ann Plast Surg.* 1984;13:396–401.

116. Dominioni L, Trocki O, Mochizuki H, et al. Prevention of severe postburn hypermetabolism and catabolism by immediate intragastric feeding. *J Burn Care Rehabil.* 1984;5:106–112.

117. Mochizuki H, Trocki O, Dominioni L, Brackett KA, Jaffe SN, Alexander JW. Mechanism of prevention of postburn hypermetabolism and catabolism by early enteral feeding. *Ann Surg.* 1984;200:297–310.

118. Carr CS, Long KD, Boulos P, Singer M. Randomised trial of safety and efficacy of immediate postoperative enteral feeding in patients undergoing gastrointestinal resection. *BMJ.* 1996;312:869–871.

119. Jenkins M, Gottschlich MM, Alexander JW, Warden GD. Enteral alimentation in the early postburn phase. In: Blackburn GL, Bell SJ, Mullen JL, eds. *Nutrition medicine: A Case Management Approach.* Philadelphia, Pa: WB Saunders Co; 1989:1–5.

120. Mochizuki H, Trocki O, Dominioni L, Alexander JW. Reduction of postburn hypermetabolism by early enteral feeding. *Curr Surg.* 1985;42:121–125.

121. Sagar S, Harland P, Shields R. Early postoperative feeding with elemental diet. *BMJ.* 1979;1:293–295.

122. Munshi IA, Steingrub JS, Wolpert I. Small bowel necrosis associated with early postoperative jejunal tube feeding in a trauma patient. *J Trauma.* 2000;49:163–165.

123. Jorba R, Fabregat J, Borobia FG, Torras J, Poves I, Jaurrieta E. Small bowel necrosis in association with early postoperative enteral feeding after pancreatic resection. *Surgery.* 2000;128:111–112.

124. Gaddy MC, Max MH, Schwab CW, et al. Small bowel ischemia: a consequence of feeding jejunostomy? *So Med J.* 1986;79:180–182.

125. Maravin RG, McKinley BA, McQuiggan M, et al. Nonocclusive bowel necrosis occurring in critically ill trauma patients receiving enteral nutrition manifests no reliable clinical signs for early detection. *Am J Surg.* 2000;179:7–12.

126. Brenner DW, Schellhammer PF. Mortality associated with feeding catheter jejunostomy after radical cystectomy. *Urology.* 1987;30:337–340.

127. Lawlor DK, Inculet RI, Malthaner RA. Small bowel necrosis associated with jejunal tube feeding. *Can J Surg.* 1998;41:459–462.

128. Myers JG, Page CP, Stewart RM, et al. Complications of needle catheter jejunostomy in 2,022 consecutive applications. *Am J Surg.* 1995;170:547–550.

129. Brotman S, Marshall WJ. Complications from needle catheter jejunostomy in post traumatic surgery. *Contemp Surg.* 1985;27:52–56.

130. Desai MH, Herndon DN, Rutan RL, et al. Ischemic intestinal complications in patients with burns. *Surg Gynecol Obstet.* 1991;172:257–261.

131. Warden GD. Burn shock resuscitation. *World J Surg.* 1992;16:16–23.

132. Gottschlich MM. Early and perioperative nutrition support. In: Matarese L, Gottschlich MM, eds. *Contemporary Nutrition Support Practice.* Philadelphia, Pa: WB Saunders Co; 1998:265–278.

133. The Veterans Affairs Total Parenteral Nutrition Cooperative Study Group: Perioperative parenteral nutrition in surgical patients. *N Engl J Med.* 1991;325:525–532.

134. Shukla HS, Rao RR, Banu N, Gupta RM, Yadav RC. Enteral hyperalimentation in malnourished surgical patients. *Indian J Med Res.* 1984;80:339–346.

135. Jenkins ME, Gottschlich MM, Warden GD. Enteral feeding during operative procedures in thermal injuries. *J Burn Care Rehabil.* 1994;15:199–205.

136. Rogers EJ, Gilbertson HR, Heine RG, Henning R. Barriers to adequate nutrition in critically ill children. *Nutrition.* 2003;19:865–868.

137. O'Neil CE, Hustler D, Hildreth MA. Basic nutritional guidelines for pediatric burn patients. *J Burn Care Rehabil.* 1989;10:278–284.

CHAPTER 30

Nutrition Support of the Premature Infant

Frank R. Greer

INTRODUCTION

Although nutrition support of the low birth weight infant has made significant advances in the past 100 years,[1] basic principles have come full cycle. At the beginning of the 20th century, breast milk was the feeding of choice. Today, breast milk is again the feeding of choice. It was once common practice to begin feeding of premature infants very soon after birth. Then came a period of time when feeds were initially withheld. Now early feeding is again recommended. In the early 1900s, the energy requirement for premature infants was reported by a number of investigators to range from 95–160 kcal/kg/day.[2] Gordon and Levine restudied the energy issue in the 1930s and determined the daily energy requirement to be 120 kcal/kg/day. This intake supports an average weight gain of 16 g/kg/day.[3] Despite this, between 1940 and the late 1960s, it was common practice to withhold nutrition support for 24–48 hours in infants with a birth weight of less than 1200 g. After reports that delayed feeding resulted in long term neurological and developmental delays and that early feedings prevented severe weight loss and reduced the incidence of hypoglycemia, hypernatremia, and hyperbilirubinemia, early feeding of premature infants was gradually reintroduced.[4]

In 1922, in the first textbook dealing exclusively with the premature infant, Julius H. Hess advocated human milk as the feeding of choice for the premature infant. Artificial milk preparations were a poor substitute and were associated with an increased mortality rate. He advocated initiating the feeding of breast milk in the second 12 hours of life with the milk supplied by a wet nurse.[5] A preference for formula feeding of preterm infants began in the 1940s following the work of Gordon and colleagues.[6] These investigators reported that premature infants (birth weights 1,000 to 2,000 g) fed a diluted half skimmed cow's milk formula gained weight more rapidly than those fed breast milk. Differences were most significant for the 49 infants with birth weights between 1,000 and 1,700 g. It was concluded that the increased protein in the cow milk based feedings promoted the increased weight gain. This study led to the widespread use of formula feedings in the premature infant. In 1943, Benjamin et al. compared premature infants fed human milk to those fed a mixture of skimmed milk and olive oil, and demonstrated that human milk, even in the presence of added vitamin D, was inadequate for the formation of the skeleton of premature infants unless supplemented with calcium and phosphorus.[7]

Since the 1940s, the ideal extrauterine rate of growth has been a subject of controversy. In 1977, Heird and Anderson stated that it was not known whether the ideal rate of weight gain for premature infants *ex utero* was the same as the *in utero* rate of weight gain.[8] In the same year, in its first statement on the nutritional needs of low-birth-weight infants, the American Academy of Pediatrics concluded that "the optimal diet for the low-birth-weight (LBW) infant may be defined as one that supports a rate of growth approximating that of the third trimester of intrauterine life, without imposing stress on the developing metabolic or excretory systems."[9]

By the beginning of the 21st century, the intrauterine rate of growth in very-low-birth-weight (VLBW) infants was achieved prior to discharge largely as a result of the improved management of acute neonatal illnesses, the introduction of total parenteral nutrition (PN), and the gradual advancement of enteral feedings to minimize the risk of feeding related complications, such as necrotizing enterocolitis (NEC). However, 90% of VLBW infants are discharged at a weight less than the 10th percentile for their postmenstrual age.[10] The ideal rate of catch-up growth for VLBW infants has yet to be established. There is little data on what constitutes ideal nutrition support of the VLBW infant after hospital discharge. An immediate goal for neonatologists in the 21st century is to establish earlier and more aggressive nutrition support of the preterm infant in the neonatal intensive care unit (NICU) and thereby obviate the need for catch-up growth.

A 1997 randomized control trial demonstrated that early, aggressive, enteral and parenteral nutrition of sick VLBW infants improves growth without increasing the risk of clinical and metabolic sequelae.[11] This chapter focuses on the methods of optimizing overall nutrition support in the VLBW infant. Specific nutrient and energy requirements have been reviewed elsewhere by this author and others.[12–14]

PARENTERAL NUTRITION SUPPORT

For the VLBW infant (birth weight < 1,500g; see Table 30-1) or the extremely-low-birth-weight infant (ELBW), initial nutrition support is almost always in the parenteral form. Parenteral administration of glucose, fat, amino acids, vitamins, and trace elements can meet most of their nutritional needs for considerable periods of time. Often, there is a delay in starting PN solutions (48 hours or longer) because of the severity of illness in the infant, the need for frequent changes in the PN solution, and the

Table 30-1 Classification of babies based on birth weight and gestational age.

Birth weight (g) or gestational age (weeks)	*Classification*	*Abbreviation*
Birth weight < 1,000	Extremely-low-birth-weight	ELBW
Birth weight < 1,500	Very-low-birth-weight	VLBW
Birth weight < 2,500	Low-birth-weight	LBW
Gestational age < 38	Preterm	Premie
Birth weight for gestational age < 10th percentile	Small-for-gestational-age	SGA
Birth weight for gestational age >10th < 90th percentile	Appropriate-for-gestational-age	AGA
Birth weight for gestational age > 90th percentile	Large-for-gestational-age	LGA
Inappropriately low weight for weeks of gestation	Intrauterine-growth-restriction	IUGR

Source: Definitions from Subcommittee on Nutritional Status and Weight Gain During Pregnancy. *Nutrition During Pregnancy.* Washington, DC: National Academy Press; 1990.

significant cost of these solutions. As will be discussed later, there is ample evidence to support the initiation of PN in the first 48 hours of life.

Protein/Amino Acids

Protein accretion rates by the fetus at 24–25 wks, 27–28 wks, and 30–32 wks of gestation are estimated to be 4.0, 3.6, and 3.3 g/kg/day, respectively.[15] In most preterm infants, 1.0–1.5 g/kg/day of intravenous amino acids along with glucose prevents catabolism.[16–26] Preterm infants are slightly anabolic even when parenteral intakes are as little as 2 g/kg/day of amino acids and 50–60 g/kg/day of energy.[25] A protein intake of 2.5 to 3.0 g/kg/day with a nonprotein energy intake of 60 kcal/kg/day results in a more positive protein balance.[20] When nonprotein energy intake is 80–85 kcal/kg/day and amino acid intake is 2.7 to 3.5 g/kg/day, nitrogen retention and growth might actually occur at the intrauterine rate.[17,18] In a recent controlled trial of 28 infants, mean birth weight of 946 g ± 40 g randomized to receive 1 g/kg/day or 3 g/kg/day of protein in PN in the first 24 hours of life, infants in the higher protein intake group had better protein accretion.[27] This presumably occurred by increasing protein synthesis and reducing protein breakdown. Furthermore, there was no difference in the degree of metabolic acidosis or blood urea nitrogen concentration between the groups, one of the main reasons that neonatologists give for not starting amino acids at higher concentrations earlier in life. Interestingly, these same investigators reported that in 99 infants (mean birth weight 1,379 g ± 600 g, mean gestational age 29.8 ± 3.9 wks), for any intake of parenteral amino acid, there was only a weakly positive correlation with serum blood urea nitrogen and amino acid intake ($p < 0.05$, $r^2 = 0.11$). There were more significant correlations between birth weight or gestational age and blood urea nitrogen.[28] Thus, it can be concluded that intravenous amino acids should be started as soon as possible after birth (within the first 24 hours). There is no evidence to support the gradual increase of total daily protein intake. An initial protein intake of 3.0 to 3.5 g/kg/day can be justified from the available literature.[15,27,29,30]

Fatty Acids

Neonatologists have been reluctant to initiate parenteral fatty acids (FAs) in the first days of life in VLBW infants because of concern about negative effects of fatty acids on pulmonary function in infants with respiratory disease, the effect FAs could have on serum bilirubin concentrations, and the possibility that FA infusions might increase the risk of infection. On the other hand, VLBW infants are deficient in essential FAs in the first 48 hours of life if provided a lipid-free diet.[31] Essential FA deficiency can be prevented by starting an infusion of FA at a rate of 1–2 g/kg/day in the first 24 hours of life.[32] The negative effects reported on pulmonary function testing, such as increased pulmonary vascular resistance, decreased arterial oxygen tension, decreased pulmonary diffusion capacity, and increased pulmonary arterial lipid deposits occurred with FA infusion rates of 2.4 to 10.8 g/kg/day given over a few hours. There is no evidence that pulmonary functions are affected at slower, 24-hour continuous infusion rates of FAs. In addition, 20% fat solutions are associated with superior lipid tolerance compared to 10% solutions.[33–35] Two of three randomized control trials involving preterm infants showed no association between infusion of FAs and chronic lung disease.[36–38] Serum triglycerides increase in the presence of bacterial sepsis and stress/trauma and serum triglyceride levels should be monitored under these conditions.[34] The risk of coagulase negative staphylococcus infection increases with FA infusions;[39] however, this risk is not reason enough to avoid FA infusions in preterm infants early in life, especially in the face of acute fatty acid deficiency. Although there is a theoretic risk that FAs might interfere with albumin binding of bilirubin and increase serum concentration of free bilirubin, randomized, controlled trials showed that in premature infants, lipid infusions at 1–4 g/kg/24 hrs have no effect on serum concentrations of total and unbound bilirubin.[40] Thus, there is no convincing evidence that FAs cannot be initiated in the first 24 hours of life at an infusion rate of at least 1.0 g/kg/day with an advancement to 3 g/kg/d during the first week of life.

Carbohydrate

There is little controversy over the use of glucose infusions after delivery of the VLBW and ELBW infant. Hyperglycemia is a common complication of PN therapy in ELBW infants; this can be explained by the fact that preterm infants have a high endogenous glucose production rate (6–8 mg/kg/min), which is not completely suppressed by glucose infusions.[41–43] Hyperglycemia, defined as serum glucose level > 180 mg/dL, can also be associated with increased production of CO2. Increased CO2 could have adverse effects on infants who have lung disease. The degree of hyperglycemia increases with decreasing birth weight and decreasing gestational age and is exaggerated by steroids and dopamine infusions (epinephrine response). Serum glucose may be increased when glucose infusion is accompanied by FA infusions.[36,43] For the VLBW infant, glucose infusions should start at a rate of 6 mg/kg/min (8.6 g/kg/day) or less. If hyperglycemia develops, the rate of the glucose infusion should be decreased. Insulin therapy may be considered if an infusion of 4–5 mg/kg/day or less of glucose results in hyperglycemia, and the total caloric intake is less than 60 kcal/kg/day. There is only a single randomized, controlled trial in preterm infants that demonstrates weight gain is improved in preterm infants treated with insulin.[44] In general, pharmacologic doses of insulin are required to achieve euglycemia, and this is associated with very high serum insulin levels. Insulin is an anabolic hormone that increases fat deposition. Hypoglycemia is a frequent complication of insulin therapy. Thus, insulin should be used with caution and only as a last resort in VLBW infants.

Complications and Monitoring of PN

There are many complications of PN therapy. These can be divided into five categories: (1) those related to the mechanical insertion and maintenance of PN central lines; (2) metabolic complications associated with delivering too much or too little of a given nutrient; (3) those associated with infection and sepsis; (4) nutrient interactions and contaminants of PN solutions; and (5) PN related cholestasis. These have been extensively reviewed elsewhere.[45,46] The number and incidence of complications increases with the duration of PN therapy as well as with decreasing birth weight and gestational age.

Metabolic bone disease in VLBW infants on PN is largely the result of calcium and phosphorus deficiency. These very small infants are on relatively low total infusion volumes and their requirements for calcium and phosphorus cannot be achieved because calcium and phosphorus precipitate in the solutions.[47] Aluminum contamination of PN solutions, due largely to the amount of aluminum in the calcium and phosphorus salts, could also contribute to bone disease.[48,49]

Cholestasis is the most significant complication of PN. It leads to liver failure and is more likely to occur in preterm infants whose bile acid pool and hepatobiliary system are immature to the point that preterm infants have a "physiologic cholestasis."[46] The incidence of cholestasis rises with decreasing birth weight and gestational age and increasing duration of PN (30–65% of all premature infants on PN for > 21 days). The most effective treatment is institution and advancement of enteral feedings if the clinical situation permits. The most sensitive measurement to monitor for PN cholestasis is a serum direct bilirubin determination made after 2 weeks of PN therapy. This should be repeated twice weekly until most nutrition is delivered enterally. It is no longer necessary to perform a metabolic chemistry panel before starting PN in VLBW infants, and one can argue that the panel does not need to be done before 2 weeks of PN therapy. In the first week of PN therapy, electrolytes and glucose must be measured at frequent intervals depending on the infant's overall fluid status.

Trophic Feedings with Parenteral Nutrition

For infants on PN who are too unstable to begin standard enteral feedings, there is a role for trophic or minimal enteral feeds, anticipating the transition from PN to EN. Both gastric emptying and intestinal transit times are slower in preterm compared to term infants. The normal pattern of gut motility is not established until 32–34 weeks postmenstrual age.

Well designed studies have documented the benefits of the early introduction of low volume, trophic feedings (1 mL every 2–4 hours, or intakes of 5–25 mL/kg/day).[50–53] Benefits include decreased incidence of indirect hyperbilirubinemia and cholestatic jaundice, increased levels of gastrin and other enteric hormones, fewer days to achieve full EN, and increased weight gain. EN enhances maturation of the motor responses of the small intestine in preterm infants when compared to preterm infants on exclusive PN.[54,55] Moreover, no study has found an increased incidence of NEC among preterm infants receiving trophic feedings, though large clinical trials are needed to confirm this observation. Evidence-based medicine supports the institution of trophic EN in VLBW infants beginning shortly after birth.

ENTERAL NUTRITION SUPPORT

When to Feed Enterally

The initiation of EN for an infant depends on many factors, including gestational age, birth weight, clinical status, and the experience of the health care providers. Decisions to be made are when to initiate, when to interrupt, method of delivery, feeding frequency, feeding volume, rate of advancement, and type of feeding (human milk, standard formula, preterm formula). Given all the decisions to be made at the time feedings are initiated, there are probably as many different ways to enterally feed a preterm infant as there are neonatologists. The route of EN is largely determined by the infant's ability to coordinate sucking, swallowing, and breathing, which occurs at 32 to 34 weeks' postmenstrual age. Infants older than 32–34 weeks can be offered a nipple or the breast. Infants who are too premature or too ill to feed by mouth are fed by nasogastric or orogastric feeding tubes. The feeds can be delivered as a bolus or continuous infusion of formula or breast milk. Except in unusual situations, transpyloric drip feedings should not be used.[56] Bolus feeds every 2 to 3 hours simulate the pattern of feeding that the infant will have when advanced to bottle or breastfeedings. One study demonstrated that preterm infants fed intermittently rather than continuously had improved feeding tolerance and increased rate of growth.[53] Other studies show no difference between these two methods of feeding.[57–59]

Full-strength breast milk or formula is preferred as the initial enteral food. There is no demonstrable advantage of diluted formula or breast milk over full strength. In fact, full strength formula more effectively promotes the development of intestinal activity than diluted formula feedings do.[60, 61]

The neonatologist's fear of NEC has had a tremendous impact on the early nutritional status of the low-birth-weight infant. The term NEC was first used in 1952;[63] it became a significant clinical problem with the improvements in neonatal intensive care of the 1960s and 1970s. No other single disease has had a greater impact on EN of premature infants, for it is the fear of NEC that governs when feedings are started, how rapidly they are advanced, what kind of feeding is used, and when they are interrupted. Although more than 40 years of research has failed to identify a feeding method that prevents NEC, most neonatologists limit the daily advancement of EN, believing that this will decrease the risk of NEC. Randomized trials have shown that fast, slow, early or delayed feedings have no effect on the incidence of NEC.[63–65] Human milk, even with fortification, is thought to decrease the incidence of NEC in LBW infants.[66] There is only 1 prospective study that shows that human milk protects against NEC.[67] In this multicenter study of 926 infants, there was no dose response to breast milk, i.e., the incidence of NEC was not different in groups exclusively fed breast milk or partially fed breast milk. The benefits of breastfeeding for the prevention of NEC were most significant for gestational ages greater than 30 weeks.

Formula Versus Breast Milk

As noted at the beginning of the chapter, starting in the 1940s, formula was preferred over breast milk for the preterm infant.[6] In the 1970s, Raiha and colleagues pointed out that protein quality, not quantity, played an important role in the feeding of the premature infant.[68] In these studies, infants were randomly assigned to pooled human milk, protein content 1.0 gm/dL, or 1 of 4 isocaloric cow milk based formulas differing in protein quantity, 1.5 or 3.0 gm/dL, and ratio of whey proteins to casein 60:40 or 18:82. Weight gain was highest in the infants receiving the high protein formula (protein intake of 4.5 gm/kg/day), but some developed azotemia, hyperammonemia, and metabolic acidosis. The intrauterine rate of weight gain was not achieved in any group. This study suggested that human milk was as adequate for LBW infants as the available formulas at that time. Another study from the early 1980s clearly established that LBW infants fed their own mother's milk had an improved growth rate compared to premature infants fed pooled, mature, donor milk.[69] This was largely thought to be due to the higher protein content of preterm breast milk compared to milk from term mothers during the first few weeks of lactation. Though this work led to a resurgence in the use of mother's own milk for preterm infants, even in Gross's study, the infants did not achieve the intrauterine rate of growth.[69]

It was known since the 1940s that the human milk concentrations of protein, calcium, phosphorus, sodium, iron, vitamins, and trace minerals would not support intrauterine growth rates for premature infants. Heird and Anderson (1977) discussed these inadequacies in their review and noted that infants fed human milk grew as well as those receiving the formulas available at that time.[8]

The 1980s saw the commercial development of special formulas for the ELBW infant.[1] Compared to standard formulas, these special formulas contained more protein (2.2 g/dL), sodium (1.5 mEq/dL), calcium (150 mg/dL), phosphorus (80 mg/dL), and vitamins per 100 mL and more closely met the needs of the growing premature infant who required smaller volumes with higher concentrations of nutrients compared to larger infants. The special formulas allowed the delivery of approximately 3 g/kg/day protein and 6.5 g/kg/day of fat with an intake of 150/mL/kg day and contained 50% of the fat as medium chain triglycerides. Clinical studies of VLBW infants showed improved growth compared to human milk without metabolic abnormalities.[70–73] Only a commercially available, sterile, ready-to-feed, liquid formula should be fed to premature infants, as powdered infant formula is not sterile. The Centers for Disease Control and Prevention recommends the use of aseptic technique during preparation of formula, which includes refrigeration of prepared formula, discarding any reconstituted formula stored for longer than 24 hours, and limiting the time the formula remains at room temperature to less than 4 hours.[74]

Commercially available human milk fortifiers became available for preterm infants in the 1990s, and fortified human milk became the preferred feeding for the LBW infant despite the observation that VLBW infants fed special formulas grew faster than those fed fortified human milk.[67,75,76] Presumed advantages of human milk in LBW infants, such as protection against infection, NEC,[67] and development of allergies, as well as the promotion of neurologic development,[77] led to its preferred status.

Human milk fortifiers contain protein, vitamins, and minerals that in theory will meet the needs to achieve intrauterine growth rates when added to human milk. Metabolic complications associated with the long term use of unsupplemented human milk in preterm infants include hyponatremia,[78] hypoproteinemia,[79] osteopenia/rickets,[80] and zinc deficiency.[81]

NUTRITION SUPPORT OF THE PRETERM INFANT AFTER HOSPITAL DISCHARGE

Feeding the preterm infant after hospital discharge presents a number of problems. First, discharges occur at a lower weight and earlier postmenstrual age than they did 20 years ago. Second, human milk is frequently a part of the diet. Third, there is no evidence-based medicine in this area, and the emphasis in the relatively few studies is on growth and not long term neurodevelopmental parameters. Even if the intrauterine rate of growth is achieved in the NICU, approximately 90% of infants with a birth weight of less than 1,500 grams are discharged at a postmenstrual weight that is less than the 10th percentile for corrected age.[10] There are no guidelines that define appropriate catch-up growth, desirable body composition, or that describe how to achieve this catch-up growth. Thus, the exact requirements for growth and development after hospital discharge can only be estimated and are largely based on expert opinion.

Human milk alone is not enough to meet the requirements for growth and development in the postdischarge preterm infant. Various amounts of powdered formula or human milk fortifiers can be added to human milk, as can supplemental vitamins and iron. Special discharge formulas are now available for preterm infants for use during the first year of life. These formulas provide a nutrient intake that is higher than that of term formulas, but less than that in the special formulas for preterm infants used in the NICU. They contain more calcium and phosphorus than term formulas, and bone mineralization is better when they are used after hospital discharge.[82,83] Three randomized, controlled studies have been done with these formulas.[84–86] In general, weight, head circumference, and length are not different for infants fed the special formula compared to infants fed the standard formula even when the preterm discharge formula was used for the first 12 months of life. There could be some advantages for special preterm formulas for SGA infants and infants with a birth weight less than 1,250 g. But the evidence for the use of special formulas for preterm infants as a group is insufficient to make a general recommendation for their use at this time. If these special discharge formulas are not used, then iron-fortified formulas and supplements of multivitamins should be given after hospital discharge.[87]

The greatest concern for feeding the preterm infant after hospital discharge is those infants who continue to receive mostly human milk. The efficacy of unfortified human milk has not been demonstrated in this population, and supplemental iron and multivitamins are needed. If breast milk is mostly consumed by these infants at 4 months corrected age, then the introduction of supplemental foods that include a supply of iron is indicated.

CONCLUSION

At the present, there is good evidence that the weight of the VLBW infant is less than the 10th percentile for corrected postmenstrual age at the time of discharge from the NICU.[10] Nutrition support in the NICU should be optimized so infants are in better nutritional health when they are discharged and there is no need or lessened need for catch-up growth. These include the early initiation of PN with FA and protein in the first 48 hours of life and the early institution of trophic EN. EN should either be the specialized formulas for VLBW infants or human milk fortified with commercially available fortifiers. Much more research is needed to determine the best nutrition support for the preterm infant after hospital discharge. There seem to be minimal indications for using the special postdischarge formulas for preterm infants at this time, and those maintained on breast milk must be supplemented with vitamins and iron and should have iron-containing complementary foods introduced at 4 months of corrected age.

REFERENCES

1. Greer FR. Feeding the premature infant in the 20th century. *J Nutri*. 2001;131:426S-430S.
2. Nichols BL. The evolution of research techniques in premature infant nutrition. In: Salle BL, Sawyer PR, eds. *Nutrition of the Low Birthweight Infant*. New York, NY: Vevy/Raven Press; 1993:31–41.
3. Gordon HH, Levine SZ, Deamer WC, McNamara H. Respiratory metabolism in infancy and in childhood: XXIII. Daily energy requirements of premature infants. *Am J Dis Child*. 1940;59:1185–1202.
4. Davies DP. The first feed of low birthweight infants: changing attitudes in the twentieth century. *Arch Dis Child*. 1978;53:187–192.
5. Hess JH. *Premature and Congenitally Diseased Infants*. Philadelphia, Pa: Lea & Ferbiger; 1922:107–204.
6. Gordon HH, Levine SZ, McNamara H. Feeding of premature infants: a comparison of human and cow's milk. *Am J Dis Child*. 1947;73:442–452.
7. Benjamin MH, Gordon HH, Marples E. Calcium and phosphorus requirements of premature infants. *Am J Dis Child*. 1943;65:412–425.
8. Heird WC, Anderson TL. Nutritional requirements and methods of feeding low birthweight infants. *Curr Probl Pediatr*. 1977;7:3–40.
9. American Academy of Pediatrics, Committee on Nutrition. Nutritional needs of low-birth-weight infants. *Pediatrics*. 1977;60:526.
10. Ehrenkranz RA, Younes N, Lemons JA, et al. Longitudinal growth of hospitalized very low birth weight infants. *Pediatrics*. 1999;104:280–289.
11. Wilson DC, Cairns P, Halliday HL, Reid M, McClure G, Dodge JA. Randomized controlled trial of an aggressive nutritional regimen in sick very low birthweight infants. *Arch Dis Child*. 1997;77:F4–F11.
12. Nutritional needs of the preterm infant. In: Kleinman RE, ed. *Pediatric Nutrition Handbook*. Elk Grove Village, Ill: American Academy of Pediatrics; 2004:23–54.
13. Tsang RC, Lucas A, Uauy R, Zlotkin S, eds. *Nutritional Needs of the Preterm Infant*. Baltimore, Md: Williams & Wilkins; 1993.
14. Cowett RM, ed. Nutrition and Metabolism of the Micropreemie. *Clinics in Perinatology*. 2000;27:1–245.
15. Ziegler EE. Protein in premature feeding. *Nutrition*. 1994;10:69–71.
16. Rubecz I, Mestyan J, Varga P, Klujber L. Energy metabolism, substrate utilization, and nitrogen balance in parenterally fed postoperative neonates and infants. *J Pediatr*. 1981;98:42–46.
17. Zlotkin SH, Bryan MH, Anderson GH. Intravenous nitrogen and energy intakes required to duplicate in utero nitrogen accretion in prematurely born human infants. *J Pediatr*. 1981;99:115–120.
18. Duffy B, Gunn J, Collinge J, Pencharz P. The effect of varying protein quality and energy intake on the nitrogen metabolism of parenterally fed very low birthweight (< 1600g) infants. *Pediatr Res*. 1981;15:1040–1044.
19. van Toledo-Eppinga L, Kalhan SC, Kulik, W, Jacobs C, LaFeber HN. Relative kinetics of phenylalanine and leucine in low birth weight infants during nutrient administration. *Pediatr Res*. 1996;40:41–46.
20. Anderson TL, Muttart CR, Bleber MA, Nicholson JF, Heird WC. A controlled trial of glucose versus glucose and amino acids in premature infants. *J Pediatr*. 1979;94:947–951.
21. Yu VYH, James B, Hendry P, MacMahon RA. Total parenteral nutrition in very low birthweight infants: a controlled trial. *Arch Dis Child*. 1979;54:653–661.
22. Saini J, MacMahon P, Morgan JB, Kovar IZ. Early parenteral feeding of amino acids. *Arch Dis Child*. 1989;64:1362–1366.
23. van Lingen RA, van Goudoever JB, Luijendijk IH, Wattimena JL, Sauer PJ. Effects of early amino acid administration during total parenteral nutrition on protein metabolism in pre-term infants. *Clin Sci*. 1992;82:199–203.
24. Rivera A Jr, Bell EF, Bier DM. Effect of intravenous amino acids on protein metabolism of preterm infants during the first three days of life. *Pediar Res*. 1993;33:106–111.
25. Kashyap S, Heird WC. Protein requirements of low birthweight, very low birthweight and small for gestational age infants. In: Raiha NC, ed. *Protein Metabolism During Infancy*. New York, NY: Raven Press; 1993:133–251.
26. van Goudoever JB, Sulkers EJ, Halliday D, et al. Whole body protein turnover in preterm appropriate for gestational age and small for gestational age infants: comparison of [15N] glycine and [1-13C] leucine administered simultaneously. *Pediatr Res*. 1995;37:381–388.
27. Thureen PJ, Melara D, Fennessey PV, Hay WW Jr. Effect of low versus high intravenous amino acid intake on very low birth weight infants in the early neonatal period. *Pediatr Res*. 2003;53:24–32.
28. Ridout E, Melara D, Thureen P. Amino acid intake is a poor predictor of blood urea nitrogen (BUN) concentrations in ventilated and ill neonates in first days of life. *Peds Res*. 2003;53:405A.
29. Ziegler EE, Thureen PJ, Carlson SJ. Aggressive nutrition of the very low birthweight infant. *Clin Perinatol*. 2002;29:225–244.
30. Thureen PJ, Hay WW Jr. Early aggressive nutrition in preterm infants. *Semin Neonatol*. 2001;6:403–415.
31. Farrell PM, Gutcher GR, Palta M, DeMets D. Essential fatty acid deficiency in premature infants. *Am J Clin Nutr*. 1988;48:220–229.

32. Gutcher GR, Farrell PM. Intravenous infusion of lipid for the prevention of essential fatty acid deficiency in premature infants. *Am J Clin Nutr*. 1991;54:1024–1028.

33. Haumont D, Richelle M, Deckelbaum RJ, Coussaert E, Carpentier YA. Effect of liposomal content of lipid emulsions on plasma lipid concentrations in low birth weight infants receiving parenteral nutrition. *J Pediatr*. 1992;121:759–763.

34. Putet G. Lipid metabolism in the micropremie. *Clin Perinatol*. 2000;27:57–70.

35. Cairns PA, Wilson DC, Jenkins J, McMaster C, McClure, BG. Tolerance of mixed lipid emulsion in neonates: effect of concentration. *Arch Dis Child*. 1996;75:F113–F116.

36. Gilbertson N, Kovar IZ, Cox DJ, Crowe L, Palmer NT. Introduction of intravenous lipid administration on the first day of life in the very low birth weight neonate. *J Pediatr*. 1991;119:615–623.

37. Hammerman C, Aramburo MJ. Decreased lipid intake reduces morbidity in sick premature neonates. *J Pediatr*. 1988;113:1083–1088.

38. Sosenko IR, Rodriguez-Pierce M, Bancalari E. Effect of early initiation of intravenous lipid administration on the incidence and severity of chronic lung disease in premature infants. *J Pediatr*. 1993;123:975–982.

39. Freeman J, Goldmann DA, Smith NE, Sidebottom DG, Epstein MF, Platt R. Association of intravenous lipid emulsion and coagulase-negative staphylococcal bacteremia in neonatal intensive care units. *N Engl J Med*. 1990;323:301–308.

40. Brans YW, Ritter DA, Kenny JD, Andrew DS, Dutton EB, Carrillo, DW. Influence of intravenous fat emulsion on serum bilirubin in very low birthweigth neonates. *Arch Dis Child*. 1987;62:156–160.

41. Cowett RM, Oh W, Schwartz R. Persistent glucose production during glucose infusion in the neonate. *J Clin Invest*. 1983;71:467–475.

42. Kalhan SC, Oliven A, King KC, Lucero C. Role of glucose in the regulation of endogenous glucose production in the human newborn. *Pediatr Res*. 1986;20:49–52.

43. Savich RD, Finley SL, Ogata ES. Intravenous lipid and amino acids briskly increase plasma glucose concentrations in small premature infants. *Am J Perinatology*. 1988;5:201–205.

44. Collins JW Jr, Hoppe M, Brown K, Edidin DV, Padbury J, Ogata ES. A controlled trial of insulin infusion and parenteral nutrition in extremely low birth weight infants with glucose intolerance. *J Pediatr*. 1991;118:921–927.

45. Shulman RJ, Phillips S. Parenteral nutrition in infants and children. *J Pediatr Gastro Nutr*. 2003;36:587–607.

46. Karpen SJ. Update on the etiologies and management of neonatal cholestasis. *Clin Perinatol*. 2002;29:159–180.

47. Greer FR. Osteopenia of prematurity. *Ann Rev Nutr*. 1994;14:169–185.

48. Committee on Nutrition. Aluminum toxicity in infants and children. *Pediatrics*. 1996;97:413–416.

49. Klein GL, Alfrey AC, Shike M, Sherrard DJ. Parenteral drug products containing aluminum as an ingredient or a contaminant: response to FDA notice of intent. ASCN/ASPEN Working Group on standards for aluminum contents of parenteral nutrition solutions. *Am J Clin Nutr*. 1991;53:399–402.

50. Berseth CL. Effect of early feeding on maturation of the preterm infant's small intestine. *J Pediatr*. 1992;120:947–953.

51. Davey AM, Wagner CL, Cox C, Kendig JW. Feeding premature infants while low umbilical artery catheters are in place: a prospective, randomized trial. *J Pediatr*. 1994;124:795–799.

52. McClure J, Newell RJ. Randomized controlled trial of trophic feeding and gut motility. *Arch Dis Child*. 1999;80:F54–F58.

53. Schanler RJ, Shulman J, Lau C, Smith EO, Heitkemper MM. Feeding strategies for premature infants: randomized trial of gastrointestinal priming and tube-feeding method. *Pediatrics*. 1999;103:434–439.

54. McClure RJ, Newell SJ. Randomized controlled study of clinical outcome following trophic feeding. *Arch Dis Child Fetal Neonatal Ed*. 2000;82:F29–F33.

55. Berseth CL, Nordyke C. Enteral nutrients promote postnatal maturation of intestinal motor activity in preterm infants. *Am J Physiol*. 1993;264:G1046–G1051.

56. MacDonald PD, Skeoch CH, Carse H, et al. Randomized trial of continuous nasogastric, bolus nasogastric, and transpyloric feeding in infants of birth weight under 1400g. *Arch Dis Child*. 1992;67:429–431.

57. McGuire W, McEwan P. Systematic review of transpyloric versus gastric tube feeding for preterm infants. *Arch Dis Child Fetal Neonatal Ed*. 2004;89:F245–F248.

58. Silvestre MA, Morbach CA, Brans YW, Shankaran SA. A prospective randomized trial comparing continuous versus intermittent feeding methods in very low birth weight infants. *J Pediatr*. 1996;128:748–752.

59. Akintorin SM, Kamat M, Pildes RS, et al. A prospective randomized trial of feeding methods in very low birth weight infants. *Pediatrics*. 1997;100:e4.

60. MacDonald PD, Skeoch CH, Carse H, et al. Randomized trial of continuous nasogastric, bolus nasogastric, and transpyloric feeding in infants of weight under 1400 g. *Arch Dis Child*. 1992;67:429–431.

61. Berseth CL, Nordyke C. Enteral nutrients promote postnatal maturation of intestinal motor activity in preterm infants. *Am J Physiol*. 1993;264:G1046–G1051.

62. Koenig WJ, Amarnath RP, Hench V, Berseth CL. Manometrics for preterm and term infants: a new tool for old questions. *Pediatrics*. 1995;95:203–206.

63. Quaiser K. Uber eine besonders schwer verlaufende Form von enteritis beim Sauling: enterocolitis ulcerosa

necroticans II. Klinische Studien. *Oesterr Z Kinderh.* 1952;8:136.

64. Rayyis SF, Ambalavanan N, Wright L, Carlo WA. Randomized trial of "slow" versus "fast" feed advancements on the incidence of necrotizing enterocolitis in very low birth weight infants. *J Pediatr.* 1999;134:293–297.
65. Kennedy KA, Tyson JE, Chamnanvanikij S. Early versus delayed initiation of progressive enteral feedings for parenterally fed low birth weight or preterm infants. Cochrane Neonatal Group. *Cochrane Database Syst Rev.* 2002(Issue 4).
66. Kennedy KA, Tyson JE, Chamnanvanikij S. Rapid versus slow rate of advancement of feeding for promoting growth and preventing necrotizing enterocolitis in parenterally fed low birth weight infants. Cochrane Neonatal Group. *Cochrane Database Syst Rev.* 2002(Issue 4).
67. Schanler RJ, Shulman R, Lau C. Feeding strategies for premature infants: beneficial outcomes of feeding fortified human milk versus preterm formula. *Pediatrics.* 1999;103:1150–1157.
68. Lucas A, Cole TJ. Breast milk and necrotising enterocolitis. *Lancet.* 1990;366:1519–1523.
69. Raiha NC, Heinonen K, Rassin DK, Gaull GE. Milk protein quantity and quality in low-birthweight infants: I. Metabolic response and effects on growth. *Pediatrics.* 1976;57:659–684.
70. Gross SJ. Growth and biochemical response of preterm infants fed human milk or modified infant formula. *N Engl J Med.* 1983;308:237–241.
71. Tyson JE, Lasky RE, Mize CE, et al. Growth metabolic response and development in very low birth weight infants fed banked human milk or enriched formula: 1. Neonatal findings. *J Pediatr.* 1983;103:95–104.
72. Schanler RJ, Oh W. Nitrogen and mineral balance in preterm infants fed human milk or formula. *J Pediat Gastroenterol Nutr.* 1985;4:214–219.
73. Cooper PA, Rothberg AD, Pettifor JM, Bolton KD, Davenhuis S. Growth and biochemical response of premature infants fed pooled preterm milk or special formula. *J Pediatr Gastronenterol Nutr.* 1984;3:749–754.
74. Greer FR, McCormick A. Improved bone mineralization and growth in premature infants fed fortified own mother's milk. *J Pediatr.* 1988;112:961–969.
75. Available at: http://www.cdc.gov/mmwr/PDF/wk/mm5114.pdf. Accessed March 9, 2006.
76. Schanler RJ, Garza C. Improved mineral balance in very low birth weight infants fed fortified human milk. *J Pediatr.* 1987;112:452–456.
77. Atkinson SA, Bryan MH, Anderson GH. Human milk feeding in premature infants: protein, fat and carbohydrate balance in the first two weeks of life. *J Pediatr.* 1981;99:617–624.
78. Morley R, Lucas A. Influence of early diet on outcome in preterm infants. *Acta Paediatr Suppl.* 1994;405:123–126.
79. Engelke SC, Shah BL, Vasan U, Raye JR. Sodium balance in very low-birth-weight infants. *J Pediatr.* 1978;93:837–841.
80. Ronnholm KA, Sipila I, Siimes MA. Human milk protein supplementation for the prevention of hypoproteinemia without metabolic imbalance in breast milk-fed, very low-birth-weight-infants. *J Pediatr.* 1982;101:243–247.
81. Greer FR, Steichen JJ, Tsang RC. Calcium and phosphate supplements in breast milk-related rickets: results in very-low-birth-weight infants. *Am J Dis Child.* 1982;136:581–583.
82. Zlotkin SH. Assessment of trace element requirements (zinc) in newborns and young infants, including the infant born prematurely. In: Chandra RK, ed. *Trace Elements in Nutrition of Children II.* New York, NY: Raven Press; 1991:49–64.
83. Bishop NJ, King FJ, Lucas A. Increased bone mineral content of preterm infants fed with a nutrient enriched formula after discharge from hospital. *Arch Dis Child.* 1993;68:573–578.
84. Chan GM. Growth and bone mineral status of discharged very low birth weight infants fed different formulas or human milk. *J Pediatr.* 1993;123:439–443.
85. Wheeler RE, Hall RT. Feeding of premature infant formula after hospital discharge of infants weighing less than 1800g at birth. *J Perinatol.* 1996;16:111–116.
86. Carver JD, Wu PY, Hall RT, et al. Growth of preterm infants fed nutrient-enriched or term formula after hospital discharge. *Pediatrics.* 2001;107:683–689.
87. Worrell LA, Thorp JW, Tucker R, et al. The effects of the introduction of a high-nutrient transitional formula on growth and development of very-low-birth-weight infants. *J Perinatol.* 2002;22:112–119.
88. Greer FR. Feeding the preterm infant after hospital discharge. *Pediatr Annals.* 2001;30:658–665.

CHAPTER 31

Nutrition Support for Inflammatory Bowel Disease

Robert M. Issenman and Tracy Hussey

INTRODUCTION

Growth is an essential part of childhood and adolescence and nutritional issues are paramount in the treatment of pediatric inflammatory bowel disease (IBD). It seems intuitive that malabsorption would explain most of the nutritional problems of the gastrointestinal tract diseases in these patients. However, research findings of the past 25 years indicate that much more complex mechanisms are involved. Loss of appetite, aberrant metabolism, exudation of nutrients, and other manifestations of inflammation also play a role and interact to varying degrees. This chapter describes the nutritional challenges, pathophysiology, and therapeutic considerations in pediatric IBD.

MECHANISMS OF DEFICIENCY

Chronic malnutrition is found in many pediatric Crohn's disease (CD) patients. Significant weight loss is seen in 85% of children with CD,[1] and 20–80% have disturbed linear growth.[2–4] In contrast, linear growth is seldom impaired in children with ulcerative colitis (UC). Common micronutrient deficiencies, particularly in CD, include those involving iron, folate, vitamins B_{12} and D, magnesium, and zinc.

Nutritional deficiencies are likely caused by an interplay of various factors. Decreased oral intake could be related to anorexia precipitated by cytokines and inflammatory mediators (see Chapter 11). Some children decrease their intake due to fear of specific foods or a generalized fear of eating.[5] Oral lesions might contribute to decreased intake in a small proportion of cases. During disease flares, oral intake is estimated to decrease by approximately 20%.[6]

Malnutrition can also be caused by excessive losses.[6] Diarrhea can increase intestinal transit interfering with absorption. Protein and blood oozing from inflamed tissue cause losses. In addition, intestinal bypass due to fistula formation can affect nutritional status. Malabsorption is most commonly seen in patients with upper small bowel involvement or those who have had bowel resections; however, malnutrition could also be due to concomitant factors that interfere with metabolism, such as infections, medications, or underlying disease of the liver, pancreas or intestine. Finally, many patients have increased nutrient requirements due to infections, fevers, and medications such as corticosteroids. Thus they are in a catabolic state at a time when their energy requirements for growth are already high.[6,7] Energy deficits are estimated to be approximately 400 kcal per day.[8]

CROHN'S DISEASE VERSUS ULCERATIVE COLITIS

There are several important distinctions in the assessment and treatment of children with CD or UC. Growth is more severely affected in children with CD,[9,10] as is bone mineralization.[11,12] Evidence of malnutrition and nutrient losses are greater in children with CD regardless of the amount of diarrhea.[13] However, lactose intolerance is reported more often in children with UC than in those with CD.[14]

The goals for treatment are similar for both entities: remission, nutrient repletion, and growth. However, nutrition support plays only an adjunctive role in UC, as there is no conclusive evidence at this time that enteral therapy induces remission in UC.[6]

NUTRITIONAL ASSESSMENT

Nutritional assessment of pediatric patients with IBD includes a history, physical exam, and laboratory testing. The history includes disease location, disease activity, stool patterns, medications, diet intake, nutritional supplements and/or complementary therapies, ongoing symptoms, and level of physical activity. Factors that affect dietary intake such as appetite, nausea, mouth lesions, and food avoidances should be reviewed. Dietary history can be examined with 3-day food records or a 24-hour recall to assess macro- and micronutrient intake deficiencies. A large proportion (70–90%) of children with IBD alter their diet after diagnosis, and this includes the exclusion of large components of a typical Western diet.[14] The exclusion of large numbers of foods or food groups puts them at risk for deficiencies. Approximately one third of pediatric patients use various vitamin and supplement preparations,[14] and the appropriateness of these supplements should be individually examined. Financial and social factors that could affect intake and access to appropriate foods need to be considered.

The physical exam includes accurate anthropometrics at each visit. Minimally, this is weight and height plotted on appropriate growth charts and weight for height or calculation of body mass index. Concerns regarding malnutrition can be confirmed using skinfold thickness and mid-arm muscle measurements, or by using subjective global assessment.[15] Tanner staging is important because it reflects delays in maturation that are most often related to nutritional status. Symptoms of various micronutrient deficiencies such as edema, pallor, clubbing, brittle hair, rashes, and hepatomegaly can be revealed through physical exam.

Laboratory testing is helpful (see Chapter 7). Serum albumin, prealbumin, and total protein can be used to determine protein (muscle) status. These should be interpreted with caution as they are affected by protein losses accompanying inflammatory processes.[16] Other tests, such as 24-hour urine urea nitrogen determination and urinary creatinine to height ratio are not routinely used clinically because it is difficult to obtain accurate specimens, and assumptions must be made in interpreting the results.

Tests for specific nutrient deficiencies should be performed on an as needed basis. Patients with severe losses, resections, or very poor oral intake, or those receiving nutritional support require closer monitoring. Routine yearly blood work for stable patients can include complete blood count, levels of vitamins A, D, E, B_{12}, folate, prothrombin time (to assess vitamin K), serum iron or ferritin, copper, calcium, alkaline phosphatase, phosphorous, magnesium, plasma zinc, and selenium.

Assessment of bone growth should be performed yearly. This assessment might include a wrist X-ray to determine bone age. If available, dual energy X-ray absorptiometry (DEXA) can be used to determine bone density and the risk of osteopenia/osteoporosis. Children with Crohn's disease and growth failure appear to be at the greatest risk of osteoporosis.[17]

GOALS AND RECOMMENDATIONS FOR NUTRITIONAL SUPPORT

There are 3 main goals of nutritional support for children with IBD: (1) remission, (2) growth, and (3) nutritional repletion. Many patients receiving nutritional support will have all 3 goals.

Macronutrients

There are many equations available to calculate energy requirements in children; however, validation with clinical outcomes for pediatric IBD patients is required. Resting energy requirements of adult IBD patients are not increased.[18] However, in calculating the energy requirements of pediatric patients, the inclusion of calories for catch-up growth is essential. Dietary energy deficits have been estimated at 400 kcal per day.[8] Children with CD generally have higher energy requirements than children with UC.[8] The energy requirement for catch-up growth is 130% of the ideal requirement (50th percentile) for chronological age[19] or 60–75 kcal/kg actual body weight.[20,21] Age is used in the equation instead of height because many children are growth delayed. When a feeding protocol is initiated, caution and careful monitoring must be used in patients who are at risk for refeeding syndrome.

Protein requirements should be assessed according to disease status and body weight. Some patients have increased requirements caused by losses from inflammation, catabolism if an infection is present, or for wound healing if surgery is required.[8] Traditional recommendations were 1–1.5 times the RDA for age for protein.[22] This protein requirement is easily met when providing the volume of commercial formula needed to provide adequate calories for catch-up growth. However, repletion studies in children with CD suggest that up to 3 grams of protein per kilogram of body weight can improve body composition.[20] Therefore, specific recommendations for protein cannot be made at this time.

Micronutrients

Vitamin and mineral deficiencies are well documented in patients with IBD.[23] In the acute disease state, dietary intake of iron, zinc, copper, and vitamin C can be 20–50% below recommendations.[8] Serum or plasma concentrations are often used to define deficiency; however, interpretation of these findings and consequent treatment guidelines are not well established.

Water Soluble Vitamins

The status of folic acid, vitamin B_{12}, and other water soluble vitamins can be altered by intake, surgical resections, inflammation, and medication interactions. Low serum folate has been described in up to 60% of patients with IBD.[12,24] Folate can be protective against colon cancer in IBD because of its role in the synthesis and repair of DNA.[25] The minimum daily folic acid requirement for adults is 50 mcg, but requirements for patients with IBD can be 6–8 times higher.[26] The conventional recommendation of 1 mg per day can be an underestimation, and so blood levels should be monitored. The best indicator of folate status is red blood cell folate.[27] Patients who are supplemented with folate must have their vitamin B_{12} monitored periodically due to the possibility of masking deficiency.

Surgical resection, gastritis, ileitis, and bacterial overgrowth can all contribute to vitamin B_{12} deficiency.[28,29] Intramuscular supplementation of vitamin B_{12} has been the treatment of choice, but evidence suggests that high doses of oral synthetic B_{12} (1,000 mcg) might be effective for some patients.[30] Although serum deficiencies in vitamin B_6, vitamin C, thiamin, riboflavin, pantothenic acid, and biotin have been reported, clinical signs of these deficiencies rarely exist.[12]

Iron and Zinc

Iron is the most common nutrient deficiency found in patients with IBD, and it is caused by blood loss and inadequate intake.[31] These losses can be difficult to replete solely with diet. Iron supplementation typically involves oral ferrous sulphate or gluconate at 300 mg 1–3 times per day. An intramuscular form is also available, but might result in "tattooing." Intravenous iron preparations are available but concern about rare anaphylactic reaction limits their widespread use. More recently, an IV preparation of iron sucrose has become available. Iron sucrose has the advantage that allergic reactions are extremely rare but it must be delivered in small doses, making multiple infusions necessary.[32] Dietary and supplemental iron absorption can be enhanced when taken with 25–50 mg of vitamin C (found in 2–3 ounces of a drink containing vitamin C).[33] Monitoring of iron status should involve the measurement of hemoglobin and ferritin. Ferritin reflects total body stores and is the best correlate of iron deficiency. But ferritin is an acute phase reactant and for this reason it can be falsely normal in the acute disease state.[34]

Zinc status is affected by stool losses, inadequate intake, increased utilization, and reduced absorption.[35] It has been estimated that up to 15 mg of zinc can be lost in each liter of stool.[15] Zinc is important for the function of more than 300 metalloenzymes that perform multiple functions, including wound healing, growth, and cytokine production. There is currently no gold standard for assessing zinc status. Reduced serum and mucosal zinc has been reported in patients with UC and CD;[36,37] however, clinical symptoms of deficiency are rarely reported. Zinc supplementation of 25 mg per day is reported to reverse acrodermatitis[38] and increase small bowel permeability.[39] Zinc supplementation and growth failure is the subject of ongoing studies. As zinc is protein bound in the serum, it is difficult to determine the presence of functionally significant deficiency. Low levels can reflect hypoproteinemia rather than low tissue zinc.[36] Therefore, supplementation should be considered in the severely malnourished patient, in the presence of suggestive clinical findings, if diarrhea is present, or if ileostomy losses are high.

Calcium, Vitamin D, and Bone Disease

Long term steroid use, avoidance of dairy products, systemic inflammation, physical inactivity, and malabsorption[40] all contribute to the reduction in bone density seen in many pediatric IBD patients.[41] Corticosteroids reduce calcium absorption, decrease calcitriol synthesis and expression of calcium binding protein, inhibit osteoblast proliferation, and stimulate osteoclastic bone resorption.[42] Significant effects on bone are seen when taken in doses greater than 7.5 mg/day, 5,000 mg lifetime dose, or more than 12 months of exposure.[43] Patients with CD are more seriously affected than are those with UC.[41]

Effective treatment of bone disease relies on treatment of the underlying inflammatory bowel disease and provision of adequate calcium and vitamin D. The Dietary Reference Intakes for adolescents are 1,300 mg calcium and 200 IU vitamin D.[44] Calcium supplementation is particularly important for patients with lactose intolerance, dietary restriction, and malabsorption.[45] Annual bone density and serum alkaline phosphatase may be considered for screening. Scrutiny for lower serum alkaline phosphatase values than expected can be a useful indicator of an evolving problem.[17] When interpreting bone density, it is useful to correct for height age, bone age, or body mass index, because growth delay increases the apparent prevalence of osteopenia/osteoporosis.[42,46]

ORAL DIETS

No specific oral diet has been found to be an effective treatment for IBD. Pediatric patients should be encouraged to follow a well-balanced, regular diet as tolerated. Patients with CD who have an ileal stricture or obstruction during flares might require low fiber intake. A high fiber diet may be recommended for patients with an element of irritable bowel syndrome accompanying quiescent colitis. Many patients also require assistance with meeting caloric requirements and could benefit from a nutritional supplement (powders or liquids). Patients and families should be discouraged from eliminating food groups or major dietary components due to the risk of causing deficiencies.

INDICATIONS FOR PARENTERAL AND ENTERAL NUTRITION SUPPORT

Adjunctive Enteral Therapy

One of the main treatment goals in pediatric IBD is to prevent growth failure and achieve catch-up growth if failure has occurred.[1] Enteral nutrition (EN) as an adjunctive therapy to medications is used to supply the additional requirements for energy. Nutritional therapy improves the weight, lean body mass, and linear growth velocity of patients with active CD and concomitant growth failure.[20,47] Long term repletion studies in pediatric CD patients have demonstrated catch-up growth in weight and height with the provision of approximately 130% of the recommended energy for ideal body weight.[19–21]

Nutritional adjunctive therapy can also increase the effectiveness of medical therapies. It can result in a significant improvement in the CD activity index and a decrease in corticosteriod requirements.[20] Use of EN can also prolong corticosteroid induced remission.[48]

There are few contraindications to EN. Short bowel syndrome, intractable disease, bowel perforation, obstruction, or toxic megacolon can preclude the use of EN.[12]

Enteral Nutrition as a Primary Therapy

Sanderson demonstrated that an elemental diet was as effective as high dose steroids in the treatment of CD of the small bowel.[49] Several studies have since demonstrated that a good therapeutic response can be elicited with EN alone. Several meta-analyses concluded that EN is inferior to steroids;[50] however, many of the failures were due to formula intolerance and high dropout rates among subjects. A meta-analysis limited to pediatric patients found exclusive EN was similar to prednisone in the effectiveness of inducing remission.[51] Since EN is also able to improve nutritional status and growth and helps avoid the side effects of corticosteroids, it might be a better first choice for therapy in the pediatric population.

This therapy is avoided in many centers because of cost restrictions, a perceived burden on the child, and the requirement for significant staffing hours for teaching and tube feeding support for families. In centers where it is used successfully, many families choose tube feeding over steroids for subsequent flares. It has been demonstrated that EN increases the quality of life of children who undergo this therapy.[52]

Parenteral Nutrition as Primary or Adjunctive Therapy

Several decades ago, total parenteral nutrition (PN) was considered the standard of care for IBD. The use of PN decreased in many pediatric centers because EN was thought to prevent bacterial translocation and promote optimal gut function (see Chapter 16). There are several serious complications associated with PN that require weighing the pros and cons of its use. The costs are higher and most of the research on the safety and efficacy of PN has been completed in adults, not in children. However, PN plays an important role in the treatment of some patients with IBD.

PN should be considered for adjunctive or primary therapy when the enteral route is not available or has not been effective. EN might be contraindicated when the disease is complicated by fistula(s), short bowel syndrome, obstruction, perforation, or toxic megacolon.[53]

PN has been used to induce remission in patients who are steroid resistant or steroid dependent, with response rates of 40–90%.[54,55] However, many of the studies are complicated by concomitant use of medications.[56] There might be more of an advantage to using PN in patients who have CD than in UC. PN does not appear to provide an advantage over steroids for UC patients, but does so for CD patients.[57] PN can, however, provide significant nutritional repletion in UC and CD patients who do not tolerate EN.[53]

PN may also be used prior to surgery in severely malnourished patients in order to reduce postsurgical complications. Preoperative and postoperative PN decreases complications by 10%.[58] The preoperative advantage holds true only for severely malnourished patients.[59,60]

FORMULA SELECTION

Controversy exists over the ideal composition of formula for EN in IBD. Manipulations of protein and fat content and sources have now been joined by the addition of various prebiotics and growth factors.

Protein Source

Trials comparing elemental, semielemental and polymeric formulas all demonstrate improvements in disease activity scores, histological and serum markers of inflammation, and growth.[20,47,61] Theoretically, elemental diets were thought to be advantageous as they might promote gut healing through gut rest. *In vitro* and small *in vivo* studies demonstrated that elemental formulas decreased enterocyte permeability.[62,63] A 2001 meta-analysis concluded that the protein source in the formula did not have a significant difference on outcomes;[64] however, the analysis included a number of subtypes of formulas in each group. The cost of polymeric formulas is typically one third of that of elemental formulas, and so if there is no benefit derived from amino acids formulas compared to intact protein, polymeric formulas will likely dominate. This lack of benefit has not been firmly established.

Fat Source and Amount

The amount and type of fatty acids supplied in formulas has also come under scrutiny. Early formulas had low fat content (5–10% of energy) because it was thought that moderate fat intake (30% of energy) would overwhelm the ability of macrophages to remove microorganisms. Boosting proinflammatory luminal leukotrienes was also theorized to result from high fat formula.[12] There is currently no consensus on the ideal percent of fat that formulas should contain.[20,61,65,66]

Evidence suggests that the type of fat contained in a formula can affect outcome. A formula that contains a higher concentration of polyunsaturated fatty acids (PUFA) such as linoleic acid (n-6) compared to oleic acid was more successful in inducing remission (52% versus 20%).[67]

There could be an immunomodulatory role for n-3 PUFAs in patients with IBD. An increased ratio of n-6:n-3 PUFAs increases the arachadonic acid concentration of cell membranes and stimulates the production of proinflammatory prostaglandins and thromboxanes. A higher ratio of n-3:n-6 inhibits the production of cytokines such as tissue necrosis factor-alpha (TNF-alpha), which has been implicated in the proinflammatory process of IBD.

Studies in adults with UC demonstrated that supplementation with doses of 2.7 to 4.2 grams of n-3 fatty acids provided some clinical improvement and reduced steroid requirements.[68] Supplemental fish oils have also reduced the rate of relapse in adults with CD.[69] To date, trials of n-3 fatty acid supplementation or its addition to formulas have not been completed in children. The use of fish oils can be limited by side effects such as increased bleeding time and unpleasant taste; although these oils available in capsule formulations have been well tolerated in adults with UC.[69]

Prebiotics

Prebiotics are nondigestible food ingredients that can beneficially affect the host by selectively stimulating the growth or activity of some bacteria (see Chapter 3 for a discussion of prebiotics).[70] Examples of prebiotics include fructooligosaccharides, inulin, and lactulose. EN products and nutritional supplements that contain these ingredients are available. Prebiotics stimulate the colonization of *Bifidobacteria* and related species and might inhibit the colonization of more proinflammatory bacteria. These ingredients can further increase the bioavailabilty of minerals such as calcium, magnesium, and zinc and improve host defenses.[71] There are no controlled studies of prebiotics in children with IBD.

Probiotics

Probiotics are living organisms that, when ingested, can exert health benefits (see Chapter 3 for a discussion of probiotics). Most probiotics are nonpathogenic, gram-positive bacteria such as *Bifidobacterium* and *Lactobacillus*. These probiotics are found in naturally fermented dairy products, vegetables, and meats. *In vitro* studies have shown that these nonpathogenic bacteria block the production of inflammatory mediators[72] and so could be useful in the treatment of IBD.

Encouraging results have been obtained in human studies of prebiotics and IBD. Probiotics have been as effective as 5-ASA therapy in the induction of remission and prevention of relapse.[73,74] Probiotics have also been used effectively in the treatment of pouchitis.[75] Further research is needed to elucidate the effect of various strains, identify mechanisms by which they induce benefits, and establish dosing and safety standards.

Bioactive Peptides and Other Factors

There are several bioactive peptides under investigation for the treatment of IBD. Transforming growth factor-β, when included in a commercially available formula and given to pediatric CD patients, decreased pro-inflammatory cytokine mRNA in the gut mucosa.[76] Glutamine supplementation decreases intestinal permeability[77] but has not been demonstrated to improve clinical outcomes.[78]

PSYCHOSOCIAL IMPACT OF NUTRITION INTERVENTIONS

IBD, like other chronic conditions, places a significant emotional and psychological burden on the child and the family.[79] However, recent data suggests that between disease flares, children and adolescents cared for in a proactive, multidisciplinary clinic can be at least as emotionally healthy and well adjusted as community controls.[80]

There is little research on the impact of nutritional interventions on quality of life in adults or children with IBD. Anecdotally, many clinicians do not offer EN as an option because they view this therapy as a large burden on the child and family. EN protocols could entail long periods of food deprivation, the disruption of family activities, and a feeding system that has to be refilled in the middle of the night. Those children who leave their feeding tubes in place over the treatment period can be exposed to ridicule at school. Some patients also have emotional reactions to the placement of feeding tubes. EN requires significant motivation and is considered unappealing by up to 40% of patients.[81] By comparison, the side effects of steroids are well known and include cushinoid features, psychological effects, acne, hypertension, osteoporosis, and growth failure.[82] When given the choice, many families chose EN as an alternative to these side effects.

CONCLUSION

Caring for pediatric patients with IBD remains a challenge. The nutritional management is critical when growth and development are ongoing. A multidisciplinary team including a nurse, social worker, and dietitian facilitates the achievement of optimum nutritional status and health of children and adolescents with IBD.

REFERENCES

1. Escher JC, Taminiau JM. Treatment of inflammatory bowel disease in childhood. *Scand J Gastroenterol.* 2001;36(suppl 234):48–50.
2. Griffiths AM, Nguyen P, Smith C, MacMillan H, Sherman PM. Growth and clinical course of children with Crohn's disease. *Gut.* 1993;34:939–943.
3. Kanof ME, Lake AM, Bayless TM. Decreased height velocity in children and adolescents before the diagnosis of Crohn's disease. *Gastroenterology.* 1988;95(6):1523–1527.
4. Motil KJ, Grand RJ, Davis-Kraft L, Ferlic LL, Smith EO. Growth failure in children with inflammatory bowel disease: a prospective study. *Gastroenterology.* 1993;105:681–691.
5. Eiden KA. Nutritional considerations in inflammatory bowel disease. *Practical Gastroenterology* [serial online]. May 2003; series 5. Available at:
6. Motil KJ, Grand RJ. Nutritional management of inflammatory bowel disease. *Pediatr Clin North Am.* 1985;32:447–469.
7. Perkal MF, Seashore JH. Nutrition and inflammatory bowel disease. *Gastroenterol Clin North Am.* 1989;18:567–578.
8. Thomas AG, Taylor F, Miller V. Dietary intake and nutritional treatment in childhood Crohn's disease. *J Pediatr Gastroenterol Nutr.* 1993;17:75–81.
9. Ruuska T, Savilahti E, Maki M, Ormala T, Visakorpi J. Exclusive whole protein enteral diet versus prednisone in the treatment of acute Crohn's disease in children. *J Ped Gastr Nutr.* 1994;19:175–180.
10. Seidman E. Inflammatory bowel disease. In: Roy CC, Silverman A, Alagille E, eds. *Pediatric Clinical Gastroenterology*. 4th ed. St. Louis, Mo: CV Mosby; 1995:417–493.

11. Ghosh S, Cowen S, Hannan WJ, Ferguson A. Low bone mineral density in Crohn's disease, but not in ulcerative colitis, at diagnosis. *Gastroenterology*. 1994;107:1031–1039.
12. Seidman EG, Lelieko N, Ament M, Berman W, Caplan D, Evans J. Nutritional issues in pediatric inflammatory bowel disease. *J Pediatr Gastroenterol Nutr.* 1991;12:424–438.
13. Jahnsen J, Falch JA, Aadland E, Mowinckel P. Bone mineral density is reduced in patients with Crohn's disease but not in patients with ulcerative colitis: a population based study. *Gut.* 1997;40:313–319.
14. Green TJ, Issenman RM, Jacobson K. Patients' diets and preferences in a pediatric population with inflammatory bowel disease. *Can J Gastroenterol.* 1998;12:544–549.
15. Jeejeebhoy KN. Clinical nutrition: management of nutritional problems of patients with Crohn's disease. *CMAJ.* 2002;166:913–918.
16. Anderson CF, Wochos DN. The utility of serum albumin values in the nutritional assessment of hospitalized patients. *Mayo Clin Proc.* 1982;57:181–184.
17. Issenman RM. Bone mineral metabolism in pediatric inflammatory bowel disease. *Inflam Bowel Dis.* 1999;5(3):192–199.
18. Schneeweiss B, Lochs H, Zauner C, et al. Energy and substrate metabolism in patients with active Crohn's disease. *J Nutr.* 1999;129:844–848.
19. Belli DC, Seidman E, Bouthillier L, et al. Chronic intermittent elemental diet improves growth failure in children with Crohn's disease. *Gastroenterology.* 1988;94:603–610.
20. Khoshoo V, Reifen R, Neuman MG, Griffiths A, Pencharz PB. Effect of low- and high-fat, peptide-based diets on body composition and disease activity in adolescents with active Crohn's disease. *JPEN.* 1996;20:401–405.
21. Polk DB, Hattner JAT, Kerner JA. Improved growth and disease activity after intermittent administration of a defined formula diet in children with Crohn's disease. *JPEN.* 1992;16:499–504.
22. American Dietetic Association. *Manual of Clinical Dietetics*. 6th ed. Chicago, Ill; 2000.
23. Graham TO, Kandil HM. Nutritional factors in inflammatory bowel disease. *Gastroenterol Clin N Am.* 2002;31:203–218.
24. Elsborg L, Larsen L. Folate deficiency in chronic inflammatory bowel diseases. *Scand J Gastroenterol.* 1979;14:1019–1024.
25. Prinz-Langenohl R, Fohr I, Pietrzik K. Beneficial role for folate in the prevention of colorectal and breast cancer. *Eur J Nutr.* 2001;40:98–105.
26. Herbert V. Making sense of laboratory tests of folate status: folate requirement to sustain normality. *Am J Hematol.* 1987;26:199–207.
27. Pitkin RM. *Dietary Reference Intakes for Thiamin, Riboflavin, Niacin, Vitamin B_6, Folate, Vitamin B_{12}, Pantothenic Acid, Biotin and Choline*. Washington, DC: National Academy Press; 2000:196–305.
28. Imes S, Pinchbeck BR, Dinwoodie A, Walker K, Thomson AB. Iron, folate, vitamin B_{12}, zinc and copper status in outpatients with Crohn's disease: effect of diet counseling. *J Am Diet Assoc.* 1987;87:928–930.
29. Harries AD, Heatley RV. Nutritional disturbances in Crohn's disease. *Postgrad Med J.* 1983;59:690–697.
30. Kuzmininski AM, Del Giacco ET, Allen RH, Stabler SP, Lindenbaum J. Effective treatment of cobalamin deficiency with oral cobalamin. *Blood.* 1998;92:1191–1198.
31. Goldschmid S, Graha M. Trace element deficiencies in inflammatory bowel disease. *Gastrenterol Clin North Am.* 1989;18:570–587.
32. Chandler G, Harchowal B, Macdougall IC. Intravenous iron sucrose: establishing a safe dose. *Am J Kidney Dis.* 2001;38(5):988–991.
33. Czajka-Narins, DM. Minerals. In: Mahan LK, Escott-Stump S, eds. *Krause's Food, Nutrition and Diet Therapy*. Philadelphia, Pa: WB Saunders Company; 1996:123–166.
34. Thomson AB, Brust R, Ali MA, Mant MJ, Valberg LS. Iron deficiency in inflammatory bowel disease: diagnostic efficacy of serum ferritin. *Am J Dig Dis.* 1978;23:705–709.
35. Solomons NW, Rosenberg IH, Sandstead HH, et al. Zinc deficiency in Crohn's disease. *Digestion.* 1977;16:87–95.
36. Solomons NW. On the assessment of zinc and copper nutriture in man. *Am J Clin Nutr.* 1979;32:856–871.
37. Lih-Brody L, Powell SR, Collier KR, Reddy GM, Cerchia R, Kahn E. Increased oxidative stress and decreased anti-oxidant defenses in mucosa of inflammatory bowel disease. *Dig Dis Sci.* 1996;41:2078–2086.
38. Heimberger DC, Tamura T, Marks RD. Rapid improvement in dermatitis after zinc supplementation in a patient with Crohn's disease. *Am J Med.* 1990;88:71–73.
39. Sturniolo GC, DiLeoV, Ferronato A, D'Odorico A, D'Inca R. Zinc supplementation tightens "leaky gut" in Crohn's disease. *Inflamm Bowel Dis.* 2001;7:94–98.
40. Arden NK, Cooper C. Osteoporosis in patients with inflammatory bowel disease. *Gut.* 2002;50:9–10.
41. Abitbol V, Roux C, Chaussade S, et al. Metabolic bone assessment in patients with inflammatory bowel disease. *Gastroenterology.* 1995;108:417–422.
42. Issenman RM, Atkinson SA, Radoja C, Fraher L. Longitudinal assessment of growth, mineral metabolism, and bone mass in pediatric Crohn's disease. *J Pediatr Gastroenterol Nutr.* 1993;17:401–406.

43. Boot AM, Bouquet J, Krenning EP, de Muinck Keizer-Schrama SM. Bone mineral density and nutritional status in children with chronic inflammatory bowel disease. *Gut.* 1998;42:188–194.

44. NIH Consensus Statement. *Osteoporosis Prev Diagn Ther*. Mar 27–29, 2000;17:1–45.

45. Silvennoinen J, Lamberg-Allardt C, Karkainen M, Niemela S, Lehtola J. Dietary calcium intake and its relation to bone mineral density in patients with inflammatory bowel disease. *J Intern Med.* 1996;240:285–292.

46. Herzog D, Bishop N, Glorieux F, Seidman EG. Interpretation of bone mineral density values in pediatric Crohn's disease. *Inflam Bowel Dis.* 1998;4:261–267.

47. Raouf AH, Hildrey V, Daniel J, et al. Enteral feeding as sole treatment for Crohn's disease: a trial of whole protein v amino acid based feed and a case study of dietary challenge. *Gut.* 1991;32:702–707.

48. Wilschanski M, Sherman P, Pencharz P, Davis L, Corey M, Griffiths A. Supplementary enteral nutrition maintains remission in paediatric Crohn's disease. *Gut.* 1996;38:543–548.

49. Sanderson IR, Udeen S, Davies PS, Savage MO, Walker-Smith JA. Remission induced by an elemental diet in small bowel Crohn's disease. *Arch Dis Child.* 1987;61:123–127.

50. Fernandez-Banares F, Cabre E, Esteve-Comas M, Gassuli MA. How effective is enteral nutrition in inducing clinical remission in active Crohn's disease? A meta-analysis of the randomized clinical trials. *JPEN.* 1995;19:356–364.

51. Heuschkel RB, Menachac L, Megerian JT, Baird AE. Enteral nutrition and corticoid steroids in the treatment of acute Crohn's disease in children. *J Ped Gastro Nutr.* 2000;31:8–15.

52. Hussey T, Issenman RM, Persad R, Otley AR, Christensen BA. Nutrition therapy in pediatric Crohn's disease improves nutritional status and decreases inflammation. *J Pediatr Gastrenerol Nutr.* 2003;37:341. Abstract 45.

53. Jeejeebhoy KN. Total parenteral nutrition: potion of poison? *Am J Clin Nutr.* 2001;74:160–163.

54. Kushner RF, Shapir J, Sitrin MD. Endoscopic, radiographic, and clinical response to prolonged bowel rest and home parenteral nutrition in Crohn's disease. *JPEN.* 1986;10:568–573.

55. Lerebours E, Messing B, Chevalier B, et al. An evaluation of total parenteral nutrition in the management of steroid-dependent and steroid-resistant patients with Crohn's disease. *JPEN.* 1986;10:274–278.

56. Ostro MJ, Greenberg GR, Jeejeebhoy KN. Total parenteral nutrition and complete bowel rest in the management of Crohn's disease. *JPEN.* 1985;9:280–284.

57. Seo M, Okada M, Yao T, et al. The role of total parenteral nutrition in the management of patients with acute attacks of inflammatory bowel disease. *J Clin Gastroenterol.* 1999;29:223–224.

58. Klein S, Kinney J, Jeejeebhoy K, et al. Nutrition support in clinical practice: review of published data and recommendations for future research directions. National Institutes of Health, American Society for Parenteral and Enteral Nutrition and American Society for Clinical Nutrition. *JPEN.* 1997;21:133–156.

59. Gouma DJ, von Meyenfeldt MF, Rouflart M, et al. Preoperative total parenteral nutrition in severe Crohn's disease surgery. *Surgery.* 1988;103:648–662.

60. Han PD, Burke A, Baldassano RN, Rombeau JL, Lichtenstein GR. Nutrition and inflammatory bowel disease. *Gastro Clin N Am.* 1999;28:423–443.

61. Royall D, Jeejeebhoy DN, Baker JP, et al. Comparison of amino acid v peptide based enteral diets in active Crohn's disease: clinical and nutritional outcome. *Gut.* 1994;35:783–787.

62. Teahon K, Smethurst P, Pearson M, Levi AJ, Biarnason I. The effect of elemental diet on intestinal permeability and inflammation in Crohn's disease. *Gastroenterology.* 1991;101:84–89.

63. Mayer L, Eisenhardt D. Lack of induction of suppressor T cells by intestinal epithelial cells from patients with inflammatory bowel disease. *J Clin Invest.* 1990;86:1255–1260.

64. Zachos M, Tondeur M, Griffiths, AM. Enteral nutrition therapy for inducing remission of Crohn's disease. *Cochrane Database of Systematic Reviews.* 2001;38: CD000542.

65. Bamba T, Shimoyama T, Sasaki M et al. Dietary fat attenuates the benefits of an elemental diet in active Crohn's disease: a randomized, controlled trial. *Eur J Gastroenterol Hep.* 2003;15:151–157.

66. Leiper K, Wooner J, Mullan MM, et al. A randomized controlled trial of high versus low long chain triglyceride whole protein feed in active Crohn's disease. *Gut.* 2001;49:790–794.

67. Gassull MA, Fernandez-Banares F, Cabre E, et al. Fat composition may be a clue to explain the primary therapeutic effect of enteral nutrition in Crohn's disease: results of a double blind randomized European trial. *Gut.* 2002;51:164–168.

68. O'Morain C, Tobin A, McColl T, Suzuki Y. Fish oil in the treatment of ulcerative colitis. *Can J Gastroenterol.* 1990;4:420–423.

69. Belluzzi A, Brignola C, Campieri M, Pera A, Boschi S, Miglioli M. Effect of an enteric-coated fish-oil preparation on relapses in Crohn's disease. *New Engl J Med.* 1996;334:1557–1560.

70. Schrezenmeir J, Vrese M. Probiotics, prebiotics and synbiotics—approaching a definition. *Amer J Clin Nutr.* 2001;73:361S–364S.

71. Sentongo TA, Semeao EJ, Stettler N, Piccoli DA, Stallings VA, Zemel BS. Vitamin D status in children,

adolescents, and young adults with Crohn's disease. *Am J Clin Nutr.* 2002;76:1077–1081.

72. Neish AS, Gewirtz AT, Zeng H, et al. Prokaryotic regulation of epithelial responses by inhibition of kappa B-alpha ubiquitination. *Science.* 2000;289:1560–1563.
73. Kruis W, Schutz E, Fric P, Fixa B, Judmaier G, Sotolte M. Double-blind comparison of an oral *Escherichia coli* preparation and mesalazine in maintaining remission of ulcerative colitis. *Aliment Pharmacol Ther.* 1997;11:853–858.
74. Rembacken B, Snelling A, Hawkey P, Chalmers D, Axon A. Non-pathogenic *Escherichia coli* versus mesalazine for the treatment of ulcerative colitis: a randomized trial. *Lancet.* 1999;354:635–639.
75. Gionchetti P, Rizzello F, Venturi A, et al. Oral bacteriotherapy as maintenance treatment in patients with chronic pouchitis: a double-blind, placebo-controlled trial. *Gastroenterology.* 2000;119:305–309.
76. Fell JM, Paintin M, Arnaud-Battandier F, Beattie RM, Hollis A, Kitching P, Donnet-Hughes A, MacDonald TT, Walker-Smith JA. Mucosal healing and a fall in mucosal pro-inflammatory cytokine mRNA induced by a specific oral polymeric diet in paediatric Crohn's disease. *Alimentary Pharmacology.* 2000;14:281–289.
77. van der Hulst RR, van Kreel BK, von Meyenfeldt MF, Brummer RJ, Arends JW, Deutz NE, Soeters PB. Glutamine and the preservation of gut integrity. *Lancet.* 1993;334:1363–1365.
78. Akobeng AK, Miller V, Stanton J, Elbadri AM, Thomas AG. Double blind randomized controlled trial of glutamine-enriched polymeric diet in the treatment of active Crohn's disease. *J Pediatr Gastroenterol Nutr.* 2000;30:78–84.
79. Engström I. Family interaction and locus of control in children and adolescents with inflammatory bowel disease. *J Am Acad Child Adolesc Psychiatry.* 1991;33:563–582.
80. Gold N, Issenman R, Roberts J, Watt S. Well-adjusted children: an alternate view of children with inflammatory bowel disease and functional gastrointestinal complaints. *Inflam Bowel Dis.* 2000;6:1–7.
81. Bouthillier L, Herzog D, Seidman EG. Acceptance and tolerance of a flavoured peptide-based formula in pediatric Crohn's disease. Poster presented at the 19th Annual Congress of the American Society for Parenteral and Enteral Nutrition. January 1995; Miami Beach, Fla.
82. Baldassano RN. Anti-TNF therapies have eliminated the need for steroids in pediatric Crohn's disease: why use steroids if safer therapies are available? *Inflam Bowel Dis.* 2001;7:338–341.

CHAPTER 32

Nutrition Support for Renal Disease

Nancy Spinozzi

INTRODUCTION

The nutritional treatment of chronic kidney disease (CKD) in pediatric patients is a challenging and dynamic task. CKD encompasses chronic renal insufficiency (CRI) when reduced kidney function can be controlled through diet and medications alone, and it includes kidney failure when the additional treatments of dialysis and/or transplantation become necessary. As patients progress from CRI to kidney failure, many changes in diet and medications need to take place and regular monitoring of patients' responses to these changes are critical. The diet must be modified according to the level of kidney function and to ensure optimal growth and development.[1] Since the advent of recombinant growth hormone use in this population, normal growth for age is possible and expected. Pediatric programs that treat children with CKD consist of a team of many specialists, and the dietitian is one of its prominent members. Because of the chronicity of the disease and the fact that currently there is no cure for kidney failure, patients are followed for long periods of time by this team of specialists.[2] Knowledge of the nutritional needs of children and young adults of all ages is necessary.

In 1997 the National Kidney Foundation, Inc (NKF) published the first set of evidence-based clinical practice guidelines: the Kidney Disease Outcomes Quality Initiative (K/DOQI). Pediatric renal nutrition guidelines were forthcoming in 2000 in the publication, *Nutrition in Chronic Renal Failure.*[3] These and all guidelines of K/DOQI can be accessed through the NKF web site, http://www.kidney.org.[4] Additional professional resources are available through NKF and the American Dietetic Association web site, http://www.eatright.org.[5]

NUTRITIONAL NEEDS AND LIMITATIONS

Attention to nutrition is important to the treatment of CKD as many patients do not follow normal growth and development patterns. Factors such as poor oral intake and decreased appetite, acidosis, renal bone disease, and growth hormone resistance contribute to poor growth. Infants and adolescents are at the greatest risk for growth failure because of their rapid growth rates. CKD presents many nutritional challenges, including the loss of protein via dialysate for peritoneal dialysis patients.[6] These patients require protein intakes in excess of the Recommended Dietary Allowance (RDA) for age.

PROTEIN AND ENERGY

Protein requirements for children with CRI/CKD should closely approximate the RDA for age. Rarely should protein be restricted below this level. It is important for children to receive at least the RDA for calories for age, based on their dry weight. In fact, it is not unusual for children to require more if there are compounding medical conditions such as prematurity or bronchopulmonary disease.

Poor appetites and complicated medication regimes often challenge caregivers to ensure optimal caloric intake. Also, many infants with CRI experience gastroesophageal reflux.[7,8] Therefore, supplemental nutrition is often indicated. Although available, intradialytic parenteral nutrition (IDPN) is used infrequently because it might not be a cost-effective method for delivering nutrition to pediatric patients on hemodialysis. On the other hand, supplemental oral nutritional products and tube feedings are highly effective in promoting optimal nutrition intake. There are several nutritional products on the market today designed specifically for CKD patients; however, almost any commercially available complete pediatric formula could be appropriate. Although some adult renal formulas can be used for children, they must be carefully considered in light of a child's needs. For example, Nepro is an excellent source of calories for dialysis patients, but its protein content (70 gm/liter) is too high for a child. In this case, Suplena (30 gm/liter) would be a better choice. The obvious drawback to most enteral supplements is their contribution to fluid intake in fluid restricted patients. If a dialysis patient is dependent on supplements to meet his or her nutritional needs, more rigorous or frequent dialysis treatments might be necessary. Calories from the glucose absorbed by patients on peritoneal dialysis might or might not be counted toward their daily caloric intake since these calories can account for as much as 7–10 kcal/kg.[9] In the case of infants requiring severe fluid limitations, it is often necessary to increase the caloric density of their formula to meet their nutritional needs.[10] Most institutions concentrate formula up to 30 calories/oz to achieve higher calories; this will also concentrate the electrolyte and mineral content of the formula. For children with renal disease, modular caloric sources, such as glucose polymers and canola oil, are preferable.[11,12] On the other hand, polyuric infants face a significant risk for dehydration and failure to thrive from severe sodium, potassium, and water wasting. In these cases, the use of high volume/low solute tube feedings is indicated.[13]

Enteral tube feeding should be considered for any patient unable to meet nutritional goals orally.[14,15] If medication is to be delivered via the tube, it is important to ensure appropriate tube placement (gastric versus jejunal) (see Chapter 20 for a discussion of tube feedings).

Despite the best attempts at ensuring adequate calorie and protein nutrition, at some point the initiation of recombinant growth hormone becomes necessary.[16] Regular assessment of growth and development should include frequent dietary interviews, at least monthly assessments of heights/lengths, dry weights, and head circumference until 3 years of age, and serum albumin, calcium, phosphorus, and parathyroid hormone (PTH) levels.[3,17] Maintaining PTH levels between 2 and 3 times normal is critical to prevent renal bone disease (renal osteodystrophy or adynamic bone disease).[18,19] Once a child has received a kidney transplant, growth hormone should be discontinued.

LIPIDS

Hyperlipidemia is common in children with CKD, particularly in those on peritoneal dialysis. However, treatment is not advised at this time.[9]

Hyperlipidemia has become more common in transplant patients due to the increased use of the immunosuppressant sirolimus. Treatment usually requires lipid-lowering medication in addition to dietary modification.

SODIUM AND FLUID

Most children with CKD require some restriction of dietary sodium to help maintain normal blood pressure. In the case of hemodialysis patients, adherence to a no added salt diet prevents excessive thirst that could result in fluid overload. Peritoneal dialysis patients might or might not require less fluid and salt restriction; therefore it is important to monitor blood pressure and weights carefully. After transplantation, children are encouraged to drink in abundance; however, sodium restriction for the short term could still be necessary to help control blood pressure.

For children who cannot concentrate their urine (such as infants with obstructive uropathy), sodium (and potassium) intake must be supplemented, and free water intake must be enough to prevent dehydration.[13]

POTASSIUM

Potassium restriction is not necessary until kidney function is less than 5% of normal. This usually coincides with the initiation of dialysis treatments. Prior to this time, a patient might be on an angiotensin converting enzyme (ACE) inhibitor to reduce proteinuria. Hyperkalemia is often a side effect of this treatment. Limiting foods that contain large amounts of potassium is usually enough to maintain a child's serum potassium within normal range. If not, then a potassium exchange resin must be prescribed. The resin is most often required for infants. Transition to an infant formula containing reduced amounts of sodium and potassium could prove helpful in this situation. However, it should be noted that the calcium and phosphorus content is also reduced in these formulas and might not be enough to sustain normal growth.[12] Attention should be given to the method of increasing caloric density of infant formulas as well.

CALCIUM AND PHOSPHORUS

In order to maintain normal calcium and phosphorus levels, several approaches are taken, usually concomitantly.[20,21] Restriction of dietary phosphorus includes the limitation of foods such as dairy products, colas, and chocolate. Since most foods contain various amounts of phosphorus, phosphate binders are often prescribed to be taken with meals and snacks. These binders usually contain calcium (as calcium carbonate or calcium acetate) and serve as calcium supplements as well, since a diet low in phosphorus is low in calcium. It is important to correct serum phosphorus levels before calcium supplementation is initiated. Finally, supplementation of the active form of vitamin D (1,25 $[OH]_2D$) is necessary for calcium absorption from the gastrointestinal tract. For patients who cannot tolerate calcium containing phosphate binders due to hypercalcemia, sevelamer hydrochloride[22] or lanthanum carbonate can be used to bind dietary phosphorus. Neither of these products come in liquid or powder form. For a list of many of the available and commonly used phosphate binders, see Tables 32-1 and 32-2.

Table 32-1 Calcium-based binders/supplements.

Compound	*Name*	*Dose*	*Elemental Ca + +*
Calcium Acetate	PhosLo Gelcap (Braintree)	667 mg	169 mg
	Hil-Cal (Hillstad)	670 mg	170 mg
Calcium Carbonate	Suspension	1,250 mg/5mL	500 mg
	Calci-Chew (Watson)	1,250 mg	500 mg
	Calci-Mix (Watson)	1,250 mg	500 mg
	Cal-100 (United Nutrition)	2,500 mg	1,000 mg
	Caltrate 600 (Whitehall-Robins)	1,500 mg	600 mg
	Nephro-Calci (Watson)	1,500 mg	600 mg
	Oscal 500 (Whitehall-Robins)	1,250 mg	500 mg
	TUMS (GlaxoSmithKline)	500 mg	200 mg
	TUMS E-X (GlaxoSmithKline)	750 mg	300 mg
	TUMS Ultra (GlaxoSmithKline)	1,000 mg	400 mg
	TUMS 500 (GlaxoSmithKline)	1,250 mg	500 mg
	Viactiv (McNeil Nutritionals)	1,250 mg	500 mg
Calcium Glubionate	Syrup	360 mg/mL	23 mg/mL

Table 32-2 Calcium-free/aluminum-free binders.

Compound	*Name brand*	*Form*
Sevelamer hydrochloride	Renagel (Genzyme)	Renagel tablets 800 mg
Lanthanum carbonate	Fosrenal (Shire)	Tablets—*chewable only!*

Children who take recombinant growth hormone should be regularly monitored for adequate calcium and phosphorus intakes to ensure optimal growth. The dose of phosphate binders can be reduced in these cases.

VITAMINS AND MINERALS

Because children with CRI/CKD experience at least occasional periods of anorexia and suboptimal nutrient intake, it is reasonable to recommend a pediatric multivitamin (see Chapter 25 for a discussion of vitamins). Once dialysis is initiated, and if the child is able to take pills, a dialysis vitamin containing water soluble vitamins and folate should be prescribed. If liquid or chewable vitamins are all a child can manage, the pediatric multivitamin should be continued either on a daily or every other day regimen, depending on the child's usual dietary intake. Folate should be supplemented to at least the RDA for age. There is limited data regarding the status of fat-soluble vitamins in pediatric patients with kidney disease, so blood levels should be measured periodically, particularly vitamin A.[23]

Secondary carnitine deficiency has been reported in adult dialysis patients.[24] Patients on maintenance hemodialysis are at high risk for deficiency because of reduced intake of meat and dairy products, reduced synthesis, and dialytic losses. Clinical conditions such as malaise, muscle weakness, cardiomyopathy, and arrhythmias could be related to carnitine deficiency. The safety and efficacy of oral carnitine have not been established, and so there is no concensus in pediatric programs regarding treating children with carnitine.

Children should take an iron supplement either orally or by periodic IV infusion, especially if they are receiving recombinant erythropoietin. In order to ensure optimal absorption, the patient might be advised to take the oral iron with a beverage high in vitamin C (and low in potassium if on dialysis).

PARENTERAL NUTRITION

In the event that parenteral nutrition becomes necessary, special attention to the patient's renal function and individual tolerance to nutrients is critical. The first consideration should be given to the allowable fluid volume. In severely fluid restricted patients, it might not be possible to achieve even close to adequate calories. Dependence on lipids is common, but in children with hypertriglyceridemia, this might not be wise. Also, hemodialysis patients might require 4–7 days of dialysis/ultrafiltration weekly instead of the usual 3. And, finally, daily monitoring of potassium, phosphorus, calcium, and magnesium is necessary and could result in constant manipulation of the solution. Initially, potassium and phosphorus content might be minimal or absent, but once a patient becomes anabolic, it is necessary to provide adequate electrolytes and minerals to support growth.

TRANSPLANTATION

Since the advent of growth hormone, children need not be transplanted early simply to avoid growth retardation. However, growth resumes normally after successful transplantation without the need for supplemental growth hormone therapy.[25,26]

There are many immunosuppression protocols being studied in pediatric transplant centers. If a patient is on a steroid free protocol, it should not be necessary to restrict sodium in the post-transplant diet, but a no–added salt diet might be prudent. Also, patients who have hypertension, whether treated with steroids or not, benefit from sodium restriction. Phosphate supplementation is indicated for many patients even with normal kidney function. Parents whose children required tube feeding prior to transplant will find the tube helpful to ensure adequate fluid intake in the months immediately after transplant. It is the experience of many programs that children begin to eat very well after transplant, and they use the tube solely to meet fluid requirements.

CONCLUSION

Nutrition therapy is an integral part of treatment for the pediatric patient with CRI/CKD. Dietary recommendations must be appropriate for the level of kidney function and must support normal growth and development. Infants especially need very close monitoring and follow-up. Each patient's nutrition plan must be individualized, assessed frequently, and modified as needed.[11]

REFERENCES

1. Rees L, Rigden SPA, Ward GM. Chronic renal failure and growth. *Arch Dis Child.* 1989;64:573–577.
2. Harvey E, Secker D, Braj B, Picone G, Balfe JW. The team approach to the management of children on chronic peritoneal dialysis. *Adv Renal Replacement Ther.* 1996;3:3–13.
3. National Kidney Foundation. K/DOQI clinical practice guidelines for nutrition in chronic renal failure. *Am J Kidney Dis*. 2000;35:S105–S136.
4. National Kidney Foundation, http://www.kidney.org/Professionals/kdoqi/index.cfm. Accessed March 14, 2006.
5. American Dietetic Association, http://www.eatright.org. Accessed March 14, 2006.
6. Quan A, Baum M. Protein losses in children on continuous cycled peritoneal dialysis. *Pediatr Nephrol.* 1996;10:728–731.
7. Ravelli AM, Ledermann SE, Bisset WM, et al. Foregut motor function in chronic renal failure. *Arch Dis Child.* 1992;67:1343–1347.
8. Ruley EJ, Boch GH, Kerzner B, Abbott AW. Feeding disorders and gastroesophageal reflux in infants with chronic renal failure. *Pediatr Nephrol.* 1989;3:424–429.
9. Secker D, Pencharz MB. Nutritional therapy for children on CAPD/CCPD: Theory and practice. In: Fine RN, Alexander SR, Warady BA, eds. *CAPD/CCPD in Children*. Boston, Mass: Kluwer Academic; 1998:567–603.
10. Yiu VWY, Harmon WE, Spinozzi N, et al. High-calorie nutrition for infants with chronic renal disease. *J Renal Nutr.* 1996;6:203–206.
11. Spinozzi NS, Nelson P. Nutrition support in the newborn intensive care unit. *J Renal Nutr.* 1996;6:188–197.
12. Spinozzi N. Chronic renal disease. In: Samour PQ, King K, eds. *Handbook of Pediatric Nutrition.* 3rd ed. Sudbury, Mass: Jones and Bartlett Publishers; 2005:381–389.
13. Parekh RS, Flynn JT, Smoyer WE, et al. Improved growth in young children with severe chronic renal insufficiency who use specified nutritional therapy. *J Am Soc Nephrol.* 2001;12:2418–2426.
14. Brewer ED. Supplemental enteral tube feeding in infants undergoing dialysis: indications and outcome. *Sem Dial.* 1994;7:429–434.
15. Ledermann SE, Spitz L, Moloney J, et al. Gastrostomy feeding in infants and children on peritoneal dialysis. *Pediatr Nephrol.* 2002;17:246–250.
16. Fine RN, Kohout EC, Brown D, Perlman AJ. Growth after recombinant human growth hormone treatment in children with chronic renal failure: report of a multicenter randomized double-blind placebo-controlled study. *J Pediatr.* 1994;124:374–382.
17. Abitol C, Chan JC, Trachtman H, et al. Growth in children with moderate renal insufficiency: measurement, evaluation, and treatment. *J Pediatr.* 1996;129:S3–S8.
18. Sanchez CP, Salusky IB. The renal bone disease in children treated with dialysis. *Adv in Renal Replacement Ther*. 1996;3:14–23.
19. Abitol CL, Zilleruelo G, Montane B, Strauss J. Growth of uremic infants on forced feeding regimens. *Pediatr Nephrol*. 1993;7:173–177.
20. Salusky IB, Goodman WG. The management of renal osteodystrophy. *Pediatr Nephrol.* 1996;10:651–653.
21. Sedman A, Friedman A, Boineau F, Strife CF, Fine R. Nutritional management of the child with mild to moderate chronic renal failure. *J Pediatr*. 1996;129:13S–18S.
22. Mahdavi H, Kuizon BD, Gales, et al. Sevelamer hydrochloride: an effective phosphate binder in dialyzed children. *Pediatr Nephrol.* 2003;18:1260–1264.

23. Warady BA, Kriley M, Alon U, Hellerstein S. Vitamin status of infants receiving long-term peritoneal dialysis. *Pediatr Nephrol.* 1994;8:354–356.

24. Eknoyan G, Latos DL, Lindberg J. Practice recommendations for the dialysis-related carnitine disorder. *AJKD.* 2003;41:868–876.

25. Harmon WE. Pediatric renal transplantation. In: Avner ED, Harmon WE, Niaudet P, eds. *Pediatric Nephrology.* 5th ed. Philadelphia, Pa: Lippincott, Williams & Wilkens; 2004:1437–1468.

26. Fine RN. Growth following solid-organ transplantation. *Pediatr Transplant.* 2002;6:47–52.

CHAPTER 33

Enteral and Parenteral Nutrition Therapy in Inherited Metabolic Disease

Steven Yannicelli and Kathryn Camp

INTRODUCTION

Inherited metabolic diseases are individually rare but collectively common. Inborn errors result in morbidity and mortality that can be ameliorated by aggressive and lifelong nutrition therapy. Nutrition management of patients with inborn errors is the first example of "nutrigenomics," that is, dietary substances interacting with a person's genotype to influence clinical outcome.

Garrod's discovery of alcaptonuria in 1908[1] was the first description of an inherited metabolic disease. Discovery of phenylketonuria (PKU) by Fölling in 1934[2] identified people in whom risk of mental retardation could be predicted by neonatal biochemical tests. Technical advances led to the description of numerous inherited metabolic diseases. Nearly one hundred inherited metabolic diseases can now be diagnosed in the neonatal period.[3] For each disorder, identification of specific abnormal metabolites leads to an understanding of the disorder and is key to clinical and nutrition management.

Expanded newborn screening programs have dramatically increased detection rates of inborn errors.[4] More cases of inherited metabolic diseases are identified by tandem mass spectroscopy screening than are diagnosed by their clinical presentation.[5] Early detection and treatment helps patients live longer. Intensive clinical and nutrition therapies are paramount for survival and quality of life.

Nutrition is an integral part of, and in many cases primary therapy for, management of patients with inherited metabolic diseases. For example, the benefit of a phenylalanine (PHE) restricted diet for PKU was described by Bickel and associates in 1953[6] after it was shown that reducing dietary PHE improved the biochemical imbalance of the patient. Studies have since revealed that early diagnosis and lifelong diet intervention results in normal intellectual development in patients with classic PKU.

Nutrition therapy for patients with inborn errors advanced our understanding of the requirements for various essential amino acids, fats, carbohydrates, vitamins, and minerals in healthy individuals, as well as in individuals with metabolic disorders. The first special dietary formulations for inherited metabolic diseases (e.g., PKU) were made from casein hydrolysates or free amino acids. It was not until several years later that special metabolic formulas (i.e., medical foods) were commercially available. Currently, a variety of commercial medical foods is available for treatment of various inherited metabolic diseases, and is used in combination with other nutrition and medical therapies (Appendix C).

The goal of this chapter is to provide a working knowledge of chronic and acute nutrition therapy for inherited defects in protein, carbo-

The views expressed in this chapter are those of the authors and do not reflect the official policy of the Department of the Army, the Department of Defense, or the U.S. Government.

hydrate, and lipid metabolism. Some inherited metabolic diseases that could respond to specific nutrition therapies are listed in Table 33-1. For a complete guide on clinical treatment and diagnostics see Suggested Reading and Resources (Appendix C).

Table 33-1 Nutrition therapies in selected metabolic disorders.

Disorder	*Nutrition therapy (other therapies)*
Aminoacidopathies	
Phenylketonuria (classic) (PKU)	Restrict phenylalanine Supplement tyrosine Tetrahydrobiopterin (?)
Hyperphenylalaninemia	Tetrahydrobiopterin Slight to moderate phenylalanine restriction
Biopterin deficiency	Slight to moderate phenylalanine restriction Tetrahydrobiopterin and dopaminergic drugs
Tyrosinemia type I	Restrict phenylalanine/tyrosine Nitisinome (NTBC)
Neonatal tyrosinemia	Low-protein diet Ascorbic acid*
Tyrosinemia type II (Richner-Hanhart)	Restrict phenylalanine and tyrosine
Maple syrup urine disease (MSD)	Restrict branched-chain amino acids (isoleucine, leucine, valine) Thiamin in thiamin-responsive MSD
Homocystinuria (HCU)	Restrict methionine Supplement cystine Supplement methyl-donors (e.g., betaine, folate) Pyridoxine* (approx. 50% of patients are responsive)
Organic acidemias	
Isovaleric acidemia (IVA)	Restrict leucine Carnitine (100–300 mg) and glycine supplementation (250 mg/kg)
Methylmalonic and propionic acidemia (MMA, PPA, respectively)	Restrict isoleucine, methionine, threonine, valine; odd-chain fatty acids Hydroxycobalamin (oral 1–2 mg/day; IM 1–2 mg/week) for defects in cobalamin metabolism (MMA disorders) Carnitine supplementation (100–300 mg/kg) D-biotin (PPA) (10–20 mg/day) (?)
Glutaric acidemia type I (GA-I)	Restrict lysine and tryptophan Riboflavin* (100–200 mg/day) Carnitine supplementation (100–300 mg/kg)
Glutaric acidemia type II (GA-II) (multiple acyl CoA dehydrogenase deficiency)	Restrict fat (20–25%) (provide sufficient essential fatty acids) Carnitine supplementation (100 mg/kg/day) Avoid fasting; offer frequent feedings Riboflavin* (100–200 mg/day)

Table 33-1 Nutrition therapies in selected metabolic disorders (continued).

Disorder	*Nutrition therapy (other therapies)*
Carbohydrate Disorders	
Galactosemia (classic)	Restrict galactose (< 50 mg/day)
Galactosemia (Duarte Variant)	Restrict galactose for at least the first year of life
Hereditary fructose intolerance (HFI)	Fructose- and sorbitol-free (< 10 mg/kg/day)
Pyruvate carboxylase (PC) deficiency	High fat, low carbohydrate, modified ketogenic diet Biotin*
Pyruvate dehydrogenase (PDH) deficiency	Same as for pyruvate carboxylase deficiency Thiamin*, lipoic acid* Alkali therapy (e.g., $NaHCO_3$)
Glycogen Storage Diseases	
Type I (glucose-6-phosphatase deficiency)	Restrict galactose and fructose Low fat, moderate protein, high complex carbohydrates (approximately 60% total energy) Frequent feedings, nocturnal feeds Uncooked cornstarch
Type III (amylo-1,6-glucosidase deficiency)	Same as for type I, except higher protein
Type IV (phosphorylase kinase deficiency)	High protein Frequent feedings
Lipid Disorders	
Medium chain acyl-CoA dehydrogenase deficiency (MCAD)	Moderate fat restriction (30%) (Avoid MCT oil) Carnitine supplementation (if indicated) Frequent feedings Avoid fasting Uncooked cornstarch (?)
Long chain hydroxyl-acyl dehydrogenase deficiency (LCHAD)	Fat-modified diet (approximately 25% total fat) Provide MCT oil (approximately 50% of fat energy) Uncooked cornstarch (?) Frequent feedings Avoid fasting
Abetalipoproteinemia	Restrict long-chain fatty acids (approximately 15% total energy) Provide adequate linoleic acid (3% total energy) Provide adequate α-linolenic acid (1% total energy) Supplement fat-soluble vitamins A, E, and K; folate; iron

Table 33-1 Nutrition therapies in selected metabolic disorders (continued).

Disorder	*Nutrition therapy (other therapies)*
Peroxisomal Disorders	
Adrenoleukodystrophy	Low fat diet Supplement with Lorenzo's oil (Nutricia North America, Gaithersburg, Md.)
Urea Cycle Disorders	Low protein diet with essential amino acids Supplement arginine except in argininemia or citrulline, except in citrullinemia Citrate supplements (esp. in argininemia)

Diets or therapies denoted by (?) indicate those that are investigative and/or questionable in regards to their effectiveness.

* Those products are prescribed in pharmacologic doses to patients who are considered clinically responsive to coenzyme therapy. Those patients who are clinically responsive might not require other nutrition therapies.

GENERAL PRINCIPLES OF METABOLISM AND NUTRITION THERAPY IN INHERITED METABOLIC DISEASES

General principles of metabolism are illustrated in Figure 33-1. Some enzymes function independently. Others require a cofactor or a coenzyme, which can be recycled by enzyme-mediated steps. Some biochemical pathways are ubiquitous; others are organ or tissue specific. Metabolic abnormalities have been associated with maturational defects in pathways. Maturation continues to occur after birth. Most inherited metabolic diseases are single gene defects with multiple mutations and are usually autosomal recessive but occasionally X-linked or autosomal dominant.

There is a wide range of clinical expression in inherited metabolic diseases due in part to polymorphism (occurrence in more than one form) in the affected gene. For this reason, a direct relationship between genotype and phenotype and phenotype and metabolite is not absolute. Polymorphism in defective genes influences enzyme activity that in turn impacts response to nutrition intervention.

Clinical symptoms are caused by abnormal metabolism. Usually, clinical expression is related to elevated or reduced concentrations of some measurable compound, but sometimes, the exact pathophysiology remains enigmatic. For most metabolic disorders, short term effects are reversible. Long term, irreversible damage occurs if the disorder is untreated. Timely treatment might lessen adverse outcomes, but permanent damage could be present at diagnosis before intervention is possible. A specific metabolite deficiency might directly or indirectly effect outcome. An example of a direct affect is the formation of cataracts by galactitol accumulation in the lens of patients with galactosemia. In galactokinase deficiency, one form of galactosemia, accumulation of galactitol accounts for most clinical manifestations. In classic galactosemia, a defect in galactose-1-phosphate uridyl-transferase, accumulation of galactitol also causes cataracts. However, these patients also have hepatic, renal, and brain involvement caused by accumulation of tissue galactose-1-phosphate and not galactitol toxicity.

In some inherited metabolic diseases secondary biochemical alterations occur. An example of an indirect effect is hyperammonemia in propionic and methylmalonic acidemia.[7,8]

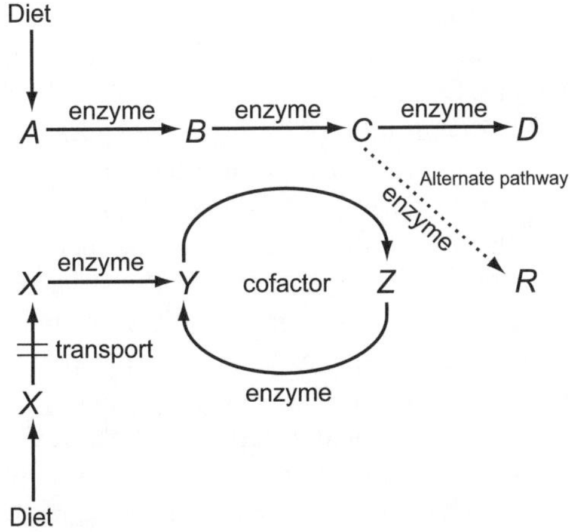

Figure 33-1 General principles of metabolism. Virtually all reactions are controlled by enzymes coded for by genes. Any product can have more than one metabolic fate or origin, and some reactions proceed in either direction depending on biochemical conditions. A transport system, enzyme, or cofactor could serve a single metabolic pathway, or it could be important for several (Y → Z). Any step that requires mediation of an enzyme is at risk for genetic error. A metabolic block could cause a decrease in concentrations of products after the enzyme defect unless there is an alternative mechanism that can produce the product. Similarly, there can be accumulation of substrate before an enzyme block depending on availability of other pathways of disposal or alternative metabolism (C → R).

Secondary nutrient deficiencies can occur as a result of a defective enzyme. In organic acidemias, secondary deficiencies in carnitine are common, resulting from the increased excretion of acylcarnitine esters (e.g., propionylcarnitine). The interconnectedness of biochemical pathways offers a challenge and opportunity to creatively manage patients.

PRINCIPLES OF NUTRITION SUPPORT

Overview of Chronic Nutrition Therapy

The goal of nutrition therapy is to correct any biochemical imbalance so that toxic concentrations of substrate or metabolite(s) are either reduced or normalized by employing the following strategies:

1. Provide all essential nutrients in quantities adequate to promote optimal physical and mental development.
2. Supply the optimal amount of any nutrient that is restricted or supplemented in order to promote growth while minimizing metabolic imbalances.

For each disease, management depends on the specific biochemistry and pathophysiology of the disease. Principle strategies of nutrition therapy are:

1. Restrict any nutrient (substrate) of toxic metabolites that accumulate as a result of defective enzyme activity. Example: restrict branched-chain amino acids, isoleucine, leucine, and valine in maple syrup disease (MSD).
2. Replenish any deficient product not adequately produced due to the affected enzyme. Examples: L-tyrosine supplementation in phenylketonuria; L-cystine in homocystinuria.
3. Supplement compounds that might combine with a toxic metabolite to promote its excretion and that could replenish a deficiency. In certain cases, these compounds are considered "conditionally essential nutrients"; for example: L-carnitine supplementation in organic acidemias.
4. Provide coenzyme in therapeutic doses to enhance residual enzyme activity if any enzyme is present. Example: hydroxycobalamin (vitamin B_{12}) responsive methylmalonic acidemia or cofactor defect.

Nutrition therapy for inherited metabolic diseases has contributed to our understanding of nutrient requirements in healthy individuals. When a specific nutrient (e.g., PHE in PKU) is overly restricted, failure to thrive and protein malnutrition result.[9]

Substrate restriction in nutrition therapy can be specific (individual amino acids, carbohydrates, or fatty acids) or general (total protein in urea cycle disorders, total carbohydrate in galactosemia, or total fat in mitochondrial fatty acid oxidation defects). When specific nutrients are restricted, it is challenging to ensure adequate intake of other related nutrients.

Diet prescriptions are calculated to provide specified amounts of protein, energy, fluid, and specific nutrients that must be restricted and/or supplemented. Depending on the disorder, a prescription could require restriction in the amount or type of carbohydrates, proteins, fats, or amino acids. In some instances, nutrition therapy might also specify avoidance of fasting, as many metabolic disorders worsen during catabolism. Guidelines for calculating specific nutrient needs for selected inherited metabolic diseases are found in Table 33-2.

The recommendation for protein intake in amino acid disorders is higher than the Dietary Reference Intakes[10,11] when most of the protein is supplied as synthetic amino acids[12] because of the difference in nitrogen retention between free amino acids and intact protein.[13,14] Differences in absorption and catabolism of amino acids between intact protein sources and free amino acids also contribute to the need for additional protein.[15–17] Adequate protein intake is essential to prevent protein insufficiency in patients with inherited metabolic diseases.[18]

Nutrition therapy for amino acids disorders requires use of synthetic amino acid-based formulas. Medical foods usually contribute 50–85% of the daily total protein requirement, depending on the type of disorder and tolerance to protein. A variety of metabolic foods are listed in Appendix A. In patients who require metabolic medical foods, intact proteins are prescribed to include a defined amount of the restricted amino acid(s). For infants who require metabolic medical foods, intact (whole) protein sources are supplied from standard infant formulas or human milk. As children get older, intact protein is supplied by low protein foods (fruits, vegetables, and some grains).

Nutritionally complete metabolic medical foods contain carbohydrates, fat, minerals, and vitamins. Other partially complete medical foods might contain little or no fat, carbohydrate, or minerals and vitamins. Medical foods have been designed in forms such as drink packets, capsules, tablets, and food bars, allowing increased flexibility and normalization of the strict diet regimen. When prescribing any diet using medical foods, clinicians must assure adequate mineral, vitamin, and essential fatty acid intake. The reliance on chemically defined metabolic formulas used in amino acid disorders can affect the bioavailability of several macroelements and trace elements, including iron, copper, selenium, and zinc. Failure to monitor nutrition status results in deficiencies.[19–21] Periodic assessment of mineral status is recommended.

Phenotypic heterogeneity requires individualized nutrition therapy and constant modification based on clinical assessment and blood/urine biochemical indices. The dietary prescription must take into account age-related normal reference values, growth, and level of stress in acute situations. Assessment of nutrition therapy includes anthropometrics and visceral protein status. Other biochemical parameters are specific to each disorder. For a number of disorders, assessment of plasma concentrations of free and acylcarnitine should be performed, and concentrations of any coenzyme (e.g., thiamin, biotin) that is supplemented should be monitored. Table 33-3 contains general nutrition assessment guidelines.

EMERGENCY NUTRITION AND MEDICAL INTERVENTION OF METABOLIC DISORDERS DURING INITIAL PRESENTATION

Categorizing metabolic disorders into groups based on therapeutic approaches to an acute life-threatening presentation or during an intercurrent illness helps define treatment.[22] All persons with inherited metabolic diseases in which illness or stress can cause metabolic decompensation must carry an emergency letter with the following information: name of disease, symptoms,

Table 33-2 Recommended nutrient intakes for inborn errors of amino acid metabolism that require specific amino acid restrictions.

Nutrients	*Age (years)*					
	0.0 < 0.5	*0.5 < 1.0*	*1 < 4*	*4 < 7*	*7 < 11*	*11 < 19*
			Inherited Disorders Of Amino Acid Metabolism			
Phenylketonuria/hyperphenylalaninemia						
PHE, mg	70–25/kg	35–15/kg	200–450/day	225–450/day	250–500/day	300–1,000/day
TYR, mg	300–250/kg	250–225/kg	1,720–3,000/day	2,250–3,500/day	2,500–4,000/day	2,100–5,500/day
Protein, g	3.5–3.0 kg	3.0–2.5/kg	≥ 30/day	≥ 35/day	≥ 40/day	50–65/day
Energy, kcal	100–125% OF NAS/FNB RDA for age					
			Branched–Chain Amino Acids			
Maple syrup disease						
ILE, mg	75–35/kg	65–30/kg	165–325/day	225–420/day	250–470/day	330–570/day
LEU, mg	100–50/kg	75–35/kg	275–535/day	360–695/day	410–785/day	540–945/day
VAL, mg	80–40/kg	70–30/kg	200–375/day	250–500/day	285–550/day	375–675/day
Protein, g	3.5–3.0/kg	3.0–2.5/kg	≥ 30/day	≥ 35/day	≥ 40/day	50–65/day
Energy, kcal	100–125% of NAS/FNB RDA for age					
			Organic Acidemias (Selected)			
Isovaleric acidemia						
LEU, mg	130–70/kg	120–50/kg	500–900/day	600–900/day	700–900/day	700–1,500/day
L-carnitine mg	50–100/kg					
GLY, mg	150–300/kg					
Protein, g	3.0–2.5/kg	3.0–2.5/kg	≥ 30/day	≥ 35/day	≥ 40/day	50–65/day
Energy, kcal	100–125% of NAS/FNB RDA for age					
Propionic acidemia and methylmalonic acidemia						
ILE, mg	110–60/kg	90–40/kg	485–735/day	630–960/day	715–1,090/day	956–1,470/day
MET, mg	50–20/kg	40–15/kg	275–390/day	360–510/day	410–580/day	550–780/day
THR, mg	125–50/kg	75–20/kg	415–600/day	540–780/day	610–885/day	830–1,200/day
VAL, mg	105–60/kg	80–40/kg	550–830/day	720–1,080/day	815–1,225/day	1105–1,655/day
D–biotin, mg	5–10/day for propionic acidemia					
Hydroxycobalamin, mg (oral)	1–2/day for cobalamin–responsive methylmalonic acidemia					
L–carnitine, mg	300–100/kg					
Protein,* g	3.0–2.5/kg	3.0–2.5/kg	≥ 30/day	≥ 35/day	~ 40/day	~ 50/day
Energy, kcal	100–125% OF NAS/FNB RDA for age					

Table 33-2 Recommended nutrient intakes for inborn errors of amino acid metabolism that require specific amino acid restrictions (continued).

Nutrients	*Age (years)*					
	0.0 < 0.5	*0.5 < 1.0*	*1 < 4*	*4 < 7*	*7 < 11*	*11 < 19*
			Urea Cycle Disorders			
Citrullinemia; argininosuccinic aciduria						
ARG, mg	700–350/kg	700–350/kg	500–250/kg	500–250/kg	500–250/kg	400–200/kg
Protein,† g	2.2–1.7/kg	1.8–1.5/kg	8–12/day	12–15/day	14–17/day	20–24/day
Energy, kcal	115–140% of NAS/FNB RDA for age					
Carbamylphosphate synthetase deficiency; ornithine transcarbamylase deficiency						
CIT, mg	700–350/kg	700–350/kg	500–250/kg	500–250/kg	500–250/kg	400–200/kg
Protein,† g	2.2–1.7/kg	1.8–1.5/kg	8–12/day	12–15/day	14–17/day	20–24/day
Energy	115–140% of NAS/FNB RDA for age					
Argininemia						
Protein,† g	2.2–1.7/kg	1.8–1.5/kg	8–12/day	12–15/day	14–17/day	20–32/day
Energy, kcal	115–140% of NAS/FNB RDA for age					

Key: ARG, arginine; CIT, citrulline; CYS, cystine; GLY, glycine; ILE, isoleucine; LEU, leucine; MET, methionine; NAS/FNB RDA, National Academy of Sciences/Food and Nutrition Board, recommended dietary allowances ; PHE, phenylalanine; THR, threonine; TYR, tyrosine; VAL, valine.

* Protein could differ if either hyperammonemia is present or renal function is impaired. For propionic and methylmalonic acidemia, approximately one half of the protein intake per day should come from intact protein.

† Total protein intake might be somewhat greater with the use of drugs that enhance waste nitrogen loss. Numbers represent total protein per day from both intact protein (50%) and essential amino acid medical foods (50%). Protein should be titrated to support normal growth and development.

Note: Requirements for children 11- < 19 years include both girls and boys and do not include requirements for pregnancy. Recommended intakes are to be used as a guide for nutrition therapy. Actual requirements might differ from data listed in the table and must be based on frequent monitoring of amino acid status, protein status, and growth. When prescribing diets based on body weight (kg), use ideal weight (50th percentile) for age to optimize intake. This is most important when calculating diets for patients who fail to thrive (Yannicelli S, Acosta PB, Velazquez A, et al. Improved growth and nutrition status in children with methylmalonic or propionic acidemia fed an elemental medical food. *Mol Genet Metab.* 2003;80:181–188).

Sources: Table modified from the following: Acosta PB, Yannicelli S. Nutrition support of inherited disorders of amino acid metabolism: Part 1. *Top Clin Nutr.* 1993;9:65–82; Acosta PB, Yannicelli S. *Nutrition Support Protocols.* 4th ed. Columbus, Ohio: Ross Products Division; 2001; Yannicelli S, Greene C. Nutrition therapies for inborn errors of metabolism. In: Hay W, ed. *Neonatal Nutrition and Metabolism.* New York, NY: Mosby Year Book; 1991:507–542; Ogier de Baulny H, Saudubray JM. Branched-chain organic aciduria. In: Fernandes J, Saudubray JM, van den Berghe G, eds. *Inborn Metabolic Diseases: Diagnosis and Treatment.* 3rd ed. Berlin, Germany: Springer-Verlag; 2000:197–212; and Food and Nutrition Board, Committee on Dietary Allowances. *Recommended Dietary Allowances.* 9th and 10th editions. Washington DC: National Academy of Sciences; 1980 and 1989.

Table 33-3 Nutrition assessment guidelines for nutrition therapy of patients with selected inborn errors of metabolism.

Assessment marker	*Specific parameters*	*Inborn error most requiring assessment*
Growth	Weight, length/height, head circumference (age-dependent)	All patients
Nutrition adequacy	3-day diet records before blood or urine collection; full nutrient analysis	All patients
Protein status indices	Total protein, albumin, transthyretin (prealbumin)	All patients
Plasma amino acids	Amino acid profile, including tryptophan and homocyste(i)ne	Disorders of amino acid metabolism; organic acidemias
Organic acids (blood, urine)	Organic acid profile, include carnitine esters	Organic acidemias, fatty acid disorders, peroxisomal disorders
Serum carnitine	Free and esters (bound)	Organic acidemias, fatty acid disorders
Essential fatty acid (EFA) profile	Blood and erythrocyte EFA	Fatty acid disorders or disorders where fat is restricted in the diet
Iron status indices	Hemoglobin, hematocrit, ferritin	All patients
Trace element status	Selenium/glutathione peroxidase, zinc	Disorders of amino acid metabolism, organic acidemias and any disorder requiring elemental medical foods

consequences of metabolic decompensation, and emergency treatment including a plan for stabilization, the type and amount of IV fluids, administration of detoxifying or coenzyme therapy, and physician contact information for transfer or consultation. Detailed information on nutrition and medical intervention during acute crisis can be found in Table 33-4.

Intoxication Disorders

Intoxication disorders are those caused by the accumulation of a toxic metabolite. They include disorders of amino acids, nitrogen, organic acid, carbohydrate, and fatty acid metabolism. Included are the urea cycle disorders, organic acidemias, aminoacidopathies, mitochondrial fatty acid oxidation defects (especially long chain fatty acid oxidation disorders), galactosemia, and hereditary fructose intolerance. Intoxication disorders typically present shortly after birth or within hours to days of life as toxic metabolites accumulate. Hereditary fructose intolerance generally presents later in infancy when solids or medications that contain fructose/sucrose are introduced into the diet. Clinical presentation is often characterized by nonspecific features including lethargy, poor feeding, vomiting, abnormal breathing, hypotonia, and seizures. Infants with intoxication disorders are often worked up for sepsis. Depending on the defect, ammonia, organic acids, amino acids, or toxic metabolites

Table 33-4 Emergency treatment of selected metabolic disorders during intercurrent illnesses.

	Major biochemical features	*Emergency treatment*
Intoxication Disorders		
Maple syrup disease • Branched-chain α-ketoacids	Hypoglycemia Ketoacidosis Elevated BCAA Elevated urine α-ketoacids	• Stop precursors (whole protein) • IV glucose + insulin • Maintain electrolytes • Treat acidosis • Na ≥ 140 mg/dL to prevent cerebral edema • Fluid restriction (100–120 mL/kg/24 hour) to reduce risk of cerebral edema Enhance protein anabolism • High energy feeds • Provide BCAA-free medical food • ILE and VAL supplements when appropriate Remove toxic metabolites • Dialysis (dependent on severity of acute illness and plasma concentration of toxins) Thiamin (5 mg/kg/d)
PPA and MMA • Methylmalonic acid • Propionyl-CoA • Propionic acid • Ammonia	Hypoglycemia Ketoacidosis Hyperammonemia Neutropenia Hyperglycinemia	• Stop precursors (whole protein) • IV glucose + insulin • Maintain electrolytes • Treat acidosis • Na ≥ 140 mg/dL Enhance protein anabolism • High energy feeds • Medical food free of ILE, MET, THR, VAL • ILE or VAL supplements, when appropriate Coenzyme supplementation • MMA, vitamin B_{12} 1–2 mg/week IM • PPA, oral biotin 10–20 mg/day Remove toxic metabolites • Metronidazole (reduces gut propionate) • IV L-carnitine (100 mg/kg/d. Titrate to normalize plasma free concentration) • Sodium benzoate (if hyperammonemia present)

Table 33-4 Emergency treatment of selected metabolic disorders during intercurrent illnesses (continued).

	Major biochemical features	*Emergency treatment*
Isovaleric acidemias	Hypoglycemia Ketoacidosis Hyperammonemia Neutropenia Hyperglycinemia	• Stop precursors (whole protein) • IV glucose + insulin • Maintain electrolytes • Treat acidosis • Na ≥ 140 mg/dL to prevent cerebral edema • Fluid restriction (10–120 mL/kg/24 hour) to reduce risk of cerebral edema Enhance protein anabolism • High energy feeds • Medical food free of LEU Remove toxic metabolites • Dialysis (if NH_3 > 600 µmol/L) • IV L-carnitine (100 mg/kg/d. Titrate to normalize plasma free concentration) • Glycine suppl. (250 mg/kg/d)
Urea cycle disorders	Hyperammonemia with normal anion gap and blood glucose Respiratory alkalosis Elevated plasma glutamine	• Stop precursors (whole protein) • IV glucose (10% with ¼ NS) + lipids High energy feeds (120–130 kcal/kg) Reverse hyperammonemia • Hemodialysis • Sodium benzoate • Sodium phenylacetate • Arginine (except in argininemia) Avoid: carnitine, IV sodium (already provided in therapies above, e.g., sodium phenylacetate, etc.)
Fasting Intolerance Disorders		
Glycogen storage disease Type 1a	Hypoglycemia Hyperlacticacidemia Hyperuricemia Hypertriacylglycerolemia Hypercholesterolemia	• IV glucose • Continuous nasogastric feedings • GIR to maintain normoglycemia: Infants 7–9 mg/kg/min • Avoid fructose and galactose Uncooked cornstarch (1.5–2.5–g/kg/ feed or as tolerated)

BCAA = branched chain amino acids, ILE = isoleucine, VAL = valine, PPA = propionic academia, MMA = methylmalonic academia, Met = methionine, Thr = threonine, GIR = glucose infusion rate

Emergency management, including nutrition intervention, must be individualized and based on degree of critical illness, concentrations of toxic compounds, and other biochemical indices. This table is to be used as a guide only and not a standard protocol for emergency management. *Sources:* Table modified from Ogier de Baulny H. Management and emergency treatments of neonates with suspicion of inborn errors of metabolism. *Semin Neonatol.* 2002;7:17–26; Summar M. Current strategies for the management of neonatal urea cycle disorders. *J Pediatr.* 2001;138:S30–S39, and Ogier de Baulny H, Saudubray JM. Branched-chain organic aciduria. In: Fernandes J, Saudubray JM, van den Berghe G, eds. *Inborn Metabolic Diseases: Diagnosis and Treatment.* 3rd ed. Berlin, Germany: Springer-Verlag; 2000:197–212.

build up as the infant is fed and from endogenous breakdown of protein or fat during the catabolic stress in the newborn period. During medical emergencies therapy must begin immediately.

Principles of acute nutrition therapy for intoxication disorders during presentation and intermittent illnesses are:

1. Remove toxic precursors from the diet (e.g., specific amino acids, intact protein).
2. Prevent cerebral edema (fatty acid oxidation disorders, isovaleric acidemia, MSD, urea cycle disorders).
3. Limit rate of catabolism and promote anabolism by providing high energy feedings and treating underlying medical conditions (e.g., infection, fever).
4. Provide electrolytes, vitamins, and minerals as clinical status dictates.
5. Provide coenzyme and alternative pathway therapy as indicated when diagnosis is established.
6. Manage acid-base status when required.
7. Prevent fasting.

Newborns with a suspected inherited metabolic disease require immediate medical and nutrition intervention even before laboratory results are available. Obtain blood and urine samples for laboratory studies before initiating therapy as biochemical derangement for some disorders might normalize rapidly with therapy. Initially, cease all sources of toxic precursors such as infant or enteral formulas or parenteral nutrition (PN). Begin IV glucose and electrolytes at approximately 150 mL/kg/24 hours to provide a glucose infusion rate (GIR) of 10 mg/kg/min. Proceed cautiously—patients with cerebral edema require fluid restriction. The aforementioned fluid intake of 150 mL/kg/24 hours supplies roughly 50 calories/kg (3.4 kcal/g IV dextrose) and can be given via peripheral line. In disorders of endogenous intoxication, such as MSD and organic acidemias, catabolism rapidly worsens, resulting in accumulation of toxic metabolites. For these conditions, aggressive nutrition intervention providing 120–150 kcal/kg/24 hours is required to promote anabolism and attenuate catabolism. Energy intakes less than 120 kcal/kg/24 hours are not sufficient to significantly reduce blood concentrations of toxic precursors. Intravenous lipids can be added via peripheral or central lines at 2–3 g/kg/24 hours (Figure 33-2). A combination of PN and enteral nutrition (EN) should be used as tolerated.

Once the neonate has been stabilized and the diagnosis confirmed, disorder-specific therapy should be initiated without delay. Peripheral PN alone will not provide sufficient nutrients to support anabolism. Small drip feeds of EN without the offending amino acids delivered into the GI tract should be provided as soon as the patient is stable. The standard EN mantra "if the gut works—use it," holds true for inherited intoxication disorders. Providing trophic feeds minimizes bacterial translocation, promotes anabolism, and allows for transition to full EN. For aminoacidopathies, organic acidemias, and urea cycle disorders, introduction of amino acids and protein should not be delayed, as this will hasten deficiency and prolong catabolism.[23]

Fasting Intolerance Disorders

Disorders of fasting intolerance are those in which glucose homeostasis cannot be maintained and include glycogen storage diseases, gluconeogenesis, and fatty acid oxidation defects since ketones cannot be synthesized via β-oxidation to provide energy. These disorders present with hypoglycemia during times of fasting or when feeding frequency decreases and circulating glucose and glycogen stores have been exhausted. Febrile illnesses exacerbate effects of fasting, causing patients to quickly decompensate.

Principles of emergency nutrition therapy for fasting intolerance disorders are to present a steady source of glucose at the rate of hepatic glucose production (5–7 mg/kg/min). Begin treatment immediately, even before laboratory results are available. Obtain blood and urine samples for laboratory studies before initiating therapy as biochemical derangement might nor-

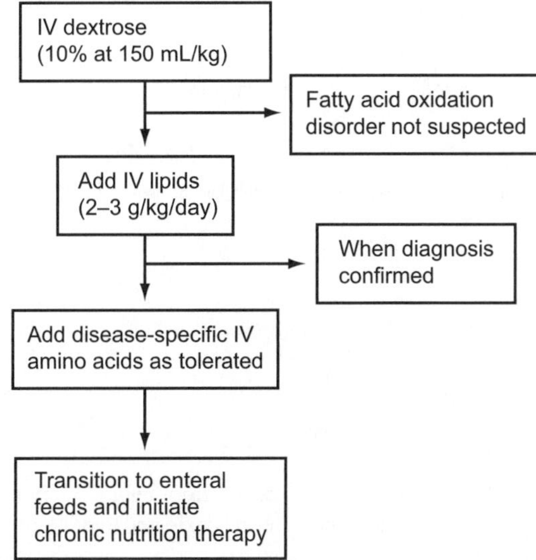

Figure 33-2 Administering intravenous nutrients in the sick newborn with suspected inherited metabolic disease.

malize quickly with therapy. Fasting intolerance disorders require cessation of sources of toxic precursors such as infant or enteral formulas or total PN and prevention of catabolism. Begin with IV glucose and electrolytes at 150 mL/kg/min to provide a GIR of 10 mg/kg/min. This can be given via a peripheral line. Begin prescribed enteral feeds when the patient is stable and transition to long term nutrition therapy.

Disorders of Energy Metabolism

Disorders of energy metabolism have defective mitochondrial function. They are a group of inherited defects in enzymes or enzyme complexes involved in the production of chemical energy (adenosine triphosphate—ATP) by oxidative phosphorylation. These disorders include defects in the pyruvate dehydrogenase complex and respiratory chain. Lactic acidosis can occur as well during periods of hypoxia, systemic disease, or intoxication from ethanol or methanol.[24] In confirmed cases of pyruvate dehydrogenase complex or respiratory chain disorders, the usually recommended rates of IV glucose administration are dangerous. The infusion of glucose should be run at 3–5 mg/kg/min and used with lipid administration at 2–6 g/kg/day.[22] Disorders of energy metabolism are rare, and patients generally have a poor prognosis. For this reason, a child with lactic acidosis should be treated with high glucose administration and careful monitoring of lactate and acid-base status[22] until diagnosis is confirmed.

Pyruvate dehydrogenase complex deficiency is treated with a ketogenic diet. During acute illness, efforts should be made to preserve ketosis by providing a ketogenic diet formula (Ketocal®, Nutricia North America, Gaithersburg, Md.) or module (RCF®, Ross Products Division, Abbott Laboratories, Columbus, Ohio) or parenterally using IV lipids, protein, and limited glucose to maintain ketosis.

SPECIFIC METABOLIC DISORDERS

Aminoacidopathies: Phenylketonuria

Classic PKU is an autosomal recessive disease; it was first described by Fölling in 1934.[2] Hyperphenylalaninemia occurs in roughly 1 of every 15,000 live births in the United States. If untreated, PKU causes severe mental retardation and neurologic problems. The defect is failure to metabolize the essential amino acid PHE to tyrosine (Figure 33-3). The cause of mental retardation in PKU is not known, but it clearly correlates with the blood concentration of PHE and is characterized by abnormal myelination in the brain. Moreover, tyrosine is a precursor to important brain chemicals, serotonin, and dopamine. Elevated plasma PHE concentrations negatively affect production of dopamine and L-DOPA.[25,26] Other mechanisms can be responsible for frontal lobe deficits in these patients.[27]

The percentage of dietary PHE that is hydroxylated to tyrosine is dependent on age, growth rate, and severity of the defect. In the rapidly growing infant, approximately 50–60% of dietary PHE is used for protein synthesis compared to 10% in the normal adult.

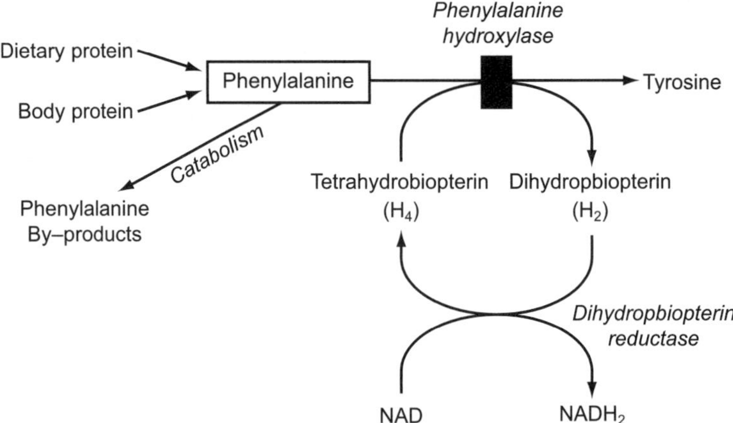

Figure 33-3 Pathway for metabolism of phenylalanine. Tetrahydrobiopterin, synthesized from neopterin by a series of reactions, is the cofactor for phenylalanine hydroxylase. The tetrahydrobiopterin is oxidized to dihydrobiopterin in the reaction and is recycled by dihydropteridine reductase.

Classic PKU is identified by state newborn screening programs. More specific biochemical tests are necessary to confirm the diagnosis. Plasma PHE concentrations greater than 1,200 µmol/L (20 mg/dL) on a normal diet are indicative of classic PKU. Mutation analysis further identifies patient-specific mutations that could help direct therapy. Recognized broad classifications of hyperphenylalaninemia at the time of diagnosis are given in Table 33-5.

Hyperphenylalaninemia could also be due to defects in the synthesis of tetrahydrobiopterin (BH_4), a coenzyme in the PHE hydroxylase enzyme complex. These disorders must be rapidly distinguished from classic PKU in the newborn period as their management and outcome are different. Research shows that a certain number of patients with hyperphenylalaninemia and milder genotypes of classic PKU respond to tetrahydrobiopterin (BH4) (10–20 mg/kg/d) by a reduction in plasma PHE concentrations.[28] This therapy is not currently available in the United States, but is under clinical investigation. Patients with mild and transient hyperphenylalaninemia usually do not require treatment, and dietary over-restriction of PHE is harmful

Table 33-5 Classification of phenylketonuria (PKU).

Classification	*Plasma phenylalanine concentration at diagnosis (µmol/L)*
Classic PKU (severe genotype)	> 1,200 (20 mg/dL)
Moderate hyperphenylalaninemia	600–1,200 (10–20 mg/dL)
Mild hyperphenylalaninemia	< 600 (< 10 mg/dL)

Sources: Blaskovics ME, Schaeffler GE, Hack S. Phenylalaninaemia: differential diagnosis. *Arch Dis Child.* 1974;49:835-843; and Guttler F. Hyperphenylalaninemia: diagnosis and classification of the various types of phenylalanine hydroxylase deficiency in childhood. *Acta Paediatr Scand Suppl.* 1980;280:46–80.

to growth and development. Overall, the most common error in nutrition therapy of PKU is the inappropriate institution of diet in a baby who does not require restriction. Mutation analysis of the PHE hydroxylase gene can help provide guidance in therapy and will become increasingly important as new treatment strategies emerge.

NUTRITION THERAPY

Early initiation of nutrition therapy and maintenance of blood PHE concentrations between 120 and 480 μmol/L (2 to 8 mg/dL) is associated with normal mental and physical development. The diet should be continued throughout life.[29–33]

Components of a PHE-restricted diet include PHE, tyrosine, protein, and energy (Table 33-2). Provision of PHE must be individualized and is determined by age, growth, and tolerance to dietary PHE. Special metabolic medical foods are supplemented with tyrosine. Additional tyrosine supplementation might be indicated if blood concentrations remain below normal (i.e., < 44 μmol/L). Because purified L-tyrosine precipitates in liquids, blood levels might remain low when liquid tyrosine supplementation is prescribed.

The basis for nutrition therapy of PKU is the availability of PHE-free metabolic medical foods (Appendix C). Throughout infancy, PHE-free medical foods supply approximately 80% of total dietary protein. Medical food is prescribed with either standard infant formulas or human milk to meet the infant's requirements for PHE. As the infant develops, natural low protein foods, including fruits, vegetables, and limited grains are introduced into the diet. With time, the entire PHE requirement is supplied by foods low in intact protein.

Blood PHE concentrations are monitored weekly in infancy and often less frequently with age. Blood tyrosine concentrations should be monitored to prevent deficiency. See Table 33-3 for general guidelines to monitoring patients with inborn errors of metabolism.

Management During Acute Illness

If sufficient calories and protein are not consumed during extended periods of fasting or acute illness, catabolism results and free amino acids are released and blood PHE concentrations increase. While blood PHE concentrations can be markedly elevated during illness, typical childhood illnesses in a well nourished patient with PKU are not life-threatening and will not cause immediate or long term neurological problems. However, during illness it is important to continue to consume the PHE-free medical food and provide sufficient energy and fluids as tolerated.

Maple Syrup Disease (Branched-Chain Ketoaciduria)

MSD is an autosomal recessive disorder of branched-chain amino acid (leucine, isoleucine, and valine) metabolism (Figure 33-4). Elevations in plasma branched-chain ketoacids correlate with clinical symptoms. Elevated plasma alloisoleucine is a specific and sensitive marker for diagnosis of MSD.[34]

Classic MSD presents in neonates who at first appear normal but within several days develop lethargy, failure to thrive, poor suck, vomiting, and ketoacidosis. Urine might smell like maple syrup. Variant forms of the disease exist. Some mild variants have symptoms only after febrile illnesses, infections, or a protein load. Early diagnosis and aggressive intervention can prevent death, severe mental retardation, and permanent neurologic deficits. Despite early treatment and diagnosis, patients are still at risk for metabolic decompensation and neurologic insult secondary to intermittent illness and injury.

Patients with MSD have a fair long term prognosis. Factors relating to outcome include age at diagnosis, peak plasma leucine concentrations, and length of time of clinical crisis during the neonatal period.[35] Long term metabolic control can also influence intelligence.[36,37] A compre-

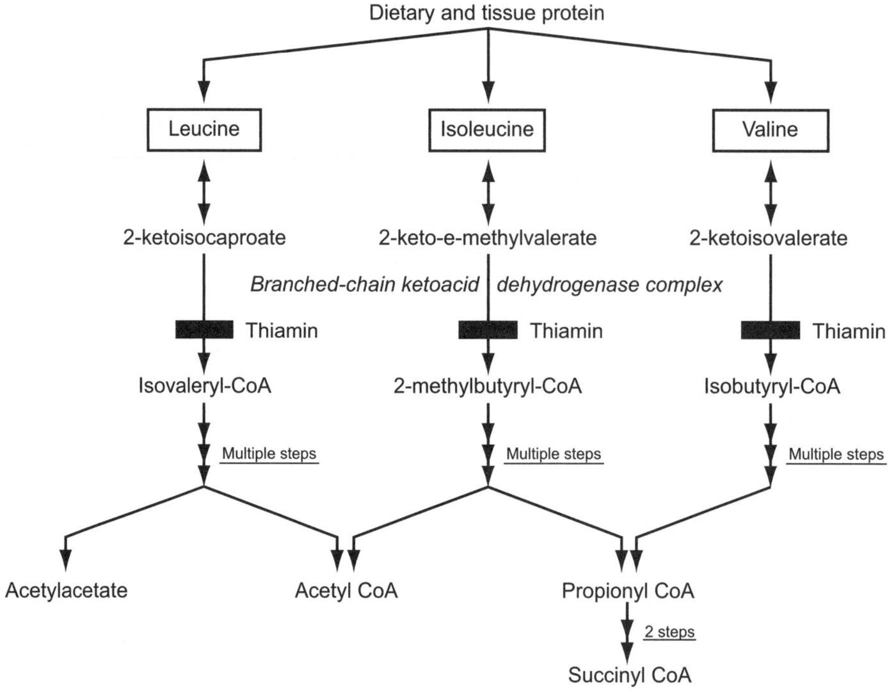

Figure 33-4 Pathway for metabolism of the branched-chain amino acids.

hensive protocol for managing patients with MSD, both acutely and chronically, can allow for normal growth and development.

Nutrition Therapy

Classic MSD must be treated aggressively during initial presentation and subsequent illnesses. Standard infant formula must not be fed to the acutely ill infant, and the infant might require dialysis if the acidosis is severe.[38] Hemodialysis is effective in rapidly reducing neurotoxic concentrations of ketoacids if the patient is critically ill with cerebral edema and coma.[39] However, aggressive nutrition intervention with intravenous therapy to normalize electrolyte status and extracellular osmolarity, without dialysis, is effective in reducing the risk of cerebral edema.[40] Insulin infusion is recommended to reduce metabolic decompensation.[41] Supplementation with L-glutamine and alanine might help normalize brain amino acid concentrations during acute crises.[40,42] Regardless of the approach, nutrition intervention is integral during acute crisis[43,40] as a catalyst for anabolism. Prevention or inhibition of catabolism is essential. If the oral route is not possible, then PN is indicated.[44,45] Parenteral amino acid solutions free of branched-chain amino acids are available (Appendix C).

Once oral feedings are tolerated, a total restriction of branched-chain amino acids might be required to normalize plasma concentrations. This can be accomplished by the use of branched-chain amino acid-free medical foods to provide the recommended amounts of protein (Table 33-2; Appendix C). Intakes of 2.5–3.0 g/kg/day of protein with high energy intakes (120–150 kcal/kg/day) supplied by medical foods and IV therapy might be needed to drive anabolism. Initial nutrition therapy with total restriction of branched-chain amino acids requires daily monitoring of plasma amino acid concentrations to prevent deficiencies. After several days of treatment, blood concentrations of valine and isoleucine normalize, but leucine levels can still be elevated. Supplementation of L-isoleucine and L-valine at approximately 40 to 45 mg/kg can normalize blood levels of all 3 branched-chain amino acids within a few days. Once the patient is stable and the plasma concentrations of branched-chain amino acids are within the therapeutic range intact protein sources such as human milk[46] or standard infant formulas can be incorporated into the diet.

Requirements for branched-chain amino acids depend on age, growth velocity, state of health, and genotype. Because most individuals with classic MSD have 0 to 2% enzyme activity, restriction of branched-chain amino acids is necessary (Table 33-2). In nature, leucine makes up a larger portion of dietary protein (8.5%) than valine and isoleucine. Tolerance to dietary leucine often decreases during later infancy, and it requires vigilance to maintain plasma leucine concentrations. Dietary restriction of leucine necessary to obtain a normal range could over-restrict dietary valine and isoleucine. Chronic supplementation of isoleucine and valine as a solution (10 mg/mL) might be necessary to normalize plasma concentrations and prevent deficiency. An excess or deficiency of any of these amino acids has clinical consequences.[47]

Analysis of plasma branched-chain amino acids should be performed at least weekly for the first year of life. Families should be instructed to daily monitor urine for presence of ketoacids using either 2, 4-dinitrophenylhydrazine (DNPH) or ketone test strips to assess health status and impending illness. Table 33-3 offers guidelines for monitoring nutrition therapy.

Organic Acidemias (Isovaleric Acidemia, Methylmalonic Acidemia, Propionic Acidemia)

Organic acidemias are a heterogeneous group of defects responsible for metabolism of one or several amino acids and odd-chained fatty acids (propionic and methylmalonic acidemia). Clinical outcomes correlate with disease severity, enzyme function, and age at presentation. For example, patients with Mut^- methylmalonic acidemia have a milder clinical course than patients with a Mut nonfunctional mutase enzyme. In addition, patients who present later in life often have a milder enzyme defect, are more clinically stable, and tolerate more dietary protein than those who present as neonates.

Patients might appear normal at birth, but within several days to weeks develop vomiting, lethargy, failure to thrive, and coma. Hyperammonemia and hypoglycemia occur. If this is not aggressively treated, death occurs, either from severe infection, ketoacidosis, or hyperammonemia. Symptoms are triggered by infections, protracted fasting, or exposure to dietary protein loads. Metabolic acidosis and decompensation occurs frequently in infancy and childhood. Mental development and cognition is wide ranging and might be normal depending on the severity of the disease.[48]

Laboratory findings include significant accumulation of organic acids relevant to each disorder in biologic fluids. Organic acids are quantified by gas chromatography/mass spectroscopy. Diagnosis is confirmed by quantitation of plasma amino acids, urinary or plasma organic acids, and cultured skin fibroblasts. In patients with isovaleric acidemia, the presence of a sweaty-feet odor is another clue to the diagnosis.

Clinical outcomes are variable and based partly on the biochemical defect and medical management during illnesses. Improvement in survival reflects early diagnosis and rapid intervention during acute crisis.[49,50] Patients who survive the neonatal course and who are under chronic management could later develop complications, such as renal insufficiency, pancreatitis, developmental delays, and cognitive impairment despite careful dietary management.

Nutrition Therapy

Offending dietary precursor amino acids (e.g., isoleucine, leucine, methionine, threonine, valine and odd-chain fatty acids) are restricted to normalize plasma and tissue concentrations and reduce accumulation of toxic organic acids. Avoidance of acidosis is key in management. The foundation of nutrition therapy is a moderate-protein, high energy diet including intact protein as a source of precursor amino acids, medical foods that are free or low in the precursor amino acids, and additional energy sources (carbohydrate and fat) to promote anabolism (Tables 33-2 and 33-4 and Appendix C). The exact amount of precursor amino acids are determined by the child's age, laboratory analyses, growth parameters, and health status. The diet must be sufficient in all nutrients, including minerals and vitamins, to prevent deficiencies.[21] Essential fatty acid deficiency has been described in patients with organic acidemias.[51]

Protein requirements of children with methylmalonic and propionic acidemias are not well established. Overrestriction of protein (intact and free amino acids from medical food) causes poor growth and nutrient deficiencies.[49,52] Treatment with medical foods in conjunction with restricted intact protein doesn't guarantee normal growth.[53] However, titration of protein and energy to levels tolerated by patients can improve growth.[54,53] Energy requirement could be lower than recommendations for age because of lower resting energy expenditure.[55,56]

Patients with failure to thrive require enough protein and energy to normalize growth. Energy from carbohydrate and fat must be supplied to protect the infant's visceral and somatic protein stores. Nocturnal infusion of a medical food is necessary for patients with organic acidemias to avoid fasting and accumulation of odd chain fatty acids from propiogenic amino acids.

Secondary carnitine deficiency occurs in organic acidemias[57,58] due to conjugation of disease-specific organic acid with carnitine for excretion (i.e., propionylcarnitine and isovalerylcarnitine). L-carnitine can conjugate with toxic acyl-CoA compounds. L-carnitine supplementation is essential for most patients with organic acidemias to replenish depleted tissue stores and as prophylactic treatment for detoxification. Recommended L-carnitine supplementation ranges from 100 to 300 mg/kg/day. Too much carnitine supplementation can cause a fishy odor secondary to overproduction of methylamines in the gastrointestinal tract. During acute crisis, intravenous L-carnitine supplementation up to 300 mg/kg/day is considered safe.

In some cases, additional therapies might include oral biotin (10–20 mg/day) for patients with propionic acidemia. However, biotin supplementation has not been shown to be clinically effective. For patients with cobalamin transport defects, a certain form of methylmalonic acidemia, hydroxycobalamin (vitamin B_{12}) (1–2 mg/day) is an essential part of therapy. For isovaleric acidemia, L-glycine (150–300 mg/kg/day) is provided. Use of sodium benzoate for management of hyperammonemia has not been shown conclusively to be beneficial but can reduce the concentrations of plasma glycine. Sodium bicarbonate is often provided to help buffer acidosis. In propionic and methylmalonic acidemia supplementation with L-isoleucine and L-valine is often required to prevent overrestriction, but does not always normalize plasma concentrations. Metronidazole (chronic or intermittent) is recommended to reduce gut propionate in patients with excessive plasma concentrations of methylmalonic and propionic acids.[59,60]

Failure to thrive and food refusal are prominent features of organic acidemias. Moreover, lifelong anorexia and oral hypersensitivity present challenges. Some children experience dysphagia and hyperactive gag reflex, both of which interfere with the provision of nutrients. Many patients are dependent on tube feeding. Patients often have a normal suck in early infancy but gradually lose it, so they cannot meet nutrient requirements later in the first year of life. Frequent monitoring of nutrition status is important because insufficient nutrient intake can quickly lead to metabolic decompensation and acute crisis.

Anorexia and food refusal might be physiologic and behavioral. The physiologic component of anorexia may be caused by altered serotonin metabolism.[61] Anorexia is exacerbated during episodes of hyperammonemia when tryptophan transport to the brain increases.[62] Anorexia is likely caused by multifactorial interactions between brain biochemistry and peripheral metabolism.[63]

Frequent infections and vomiting make it difficult to provide optimal nutrients for any extended period of time. Children are prone to recurrent infections and illness.[64,65] During acute intermittent illnesses, correction of acidosis and provision of high energy feedings of medical food without the precursor amino acids (i.e., intact protein) are essential to help correct metabolic decompensation. Maintenance of hydration status is important. Mild acidosis or illness can be successfully managed at home. During the initial stages of illness, dietary protein intake should be stopped and nasogastric feedings of electrolytes and glucose polymers (20 kcal per fluid ounce) should be given. If illness escalates to acute crisis and enteral feeds are not tolerated, parenteral nutrition might be needed.[66,67] Continuous insulin infusion could be helpful in promoting anabolism and reducing severity of metabolic acidosis and hyperammonemia.[67] Additional therapies, including L-carnitine, must be maintained and given by infusion if required. As tolerated, medical food and protein sources can be slowly reintroduced while maintaining optimal energy intake.

Urea Cycle Disorders

Urea cycle disorders (Figure 33-5) are a variety of enzymatic defects in the production of urea, the end product of nitrogen metabolism. The enzyme defects include defects in: (1) carbamyl-phosphate synthetase (CPS), (2) ornithine transcarbamylase (OTC), (3) argininosuccinic acid synthase (citrullinemia), (4) argininosuccinic acid lyase, (5) arginase (argininemia) and (6) N-acetylglutamate synthetase. A defect in any of these enzymes results in life-threatening ammonia toxicity.[68] Hyperammonemia is a

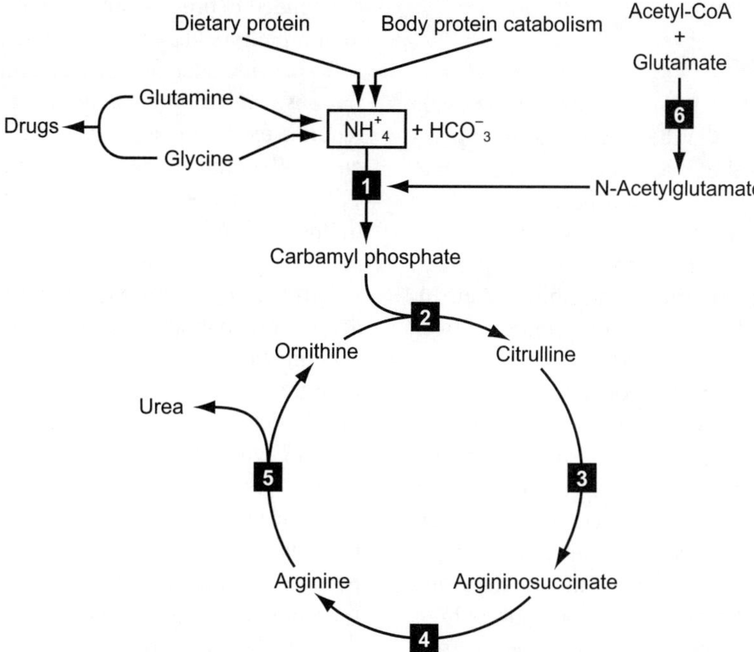

Figure 33-5 Urea cycle.

pathognomonic biochemical finding in all urea cycle disorders, except arginase deficiency, and is responsible for the severe neuropathology.[69,70] Plasma amino acids show low arginine concentrations and significantly elevated glutamine. Typical neonatal clinical features include vomiting, poor feeding, lethargy, respiratory distress, seizures, and coma. Without early diagnosis and aggressive nutrition intervention during episodes of hyperammonemia, outcomes are poor and include mental retardation.[71] Patients with arginase deficiency have a later onset disorder and a more progressive neurologic disorder. Hyperammonemia is rare.

Survival depends on the age at diagnosis, the enzyme defect, degree of severity, peak plasma ammonia concentration, and time of intervention. In general, patients who have defects that occur early in the cycle and patients with lower enzyme activity have the highest mortality. Mortality is highest for patients who have CPS deficiency, for boys who have classic OTC deficiency, and any patient who responds poorly to therapy. For some patients, liver transplantation might be necessary.[72]

Nutrition Therapy

Management of patients with a urea cycle disorder requires (1) the use of alternate pathways for removal of waste nitrogen by pharmacologic agents (e.g., sodium benzoate, sodium phenylacetate, and/or sodium phenylbutyrate); (2) the restriction of amino acids and protein; and (3) supplementation of arginine or citrulline to prevent deficiency and promote nitrogen excretion.

During acute hyperammonemic episodes, the goal is to immediately reduce plasma ammonia concentrations. Aggressive measures using peritoneal dialysis, hemodialysis, or exchange transfusion might be necessary. Hemodialysis and continuous arteriovenous hemofiltration are effective.[73,74] Enteral feeding cannot be given during this time, and the risk of infection is high. Intravenous L-arginine at doses ranging from 250 to 500 mg/kg should be given, except for patients who have arginase deficiency.

During acute crises, all exogenous protein sources are stopped. Nonprotein energy sources, intravenous or enteral, are necessary to prevent catabolism. A protein-free carbohydrate and fat module is useful if enteral feeds are tolerated. Reintroduction of protein should be performed slowly, starting at 0.5 g/kg/day and increased to approximately 1.0 to 1.25 g/kg/day.

To promote anabolism, 145 kcal/kg/day and 1.0 to 1.5 g protein/kg/day is recommended. Initially, restricting protein intake to a minimum daily requirement might be sufficient to support protein synthesis and growth, but only if optimal calories from fat and carbohydrates are provided to inhibit gluconeogenesis.

The use of a mixture of essential L-amino acids prescribed as a percent of the total protein might improve nitrogen retention and reduce waste nitrogen. Low intact protein diets alone could result in essential amino acids deficiencies and growth retardation. Medical foods that contain essential and conditionally essential amino acids (see Chapter 24 for an explanation of conditionally essential amino acids) are recommended to provide approximately 50% of the total protein intake per day (Table 33-1).

To provide adequate plasma arginine concentrations, oral supplementation of L-arginine is required except in the treatment of arginase deficiency. Recommended intakes for L-arginine are 175 to 250 mg/kg/day. Actual supplementation might need to be adjusted to maintain adequate plasma concentrations.

Nitrogen excretion is important in the management of patients with urea cycle disorders. Sodium benzoate and phenylbutyrate in conjunction with nutrition therapy can improve metabolic control. These compounds act by conjugating with nitrogen from either glycine or glutamine, respectively, and excreting them in the urine. Scaglia and colleagues[75] noted that plasma branched-chain amino acid concentrations could become deficient in patients on compounds that remove nitrogen by alternative pathways.

Secondary carnitine deficiency could occur in patients with urea cycle disorders.[76] The deficiency might be more pronounced during hyperammonemic episodes. Supplementation of oral L-carnitine (100 mg/kg/day) should be considered.

Patients with urea cycle disorder often have anorexia and avoid certain foods. This makes it challenging to support normal nutrition status. Patients should be monitored to ensure adequate growth and protein status. See Table 33-3 for further guidelines to nutrition assessment.

CONCLUSION

Collectively inherited metabolic diseases are relatively common, although each individual disease is rare. Nutrition is an important part of treatment and in many cases is primary therapy for these diseases. Aggressive lifelong nutrition therapy can attenuate morbidity and in some cases prevent mortality.

REFERENCES

1. Garrod AE. Inborn errors of metabolism (Croonian lectures). *Lancet.* 1908;2:1–7,73–79, 142–148.
2. Fölling A. Uber ausscheidung von phenlbrenztraub en saure in den harn als stoffwechsel anomalie in verbindemgmit imbezillitat. *Hoppe-Seylers Z Physiol Chem.* 1934;277:169–176.
3. Saudubray JM, Nassogne MC, DeLonlay P, Touati G. Clinical approach to inherited metabolic disorders in neonates: an overview. *Semin Neonatol.* 2002;7:3–15.
4. Schulze A, Lindner M, Kohlmuller D, Olgemoller K, Mayatepek E, Hoffmann GF. Expanded newborn screening for inborn errors of metabolism by electrospray ionization-tandem mass spectrometry: results, outcome, and implications. *Pediatrics.* 2003;111:1399–1406.
5. Wilcken B, Wiley V, Hammond J, Carpenter K. Screening newborns for inborn errors of metabolism by tandem mass spectrometry. *N Engl J Med.* 2003;348:2304–2312.
6. Bickel H, Gerrard J, Hickmans EM. Influence of phenylalanine intake on phenylketonuria. *Lancet.* 1953;812–813.
7. Coude FX, Sweetman L, Nyhan WL. Inhibition by propionyl-coenzyme A of N-acetylglutamate synthetase in rat liver mitochondria: a possible explanation for hyperammonemia in propionic and methylmalonic acidemia. *J Clin Invest.* 1979;64(6):1544–1551.
8. Stewart PM, Walser M. Failure of the normal ureagenic response to amino acids in organic acid loaded rats: a proposed mechanism for the hyperammonemia of propionic and methylmalonic acidemia. *J Clin Invest.* 1989;66:484–492.
9. Hanley WB, Linsao L, Davidson W, Moes CAF. Malnutrition with early treatment of phenylketonuria. *Pediatr Res.* 1970;4:318–327.
10. Institute of Medicine. *Dietary Reference Intakes for Energy, Carbohydrate, Fiber, Fat, Fatty Acids, Cholesterol, Protein, and Amino Acids.* Washington, DC: National Academy Press; 2002.
11. Trumbo P, Schlicker S, Yates AA, Poos M. Dietary reference intakes for energy, carbohydrate, fiber, fat, fatty acids, cholesterol, protein, and amino acids. *J Am Diet Assoc.* 2002;102:1621–1630.
12. Acosta PB, Yannicelli S, Singh R, et al. Nutrient intakes and physical growth of children with phenylketonuria undergoing nutrition therapy. *J Am Diet Assoc.* 2003;103:1167–1173.
13. Herrmann ME, Brosicke HG, Keller M, Monch E, Helge H. Dependence of the utilization of a phenylalanine-free amino acid mixture on different amounts of single dose ingested: a case report. *Eur J Pediatr.* 1994;153:501–503.
14. Schoeffer A, Herrmann ME, Broesicke HG, Moench E. Effect of dosage and timing of amino acid mixtures on nitrogen retention in patients with phenylketonuria. *J Nutr Med.* 1994;4:415–418.
15. Gropper SS, Gropper DM, Acosta PB. Plasma amino acid response to ingestion of L-amino acids and whole protein. *J Pediatr Gastroenterol Nutr.* 1993;16:143–150.
16. Gropper SS, Acosta PB. Effect of simultaneous ingestion of L-amino acids and whole protein on plasma amino acid and urea nitrogen concentrations in humans. *JPEN.* 1991;15:48–53.
17. Jones BJ, Lees R, Andrews J, Frost P, Silk DB. Comparison of an elemental and polymeric enteral diet in patients with normal gastrointestinal function. *Gut.* 1983;24:78–84.
18. Arnold GL, Vladutiu CJ, Kirby RS, Blakely EM, Deluca JM. Protein insufficiency and linear growth restriction in phenylketonuria. *J Pediatr.* 2002;141:243–246.
19. Gropper SS, Acosta PB, Clarke-Sheehan N, Wenz E, Cheng M, Koch R. Trace element status of children with PKU and normal children. *J Am Diet Assoc.* 1988;88:459–465.
20. Reilly C, Barrett JE, Patterson CM, Tinggi U, Latham SL, Marrinan A. Trace element nutrition status and dietary intake of children with phenylketonuria. *Am J Clin Nutr.* 1990;52:159–165.
21. Yannicelli S, Hambidge KM, Picciano MF. Decreased selenium intake and low plasma selenium concentrations leading to clinical symptoms in a child with propionic acidaemia. *J Inherit Metab Dis.* 1992;15:261–268.

22. Prietsch V, Lindner M, Zschocke J, Nyhan WL, Hoffmann GF. Emergency management of inherited metabolic diseases. *J Inherit Metab Dis.* 2002;25:531–546.
23. Acosta PB. Nutrition support of inborn errors of metabolism. In: Queen Samour P, Helm KK, and Lang CE, eds. *Handbook of Pediatric Nutrition.* 2nd ed. Rockville, Md: Aspen Publishers; 1999:243–292.
24. Clarke S. Tandem mass spectrometry: the tool of choice for diagnosing inborn errors of metabolism? *Br J Biomed Sci.* 2002;59:42–46.
25. Krause W, Halminski M, McDonald L, et al. Biochemical and neuropsychological effects of elevated plasma phenylalanine in patients with treated phenylketonuria: a model for the study of phenylalanine and brain function in man. *J Clin Invest.* 1985;75:40–48.
26. Diamond A, Prevor MB, Callender G, Druin DP. Prefrontal cortex cognitive deficits in children treated early and continuously for PKU. *Monogr Soc Res Child Dev.* 1997;62:1–208.
27. Luciana M, Hanson KL, Whitley CB. A preliminary report on dopamine system reactivity in PKU: acute effects of haloperidol on neuropsychological, physiological, and neuroendocrine functions. *Psychopharmacology (Berl).* 2004;175:18–25.
28. Blau N, Erlandsen H. The metabolic and molecular bases of tetrahydrobiopterin-responsive phenylalanine hydroxylase deficiency. *Mol Genet Metab.* 2004;82:101–111.
29. Koch R, Friedman EG, Azen CG, et al. Report from the United States collaborative study of children treated for phenylketonuria (PKU). In: Bickel H, Wachtel U, eds. *Inherited Diseases of Amino Acid Metabolism.* Stuttgart, Germany: George Thieme; 1985:134–150.
30. Azen CG, Koch R, Friedman EG, et al. Intellectual development in 12-year-old children treated for phenylketonuria. *Am J Dis Child.* 1991;145(1):35–39.
31. Rouse B, Azen C, Koch R, et al. Maternal Phenylketonuria Collaborative Study (MPKUCS) offspring: facial anomalies, malformations, and early neurological sequelae. *Am J Med Genet.* 1997;69:89–95.
32. Waisbren SE, Hanley W, Levy HL, et al. Outcome at age 4 years in offspring of women with maternal phenylketonuria: the Maternal PKU Collaborative Study. *JAMA.* 2000;283:756–762.
33. Matalon KM, Acosta PB, Azen C. Role of nutrition in pregnancy with phenylketonuria and birth defects. *Pediatrics.* 2003;112(6 Pt 2):1534–1536.
34. Schadewaldt P, Bodner-Leidecker A, Hammen HW, Wendel U. Significance of L-alloisoleucine in plasma for diagnosis of maple syrup urine disease. *Clin Chem.* 1999;45:1734–1740.
35. Yoshino M, Aoki K, Akeda H, et al. Management of acute metabolic decompensation in maple syrup urine disease: a multi-center study. *Pediatr Int.* 1999;41:132–137.
36. Hilliges C, Awiszus D, Wendel U. Intellectual performance of children with maple syrup urine disease. *Eur J Pediatr.* 1993;152:144–147.
37. Kaplan P, Mazur A, Field M, et al. Intellectual outcome in children with maple syrup urine disease. *J Pediatr.* 1991;119:46–50.
38. Puliyanda DP, Harmon WE, Peterschmitt MJ, Irons M, Somers MJ. Utility of hemodialysis in maple syrup urine disease. *Pediatr Nephrol.* 2002;17:239–242.
39. Hmiel SP, Martin RA, Landt M, Levy FH, Grange DK. Amino acid clearance during acute metabolic decompensation in maple syrup urine disease treated with continuous venovenous hemodialysis with filtration. *Pediatr Crit Care Med.* 2004;5:278–281.
40. Morton DH, Strauss KA, Robinson DL, Puffenberger EG, Kelley RI. Diagnosis and treatment of maple syrup disease: a study of 36 patients. *Pediatrics.* 2002;109:999–1008.
41. Biggemann B, Zass R, Wendel U. Postoperative metabolic decompensation in maple syrup urine disease is completely prevented by insulin. *J Inherit Metab Dis.* 1993;16:912–913.
42. Yudkoff M, Daikhin Y, Nissim I, et al. Brain amino acid requirements and toxicity: the example of leucine. *J Nutr.* 2005;135:1531S–1538S.
43. Jouvet P, Jugie M, Rabier D, et al. Combined nutritional support and continuous extracorporeal removal therapy in the severe acute phase of maple syrup urine disease. *Intensive Care Med.* 2001;27:1798–1806.
44. Townsend I, Kerr DS. Total parenteral nutrition therapy of toxic maple syrup urine disease. *Am J Clin Nutr.* 1982;36:359–365.
45. Berry GT, Heidenreich R, Kaplan P, et al. Branched-chain amino acid-free parenteral nutrition in the treatment of acute metabolic decompensation in patients with maple syrup urine disease. *N Engl J Med.* 1991;324:175–179.
46. Huner G, Baykal T, Demir F, Demirkol J. Breastfeeding experience in inborn errors of metabolism other than phenylketonuria. *J Inherit Metab Dis.* 2005;28:457–465.
47. Tornqvist K, Tornqvist H. Corneal deepithelialization caused by acute deficiency of isoleucine during treatment of a patient with maple syrup urine disease. *Acta Ophthalmol Scand Suppl.* 1996;48–49.
48. Varvogli L, Repetto GM, Waisbren SE, Levy HL. High cognitive outcome in an adolescent with mut$^-$ methylmalonic acidemia. *Am J Med Genet.* 2000;96(2):192–195.
49. Baumgarter ER, Viardot C. Long-term follow-up of 77 patients with isolated methylmalonic acidaemia. *J Inherit Metab Dis.* 1995;18:138–142.
50. Ogier de Baulny H, Benoist JF, Rigal O, Touati G, Rabier D, Saudubray JM. Methylmalonic and propionic acidaemias: management and outcome. *J Inherit Metab Dis.* 2005;28:415–423.

51. Sanjurjo P, Ruiz JI, Montejo M. Inborn errors of metabolism with a protein-restricted diet: effect on polyunsaturated fatty acids. *J Inherit Metab Dis.* 1997;20:783–789.

52. Sequeira JSS, Dixon MA, Leonard JF. Growth in disorders of propionate metabolism. *J Inherit Metab Dis.* 1996;19(suppl 1):44A.

53. Yannicelli S, Acosta PB, Velazquez A, et al. Improved growth and nutrition status in children with methylmalonic or propionic acidemia fed an elemental medical food. *Mol Genet Metab.* 2003;80:181–188.

54. North KN, Korson MK, Yasodha RG. Neonatal-onset propionic academia: neurologic and developmental profiles, and implications for management. *J Pediatr.* 1995;126:916–922.

55. Feillet F, Bodamer OAF, Dixon MA, Sequeira S, Leonard JV. Resting energy expenditure in disorders of propionate metabolism. *J Pediatr.* 2000;136:659–663.

56. Thomas JA, Bernstein LE, Greene CL, Koeller DM. Apparent decreased energy requirements in children with organic acidemias: preliminary observations. *J Am Diet Assoc.* 2000;100:1074–1076.

57. Chalmers RA, Stacey TE, Tracey BM, et al. L-carnitine insufficiency in disorders of organic acid metabolism: response to L-carnitine by patients with methylmalonic aciduria and 3-hydroxy-3-methylglutaric aciduria. *J Inherit Metab Dis.* 1984;7(suppl 2):109–110.

58. DiDonato S, Rimoldi M, Garavaglia B, Uziel G. Propionylcarnitine excretion in propionic and methylmalonic acidurias: a cause of carnitine deficiency. *Clin Chim Acta.* 1984;139:13–21.

59. Bain MD, Jones M, Borriello SP, et al. Contribution of gut bacterial metabolism to human metabolic disease. *Lancet.*1988;14(18594):1078–1079.

60. Thompson GN, Walter JH, Bresson JL, et al. Sources of propionate in inborn errors of propionate metabolism. *Metabolism.* 1990;39:1133–1137.

61. Hyman SL, Porter CA, Page TJ, Iwata BA, Kissel R, Batshaw ML. Behavior management of feeding disturbances in urea cycle and organic acid disorders. *J Pediatr.* 1987;111:558–562.

62. Rossi-Fanelli F, Laviano A. Role of brain tryptophan and serotonin in secondary anorexia. *Adv Exp Med Biol.* 2003;527:225–232.

63. Plata-Salaman CR. Central nervous system mechanisms contributing to the cachexia-anorexia syndrome. *Nutrition.* 2000;16:1009–1012.

64. Inoue S, Krieger I, Sarnaik A, Ravindranath Y, Fracassa M, Ottenbreit MJ. Inhibition of bone marrow stem cell growth in vitro by methylmalonic acid: a mechanism for pancytopenia in a patient with methylmalonic acidemia. *Pediatr Res.* 1981;15:95–98.

65. Stork LC, Ambruso DR, Wallner SF. Pancytopenia in propionic acidemia: hematologic evaluation and studies of hematopoiesis in vitro. *Pediatr Res.* 1986;20:783–788.

66. Kahler SG, Millington DS, Cederbaum SD. Parenteral nutrition in propionic and methylmalonic acidemia. *J Pediatr.* 1989;115:235–241.

67. Kalloghlian A, Gleispach H, Ozand PT. A patient with propionic acidemia managed by continuous insulin infusion and total parenteral nutrition. *J Child Neurol.* 1992;7:S88–S91.

68. Burton BK. Urea cycle disorders. *Clin Liver Dis.* 2000;4:815–830.

69. Cohn RM, Roth KS. Hyperammonemia, bane of the brain. *Clin Pediatr (Phila).* 2004;43:683–689.

70. Felipo V, Butterworth RF. Neurobiology of ammonia. *Prog Neurobiol.* 2002;67:259–279.

71. Bachmann C. Outcome and survival of 88 patients with urea cycle disorders: a retrospective evaluation. *Eur J Pediatr.* 2003;162:410–416.

72. Whitington PF, Alonso EM, Boyle JT, et al. Liver transplantation for the treatment of urea cycle disorders. *J Inherit Metab Dis.* 1998;21(suppl 1):112–118.

73. Schaefer F, Straube E, Oh J, et al. Dialysis in neonates with inborn errors of metabolism. *Nephrol Dial Transplant.* 1999;14:910–918.

74. Mathias RS, Kostiner D, Packman S. Hyperammonemia in urea cycle disorders: role of the nephrologist. *Am J Kidney Dis.* 2001;37:1069–1080.

75. Scaglia F, Carter S, O'Brien WE, Lee B. Effect of alternative pathway therapy on branched chain amino acid metabolism in urea cycle disorder patients. *Mol Genet Metab.* 2004;81(suppl 1):S79–S85.

76. Matsuda I, Ohtani Y, Ohyanagi K, Yamamoto S. Hyperammonemia related to carnitine metabolism with particular emphasis on ornithine transcarbamylase deficiency. *Enzyme.* 1987;38:251–255.

ACKNOWLEDGMENTS

The authors would like to thank Drs. Gerard Berry and Alan Ryan for their expertise and editorial comments, and Ms. Christine Downs for her technical services.

Chapter 34

Oncology and Stem Cell Transplantation

Lori J. Bechard and Tara C. McCarthy

INTRODUCTION

Cancer in children is expected to affect approximately 1 in 300 newborns,[1] and the disease has significant implications for nutrition support. Many treatments for pediatric cancer cause gastrointestinal toxicities that reduce or preclude normal oral intake. The tumor burden alone could interfere with adequate nutrition due to its location or physical proximity to the gastrointestinal tract. Furthermore, the psychological impact of life threatening illness can negatively affect the social and behavioral eating patterns of children. The background, methodologies, and future directions for nutrition support in children with cancer will be reviewed in this chapter.

Advances in therapy for pediatric malignancies have led to substantially greater survival rates. More children live through and beyond cancer diagnosis and treatment. Nutrition support is known to be an essential component of cancer treatment and could also play a key role in the quality of life for long term childhood cancer survivors.

NUTRITION RISK IN PEDIATRIC CANCER

There are many circumstances in which nutrition support is indicated. It is important to carefully examine the rationale for each method and make the best choice for each individual. The process of evaluation includes nutrition assessment, and at varying intervals, reassessment. Different types of cancer are more likely to elevate nutritional risk and lead to malnutrition (Table 34-1). Higher risk diagnoses require more frequent, more aggressive nutrition intervention. Good nutrition monitoring and services are essential to the prevention and treatment of malnutrition in children with cancer. A summary of the rationale for such care is summarized in Table 34-2.

Pediatric cancer treatment includes chemotherapy, radiation, and surgery. Most malignant diseases require chemotherapy. More aggressive malignancies require the use of multiple treatment modalities. Stem cell transplantation (SCT) is reserved for those cases without other reasonable options, since it is known to be a high risk, highly toxic treatment (see Table 34-3). Graft versus host disease (GVHD), a condition involving the attack of newly engrafted cells on the host recipient, can occur following allogeneic SCT. Acute gastrointestinal GVHD can cause symptoms ranging from mild nausea and anorexia to profuse, bloody diarrhea. The manifestation of acute skin GVHD varies from a mild rash to severe epithelial sloughing, akin to a burn injury. Chronic GVHD occurs more than 100 days following transplant, and while its symptoms tend to be less severe initially, it is associated with significant long term morbidity and mortality.[1–4] Treatment for both types of GVHD often involves the use of steroids for their immunosuppressive effects.

Table 34-1 Risk factors for malnutrition in pediatric cancer patients.

High Nutritional Risk

- Advanced stage diseases during initial intense treatment:
  - Wilms' tumor
  - Neuroblastoma
  - Rhabdomyosarcoma
  - Ewing's sarcoma
  - Non-Hodgkin's lymphoma
  - Acute lymphoblastic leukemia
- Tumors of the head and neck (e.g., nasopharyngeal carcinomas)
- Acute myelogenous leukemia
- Multiply relapsed leukemia
- Medulloblastoma and other high grade brain tumors

Low Nutritional Risk

- Good prognosis acute lymphoblastic leukemia
- Nonmetastatic solid tumors
- Other diseases in remission

Adapted from Mauer AM, Burgess JB, Donaldson SS, et al. Special nutritional needs of children with malignancies: a review. *Jpen: Journal of Parenteral & Enteral Nutrition.* 1990;14(3):315-324, Rickard K, Grosfeld J, Coates T, Weetman R, Baehner R. Advances in nutrition care of children with neoplastic diseases: a review of treatment, reseach, and application. *J Am Diet Assoc.* 1986;86:1666-1676, Yu C. Nutrition and Childhood Malignancies. In: Suskind R, Lewinter-Suskind L, eds. *Textbook of Pediatric Nutrition.* 2nd ed. New York: Raven Press, Ltd.; 1993.

Table 34-2 importance of identifying, treating, and preventing malnutrition in pediatric cancer patients.

1) Malnutrition is common among children with cancer.
   - weight loss or poor weight gain
   - poor linear growth
2) Symptoms of malnutrition may be obscure in the absence of obvious wasting or stunting.
   - changes in body composition [a]
   - alterations in substrate metabolism [b,c]
3) Malnutrition is associated with increased morbidity and mortality [d-i].
   - decreased immune competence, increased infections
   - delayed wound healing
   - reduction in muscle strength
   - increased hospitalization time
   - developmental delay
4) Pediatric cancer patients with malnutrition have lower tolerance to chemotherapy [j,k] and higher mortality rates [l-n].
5) Early identification of the patient at risk for malnutrition can obviate the need for more aggressive nutritional support later.
   - anticipatory guidance
   - oral or enteral supplements [o]
6) Successful nutritional support may enhance therapy, decrease complications, improve immunologic status, and perhaps improve survival.

Adapted from Bechard et al[p].

References

a. Smith D, Stevens M, Booth I. Malnutrition at diagnosis of malignancy in childhood: common but mostly missed. *Eur J Pediatr.* 1991;150:318–322.

b. Burt M, Stein T, Schwade J, Brennan M. Whole-body protein metabolism in cancer-bearing patients: effect of total parenteral nutritionand associated serum insulin response. *Cancer.* 1984;53:1246–1252.

c. Kern K, Norton J. Cancer cachexia. *Journal of Parenteral and Enteral Nutrition.* 1988;12:286–298.

d. Bistrian BR, Blackburn GL, Scrimshaw NS, Flatt JP. Cellular immunity in semi-starved states in hospitalized adults. *Am J Clin Nutr.* 1975;28:1148.

e. Naber TH, Schermer T, de Bree A, et al. Prevalence of malnutrition in nonsurgical hospitalized patients and its association with disease complications. *Am J Clin Nutr.* 1997;66(5):1232–1239.

f. Martyn CN, Winter PD, Coles SJ, Edington J. Effect of nutritional status on use of health care resources by patients with chronic disease living in the community. *Clin Nutr.* 1998;17(3):119–123.

g. Chima CS, Barco K, Dewitt ML, Maeda M, Teran JC, Mullen KD. Relationship of nutritional status to length of stay, hospital costs, and discharge status of patients hospitalized in the medicine service. *J Am Diet Assoc.* 1997;97(9):975–978.

h. Sommer A, Loewenstein M. Nutritional status and mortality: a prospective evaluation of the QUAC stick. *Am J Clin Nutr.* 1975;28:287–292.

i. Galler J, Ramsey F, Soliman G, et al. The influence of early malnutrition on subsequent behavioral development: 1. Degree of impairment in intellectual performance. *J Am Acad Child Adolesc Psychiatry.* 1983;22:8.

j. Rickard K, Detamore C, Coates T, et al. Effect of nutrition staging on treatment delays and outcome in stage IV neuroblastoma. *Cancer.* 1983;52:587–598.

k. Rickard K, Loghmani E, Gorsfeld J, et al. Short- and long-term effectiveness of enteral and parenteral nutrition in reversing or preventing protein energy malnutrition in advanced neuroblastoma: a prospective randomized study. *Cancer.* 1985;56:2881–2897.

l. Donaldson S, Wesley M, DeWys W, et al. A study of the nutritional status of pediatric cancer patients. *Am J Dis Child.* 1981;135:1107.

m. Viana M, Murao M, Ramos G, et al. Malnutrition as a prognostic factor in lymphoblastic leukaemia: a multivariate analysis. *Arch Dis Child.* 1994;71:304–310.

n. Lobato-Mendizabal E, Lopez-Martinez B, Ruiz-Arguelles GJ. A critical review of the prognostic value of the nutritional status at diagnosis in the outcome of therapy of children with acute lymphoblastic leukemia. *Rev Invest Clin.* Jan–Feb 2003;55(1):31–35.

o. Souba W. Nutritional support. *New Engl J Med.* 1997;336:41–48.

p. Bechard L, Eshach-Adiv O, Jaksic T, Duggan C. Nutritional Supportive Care. In: Pizzo P, Poplack D, eds. *Principles and Practice of Pediatric Oncology.* 4th edition ed. Philadelphia: Lippincott Williams and Wilkins; 2002.

Table 34-3 Indications for hematopoietic stem cell transplantation in childhood.

Malignant diseases	*Nonmalignant conditions*
Acute myeloid leukemia	Aplastic anemia
Acute lymphocytic leukemia	Fanconi's anemia
Chronic myelogenous leukemia	Diamond-Blackfan anemia
Advanced stage neuroblastoma	Severe combined immunodeficiency (SCID)
Refractory Ewing's sarcoma	Wiskott-Aldrich syndrome
Advanced stage Wilms' tumor	Other cellular immunodeficiencies
Myelodysplastic syndrome	Mucopolysaccharidoses (Hurler's, Hunter's)
Lymphoma	Osteopetrosis

Source: Adapted from Charuhas PM. Pediatric hematopoietic stem cell transplantation. In: Hasse JM, Blue LS, eds. *Comprehensive guide to transplant nutrition.* Chicago, Ill: American Dietetic Association; 2002.

NUTRITIONAL EFFECTS OF TREATMENT

Cancer treatment can have a considerable effect on a child's nutritional status. Frequently occurring nutritional problems with malignancy and their associated treatments are listed in Table 34-4. Medical therapies, particularly prolonged courses of chemotherapy (see Table 34-5 for nutritional side effects of chemotherapy), often cause patients to receive less than optimal nutrition. SCT involves a time course of events that commonly leads to nutritional aberrations. A depiction of these associated events is shown in Figure 34-1. Proposed strategies for managing nutrition related side effects are presented in Table 34-6.

Chemotherapy is the principal cause of most nausea and vomiting in children with cancer.[5] The severity of nausea and vomiting depends on the dose, administration method, and the agent prescribed. Mucositis can cause nausea and vomiting. Oral mucositis is a major nonhematologic complication of cytotoxic chemotherapy and radiotherapy and is associated with morbidity, pain, and odynophagia.[6] Mucositis might lead to decreased intake of liquids and solids. Food aversion could develop. Nasogastric or gastrostomy tube feeding may be an option for children with severe mucositis. If enteritis is severe, enteral feeds (EN) might not be an option and parenteral nutrition (PN) support might be needed.

Diarrhea and constipation or a combination of the 2 can occur with treatment. Diarrhea can result from chemotherapy, radiation, prolonged antibiotic use, or infections. Narcotics and some chemotherapeutic agents decrease intestinal motility and cause constipation. Stool softeners can be effective in lessening symptoms.

Radiation therapy, depending on the amount, the location and the extent of the field, can have a significant impact on nutritional symptoms.[7] Radiation to the head, neck, and chest causes mucositis, altered taste perception, anorexia, and dysphagia. When the radiation field includes the abdomen or pelvis, gastrointestinal side effects including nausea, vomiting, or radiation enteritis occur.[7]

Nutritional status can be affected by surgical treatments and depends on the site of the tumor and the extent of the resection.[7] The efficient ingestion, digestion, absorption, and utilization of food are a complex process.

Table 34-4 Nutritional problems in pediatric cancer treatment.

	Malignancy	*Chemotherapy*	*Radiation*	*Surgery*	*SCT*
Anorexia	X	X	X		X
Infection		X	X	X	X
Diarrhea	X	X	X		X
Nausea and vomiting		X	Depends on site		X
Malabsorption	X	X	Depends on site	Depends on site	X
Blood loss	X	X		X	X
Renal damage		X	Depends on site		X
Ileus	X	X	Depends on site	X	

SCT = stem cell transplant

Table 34-5 Nutritional side effects of treatments used in pediatric oncology.

Category	*Examples*	*Side effects*
Chemotherapy	Busulfan	N&V, mucositis, hepatic toxicity (high dose)
	Cisplatin	N&V, anorexia, diarrhea, altered taste/smell
	Cyclophosphamide	N&V, altered taste/smell
	Cytarabine	N&V, mucositis, diarrhea
	Dactinomycin	N&V, mucositis, hepatic toxicity, diarrhea
	Doxorubicin	Severe mucositis, N&V, diarrhea
	Etoposide	Anorexia, N&V
	L-asparaginase	Pancreatitis, hepatic toxicity, hyperglycemia, altered taste/smell
	Melphalan	N&V, mucositis, diarrhea
	Methotrexate	Mucositis, diarrhea, hepatic toxicity, pancreatitis
	Vincristine	Ileus, constipation
Corticosteroids	Prednisone, dexamethasone	Hyperglycemia, fluid and salt retention, muscle wasting, osteoporosis, cushnoid features, acne, hypertension, psychologic effects, cataracts
Antimicrobials	Augmentin, erythromycin, clindamycin, amphotericin, acyclovir	Diarrhea/upset stomach, renal toxicity with cation losses
Narcotics	Codeine, morphine	Ileus, constipation
Radiation	Total body irradiation, focal irradiation	Mucositis, radiation enteritis (depending on site)

N&V = nausea and vomiting

Source: Adapted from Bechard L. Oncology and bone marrow transplantation. In: Hendricks K, Duggan C, Walker W, eds. *Manual of Pediatric Nutrition.* 3rd. ed. Hamilton, Ontario: Decker; 2000:490–502.

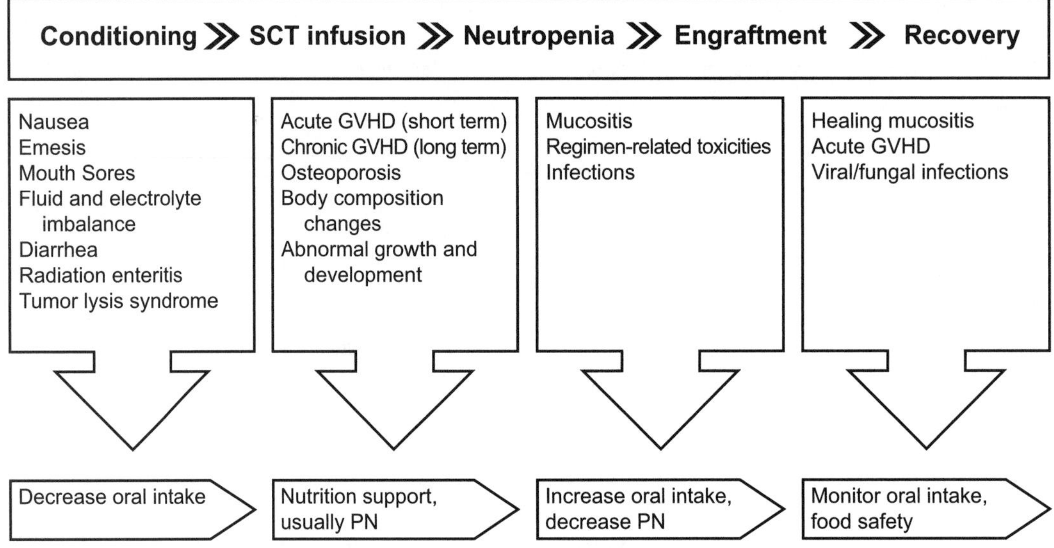

Figure 34-1 Continuum of nutritional effects of stem cell transplantation. SCT = stem cell transplant, GVHD = graft versus host disease, PN = parenteral nutrition

Table 34-6 Strategies for coping with side effects during cancer treatment.

Loss of Appetite
- Small, frequent feedings (6–8 meals/snacks per day)
- Encourage nutrient-dense beverages between meals
- Offer favorite nutritious foods during treatment free periods to prevent learned food aversions

Nausea and Vomiting
- Optimize antiemetic therapy
- Offer small amounts of cool foods and encourage slow eating; avoid strong odors
- Offer clear liquids between meals
- Offer liquids with a straw in a covered cup

Mouth Sores
- Serve soft or pureed bland food or liquids
- Add butter, gravy, sauce, or salad dressing to moisten foods
- Avoid highly seasoned or hard, rough foods

Altered Taste Perception
- Use stronger seasonings; avoid excessively sweet foods
- Offer salty or sour foods; try new flavors

Diarrhea and Constipation
- Increase fiber and fluids
- Assure adequate hydration

Source: Adapted from Bechard L. Oncology and bone marrow transplantation. In: Hendricks K, Duggan C, Walker W, eds. *Manual of Pediatric Nutrition.* 3rd. ed. Hamilton, Ontario: Decker; 2000:490–502.

Surgical disruption such as impaired swallowing, decreased gastric reserve or intestinal length can result in decreased oral intake and malabsorption.[8]

NUTRITION SUPPORT METHODOLOGIES

Food Safety

Because cancer and its treatment cause immunosuppression, low microbial diets are used to minimize risk of illness from food borne pathogens.[9] There is little evidence to support efficacy of these regimens in preventing clinical infections. Nevertheless, they make intuitive sense and are harmless. Table 34-7 reviews principles of food safety recommended for children with cancer and other causes of immune compromise.

Table 34-7 Sanitary food practices for immunocompromised patients.

- Good hand washing before and after preparing and eating meals
- Do not share food with others
- Avoid foods from street vendors, salad bars, shared bins of foods in grocery stores
- Wash raw foods well prior to eating
- Cook meat until well done
- Avoid raw eggs
- Keep foods at < 40 degrees F or > 140 degrees F to minimize growth of bacteria
- Clean all preparation items thoroughly before and after use to avoid cross-contamination
- Keep refrigerated leftovers for no more than 3 days

Source: Adapted from Bechard L. Oncology and bone marrow transplantation. In: Hendricks K, Duggan C, Walker W, eds. *Manual of Pediatric Nutrition.* 3rd. ed. Hamilton, Ontario: Decker; 2000:490–502.

Enteral Feeding

Volitional oral feeding is the ultimate goal of nutrition care of the pediatric cancer patient; more aggressive measures of nutrition support are often needed for short term and, occasionally, long term nutrition. Tube feedings are used to treat and prevent malnutrition in children with neoplastic disease. Outcomes vary. Several authors examined the use of gastrostomy feedings in children with a variety of cancers, many of whom developed malnutrition during treatment. Children on treatment for cancer who receive EN through gastrostomy tubes maintained or gained weight and had fewer infections and less cost associated with their care compared to children who received PN.[10–12] EN for children undergoing SCT has mixed success. Papadopoulou et al. found that 8 of 21 children undergoing SCT were unable to tolerate EN for greater than 8–10 days of their hospitalization, although those who did tolerate tube feeding gained weight.[13] In a more recent report from Ireland, 86% of children receiving nasogastric feedings were maintained exclusively on EN; energy intake was < 50% of estimated requirements throughout the peritransplant period, although weight was unchanged in most patients.[14] Further outcome data are needed to support the routine use of tube feedings, especially in SCT recipients. EN in children with cancer is feasible and effective; nevertheless, some children require PN during particularly toxic therapies.

For EN a standard, age appropriate formula is the first choice for children with cancer. Recent additions to the formula market include high protein, cancer-specific formulas with added omega-3 fatty acids. Omega-3 fatty acids increase lean body mass in adults with aggressive solid tumors.[15,16] No clinical trials document benefits of these formulas in children. While most children tolerate intact protein formulas, some could benefit from semielemental formulas, especially when gastrointestinal function is impaired. Table 34-8 describes features of formulas for use in pediatric oncology and SCT patients.

Table 34-8 Formulas used for children with cancer.

Formula	*Kcal/mL Type*	*Features*
For older children and adults		
Resource Breeze‡	1.06 O	Clear liquid, fat-free supplement with 14% kcal from whey protein; wild berry, orange, and peach flavors
Carnation Instant Breakfast Juice Drink§	1.0 O	Clear liquid, fat-free juice drink with 16% kcal from whey protein; sweet berry and orange flavors
Boost‡	1.01 O/C	Milk-based, lactose-free liquid; 6 flavors; also available with fiber, increased calories, increased protein, and as pudding
Ensure†	1.06 O/C	Liquid nutrition with casein, soy, and whey protein; 7 flavors; also available with fiber/FOS, varied calories, high protein or calcium, bars, pudding, and powder
Prosure†	1.27 O	Casein-based supplement for cancer cachexia; contains 1 g EPA, 3 g fiber per 8 oz. serving from FOS, 23% protein, 21% fat; 2 flavors
Resource Support‡	1.5 O	Casein and amino acid-based supplement with EPA for cancer cachexia; 3 g fiber per 8 oz.; 23% protein, 30% fat; in Brik paks
Peptamen§	1.0 O/C	Semi-elemental nutrition with hydrolyzed whey, 70% fat as MCT; also available with FOS/inulin; 1.5 kcal/mL; high protein
For children ages 1–10 yrs.		
Kindercal (TF)*	1.06 O/C	Milk-based, lactose-free liquid; meets RDA for 7–10 yrs. in 1,000 mL; with or without fiber; vanilla and chocolate flavors
PediaSure (Enteral)†	1.0 O/C	Milk-based, lactose-free liquid; meets RDA in 1,000 mL (1–6 yrs.); 1,300 mL (7–10 yrs.); available with or without fiber; 5 flavors
Resource Just for Kids‡	1.0 O/C	Casein and whey protein-based liquid in Brik paks; also available with fiber, increased calories; meets RDA in 1,000 mL; 3 flavors
Peptamen Jr.§	1.0 O/C	Semielemental nutrition with hydrolyzed whey, 60% fat as MCT, isotonic (unflavored only); meets RDA in 1,000 mL, flavor packets; available with FOS/inulin
Nutren Jr.§	1.0 O/C	Whey- (50%) and casein- (50%) based liquid; 21% fat as MCT; meets RDA in 1,000 mL; with or without fiber; 10 flavor packets

* Mead Johnson Nutritionals
† Ross Products, a division of Abbott Laboratories
‡ Novartis Nutrition
§ Nestle Clinical Nutrition
O = oral supplement
C = complete feeding
MCT = medium chain triglycerides
FOS = fructo-oligosaccharides
EPA = eicosapentaenoic acid
RDA = Recommended Dietary Allowance

Sources: From product information.

PARENTERAL NUTRITION

The efficacy of PN in supporting children with cancer has been established in SCT recipients.[17,18] Positive outcomes for PN during standard cancer treatment in children have not been documented. Indications for PN include severe mucositis with anorexia, prolonged ileus, and severe malabsorption, as seen with GVHD. While the use of PN support during disease or treatment-related gastrointestinal failure could prevent the exacerbation of malnutrition, PN can be associated with hepatotoxicity, metabolic abnormalities, suppression of oral intake, and infections. Moreover, the appropriate PN prescription specific for children with cancer remains unclear.

Most children require central venous catheters for administration of chemotherapy, so hyperosmolar PN can be infused without an additional surgical procedure. However, 2.4 times greater risk of infections is seen in children receiving PN.[19] Delayed resumption of oral intake,[20] nausea, and vomiting[21] are observed in children receiving PN at home.

Chemotherapy and radiation cause severe muscle catabolism, and especially high doses are used in preparation for SCT. Body composition can be altered as a result. Therefore, standard equations for predicting energy expenditure and protein requirements might be inaccurate.[22] Conflicting reports exist as to the appropriate level of energy intake for these children. A retrospective review of 20 children undergoing allogeneic and autologous SCT suggested that less energy was delivered than was calculated and that caloric intake and time to engraftment were correlated.[23] Expected energy intake was defined as 1.2–1.5 times basal metabolic rate as calculated by the World Health Organization (WHO) equation.[24] A prospective study of 34 children measured energy expenditure by weekly indirect calorimetry, from pretransplant through day 21 posttransplant. Results showed a lower than predicted energy expenditure compared to the WHO equation at all times except day 14 after SCT.[25] Another report described a significant decline in measured resting energy expenditure of pediatric allogeneic SCT recipients over time. Indirect calorimetry was used to measure energy expenditure weekly from baseline through 5 weeks after SCT. Baseline values were near those estimated by the WHO equation. A slight increase in energy expenditure was noted between weeks 4 and 5, suggesting that energy requirements decline during SCT, but might rebound following engraftment.[26] Further studies of body composition and its effects on nutrient requirements during SCT in children are warranted. PN prescriptions should be individually considered; the use of indirect calorimetry can be more helpful than standard equations to estimate calorie requirements in children undergoing oncologic treatment.

Conventional recommendations for starting and monitoring PN are applicable for children with cancer (Tables 34-9 and 34-10). Attention to electrolyte and mineral requirements is particularly important in the setting of organ dysfunction related to treatment and/or disease. Tumor lysis syndrome, a metabolic complication wherein destruction of tumor mass causes

Table 34-9 Initiation of parenteral nutrition in children with cancer.

Nutrient	*Start with*	*Advance by*	*Goal*
Dextrose	3–4 mg/kg/hr	2–3 mg/kg/hr	8–18 mg/kg/hr
Amino acids	1 g/kg/d	0.5–1 g/kg/d	1.5–3 g/kg/d
Lipids	1 g/kg/d	0.5–1 g/kg/d	1–3 g/kg/d

Table 34-10 Nutritional monitoring of children undergoing oncologic treatment.

Parameter	*Hospitalized patients on parenteral nutrition*	*Hospitalized patients on oral/ tube feedings*	*Outpatients on parenteral nutrition*	*Outpatients on oral/tube feedings*
Weight	Daily	Daily	Weekly	Monthly
Height	Monthly	Monthly	Monthly	Monthly
Head circumference (< 36 months)	Weekly	Weekly	Monthly	Monthly
Arm anthropometrics	Monthly	As indicated	Monthly	As indicated
Intake/output	Daily	Daily	Daily to weekly	Weekly to monthly
Electrolytes, glucose	Daily	Weekly	Weekly	Monthly
BUN, creatinine	Weekly	Weekly	Weekly	Monthly
Calcium, phosphorus, magnesium	Daily to weekly	Weekly	Weekly	Monthly
Triglyceride	Weekly	Monthly	Weekly	As indicated
Liver function tests	Weekly	Weekly	Monthly	Monthly
Trace elements	Monthly	As indicated	Biannually	As indicated
Carnitine	Monthly	As indicated	Biannually	As indicated
Vitamin levels	Monthly	As indicated	Biannually	As indicated

a massive release of cell contents, can occur as a consequence of initial chemotherapy. Life threatening electrolyte abnormalities can result from untreated tumor lysis syndrome; the standard of care for most newly diagnosed children involves prophylaxis with allopurinol, hyperhydration, and intravenous bicarbonate solutions.

Several investigators have found conflicting results with the use of glutamine, primarily in adults, during SCT. Glutamine supplemented PN is associated with shorter lengths of hospital stay, better nitrogen balance, and fewer clinical infections.[27,28] Trials using oral glutamine show lessened symptoms of mucositis with a swish and swallow regimen.[29,30] More recent controlled trials, however, showed no significant positive outcomes with oral or intravenous glutamine supplementation.[31,32] To date, convincing results for children have not been reported; consequently, clinical use of glutamine cannot be routinely recommended.

LONG TERM NUTRITIONAL SIDE EFFECTS OF TREATMENT

Treatments and therapies for childhood cancers, including SCT, are continuously evolving. Improvements in survival rates have led to greater interest in long term quality of life and reduction of late morbidity and mortality. As a result, the long term side effects of treatment are increasingly relevant to nutrition care. Obesity, cardiovascular disease, and osteoporosis are found in survivors of childhood cancers.[33–37] Effects from SCT include late toxicities from the treatment regimen, frequent infections caused by treatment-induced immunodeficiency, endocrine disturbances, growth impairment, psychosocial adjustment disorders, secondary malignancies, and chronic GVHD.[38,39]

Numerous risk factors, including glucocorticoid treatment, chemotherapy, cranial radiation, and psychosocial stress are implicated in the pathogenesis of obesity in children who have cancer. Survivors of the 2 most common pediatric cancers, acute lymphoblastic leukemia (ALL), and brain tumors are at high risk for developing obesity.[34,35] Nysom et al. concluded that a higher percent of body fat in ALL survivors compared to controls was related to cranial radiation or growth hormone insufficiency, but not to gender, cumulative doses of anthracyclines or corticosteroids, or type of corticosteroid.[40] Lustig et al. suggested hypothalamic damage caused by surgery, tumor location, or radiation treatment is the major cause of intractable weight gain in children who survive brain tumors.[34] Long term survivors of childhood brain cancers who received cranial radiation had greater dyslipidemia, central obesity, and higher blood pressure measurements compared to age-matched, normal controls in one study from the Netherlands.[41] These findings were more pronounced in the subgroup of patients with growth hormone deficiency. Taskinen et al. found that long term survivors of SCT are at risk for insulin resistance, impaired glucose tolerance, type 2 diabetes, dyslipidemia, and abdominal obesity or some combination of these. These complications could heighten later risk of cardiovascular disease in former SCT patients.[39] Poor nutrition, decreased physical activity during treatment, corticosteroids, and cranial radiation have been associated with bone loss. Recent changes in treatment regimes are associated with fewer bone abnormalities.[41,42] It is important to screen and monitor long term childhood cancer survivors for growth and nutrition-related late effects of treatment. Patients should be encouraged to follow guidelines for a heart-healthy lifestyle (see Table 34-11).

Table 34-11 Healthy lifestyle guidelines for childhood cancer survivors.

Aim for Fitness

- Aspire to a healthy weight
- Be active each day within personal limitations

Build a Healthy Base

- Include moderate amounts of foods from the 5 food groups
- Eat a variety of whole grains, fruits, and vegetables each day

Choose Sensibly

- Select a diet low in saturated fat and cholesterol
- Limit sugary foods and beverages
- Choose and prepare foods with less salt.

Source: Adapted from USDA. Dietary Guidelines for Americans. United States Department of Agriculture; 2000. Available at: http://www.health.gov/dietaryguidelines/dga2000/document/contents.htm.

CONCLUSION

Nutritional ramifications of pediatric cancer are numerous. The effects of the disease and its treatment have consequences on the selection of nutrition support for children and their families. The preferred approach to nutritional care is multidisciplinary and family focused. Short term concerns include prompt and continual nutrition assessment, suitable nutrition intervention and effective nutrition monitoring during diagnosis and treatment. Awareness of long term problems during this time allows anticipatory guidance to be provided to children at high risk for long term nutritional side effects. Finally, attention to healthy lifestyle choices is imperative in post-treatment survival.

REFERENCES

1. Ries L, CL P, Bunin G. Introduction. In: Ries L, Smith M, Gurney J, et al., eds. *Cancer Incidence and Survival among Children and Adolescents: United States SEER*

Program 1975–1995. NIH Pub. No. 99–4649. Bethesda, Md: National Cancer Institute, SEER Program; 1999.

2. Wingard JR, Piantadosi S, Vogelsang GB, et al. Predictors of death from chronic graft-versus-host disease after bone marrow transplantation. *Blood*. 1989;74(4):1428–1435.
3. Stern JM, Chesnut CH, 3rd, Bruemmer B, et al. Bone density loss during treatment of chronic GVHD. *Bone Marrow Transplant*. 1996;17(3):395–400.
4. Jacobsohn DA, Margolis J, Doherty J, Anders V, Vogelsang GB. Weight loss and malnutrition in patients with chronic graft-versus-host disease. *Bone Marrow Transplant*. 2002;29(3):231–236.
5. Davis MP, Walsh D. Treatment of nausea and vomiting in advanced cancer. *Support Care Cancer*. 2000;8(6):444–452.
6. Kostler WJ, Hejna M, Wenzel C, Zielinski CC. Oral mucositis complicating chemotherapy and/or radiotherapy: options for prevention and treatment. *CA Cancer J Clin*. 2001;51(5):290–315.
7. Donaldson SS. Effects of therapy on nutritional status of the pediatric cancer patient. *Cancer Res*. 1982;42(suppl 2):729s–736s.
8. Sheard N, Clark N. Nutritional management of pediatric oncology patients. In: Baker S, Baker R, Davis A, eds. *Pediatric Enteral Nutrition*. New York, NY: Chapman & Hall; 1994:387–398.
9. Aker SN, Cheney CL. The use of sterile and low microbial diets in ultraisolation environments. *J Parenter Enter Nutr*. 1983;7:390–397.
10. Pedersen A-MB, Kok K, Petersen G, Nielsen O, Michaelsen K, Schmiegelow K. Percutaneous endoscopic gastrostomy in children with cancer. *Acta Paediatr*. 1999;88:849–852.
11. Mathew P, Bowman L, Williams R, et al. Complications and effectiveness of gastrostomy feedings in pediatric cancer patients. *J Pediatr Hematol Oncol*. 1996;18(1):81–85.
12. Aquino VM, Smyrl CB, Hagg R, McHard KM, Prestridge L, Sandler ES. Enteral nutritional support by gastrostomy tube in children with cancer. *J Pediatr*. 1995;127:58–62.
13. Papadopoulou A, MacDonald A, Williams MD, Darbyshire PJ, Booth IW. Enteral nutrition after bone marrow transplantation. *Arch Dis Child*. 1997;77(2):131–136.
14. Langdana A, Tully N, Molloy E, Bourke B, O'Meara A. Intensive enteral nutrition support in paediatric bone marrow transplantation. *Bone Marrow Transplant*. 2001;27(7):741–746.
15. Barber MD, Ross JA, Voss AC, Tisdale MJ, Fearon KC. The effect of an oral nutritional supplement enriched with fish oil on weight-loss in patients with pancreatic cancer. *Br J Cancer*. 1999;81(1):80–86.
16. Barber MD, Fearon KC, Tisdale MJ, McMillan DC, Ross JA. Effect of a fish oil-enriched nutritional supplement on metabolic mediators in patients with pancreatic cancer cachexia. *Nutr Cancer*. 2001;40(2):118–124.
17. Weisdorf S, Hofland C, Sharp H, et al. Total parenteral nutrition in bone marrow transplantation: a clinical evaluation. *J Pediatr Gastroenterol Nutr*. 1984;3:95–100.
18. Weisdorf S, Lysne J, Wind D, et al. Positive effect of prophylactic total parenteral nutrition on long-term outcome of bone marrow transplantation. *Transplantation*. 1987;43(6):833–838.
19. Christensen ML, Hancock ML, Gattuso J, et al. Parenteral nutrition associated with increased infection rate in children with cancer. *Cancer*. 1993;72(9):2732–2738.
20. Charuhas P, Fosberg K, Bruemmer B, et al. A double-blind randomized trial comparing outpatient parenteral nutrition with intravenous hydration: effect on resumption of oral intake after marrow transplantation. *J Parenter Enter Nutr*. 1997;21(3):157–161.
21. Nicol J, Hoagland R, Heitlinger L. The prevalence of nausea and vomiting in pediatric patients receiving home parenteral nutrition. *Nutr Clin Pract*. 1995;10(5):189–192.
22. Schloerb PR, Bodanszky HE. Body cell mass as a reference for nutritional support in pediatric cancer patients. *Ann N Y Acad Sci*. 1997;824:234–236.
23. Forchielli ML, Azzi N, Cadranel S, Paolucci G. Total parenteral nutrition in bone marrow transplant: what is the appropriate energy level? *Oncology*. 2003;64(1):7–13.
24. World Health Organization. Report of a Joint FAO/WHO Ad Hoc Expert Committee. *Energy and Protein Requirements*. Geneva, Switzerland: WHO; 1973. WHO Technical Report No. 522.
25. Ringwald-Smith KA, Heslop HE, Krance RA, et al. Energy expenditure in children undergoing hematopoietic stem cell transplantation. *Bone Marrow Transplant*. 2002;30(2):125–130.
26. Duggan C, Bechard L, Donovan K, et al. Changes in resting energy expenditure among children undergoing allogeneic stem cell transplantation. *Am J Clin Nutr*. 2003;78(1):104–109.
27. Ziegler TR, Young LS, Benfell K, et al. Clinical and metabolic efficacy of glutamine-supplemented parenteral nutrition after bone marrow transplantation: a randomized, double-blind, controlled study. *Ann Intern Med*. 1992;116(10):821–828.
28. Schloerb PR, Amare M. Total parenteral nutrition with glutamine in bone marrow transplantation and other clinical applications (a randomized, double-blind study). *JPEN*. 1993;17(5):407–413.
29. Skubitz KM, Anderson PM. Oral glutamine to prevent chemotherapy induced stomatitis: a pilot study. *J Lab Clin Med*. 1996;127(2):223–228.

30. Anderson PM, Ramsay NK, Shu XO, et al. Effect of low-dose oral glutamine on painful stomatitis during bone marrow transplantation. *Bone Marrow Transplant.* 1998;22(4):339–344.
31. Coghlin Dickson T, Wong R, Negrin R, et al. Effect of oral glutamine supplementation during bone marrow transplantation. *JPEN.* 2000;24:61–66.
32. Schloerb PR, Skikne BS. Oral and parenteral glutamine in bone marrow transplantation: a randomized, double-blind study. *JPEN.* 1999;23(3):117–122.
33. Gurney JG, Kadan-Lottick NS, Packer RJ, et al. Endocrine and cardiovascular late effects among adult survivors of childhood brain tumors: Childhood Cancer Survivor Study. *Cancer.* 2003;97(3):663–673.
34. Lustig RH, Post SR, Srivannaboon K, et al. Risk factors for the development of obesity in children surviving brain tumors. *J Clin Endocrinol Metab.* 2003;88(2):611–616.
35. Oeffinger KC, Mertens AC, Sklar CA, et al. Obesity in adult survivors of childhood acute lymphoblastic leukemia: a report from the Childhood Cancer Survivor Study. *J Clin Oncol.* 2003;21(7):1359–1365.
36. Oeffinger KC, Buchanan GR, Eshelman DA, et al. Cardiovascular risk factors in young adult survivors of childhood acute lymphoblastic leukemia. *J Pediatr Hematol Oncol.* 2001;23(7):424–430.
37. Haddy TB, Mosher RB, Reaman GH. Osteoporosis in survivors of acute lymphoblastic leukemia. *Oncologist.* 2001;6(3):278–285.
38. Wingard JR, Vogelsang GB, Deeg HJ. Stem cell transplantation: supportive care and long-term complications. *Hematology (Am Soc Hematol Educ Program).* 2002:422–444.
39. Taskinen M, Saarinen-Pihkala U, Hovi L, Lipsanen-Nyman M. Impaired glucose tolerance and dyslipidemia as late effects after bone marrow transplantation in childhood. *Lancet.* 2000;356:993–997.
40. Nysom K, Holm K, Michaelsen KF, Hertz H, Muller J, Molgaard C. Degree of fatness after treatment for acute lymphoblastic leukemia in childhood. *J Clin Endocrin Metabol.* 1999;84(12):4591–4596.
41. Heikens J, Ubbink MC, van der Pal HP, et al. Long term survivors of childhood brain cancer have an increased risk for cardiovascular disease. *Cancer.* 2000;88(9):2116–2121.
42. Kadan-Lottick N, Marshall JA, Baron AE, Krebs NF, Hambidge KM, Albano E. Normal bone mineral density after treatment for childhood acute lymphoblastic leukemia diagnosed between 1991 and 1998. *J Pediatr.* 2001;138(6):898–904.

Chapter 35

Nutrition Support for Cystic Fibrosis

Nancy Ann Garrison, Chris Coburn-Miller, and Robert D. Baker

INTRODUCTION

Children and adolescents with cystic fibrosis (CF) should grow normally. Still, suboptimal growth occurs, and is due, in part, to chronic infection with subsequent poor appetite and cytokine-induced catabolism.[1] Chronic, progressive pulmonary damage can lead to increased work of breathing and higher than expected nutrient needs.[2] Despite these non-GI reasons for poor growth, nutrient delivery, digestion, and absorption are necessary to achieve normal growth, thus allowing optimal pulmonary function and prolonging life.

The CF Foundation (CFF) patient registry has documented impressive improvement in life expectancy of patients with CF.[3] To a large degree, the longer life achieved by patients with CF can be ascribed to improved treatment of lung disease, pulmonary toilet, potent and tailored antibiotics, DNAse, and lung transplantation. However, little has changed in the nutritional therapy of CF since it was recognized that fat-restricted diets do not improve outcomes.[4] Pancreatic enzyme replacement (PET) with dietary advice remains the most commonly used form of nutritional therapy in CF. The CFF, recognizing the need and the opportunity to improve nutritional therapy in CF, has convened 2 groups of experts to address nutrition in CF. These conferences resulted in a consensus report on nutrition in pediatric cystic fibrosis[5] and a more theoretic report on gastrointestinal outcomes and confounders in cystic fibrosis.[6]

CF is due to a defect in a transmembrane conductance regulator of cell membranes that regulates a chloride channel.[7] More than 100 mutations in the gene coding for cystic fibrosis transmembrane conductance regulator (CFTR) are described, and it is clear that CF represents a spectrum of disease, varying according to the genotype and with individual and environmental factors. This spectrum has profound implications for nutritional intervention. Approximately 11% of CF patients are pancreatic sufficient (PS).[8] PS patients do not require PET; they tend to have less severe lung disease, and their nutritional status is better than their pancreatic insufficient (PI) counterparts. PS versus PI status can be relatively simply determined by measuring the fecal elastase.[8] This test should be done on each patient with CF to determine the need for PET.

Pancreatic enzymes are extracts of porcine pancreas. Most enzyme preparations used in CF are granules or microspheres that are coated with a pH-sensitive material that protects the enzyme from destruction by acid in the stomach (see Table 35-1). The coating dissolves in the alkaline milieu of the duodenum, releasing the enzyme.[9] Although specific information is lacking, the pH of the GI tract in CF probably varies from patient to patient and from time to time in the same patient. Thus there is concern about matching enzyme release to the digestive needs of individual patients. The 72-hour fecal fat determination is the only current clinical method of quantifying fat malabsorption. It is tedious, inaccurate, and

Table 35-1 Oral pancreatic enzymes.*

Product	*Form*	*Lipase*	*Protease*	*Amylase*
Cotazyme-S-Forte†	Enteric coated microspheres	10,000	7,700	750
Pancrease	Enteric coated microtablets	4,500	25,000	20,000
Pancrease MT4		4,000	12,000	12,000
Pancrease MT10		10,000	30,000	30,000
Pancrease MT16		16,000	48,000	48,000
Pancrease MT20		20,000	44,000	56,000
Creon 5	Enteric coated microspheres in capsules	5,000	18,750	16,600
Creon 10		10,000	37,500	33,200
Creon 20		20,000	75,000	66,400
Ultrase	Enteric coated minitablets	4,500	25,000	20,000
Ultrase 12		12,000	39,500	39,500
Ultrase 18		18,000	58,500	58,500
Ultrase 20		20,000	65,000	65,000
Viokase	Powder (1/4 tsp)	16,800	70,000	70,000
Viokase 8	Tablet	8,000	30,000	30,000
Viokase 16	Tablet	16,000	60,000	60,000
Zymase	Enteric coated spheres	12,000	24,000	24,000
Pancrecarb MS4	Enteric coated microspheres with bicarbonate	4,000	25,000	25,000
Pancrecarb MS8		8,000	45,000	40,000
Pancrecarb MS16		16,000	52,000	52,000

* Information obtained from suppliers.
† Not available in the United States.

odious, and therefore is seldom used. PET, for the most part, is guided by patient-reported symptoms of malabsorption such as diarrhea; foul smelling, greasy, bulky stools; bloating; gassiness; and abdominal pain. These symptoms might not correlate with PET therapy.[10] So at present there is no accurate and practical method of deciding on the amount of PET needed.

ASSESSING AND MONITORING NUTRITION

The key to maintaining good nutrition status in cystic fibrosis, as in other chronic diseases, is to prevent suboptimal nutrition from occurring. Early detection of impending nutritional deterioration depends on careful and repeated nutritional assessment. The CFF recommends that children with CF be seen at 3 monthly intervals. A thorough dietary history and nutritional assessment should be a part of each of those visits. Table 35-2 gives the recommended nutritional assessment for routine CF center care.

The 2000 edition growth charts (http://www.cdc.gov/growthcharts) should be used for CF clinical care and have been used in calculation of the CFF patient registry data beginning with the 1999 annual report. One strong indicator of overall nutritional sufficiency is if patients are growing in height to their full genetic potential.[11] The genetic potential for height of each patient can be estimated by a variety of methods.[12,13] Genetic potential for height should be determined for each patient and the target height range (genetic potential related to biological parental height) should be noted on each patient's

Table 35-2 Nutritional assessment in routine CF center care.

	At diagnosis	*Every 3 months birth to 24 months*	*Every 3 months*	*Annually*
Head circumference	x*	x		
Weight (to 0.1 kg)	x	x	x	
Length (to 0.1 cm)	x	x		
Height (to 0.1 cm)	x		x	
Mid-arm circumference (to 0.1 cm)	x			x
Triceps skinfold (to 1.0 mm)	x†			x
Mid-arm muscle area, mm^2 (calculated from MAC and TSF)	x†			x
Mid-arm fat area, mm2 (calculated from MAC and TSF)	x†			x
Biological parents height‡	x			
Pubertal status, female				x§
Pubertal status, male				x‖
24-hour diet recall				x
Nutritional supplement intake¶				x
Anticipatory dietary and feeding behavior guidance		x	x#	x

* If less than 24 months of age at diagnosis.
† Only in patients over 1 year of age.
‡ Record in cm and gender-specific height percentile; note patient's target height percentile on all growth charts.
§ Starting at age 9 years, annual pubertal self-assessment form (patients or parent and patient) or physician examination for breast and pubic hair, Tanner stage determination; annual question as to menarchal status. Record month and year of menarche on all growth charts.
‖ Starting at age 12 years, annual pubertal self-assessment form (patients or parent and patient) or physician examination for genital development and pubic hair, Tanner stage determination.
¶ A review of enzymes, vitamins, minerals, oral or enteral formulas; herbal, botanical, and other CAM products.
# Routine surveillance may be done informally by other team members, but the annual assessment and q 3 monthly visits in the first 2 years of life and q 3 monthly visits for patients at nutritional risk should be done by the center dietician.

Source: Pediatric Nutrition for Patients with Cystic Fibrosis. *Consensus Conferences; Concepts in CF Care.* 2001;10(1):25.

growth chart. A definition of nutritional status in CF is given in Table 35-3.

NUTRITIONAL REQUIREMENTS

In the past, the caloric requirement of a CF patient was estimated at 130% of RDA calories.[14] This is now an unwarranted simplification. Each patient with CF should have a tailored nutritional regimen, based on the genetic defect,[15] the past medical history, and the degree of lung involvement. Ideally, energy expenditure should be measured for each individual; however, especially in CF, techniques of

Table 35-3 Definition of nutritional failure in patients with CF and those at risk.

Nutritional status	*Length or height*	*Weight-for-length percentile* 0 to 2 years*	*BMI percentile† 2 to 20 years*	*Action*
Acceptable	Normal growth	> 25th	> 25th	Continue to monitor with usual care
At-risk‡	Not at genetic potential	10 to 25th	10 to 25th	Consider nutritional and medical evaluation; some but not all patients in this category are at risk for nutritional failure
Nutritional failure§	< 5%	< 10th	< 10th	Treat nutritional failure

* From 2000 NCHS/CDC growth charts (weight-for-length) available for children, ages 0 to 2 years

† From 2000 NCHS/CDC growth chart, available for children and adolescents, ages 2 to 20 years.

‡ Delayed puberty should also be considered a marker of patients at risk for nutritional failure (no breast development past age 13 in girls; no menarche by age 16 or more than 5 years after the start of breast development in girls; no testicular enlargement or genital changes by age 14 in boys).

§ Weight plateau is defined as no increase in weight for > 3 months in a patient under 5 years of age, or no increase in weight for > 6 months in a patient over 5 years of age.

Source: Pediatric Nutrition of Patients with Cystic Fibrosis. *Consensus Conference:Concepts in CF Care.* 2001;10(1):24.

determining energy expenditure could be problematic. The metabolic cart requires either endotracheal intubation or a tight fitting hood to collect expired gases. CF patients will not tolerate either method. A handheld apparatus for measuring resting energy expenditure is available.[16] To date, this has not been used in CF patients and its use could be limited by chronic cough and by problems with contamination. Yet, if feasible, its use could allow more exact matching of patients' needs with nutritional recommendations.

PULMONARY FUNCTION TESTING

Pulmonary function testing (PFT) is not a measure of nutritional status; however, there is a very tight correlation between PFT and nutritional status. It is unclear whether worsening lung function causes nutritional deterioration (by decreasing intake or by increasing requirements) or whether deteriorating nutritional status causes poor performance on PFT testing (by weakening respiratory musculature or other mechanisms).[17–19] However, the 2 are so closely linked that any child with worsening PFTs should be carefully evaluated for nutritional inadequacies.

BLOOD TESTS

As a part of monitoring for nutritional status, laboratory determinations are recommended. Table 35-4 lists the CFF-recommended laboratory tests and the frequency with which these tests should be done.

Table 35-4 Laboratory monitoring of nutritional status.

	How often to monitor			
	At diagnosis	*Annually*	*Other*	*Tests*
Beta carotene			At physician's discretion	Serum levels
Vitamin A	x*	x		Vitamin A (retinol)
Vitamin D	x*	x		25-OH-D
Vitamin E	x*	x		α-tocopherol
Vitamin K	x*		If patient has hemoptysis or hematemesis; in patients with liver disease	PIVKA-II (preferably) or prothrombin time
Essential fatty acids			Consider checking in infants or those with FTT†	Triene: tetraene
Calcium/ bone status			> age 8 years if risk factors are present (see text)	Calcium, phosphorus, intact PTH,‡ DEXA§ scan
Iron	x	x	Consider in-depth evaluation for patients with poor appetite	Hemoglobin, hematocrit
Zinc			Consider 6-month supplementation trial and follow growth	No acceptable measurement
Sodium			Consider checking if exposed to heat stress and becomes dehydrated	Serum sodium; spot urine sodium if total body sodium depletion suspected
Protein stores	x	x	Check in patients with nutritional failure or those at risk	Albumin

* Patients diagnosed by neonatal screening do not need these measured.
† FTT = failure to thrive.
‡ Intact PTH = intact parathyroid hormone.
§ DEXA = dual energy x-ray absorptometry.
PIVKA-II = Protein induced by vitamin K absence (des-carbohydrate prothrombin)

Source: Pediatric Nutrition for Patients with Cystic Fibrosis. *Consensus Conference: Concepts in CF Care.* 2001;10:32.

SCREENING FOR CF-RELATED DIABETES

Approximately 5–6% of patients with CF suffer from CF-related diabetes (CFRD),[20,3] and there is an increase in incidence with age such that only 3% of CF patients less than 10 years of age have diabetes,[21] but 32% of those over 25 years of age have diabetes.[22] CF diabetes mellitus (CFDM) is associated with clinical deterioration including poor growth, decrease in nutritional status, worsening lung function, and early death. Deterioration in clinical status might be apparent 2–4 years before the diagnosis of CFDM is made.[23] To avoid clinical deterioration and death, timely diagnosis and intervention is required. The CFF recommends a yearly random blood glucose determination and follow-up of any level greater than 126 mg/dl. However, in a small series of patients (unpublished) who underwent oral glucose tolerance testing (OGTT), it was found that the CFF approach would have missed 7 out of 16 patients screened. Therefore, in addition it to random glucose testing and Hb A1C, all CF patients over 10 years of age should have OGTTs performed every 2 years. After 16 years of age, the OGTT should be done every year. Continuous glucose monitoring is a new technique that might be more sensitive than OGTT for detecting abnormal hyperglycemia.[24]

SCREENING FOR BONE DISEASE

Patients with CF could have multiple risk factors for developing bone disease: (1) failure to thrive, (2) delayed pubertal development; (3) malabsorption of calcium, magnesium, vitamin D, and vitamin K; (4) hepatobiliary disease; (5) reduced weight-bearing activity; and (6) chronic corticosteroid use.[25] Children at risk for bone disease should have yearly determination of calcium, phosphorus, intact parathyroid hormone, and 25 hydroxyvitamin D levels. Dual-energy X-ray absorptometry (DEXA) is now widely available, and there are pediatric age group specific standards.[26] Children over age of 8 years should have a DEXA scan. If the scan shows low density, corrective treatment with vitamin D, vitamin K, calcium, and phosphorus should be undertaken. Low impact, weight-bearing exercise should be encouraged, and DEXA scans should be repeated on a yearly basis. If the DEXA scan shows bone density within the normal range, repeat scans should be done every 2 years. Requirements for calcium, phosphorus, vitamin D, and vitamin K are listed in Table 35-5.

ORAL NUTRITION SUPPORT

Oral nutrition support usually begins by attempting to increase oral intake with food. There are a number of studies that support this approach claiming nutritional benefit through behavior modification.[27–31] The second approach to

Table 35-5 Dietary requirements relevant for bone health in cystic fibrosis.

	Dietary Reference Adequate Intake			
Age	*Calcium**	*Phosphorus**	*Vitamin D*	*Vitamin K*
0–6 months	210 mg	100 mg	400 IU	300–500 μg
7–12 months	270 mg	275 mg	400 IU	300–500 μg
1–3 years	500 mg	460 mg	400–800 IU	300–500 μg
4–8 years	800 mg	500 mg	400–800 IU	300–500 μg
9–13 years	1,300 mg	1,250 mg	400–800 IU	300–500 μg
14–18 years	1,300 mg	1,250 mg	400–800 IU	300–500 μg

Sources: Institute of Medicine. *Dietary Reference Intakes for Calcium, Vitamin D and Fluoride.* Washington, DC: National Academies Press; 1997. Institute of Medicine. *Dietary Reference Intakes for Vitamin A, Vitamin K, Boron, Chromium, Copper, Iodine, Iron, Manganese, Molybdenum, Nickel, Vanadium, and Zinc.* Washington, DC: National Academy Press; 2001.

oral NS is supplemental feeds. Table 35-6 gives CFF recommendations for vitamin supplementation and the composition of some commercially available multivitamins. Table 35-7 lists

Table 35-6 Fat soluble vitamins.

Age	*CFF recommendations*	*ADEK drops/ chewable*	*Source ABDEK*	*Vitamax Chewable*	*Centrum Chewable/ tablet*
		Total Vitamin A (IU) (Retinol and β-Carotene)			
0–12 months	1,500				
1–3 years	5,000 (retinol)	6,340/2 mL			
4–8 years	5,000–10,000 (retinol)	9,000/tab, 60% β-carotene	9,000/cap, 60% β-carotene	5,000/tab	5,000/ chewable, 20% β-carotene
9–18 years	10,000 (retinol)	18,000/2 tabs, 60% β-carotene	18,000/2 caps, 60% β-carotene	10,000/2 tabs	10,000/2 tabs, 20% β-carotene
> 18 years	8,000 (retinol)	18,000/2 tabs, 60% β-Carotene	18,000/2 caps, 60% β-carotene	10,000/2 tabs	10,000/2 tabs, 20% β-carotene
		Vitamin E (IU)			
0–12 months	40–50				
1–3 years	80–150	800/2 mL drops			
4–8 years	100–200	400/tab	400/cap	400/tab	400/chewable
9–18 years	200–400	800/2 tabs	800/2 caps	800/2 tabs	800/2 chewable
> 18 years	200–400	800/2 tabs	800/2 caps	800/2 tabs	800/2 chewable
		Vitamin D (IU)			
0–12 months	400				
1–3 years	400–800	800/2 mL drops			
4–8 years	400–800	400/tab	400/cap	400/tab	400/chewable
9–18 years	400–800	800/2 tabs	800/2 caps	800/2 tabs	800/2 chewable
> 18 years	800	800/2 tabs	800/2 caps	800/2 tabs	800/2 chewable

Table 35-6 Fat soluble vitamins (continued).

Age	*CFF recommendations*	*ADEK drops/ chewable*	*Source ABDEK*	*Vitamax Chewable*	*Centrum Chewable/ tablet*
		Vitamin K (mcg)			
0–12 months	300–500				
1–3 years	300–500	200/2 mL drops			
4–8 years	300–500	150/tab	500/cap	150/tab	10/chewable
9–18 years	300–500	300/2 tabs	1,000/2 caps	300/2 tabs	50/2 tabs
> 18 years	1,000–1,500	300/2 tabs	1,000/2 caps	300/2 tabs	50/2 tabs

Source: Pediatric Nutrition for Patients with Cystic Fibrosis. *Consensus Conference: Concepts in CF Care.* 2001;10:31.

Table 35-7 Oral supplements.

Supplement	*Company*	*Fat (grams)*	*Type of Fat*	*Kcal/ml*
Ensure	Ross	6.1 g/8 oz	High oleic safflower, canola, corn oil	1.06
Boost	Novartis	4 g/8 oz	Canola, high oleic sunflower, corn oil	1.01
Resource	Novartis	6 g/8 oz	High oleic sunflower, corn oil	1.06
Pediasure	Ross	11.8 g/8 oz	High oleic safflower, soy, MCT oil	1.0
Carnation Instant Breakfast (powder)	Nestle	7.1g/8 oz	Butter fat	1.05
Ensure Plus	Ross	11.4 g/8 oz	High oleic safflower, canola, corn oil	1.5
Boost Plus	Novartis	14 g/8 oz	Canola, high oleic sunflower, corn oil	1.52
Resource Plus	Novartis	11 g/8 oz	High oleic sunflower, corn oil	1.5
Resource Just of Kids 1.5	Novartis	18 g/8 oz	High oleic sunflower, soybean, MCT oil	1.5
Carnation Instant Breakfast Lactose free Plus	Nestle	17 g/8 oz	Canola, corn oil	1.5
Carnation Instant Breakfast Lactose free VHC	Nestle	30.6 g/8 oz	Canola, corn oil	2.25
Scandishake	Axcan	24 g/8 oz	Partially hydrogenated vegetable oil, butter fat	2.0
Boost Breeze	Novartis	0		0.68
Resource fruit beverage	Novartis	0		1.06

Source: Pediatric Nutrition for Patients with Cystic Fibrosis. *Consensus Conference; Concepts in CF Care.* 2001;10:31.

available supplements used in CF. Supplements are often less efficacious than expected because the supplements tend to replace ordinary food rather than being taken in addition to a usual diet.[32] Patients also often complain of taste fatigue with these oral supplements.

ENTERAL TUBE NUTRITION SUPPORT

When oral NS fails, EN tube feeding should be employed. A Cochrane Database analysis of enteral tube feeding in CF found 13 studies, but no randomized studies, and thus was unable to conclude that EN was beneficial.[33] Nevertheless, EN is widely used and perceived as being helpful.[34–36] In CF, the G-tube route is favored as NG-tubes are poorly tolerated due to chronic cough, nasal polyps, and the sensation of suffocating. G-J feeding and J-tube feeding are possible, but these tubes are more difficult to place and maintain in position. Additionally, this type of EN requires continuous delivery of formula, making it inconvenient for ambulatory patients. G-tubes can be placed surgically, endoscopically (PEG), or by an interventional radiologist, with minimal risk. If anesthesia is not advisable, G-tubes can be inserted with sedation and local anesthesia.

Schedules for tube feeding vary and should take into account the patient's activities and other therapies. In general, tube feeding can be continuous, bolus, or a combination of these 2 regimens. For the school-age child, a frequently employed schedule is to supply approximately 40% of daily requirements via a slow infusion overnight; the remainder of the requirements are taken as regular meals during the day. If the child is unable to meet the daily requirements, the nighttime infusions can be lengthened, or the rate of infusion increased so that a greater percent of daily requirements are delivered overnight. For the younger patient, nighttime continuous feeds can be combined with daytime meals calculated to supply a given amount of nutrition. If the child fails to ingest the prescribed amount at a sitting, the meal is completed with a bolus feed to compensate. CF patients are often on many medications as well as doing frequent pulmonary therapy. Feeding schedules should take these other elements of therapy into account.

A variety of formulas have been used for CF patients, and there is no one class of formula that has been shown to be superior to another. In one study, a nonelemental formula plus PET was as well absorbed as a semielemental formula without PET.[37] Concentrated formulas with 1.5 to 2.0 Kcal/ml have the advantage of delivering more calories in a smaller volume. Since nighttime urination is a problem when giving overnight feeds, this smaller volume might make the feeding schedule more tolerable. Using the more concentrated formulas risks carbohydrate overload and possible inadequate supply of free water. Table 35-8 lists some formulas that are commonly used for CF patients receiving tube feeds.

As with other aspects of EN in CF, there is little information on the best way to administer PET. With no guidance available, the following suggestions seem to make sense: start by calculating the grams of long chain triglycerides (LCT) being administered. While medium chain triglyceride (MCT) does require lipase to hydrolyze the fatty acids from the glycerol backbone, the amount of lipase is much less than that needed for LCT. It appears the MCT accounts for little of the fat malabsorption in CF. Supply 1,600–2,000 lipase units per gram LCT. For cycled, continuous overnight feeds, administer three fourths of the enzymes at the beginning of the tube feeding and one fourth of the enzymes at the end of the tube feeding. For bolus feedings, administer the calculated amount of enzymes just prior to the bolus feeding. For continuous 24-hour feedings, divide the total calculated lipase into 6 doses to be given every 4 hours.

Although there have been no randomized trials of EN in CF, there have been a number of studies that point to improved nutritional status and stabilization of lung functions. Levy et al.[38] studied 14 patients with moderate to severe lung disease. Mean follow-up was for 1.1 years. Age- and disease-matched contemporary controls were retrospectively compared. The patients

Table 35-8 Enteral formulas.

Formula	*Company*	*MCT (% fat Kcal)*	*Kcal/mL*	*Protein source*	*mOsm*
Pregistimil	Mead-Johnson	55	0.67	Hydorlyzed casein	330
Peptamen Junior	Nestle	60	1.0	Hydrolyzed whey	260
Peptamen	Nestle	70	1.0	Hydrolyzed whey	300
Nutren 1.5	Nestle	50	1.5	Caseinate	430
Nutren 2.0	Nestle	75	2.0	Caseinate	745
Elecare 20	Ross	33	0.67	Amino acids	335
Elecare 30	Ross	33	1.0	Amino acids	551
Vivonex pediatric	Novartis	68	1.0	Amino acids	360
Peptinex DT	Novartis	50	1.0	Peptides	290
Vital HN	Ross	45	1.0	Peptides	500
Peptamen 1.5	Nestle	70	1.5	Hydrolyzed whey	550

Source: Pediatric Nutrition for Patients with Cystic Fibrosis. *Consensus Conference: Concepts in CF Care.* 2001;10:31.

receiving EN experienced a weight percentile increase while the controls fell off their growth percentile. The Forced Expiratory Volume (FEV1) in the EN group did not change while the FEV1 of the controls worsened. Steinkamp and others[39] studied a similarly small number of patients, while Williams et al.[35] followed 53 patients with CF (only 10 were children). Neither of the latter 2 studies included controls, but both found similar results; that is, increase in expected weight and stabilization of lung function.

PARENTERAL NUTRITION SUPPORT (PN)

PN should be prescribed for CF patients when GI function is inadequate to supply complete nutrition. This could occur during times of extreme metabolic stress, such as posttransplantation or following GI surgical procedures. The PN solution should contain a balance of amino acids, dextrose, lipids, vitamins, and trace elements to provide appropriate nutrition. One study observed that CF patients receiving PN had higher sepsis rates, and that once PN was discontinued, weight dropped and no long term gain was achieved.[40] PN should not be a part of palliative care.

CONCLUSION

The present approach to nutrition in CF is focused on pancreatic insufficiency and PET. The chloride channel regulator is ubiquitous. It is present in the liver, gallbladder, the small bowel, and the colon as well as in the lungs, the nasal passages, the rectal mucosa, and the sweat glands. Supplying exogenous lipase addresses only 1 facet of the problem. Clearly there is a need for better tools to investigate and manage nutrition therapy in CF. Still, there is much to be gained by maximizing the nutritional modalities presently available.

REFERENCES

1. Reilly JJ, Edwards CA, Weaver LT. Malnutrition in children with cystic fibrosis: the energy-balance equation. *J Pediatr Gastroenterol Nutr.* 1997;25(2):127–136.

2. Zemel BS, Jawad AF, FitzSimmons S, Stallings VA. Longitudinal relationship among growth, nutritional status, and pulmonary function in children with cystic fibrosis: analysis of the Cystic Fibrosis Foundation National CF patient registry. *J Pediatr.* 2000;137(3):374–380.
3. Cystic Fibrosis Foundation. *Patient Registry 2003 Annual Report.* Bethesda, Md; 2004.
4. Corey M, McLaughlin FJ, Williams M, Levison H. A comparison of survival, growth, and pulmonary function in patients with cystic fibrosis in Boston and Toronto. *J Clin Epidemiol.* 1988;41(6):583–591.
5. Borowitz D, Baker RD, Stallings V. Consensus report on nutrition for pediatric patients with cystic fibrosis. *J Pediatr Gastroenterol Nutr.* 2002;35(3):246–259.
6. Borowitz D, Durie PR, Clarke LL, et al. Gastrointestinal outcomes and confounders in cystic fibrosis. *J Pediatr Gastroenterol Nutr.* 2005;41(3):273–285.
7. Riordan JR, Rommens JM, Kerem B, et al. Identification of the cystic fibrosis gene: cloning and characterization of complementary DNA. *Science.* 1989;245(4922):1066–1073.
8. Borowitz D, Baker SS, Duffy L, et al. Use of fecal elastase-1 to classify pancreatic status in patients with cystic fibrosis. *J Pediatr.* 2004;145(3):322–326.
9. Kraisinger M, Hochhaus G, Stecenko A, Bowser E, Hendeles L. Clinical pharmacology of pancreatic enzymes in patients with cystic fibrosis and in vitro performance of microencapsulated formulations. *J Clin Pharmacol.* 1994;34(2):158–166.
10. Baker SS, Borowitz D, Duffy L, Fitzpatrick L, Gyamfi J, Baker RD. Pancreatic enzyme therapy and clinical outcomes in patients with cystic fibrosis. *J Pediatr.* 2005;146(2):189–193.
11. Wright CM, Cheetham TD. The strengths and limitations of parental heights as a predictor of attained height. *Arch Dis Child.* 1999;81(3):257–260.
12. Garn SM, Rohmann CG. "Midparent" values for use with parent-specific, age-size tables when paternal stature is estimated or unknown. *Pediatr Clin North Am.* 1967;14(1):283–284.
13. Himes JH, Roche AF, Thissen D, Moore WM. Parent-specific adjustments for evaluation of recumbent length and stature of children. *Pediatrics.* 1985;75(2):304–313.
14. Roy CC, Darling P, Weber AM. A rational approach to meeting macro- and micronutrient needs in cystic fibrosis. *J Pediatr Gastroenterol Nutr.* 1984;3(suppl 1): S154–162.
15. Drumm ML, Konstan MW, Schluchter MD, et al. Genetic modifiers of lung disease in cystic fibrosis. *New Engl J Med.* 2005;353(14):1443–1453.
16. Novitsky S, Segal KR, Chatr-Aryamontri B, Guvakov D, Katch VL. Validity of a new portable indirect calorimeter: the AeroSport TEEM 100. *European J Appl Physiol Occup Physiol.* 1995;70(5):462–467.
17. Zemel BS, Kawchak DA, Cnaan A, Zhao H, Scanlin TF, Stallings VA. Prospective evaluation of resting energy expenditure, nutritional status, pulmonary function, and genotype in children with cystic fibrosis. *Pediatr Res.* 1996;40(4):578–586.
18. Peterson ML, Jacobs DR Jr, Milla CE. Longitudinal changes in growth parameters are correlated with changes in pulmonary function in children with cystic fibrosis. *Pediatrics.* 2003;112(3 Pt 1):588–592.
19. Steinkamp G, Wiedemann B. Relationship between nutritional status and lung function in cystic fibrosis: cross sectional and longitudinal analyses from the German CF quality assurance (CFQA) project. *Thorax.* 2002;57(7):596–601.
20. Rosenecker J, Eichler I, Barmeier H, von der Hardt H. Diabetes mellitus and cystic fibrosis: comparison of clinical parameters in patients treated with insulin versus oral glucose-lowering agents. *Pediatr Pulmonol.* 2001;32(5):351–355.
21. Rosenecker J, Eichler I, Kuhn L, Harms HK, von der Hardt H. Genetic determination of diabetes mellitus in patients with cystic fibrosis. Multicenter Cystic Fibrosis Study Group. *J Pediatr.* 1995;127(3):441–443.
22. Lanng S, Thorsteinsson B, Erichsen G, Nerup J, Koch C. Glucose tolerance in cystic fibrosis. *Arch Dis Child.* 1991;66(5):612–616.
23. Lanng S, Thorsteinsson B, Nerup J, Koch C. Diabetes mellitus in cystic fibrosis: effect of insulin therapy on lung function and infections. *Acta Paediatrica.* 1994;83(8):849–853.
24. Jefferies C, Solomon M, Perlman K, Sweezy N, Daneman D. Continuous glucose monitoring in adolescents with cystic fibrosis. *J Pediatr.* 2005;147(3):396–398.
25. Bhudhikanok GS, Wang MC, Marcus R, Harkins A, Moss RB, Bachrach LK. Bone acquisition and loss in children and adults with cystic fibrosis: a longitudinal study. *J Pediatr.* 1998;133(1):18–21.
26. Simpson DE, Dontu VS, Stephens SE, et al. Large variations occur in bone density measurements of children when using different software. *Nucl Med Commun.* 2005;26(6):483–487.
27. Singer LT, Nofer JA, Benson-Szekely LJ, Brooks LJ. Behavioral assessment and management of food refusal in children with cystic fibrosis. *J Dev Behav Pediatr.* 1991;12(2):115–120.
28. Stark LJ, Bowen AM, Tyc VL, Evans S, Passero MA. A behavioral approach to increasing calorie consumption in children with cystic fibrosis. *J Pediatr Psychol.* 1990;15(3):309–326.
29. Stark LJ, Knapp LG, Bowen AM, et al. Increasing calorie consumption in children with cystic fibrosis: replication with 2-year follow-up. *J Appl Behav Anal.* 1993;26(4):435–450.

30. Stark LJ, Jelalian E, Mulvihill MM, et al. Eating in preschool children with cystic fibrosis and healthy peers: behavioral analysis. *Pediatrics.* 1995;95(2):210–215.
31. Jelalian E, Stark LJ, Reynolds L, Seifer R. Nutrition intervention for weight gain in cystic fibrosis: a meta analysis. *J Pediatr.* 1998;132(3 Pt 1):486–492.
32. Kalnins D, Corey M, Ellis L, Pencharz PB, Tullis E, Durie PR. Failure of conventional strategies to improve nutritional status in malnourished adolescents and adults with cystic fibrosis. *J Pediatr.* 2005;147:399–401.
33. Conway SP, Morton A, Wolfe S. Enteral tube feeding for cystic fibrosis. *Cochrane Database of Systematic Reviews;* 2005;(2):3.
34. Walker SA, Gozal D. Pulmonary function correlates in the prediction of long-term weight gain in cystic fibrosis patients with gastrostomy tube feedings. *J Pediatr Gastroenterol Nutr.* 1998;27(1):53–56.
35. Williams SG, Ashworth F, McAlweenie A, Poole S, Hodson ME, Westaby D. Percutaneous endoscopic gastrostomy feeding in patients with cystic fibrosis. *Gut.* 1999;44(1):87–90.
36. Akobeng AK, Miller V, Thomas A. Percutaneous endoscopic gastrostomy feeding improves nutritional status and stabilizes pulmonary function in patients with cystic fibrosis. *J Pediatr Gastroenterol Nutr.* 1999;29(4):485–486.
37. Erskine JM, Lingard CD, Sontag MK, Accurso FJ. Enteral nutrition for patients with cystic fibrosis: comparison of a semi-elemental and nonelemental formula. *J Pediatr.* 1998;132(2):265–269.
38. Levy LD, Durie PR, Pencharz PB, Corey ML. Effects of long-term nutritional rehabilitation on body composition and clinical status in malnourished children and adolescents with cystic fibrosis. *J Pediatr.* 1985;107(2):225–230.
39. Steinkamp G, Rodeck B, Seidenberg J, Ruhl I, von der Hardt H. [Stabilization of lung function in cystic fibrosis during long-term tube feeding via a percutaneous endoscopic gastrostomy]. [German] *Pneumologie.* 1990;44(10):1151–1153.
40. Munck A, Malbezin S, Bloch J, et al. Follow-up of 452 totally implantable vascular devices in cystic fibrosis patients. *Eur Respir J.* 2004;23(3):430–434.

Chapter 36

Nutrition Support in Children with Liver Disease

Renee A. Wieman and William F. Balistreri

INTRODUCTION

The liver plays a fundamental role in all nutritional processes. Hepatic dysfunction disrupts the absorption and metabolism of all major nutrients, causing significant nutritional problems. This is especially true for cholestatic liver disease, in which impaired bile flow leads to reduced output of bile acids into the intestinal lumen, and so impedes fat digestion and absorption. In addition, retained bile acids cause liver cell injury. Infants and children with chronic liver disease are at high risk of nutritional compromise and malnutrition as the disease progresses. Children with chronic liver disease, like adults, suffer from ascites, pruritus, encephalopathy, and the consequences of portal hypertension, but the impact of liver disease on growth failure and development is unique to children.[1] Some of the mechanisms leading to nutritional deficiencies in various liver diseases, as well as our recommendations for metabolic management and maintenance of nutritional status, are discussed in this chapter.

OVERVIEW

Childhood is a time of rapid growth and development; unimpeded progression through this phase of life is vital to future health and well being. Undernutrition leads to stunted growth and development and has a negative impact on the prognosis of children with liver disease. This emphasizes the critical importance of timely and adequate nutritional assessment and initiation of therapy for children with liver disease of any nature.

SPECTRUM OF PEDIATRIC LIVER DISEASES

Liver diseases that cause chronic cholestasis present difficult nutritional challenges. In pediatric patients, the most common chronic cholestatic disease is biliary atresia, which has an incidence of approximately 1 in 8,000 to 15,000 births.[2] Initially, children are managed surgically with a hepatoportoenterostomy. One half to two thirds have poor postoperative bile drainage with persistent cholestasis or have partial resolution of their jaundice but have continued hepatocellular injury.[3] Other less common chronic cholestatic diseases in children include Alagille syndrome, which is defined by intrahepatic bile duct paucity, often in association with other nonhepatic abnormalities such as cardiac disease, skeletal abnormalities, ocular abnormalities, and a characteristic facial phenotype.[4,5] The estimated incidence of Alagille syndrome is 1 per 70,000 births. Progressive familial intrahepatic cholestasis (PFIC) and neonatal hepatitis are less common cholestatic liver diseases.[6]

Metabolic liver diseases cause liver injury, often with cholestasis, in a considerable number of infants and children. In many cases, the liver is the only organ affected, but in some diseases, other organs are affected. However, liver disease is the major cause of morbidity and mortality. Taken together, genetic and metabolic liver disease account for approximately 30% of children who undergo liver transplantation.[7] Alpha-1-antitrypsin deficiency, the most common metabolic liver disease in children, affects approximately 1 in 1,800 live births.[8] It is an autosomal recessive disease in which affected infants might present with cholestasis, failure to thrive, and hepatomegaly. It was originally believed that only 2–8% of patients who have cystic fibrosis develop liver disease and portal hypertension. As patients with cystic fibrosis survive longer, it is likely the prevalence of liver disease will be as high as 15%.[9] Hereditary tyrosinemia is caused by mutations in fumaryl acetoacetate hydrolase, an enzyme on the tyrosine degradation pathway, and leads to progressive liver failure, renal tubular dysfunction, and hypophosphatemic rickets. Neonatal hemochromatosis or neonatal iron storage disease is also a rare disorder of unknown etiology in which hemosiderin deposits in the liver lead to liver failure within days to weeks of birth from liver fibrosis and extrahepatic siderosis.[10] Glycogen storage diseases (GSD) are associated with glycogen accumulation in the liver and other tissues due to a specific defect in glycogenolysis. Patients with GSD type Ia have hypoglycemia, developmental delays, metabolic acidosis, serum triglyceride and uric acid elevation, hepatomegaly, hepatic adenomas, and hepatocellular carcinoma caused by defects in glucose-6-phosphatase pathways. This type is nutritionally managed with dietary cornstarch supplementation. In GSD type Ib, patients also have neutrophil dysfunction and recurrent infections caused by a primary defect in a microsomal glucose-6-phosphate transporter. GSD III is characterized by hepatomegaly, but liver dysfunction is rare. In GSD type IV, a deficiency in the debrancher enzyme, there is progressive liver dysfunction and liver failure.[9]

Another group of patients who often develop cholestasis and possibly end-stage liver disease are those patients who require long term total parenteral nutrition (PN) support. PN associated liver disease in children is most commonly seen in patients who have undergone massive intestinal resections and/or have had intestinal failure. PN-associated liver disease develops in 40–60% of children who require long term (PN) support.[11] The clinical spectrum of this disease includes cholestasis, cholelithiasis, hepatic fibrosis with progressive biliary cirrhosis, and the development of portal hypertension and liver failure. Risk factors include prematurity, duration of enteral starvation, duration of PN, and the history of major insults during the neonatal period such as sepsis, severe hypotension, or hypoxia and major surgeries. Speculated etiologies include antioxidant/oxidant imbalance, excessive dextrose and/or amino acid infusion, methionine toxicity, magnesium toxicity, taurine deficiency, and carnitine deficiency.[12,13] The incidence or severity of cholestasis can be reduced by enteral nutrition to promote enterohepatic circulation of bile acids, antibiotics to control bacterial overgrowth, and aggressive management of sepsis. Ursodeoxycholic acid (15–20 mg/kg/day) in children and adults is effective in reducing liver enzymes and serum bilirubin levels. Even with optimal medical management, many progress to intestinal and/or liver transplantation.

THERAPEUTIC OPTIONS FOR LIVER DISEASES IN CHILDREN

Recent important research has clearly furthered our understanding of the pathogenesis of specific metabolic diseases that lead to cholestasis so that nontransplant therapeutic options can be specifically tailored to a disease. For example, pharmacologic treatment for tyrosinemia and cholestasis such as ursodeoxycholic acid for children with defects in bile acid metabolism have been highly successful. These therapeutic agents reverse liver injury, halt the progression of liver disease, and obviate the need for liver transplantation.[14] Unfortunately, there is no curative therapy for most children with cholestatic disease such as biliary atresia and intrahepatic cholestasis. The ultimate goal in the management of the child with hepatic dysfunction is to prevent end-stage liver disease and to promote growth and development. Many pediatric liver diseases can progress to end-stage liver disease. Complications such as portal hypertension, varices, ascites, and recurrent spontaneous bacterial peritonitis can interfere with the provision of adequate nutritional support.

NUTRITIONAL MANAGEMENT AS A COMPONENT OF CARE

The nutritional management of infants and children with liver disease is a complex yet critical portion of the care required for optimal support and metabolic control of these patients. Nutritional requirements are dependent upon the nature of the disease process and whether the course is acute or chronic. Acute liver disease, such as viral hepatitis or acute liver failure, generally requires no specific nutritional modifications except for the occasional need to limit or modify protein intake. In acute liver disease, factors contributing to the worsening of nutritional status and loss of lean body mass include anorexia, emesis, diarrhea from lactulose therapy, and altered protein metabolism.[15] The clinical features of hepatic encephalopathy are well defined in the adult literature, but not so for children. Elevation of the serum ammonia levels remains an important marker for encephalopathy in pediatrics. The treatment of encephalopathy can involve reduction or removal of enteral or parenteral protein and the inhibition of intestinal absorption of ammonia with oral lactulose and/or neomycin.[16]

On the other hand, chronic liver disease in infants and children affects the nutritional status of most patients, especially those who are cholestatic.[17] In cholestatic liver disease, the bile acid concentration in the intestinal lumen is decreased. Protein energy malnutrition leading to growth failure is a nearly inevitable consequence of chronic liver disease.[18] In pediatric patients with chronic liver disease, there are numerous factors that contribute to the development of malnutrition: (1) decreased dietary intake from anorexia, nausea, and vomiting; (2) ascites, which can cause early satiety; (3) malabsorption of dietary proteins and fats that contributes to the poor nutritional status seen in the early stages of liver disease in the rapidly growing infant and deprives them of sustenance needed to maximize normal development; and (4) unpalatability of diets rich in medium chain triglycerides (MCTs) and often low in sodium. MCT containing formulas are frequently offered to patients with chronic cholestasis because MCT oil is directly absorbed without bile acid emulsification. Caloric intake can be improved by supplemental nasogastric tube feedings with high calorie formulas. MCT containing formulas, such as Pregestimil, Alimentum, or Peptamen Jr, are used to improve fat absorption. Initially, formula can be concentrated to 24 cal/oz. Thereafter, addition of MCT and carbohydrate to a maximum of 30 cal/oz is a common strategy. By not concentrating the formula base to 30 cal/oz, adequate free water is provided to allow excretion of the solute load, and a lower osmolality can be maintained.

Liver disease has also been shown to increase energy requirements secondary to both the disease itself and to complicating factors of infection. The resting energy expenditure (REE) of some pediatric patients with liver disease is 127–140% of predicted REE.[19,20] For this reason, aggressive nutritional support to replace losses and offset increased energy expenditure is the primary focus of care providers.

Cholestasis also leads to malabsorption of fat-soluble vitamins. Fat-soluble vitamin deficiency is common among children with chronic liver disease, and vitamins A, D, E, and K are routinely supplemented in these patients (Table 36-1).[21] Close monitoring of serum vitamin and mineral levels is necessary to prevent deficiency and to recognize vitamin toxicity as discussed in Vitamins and Minerals section, later in this chapter.

NUTRITIONAL ASSESSMENT

A thorough nutritional assessment should be a component of the initial management of infants and children with liver disease, and routine periodic assessments should be conducted throughout the course of this disease. These assessments

Table 36-1 Fat-soluble vitamin recommendations.

Vitamin	*Amount given*
Vitamin A (aqueous)	1,000 IU/kg/day up to 25,000 IU
25-OH vitamin D	3–5 mcg/kg/d
Vitamin E	20–25 IU /kg/d as TPGS
Vitamin K	2.5–5 mg/d 3 times per week

TPGS = tocopheryl polyethylene glycol-1,000 succinate.

are used to identify the degree of malnutrition and initiate a nutritional care plan tailored to preserve lean body mass while minimizing the potential complications of metabolic disturbances seen with progressive disease. The assessment should include a complete medical and diet history, physical examination, and evaluation of laboratory tests. A detailed history of usual caloric, fat, and protein intake; weight changes; as well as a thorough evaluation of nutrition related problems such as nausea, vomiting, diarrhea, early satiety from ascites, and dietary restrictions is essential.

The usual markers of nutritional status are not reliable in the assessment of patients with liver disease. Body weight is not a reliable measure because ascites, edema (depleted visceral protein stores cause increased total body water and salt retention), and hepatosplenomegaly can mask weight loss.[22] Height changes are a more reliable marker of chronic malnutrition for infants and children. Acute malnutrition is best evaluated through upper extremity triceps skinfold (TSF) thickness and measurement of mid-arm muscle circumference (MAMC). The arm is less prone to fluid accumulation than the lower extremities and can provide an indirect assessment of body adipose and somatic muscle stores.[23] TSF measures provide an estimate of energy reserves (fat), and MAMC estimates somatic muscle reserves. The early depletion of fat and muscle stores signals the preferential utilization of adipose reserves as an energy source to spare somatic protein stores in malnourished patients.[24] To assure accuracy of anthropometric measures, they should be performed serially, by a single observer, using a standardized technique.[25] Anthropometric measures are simple to perform, noninvasive, inexpensive, and can provide a means for early detection of nutritional depletion.

Plasma proteins measured for nutritional assessment (albumin, prealbumin, retinol-binding protein, and transferrin) are synthesized in the liver. These proteins are decreased in liver disease and will not accurately measure visceral protein status. The plasma concentrations of these proteins correlate more with the severity of the liver injury than the degree of malnutrition.[26]

Medications commonly used in treating chronic liver disease can have significant adverse effects on nutritional status. Cholestyramine can cause fat and fat-soluble vitamin malabsorption. Neomycin can cause steatorrhea, carbohydrate malabsorption, and vitamin B_{12} deficiency. Lactulose can cause osmotic diarrhea, leading to malabsorption of nutrients as well as hyponatremia and hypokalemia from electrolyte losses in the stool.[27]

The subjective global assessment of a patient's nutritional status is one of the most reliable and acceptable standards of assessment when compared with other objective measures.[28,29] The subjective global assessment, the anthropometric assessment, signs and symptoms of vitamin and mineral deficiency, and laboratory tests lay the foundation for early detection and treatment of nutrition problems in liver disease. Based on this assessment, patients can be grouped as to those who need immediate nutritional intervention, those at risk of protein-energy malnutrition, and those who probably will do well without nutritional intervention. Patients at risk for nutritional deterioration require intensive surveillance. Aggressive nutritional management of patients at risk ensures optimal growth and development, minimizes the complications associated with the underlying disease, and contributes to the successful outcome of liver transplantation.

MANAGEMENT GOALS

The nutritional management goals for pediatric patients with cholestatic disease or end-stage liver disease are: optimize growth and development, prevent further liver injury, and if possible, promote liver regeneration, slow the deterioration of the patient, minimize the risk of infection, and avoid vitamin and mineral deficiency.[30] This involves detailed attention to all of the components of nutritional support.

Energy Requirements

Energy needs vary with age, nutritional status, and degree of malabsorption. Children with end-stage liver disease require 130–150% of the Recommended Daily Intake (RDA) for energy based on ideal body weight.[31] In general, infants with cholestatic liver disease require 120–150 kcal/kg/d based on dry weight.[32] For infants, formula should contain > 50% of the fat as MCT. Care should be taken to maintain the intake of long chain fatty acids at ~ 10% of total energy intake to prevent essential fatty acid (EFA) deficiency. The caloric density of the formula should be progressively increased as tolerated to a goal of 30 calories/oz (1 kcal/mL). This can be achieved by concentrating the formula and/or adding modular nutrients such as glucose polymers or MCT oil. Infants can be breastfed, but if an infant cannot maintain adequate growth, then mother's milk can be fortified and fed to the baby in a bottle. There are several pediatric formulas that can be prepared as a 1 kcal/mL product containing > 50% of the fat as MCT oil (see Table 36-2).[33] These formulas offer an option to supplement children > 1 year of age who have inadequate oral intake.

Protein Intake

Protein requirements and the amino acid composition of the diet have been controversial in chronic or end-stage liver disease. Enough protein must be provided to prevent catabolism, but not so much that it contributes to hyperammonemia. When protein is restricted, lean body mass provides a protein source and the catabolism of lean body mass increases serum ammonia. Infants require at least 3 g/kg/day protein and can tolerate up to 4 g/kg/day without encephalopathy.[31,34] Studies of adult patients with liver disease show the protein RDA maintains nitrogen balance. Whole protein is preferred because it is more palatable. The use of branched-chain amino acid (BCAA) enriched diets (see Chapter 24) for infants and children with end-stage liver disease is controversial. In liver disease, an imbalance of BCAA and aromatic amino acids (AAA) occurs so that cerebral uptake of AAA increases, and this contributes to encephalopathy. In some studies in children, BCAA-enriched formulas are associated with improvement in nutritional status compared to semielemental formulas.[35,36] The overall lack of studies and questions about the cost-benefit ratio have limited the use of BCAA-enriched diets in the nutritional support of children with hepatic dysfunction.[37,38]

Lipids

There is no reason to restrict lipids in pediatric patients with liver disease. Restricting fat intake can adversely affect overall caloric intake and hasten the development of malnutrition. Increasing fat intake, despite some increase in steatorrhea, could increase the overall amount of calories absorbed. Approximately 90% of MCT can be absorbed even in advanced cholestatic disease. Thirty to fifty percent of fat should be provided as MCT in order to improve nutritional status.[39,40] MCT is beneficial in liver disease because intestinal absorption does not depend on incorporation into bile acid containing mixed micelles as does long chain fatty acids. Fecal studies that differentiate between medium chain and long chain triglyceride in fecal specimens indicate that 90% of MCT is absorbed compared to only 50–60% absorption of long chain fats.[41] MCT oil can be added to infant formula easily to increase the caloric content. This modification in diet is well tolerated by infants but

Table 36-2 Enteral Formulas for Liver Disease.

Formula	Nutrient source: Protein	Nutrient source: Fat	Nutrient source: Carbohydrate	kcal/mL	g/mL: Protein	g/mL: Fat	g/mL: Carbohydrate	mOsm/Kg H_2O	% H_2O	Comments
For Infants with Protein Maldigestion or Fat Malabsorption										
Alimentum® (Ross)	Hydrolyzed casein, free amino acids	33% MCT oil, safflower oil, soy oil	Modified tapioca starch, sucrose	0.67	0.018	0.037	0.069	370	90	• For severe food allergies, protein maldigestion or fat malabsorption • Contains hydrolyzed milk proteins • Ready to feed only
Pregestimil® (Mead Johnson)	Hydrolyzed casein, free amino acids	55% MCT oil, corn oil, soy oil, high oleic safflower or sunflower oil	Corn syrup solids, dextrose, modified cornstarch	0.67	0.019	0.038	0.069	320	89	• For severe or multiple food allergies (sensitive to milk protein) • For fat-malabsorption • Hypoallergenic, isotonic formula • Contains hydrolyzed milk protein
Portagen® (Mead Johnson)	Sodium caseinate	86% MCT oil, 15% corn oil	Corn syrup solids, sucrose	0.67	0.023	0.032	0.077	233	89	• For patients who do not efficiently digest or absorb conventional fats and long chain fatty acids

Table 36-2 Enteral Formulas for Liver Disease (continued).

Elemental and Semielemental Pediatric Enteral Products

Designed for Children with Significantly Impaired Gastrointestinal Function Ages 1-10 Years

	Nutrient source				g/mL					
Formula	*Protein*	*Fat*	*Carbohydrate*	*kcal/mL*	*Protein*	*Fat*	*Carbohydrate*	*mOsm/Kg H_2O*	*% H_2O*	*Comments*
Peptamen Junior® (Nestle)	Enzymatically hydrolyzed whey	60% MCT oil, soy oil, canola oil	Maltodextrin, cornstarch	1	0.03	0.038	0.138	260–360	85	• Ready to feed and powder available • Contains glutamine • Vanilla and unflavored
Vivonex Pediatric® (Novartis)	Amino acids	68% MCT oil, soybean oil	Maltodextrin, modified corn-starch	.8	0.024	0.024	0.13	360	89	• Powder • Standard 24 cal/oz concentration • Can be concentrated up to 30 cal/oz • Contains glutamine
Neocate One +® (SHS)	Amino acids	Fractionated coconut oil, canola oil, high oleic safflower oil, 35% MCT, 65% LCT	Corn syrup solids	1	0.025	0.035	0.0146	powder 610	80	• Protein hypersensitivity and allergy • Tube feeding—unflavored powder • Contains free glutamine • Flavor packets available
Elecare® (Ross)	Free L-amino acids	33% MCT oil, high oleic safflower oil, soy oil	Corn syrup solids	1	0.03	0.046	0.107	551	83	• Free amino acids • Powder only
Neocate Jr ® (SHS)	Free amino acids	Fractionated coconut oil, canola oil, high oleic safflower oil 35% MCT, 65% LCT	Corn syrup solids	1	0.03	0.05	0.104 tropical 0.109	Unflavored—607 tropical flavor 690		• Powder only • Flavored/ unflavored

Table 36-2 Enteral Formulas for Liver Disease (continued).

Adult Elemental and SemiElemental Enteral Products

Designed for Children Ages > 10 Years with Significantly Impaired Gastrointestinal Function

	Nutrient source				*g/mL*					
Formula	*Protein*	*Fat*	*Carbohydrate*	*kcal/ mL*	*Protein*	*Fat*	*Carbohydrate*	*mOsm/ Kg H_2O*	*% H_2O*	*Comments*
Peptamen® (Nestle)	Enzymatically hydrolyzed whey protein	70% MCT oil, soy oil	Maltodextrin, cornstarch	1	0.04	0.039	0.127	270-380	85	• Peptide based • Contains glutamine • Unflavored—flavor packets available • Ready to feed
Peptamen 1.5® (Nestle)	Enzymatically hydrolyzed whey protein	70% MCT oil, soy oil	Maltodextrin, cornstarch	1.5	0.06	0.056	0.19	550	77	• Higher calories than standard Peptamen • Contains glutamine • Unflavored—flavor packets available • Ready to feed

sometimes poses a challenge for the older child. MCT oil does not contain essential fatty acids (EFA), therefore the diet should be carefully monitored to ensure that enough EFAs are consumed. The actual requirement for EFAs (linoleic and linolenic acids) in children with liver disease is not known. The current minimal intake of linoleic acid recommended for young infants is 2.7–4.5% of energy. The ratio of linoleic to linolenic acid should be 5:1.[42] Hypercholesterolemia occurs in some patients with cholestatic liver disease, but much of the cholesterol is in the form of lipoprotein-X, which is not a risk for vascular disease because it cannot react with vascular epithelium. Therefore, it is not necessary to restrict dietary fat and cholesterol.[43]

Vitamins and Minerals

Vitamin A deficiency, found in 20–50% of children with chronic cholestatic diseases,[44] can be associated with xerophthalmia and immune deficiency. Plasma retinol levels are used to monitor vitamin A status; however, in the presence of compromised hepatic synthetic function, retinol-binding protein (RBP) levels can be low, but retinol might not be deficient. The retinol: RBP molar ratio is helpful. A ratio of < 0.8 suggests vitamin A deficiency. Side effects of vitamin A supplementation are seen only when doses exceeding physiologic replacement are administered. These include visual disturbances, irritability, increased intracranial pressure, vomiting, and diarrhea.

Vitamin D deficiency leads to hepatic osteodystrophy characterized by osteoporosis, rickets, and fractures. The precise cause is unknown. Hepatic osteodystrophy might not be responsive to large doses of vitamin D supplementation and sunlight exposure. Both calcium and magnesium deficiency have been implicated in the pathophysiology of this disorder. The serum 25 (OH) D concentration is the best biologic marker of vitamin D status.[45,46]

Vitamin E deficiency leads to a neuromuscular disease consisting of truncal ataxia, hyporeflexia, or areflexia. These abnormalities are reversible if adequate vitamin E supplementation is instituted prior to the age of 3 years.[47] Children with cholestasis might require high doses of α-tocopherol. Monitoring is problematic because high plasma lipid levels are associated with a false elevation in the serum α-tocopherol level.[48] Therefore, vitamin E status can be more reliably evaluated by measuring the ratio of serum vitamin E levels to total lipids. The total serum lipid concentration is the sum of serum cholesterol, triglyceride and phospholipids. A vitamin E: total serum lipid ratio of ≤ 0.8 total tocopherol per gram of total lipid indicates vitamin E deficiency in adolescents and adults. For children less than 12 years, a ratio of ≤ 0.6 indicates vitamin E deficiency.[49]

Vitamin K deficiency leads to a coagulopathy manifested as easy bruising or bleeding. Measurement of the prothrombin time provides an assessment of vitamin K status. Liver disease could prolong the prothrombin time because of impaired synthesis of clotting factors active in the coagulation pathway.[50–52] Vitamin K is required for posttranslational carboxylation of vitamin K-dependent proteins such as prothrombin.

Fat-soluble vitamins should be supplemented individually to maximize the doses and absorption. Admixture with D-alpha-tocopheryl polyethylene glycol-1,000 succinate (TPGS), a water-soluble preparation of vitamin E, can improve the absorption of other water-soluble vitamins.[21,53] A commercial fat-soluble vitamin preparation, ADEK, is available. Each tablet contains 9,000 IU vitamin A, 400 IU vitamin D, 150 IU vitamin E, and 10 mg vitamin K. One mL of liquid ADEK contains 3,170 IU vitamin A, 400 IU vitamin D, 40 IU vitamin E, and 100 mcg vitamin K. Generally 1 mL is prescribed for children ≤ 1 year, 2 mL for children up to 3 years. Older children (ages 4–11) can receive 1 tablet, while adults can take 2 tablets daily.

Although patients with childhood liver disease are at risk for water-soluble vitamin deficiencies secondary to inadequate dietary intake and malabsorption, there are no studies available that address the true incidence or the need for supplementation.

Mineral supplementation with calcium, zinc, and sometimes iron might be required. Calcium absorption, although not significantly impaired in children with chronic cholestatic disease when compared with control children, can be improved by vitamin D administration.[54,55] However, bile acid supplementation commonly used in patients with cholestasis decreases calcium absorption. Supplemental enteral formula improves calcium intake and allows for positive calcium balance. Calcium-fortified foods such as orange juice, waffles, or supplements that taste good, like Tums and Viactiv, can be used to provide extra calcium. Magnesium repletion can improve bone mineral density in cholestatic children.

Zinc deficiency is fairly common and is required for the crucial enzymatic processes that affect liver metabolism.[56] Hambidge et al. noted that infants and children with biliary atresia had plasma zinc concentrations lower than control subjects.[57] The usual zinc dose is 1–2 mg/kg/day of elemental zinc. Iron deficiency can develop because of recurrent gastrointestinal bleeding and malnutrition. Iron supplementation might be required. Copper, on the other hand, is excreted via the biliary route. In patients who have cholestatic disease, copper might be retained in potentially toxic amounts. For patients receiving PN, copper should be carefully monitored and the amount provided might need to be reduced.

NUTRITION IN THE PEDIATRIC LIVER TRANSPLANTATION CANDIDATE

Poor growth, deterioration of nutritional status, and other complications of end-stage liver disease make the timing of the liver transplant evaluation important. Malnutrition is one of the major factors adversely affecting the survival of infants and children awaiting transplantation.[58] The goals of nutrition support in this pretransplant phase of care are focused on the prevention, if possible, of further liver injury, possible liver tissue regeneration, maintenance of growth and development, prevention of nutrient depletion, and disease related complications. It is recommended that patients with arm muscle circumferences below the fifth percentile have nutritional support implemented prior to transplantation.[59]

Nutrition in the Pretransplant Period

The first successful pediatric liver transplant was performed in 1967. Improvements in surgical techniques and the development of long term immunosuppressant medications make liver transplantation a valid therapy for children with advanced liver disease.[60] Liver transplantation is a legitimate goal for most cases of end-stage liver disease. Previously, requirements for a size-matched cadaveric liver severely limited pediatric transplantation and led to high death rates among patients awaiting transplantation. The use of reduced-size cadaveric grafts and living related donors increased the availability of donor organs. Survival rates after pediatric liver transplantation have reached 85–90%, and the quality of life for most patients after transplant is improved.[61] These advances caused pediatric gastroenterologists and dietitians to shift their primary focus of care from purely supportive to treatments that improve the clinical status before transplantation. Malnutrition adversely affects the outcome of orthotopic liver transplantation and is the primary area of care where the greatest improvements can be made. Optimal nutritional status prior to transplantation decreases surgical risk, increases the chances of survival, and ultimately improves the quality of life.

The keys to pretransplant management in pediatric patients are aggressive medical management of the complications of end-stage liver disease, prolonging the growth period, and timing the transplant. A child who is experiencing growth failure due to progressive liver disease cannot improve prior to transplantation.[62]

Many children can maintain good dietary intake and growth with oral intake of an age-appropriate diet during the early stages of progressive liver disease even if cholestasis is present. As the liver disease advances and complications arise, more aggressive nutrition support becomes necessary. During advanced liver disease, even with nutrient intakes above normal, nutritional status cannot be maintained because of increased energy requirements, disruption of intermediary metabolism of nutrients, and the effects of vitamin and mineral deficiencies.[27] Elemental infant formulas can be concentrated as tolerated to 30 calories/oz by concentrating infant formula and adding nutrients such as modular glucose polymers and MCT. Children over the age of 1 year can receive MCT oil-containing pediatric formulas and modular caloric additives to foods for additional calories. When patients are unable to consume adequate calories to maintain appropriate lean body mass, tube feedings should be initiated. Nasogastric tubes are preferred if patients can tolerate adequate formula volume to achieve goals. However, in many instances, nasojejunal placement of feeding tubes is necessary because of emesis and intolerance to large volumes. These problems arise because of abdominal distension caused by ascites or organomegaly. Continuous nocturnal feedings are commonly used so that oral feeding skills can be maintained during the day. This feeding schedule might also be beneficial for patients with end-stage liver disease who are unable to maintain blood glucose levels in the normal range overnight. In many instances, these patients progress to 24-hour continuous tube feeding infusions to achieve the increased intakes required to maintain nutritional status.

Maintaining oral motor function is essential to ensure proper transition to normal feeding posttransplantation. Tube feeding supplementation might also be required for a short period of time after transplantation until normal oral feeding patterns can resume and the added effects of appetite stimulation from higher dose steroids are seen.

PN is used pretransplant only when disease complications such as severe varices and GI bleeding, excessive emesis, or recurrent complications make it unsafe or impossible to feed enterally. PN is sometimes used as an adjunctive nutritional therapy in patients who are severely malnourished and in whom the ability to achieve full enteral nutritional support is unattainable. A balance of standard amino acids, dextrose, lipids, electrolytes, and minerals are patient specific and designed to meet nutritional needs while minimizing metabolic complications. Amino acid mixtures enriched in BCAAs and made specifically for patients with liver disease have not been found to be beneficial in pediatric patients.[63] Whatever the modality of nutritional support, serial anthropometric measurements are recommended to follow the effectiveness and adequacy of nutritional interventions.[64]

Nutrition in the Posttransplant Period

In the immediate posttransplant period, nutrition support is important to manage the catabolic effect of the surgery, facilitate weaning from the ventilator, reduce the possibility of infection, improve wound repair, and anticipate and treat nutrition and metabolic problems that arose in the pretransplant period, such as refeeding syndrome. Refeeding syndrome (see Chapter 25) is a serious complication associated with aggressive nutritional rehabilitation of malnourished patients, and it is characterized by hypokalemia, hypophosphatemia, and hypomagnesemia, glucose and fluid intolerance, and possible cardiac and pulmonary dysfunction.[65] PN via a central venous catheter is generally started within 24–48 hours posttransplant after hemostasis is achieved with aggressive intravenous electrolyte and mineral replacement. PN is maintained until the patient is able to take 50–75% of the total caloric requirements by mouth.[66] If the patient is unable to achieve the above goals orally with the use of high calorie supplements or infant formula, PN may be used as a supplement to tube feeding support. Enteral feeding should be instituted as soon as gut function is restored. When oral intake improves, tube feedings can be weaned and eventually discontinued. Persistent inadequate oral intake posttransplant can be a significant factor in patients with hepatic dysfunction, rejection, or surgical complications. Feeding problems caused by behavorial issues are common, but not clearly defined. Contributing factors include anorexia, vomiting, and unpalatable foods. Many infants and younger children who received tube feeds supplementation pretransplant might not develop normal feeding skills because they missed developmental milestones for chewing and swallowing. These feeding problems can contribute to growth failure that occurs in 10% of children after transplant because of inadequate intake.[67] Recent studies indicate that 80% of children who survive liver transplantation achieve normal growth patterns and body habitus. Weight, midarm circumference, and triceps skinfolds returned to normal within 1 year of the transplant. Initial catch-up growth in height was slower, possibly caused by the growth effects of corticosteroids used in the first 3 to 6 months after transplant. By 4 years, all children had satisfactory height standard deviation score.[68,69] Most children will resume a normal diet before discharge from the hospital, although some might require additional oral supplements to achieve catch-up growth. A small portion of infants and children, particularly those with behavioral feeding issues, might require supplemental tube feedings for several months to years.

Along with surgical, medical, and behavioral complications, iatrogenic factors such as immunosuppressive drugs, carry significant side effects that could affect nutrition (Table 36-3). These medications can cause long term nutrition problems that must be managed throughout the posttransplant and recovery phase.

Posttransplant quality of life issues are pivotal. Long term goals focus on maximizing linear growth and cognitive, physical, and emotional states.[70] Optimal nutritional support can improve long term quality of life in pediatric patients by reducing or avoiding the incidence of linear growth failure, rickets from osteomalacia with related pathologic fractures, and neurodevelopmental delay.[71] Clearly, reaching normal height is an important aspect of quality of life because it impacts social reintegration and self-esteem. The causes of poor growth after liver transplantation include pretransplant growth failure, poor graft function, and the long term use of glucocorticoid therapy. The efficacy and safety of recombinant growth hormone (rhGH) as a treatment of linear growth failure for liver transplant patients is presently under investigation. It has been used successfully to treat children after renal transplantation.[72] One of the primary goals after transplantation is to minimize the complications associated with chronic use of immunosuppressive drugs while achieving optimal protection of the organ graft. Reduced drug doses are the key to minimizing the potential for complications. Target blood levels of cyclosporine or tacrolimis are usually reduced within the first 1–2 years, depending on episodes of acute rejection. Aggressive corticosteroid wean is attempted over the first 3–6 months after transplantation.

Complications for younger children are primarily related to growth impairment and osteopenia from steroid use and are more serious than those observed in older children. Multiple factors contribute to the development of osteopenia in patients with chronic liver disease awaiting liver transplantation, including immobility, malnutrition, poor muscle mass, poor renal function, and cholestasis. In the posttransplant period, high-dose corticosteroid therapy is the main cause of bone loss. In a retrospective study of children with end-stage liver disease who underwent orthotopic liver transplantation, 16% had bone fractures in the postoperative period. In our center, osteopenia associated with cholestatic disease improved after transplantation.[73]

Irrespective of the postoperative bone density, most liver transplant recipients lose bone mass for 3–6 months after transplantation, but by 6 months, the bone loss ceases in patients with normal allograft function, then stabilizes or increases.[74] Adequate calcium and vitamin D supplementation in the pretransplant and posttransplant phases, as well as the promotion of physical activity and the minimized use of osteopenia-producing medications are keys in the preservation of bone mass during the early posttransplant phase.

Nephrotoxicity and abnormal renal function characterized by decreased glomerular filtration rate have been associated with the long-term use of immunosuppressive drugs such as cyclosporine and tacrolimus, other nephrotoxic drugs, and episodes of rejection

Table 36-3 Most common posttransplant medications and nutrition-related side effects.

Primary Immunosuppressant

	Description	*Warnings/adverse reactions*
Cyclosporine (Sand immune, Neural, Sancta)	Immunosuppressant used in the prophylaxis of graft rejection.	Nephrotoxicity, hepatotoxicity, increased susceptibility to infection and lymphoma, hypertension, and gum hyperplasia.
Methylprednisolone (Solu-medrol)	Immunosuppressive adjunct for the prevention and treatment of solid organ rejection.	Increased calcium excretion leading to osteoporosis, sodium and fluid retention leading to cushingoid state, hypertension, suppression of growth in children, secondary decreased carbohydrate tolerance, impaired wound healing, peptic ulcers, pancreatitis, muscle weakness, steroid myopathy, subcapsular cataracts, and glaucoma.
Tacrolimus (Prograf, FK-506)	Immunosuppressant. Prophylaxis of graft rejection in liver and kidney transplants.	Increased incidence of posttransplant diabetes mellitus, neurotoxicity, nephrotoxicity, hyperkalemia, increased risk of infection and lymphomas, hypertension that might require treatment with antihypertensive agents, and headaches. Increased magnesium losses.
Immunosuppressants Used to Treat Acute Rejection		
Muromonab-CD3 (OKT3)	Treatment of steroid-resistant allograft rejection.	Cytokine release syndrome leading to flulike symptoms, nausea and vomiting with the first few doses administered.
Mycophenolate mofetil	Prophylaxis of graft rejection.	Increased susceptibility to infection and lymphoma, neutropenia, and gastrointestinal hemorrhage might occur.
Rapamycin (sirolimus, Rapamune)	Prevention and treatment of allograft rejection.	Thrombocytopenia and hyperlipidemia.

and hypertension. Abnormal renal function occurs in approximately one third of all children at any given time posttransplant.[75] Hypertension remains a serious posttransplant complication; 10–28% of children require long term antihypertensive treatment.[76] Blood pressure should be routinely monitored.

Hyperlipidemia in some pediatric patients following liver transplantation is associated with the use of cyclosporine, high-dose corticosteroid therapy, obesity, and diabetes mellitus. Prepubertal children and adolescents seem to have more complications with diabetes mellitus, hyperlipidemia, and obesity. A family history of hyperlipidemia is a contributing factor. Tacrolimus is used as the primary immunosuppressive drug and has less of an effect on serum lipid levels.[77,78] One of the major focuses of treatment remains dietary intervention. Patient and family education on menu planning, food purchasing, and preparation techniques and lifestyle modifications that include an exercise regimen are recommended.

Diabetes mellitus is sometimes seen in children after liver transplantation. Hyperglycemia could occur in some children on tacrolimus in combination with high-dose corticosteroids. In most instances, hyperglycemia resolves when corticosteroid doses are reduced. Insulin injections are required when hyperglycemia is sustained. Patients with a family history of diabetes mellitus or a diagnosis of autoimmune liver disease appear to be at risk of developing diabetes mellitus in the postoperative period.[79] Obesity after liver transplantation occurs more frequently in adults than children, but it can affect adolescents and children. The goal of treatment should focus on lifestyle changes and behavior modification rather than calorie-restricted diets as the tendency for weight gain will be present throughout life.

CONCLUSION

The goal of nutrition support in infants and children with liver disease is to optimize growth, preserve lean body mass, and manage complications associated with the primary disease process. Aggressive nutrition support and metabolic dietary management during all phases of the disease are essential in preparing patients for transplantation. Transplantation offers a therapeutic option for infants and children who have otherwise fatal hepatic disease.

REFERENCES

1. Squires RH. End-stage liver disease in children. *Curr Treat Options Gastroenterol.* 2001;4(5):409–421.
2. Shneider B, Alonso EM, Narkewicz MR. Research agenda for pediatric gastroenterology, hepatology and nutrition: hepatobiliary disorders. Report of the North American Society for Pediatric Gastroenterology, Hepatology and Nutrition for the Children's Digestive Health and Nutrition Foundation. *J Pediatr Gastroenterol Nutr.* 2002;35(suppl 3):S268–274.
3. Heubi JE, Heyman MB, Shulman RJ. The impact of liver disease on growth and nutrition. *J Pediatr Gastroenterol Nutr.* 2002;35(suppl 1):S55–59.
4. Alagille D, Odieve M, Gautier M, Dommergus JP. Hepatic ductular hypoplasia associated with characteristic facies, vertebral malformations, retarded physical, mental and sexual development, and cardiac murmur. *J Pediatr.* 1975;86:63–71.
5. Krantz ID, Piccoli DA, Spinner NB. Alagille syndrome. *J Med Genet.* 1997;34:152–157.
6. Suchy FJ, Burdelski M, Tomar BS, Sokol RJ. Cholestatic liver disease: working group report of the First World Congress of Pediatric Gastroenterology, Hepatology, and Nutrition. *J Pediatr Gastroentrol Nutr.* 2002;35(suppl 2): S89–97.
7. Perlmutter D, Azevedo R, Kelly D, Sheperd R, Tazawa Y. Metabolic liver disease: working group report of the First World Congress of Pediatric Gastroenterology, Hepatology, and Nutrition. *J Pediatr Gastroenterol Nutr.* 2002;35(suppl 2):S180–186.
8. Sveger T. Liver disease in alpha-1-antitrypsin deficiency detected by screening of 200,000 infants. *N Engl J Med.* 1976;294:1216–1221.
9. Perlmutter D, Azevedo RA, Kelly D, Shepard R, Tazawa Y. Metabolic liver disease: working group report of the First World Congress of Pediatric Gastroenterology, Hepatology, and Nutrition. *J Pediatr Gastroenterol Nutr.* 2002;35(suppl 2):S180–186.
10. Sigurdsson L, Reyes J, Kocoshis, SA, et al. Neonatal hemochromatosis: outcomes of pharmacologic and surgery therapies. *J Pediatr Gastroenterol Nutr.* 1998;26:85–89.
11. Kelly DA. Liver complications of pediatric parenteral nutrition: epidemiology. *Nutrition.* 1998;14:153–157.

12. Btaiche IF, Khalidi N. Parenteral nutrition-associated liver complications in children. *Pharmacotherapy.* 2002;22(2):188–211.
13. Bell R, Ferry G, Smith E. Total parenteral nutrition-related cholestasis in infants. *JPEN.* 1986;10:356–359.
14. Balistreri WF. Non-transplant options for the treatment of metabolic liver disease: saving livers while saving lives (editorial). *Hepatology.* 1994;19:782–787.
15. Chin SE, Shepard RW, Thomas BJ, et al. Nutritional support in children with end-stage liver disease: a randomized crossover trial of a branched-chain amino acid supplement. *Am J Clin Nutr.* 1992;56:158–163.
16. Riordan SM, Williams R. Treatment of hepatic encephalopathy. *N Engl J Med.* 1997;350:1309–1315.
17. Novy MA, Schwartz KB. Nutritional considerations and management of the child with liver disease. *Nutrition.* 1997;13(3):177–184.
18. Beath S, Pearmain G, Kelly D, McMaster P, Mayer A, Bukels J. Liver transplant in babies and children with extra hepatic biliary atresia: pre-operative condition, complications, survival and outcome. *J Pediatr Surg.* 1993;28:1044–1047.
19. Greer R, Lehnert M, Lewindon P, Cleghorn GJ, Shepherd RW. Body composition and components of energy expenditure in children with end-stage liver disease. *J Pediatr Gastroenterol Nutr.* 2003;36:358–363.
20. Pierro A, Koletzko B, Carnelli V, et al. Resting energy expenditure is increased in infants with extra hepatic biliary atresia and cirrhosis. *J Pediatric Surg.* 1989;24:534–538.
21. Sokol RJ, Butler-Simon N, Conner C, et al. Multicenter trial of d-alpha-tocopheryl polyethylene glycol 1000 succinate for the treatment of vitamin E deficiency in children with chronic cholestasis. *Gastroenterology.* 1993;104:1727–1735.
22. Sokol RJ, Stall C. Anthropometric evaluation of children with chronic liver disease. *Am J Clin Nutr.* 1990;52:203.
23. Chin SE, Sheperd RW, Thomas BJ, et al. The nature of malnutrition in children with end-stage liver disease awaiting orthotopic liver transplantation. *Am J Clin Nutr.* 1992;56:164.
24. Schneeweiss B, Graninger W, Ferenci P, et al. Energy metabolism in patients with acute and chronic liver disease. *Hepatology.* 1990;11:387.
25. Hall JC, O'Quigley J, Giles GR, Appleton N, Stocks H. Upper limb anthropometry: the value of measure variance studies. *Am J Clin Nutr.* 1980;33:1846–1847.
26. Merli M, Romiti A, Riggio O, et al. Optimal nutritional indexes in chronic liver disease. *JPEN.* 1987;11:130S.
27. Kleinman R, Warman KY. Nutrition in liver disease. In: Baker SB, Baker RD, Davis A, eds. *Pediatric enteral nutrition.* New York: Chapman and Hall, Inc; 1994:261–279.
28. Detsky AS, Baker JP, O'Rourke K, et al. Predicting nutrition-associated complications of patients undergoing gastrointestinal surgery. *JPEN.* 1987;11(5):440.
29. Hasse J, Strong S, Gorman MA, Liepa G. Subjective global assessment: alternative nutrition assessment technique for liver transplant candidates. *Nutrition.* 1993;339–343.
30. Ramaccioni V, Soriano HE, Arumugam R, Klish WJ. Nutritional aspects of chronic liver disease and liver transplant in children. *J Pediatr Gastroenterol Nutr.* 2000;30(4):361–367.
31. Kaufman SS, Scrivner DJ, Guest JE. Preoperative evaluation, preparation, and timing of orthotopic liver transplantation in children. *Semin Liver Dis.* 1989;3:176–183.
32. Kaufman SS, Murray ND, Wood RP, Shaw BW Jr, Vanderhoof JA. Nutritional support for the infant with extrahepatic biliary atresia. *J Pediatr.* 1987;110(5):679.
33. The Nutrition Therapy Division of Cincinnati Children's Hospital Medical Center. *Pediatric Nutrition Handbook.* Cincinnati Children's Hospital, Cincinnati, OH 2001.
34. Charlton CP, Buchanan E, Holden CE, et al. Intensive enteral feeding in advanced cirrhosis: reversal of malnutrition without precipitation of hepatic encephalopathy. *Arch Dis Child.* 1992;67:603–607.
35. Chin SE, Shepard RW, Cleghorn GJ, et al. Pre-operative nutritional support in children with end-stage liver disease accepted for liver transplantation: an approach to management. *J Gastroenterol Hepatol.* 1990;5:566–572.
36. Chin SE, Shepard RW, Thomas BJ, et al. Nutritional support in children with end-stage liver disease: a randomized crossover trial of a branched-chain amino acid supplement. *Am J Clin Nutr.* 1992;56:158–163.
37. Novy MA, Schwartz KB. Nutritional considerations and management of the child with liver disease. *Nutrition.* 1997;13(3):177–184.
38. Setty AK, Schmidt-Sommerfeld E, Udall JN Jr. Nutritional aspects of liver disease in children. *Nutrition.* 1999;15(9):727–729.
39. Beath S, Hooley I, Willis K, Johnson S, Booth I. Long chain triacylglycerol malabsorption and pancreatic function in children with protein energy malnutrition complicating severe liver disease. *Proc Nutr Soc.* 1993;52:252A.
40. Cohen MI, Gartner LM. The use of medium-chain triglycerides in the management of biliary atresia. *J Pediatr.* 1971;79:379–384.
41. Beath S, Johnson T, Willis K, et al. Superior absorption of medium chain triglycerides compared with conventional dietary long chain fat in children with chronic liver disease. *Proc Nutr Soc.* 1993;52:252.
42. Aggett PJ, Haschke F, et al. ESPGAN committee on nutrition: comment on the content and composition

of lipids in infant formula. *Acta Paediatr (Scand)*. 1991;80:887–896.

43. Whitington PF. Chronic cholestasis of infancy. *Pediatr Clin North Am*. 1996;43:1–25.
44. Kaplan MM, Elta GH, Furie B, Sadowski JA, Russell RM. Fat soluble vitamin nutriture in primary biliary cirrhosis. *Gastroenterology*. 1988;95:787–792.
45. Heubi JE, Higgins JV, Argao EA, et al. The role of magnesium in the pathogenesis of bone disease in childhood cholestatic liver disease: a preliminary report. *J Pediatr Gastroenterol Nutr*. 1997;25:301–306.
46. Klein GL, Soriano H, Shulman RJ, et al. Hepatic osteodystrophy in chronic cholestasis: evidence for a multifactorial etiology. *Pediatr Transplant*. 2002;6:136–140.
47. Sokol RJ, Heubi JE, McGraw C, et al. Correction of vitamin E deficiency in children with chronic cholestasis: II. Effect on gastrointestinal and hepatic function. *Hepatology*. 1986;6:1263–1269.
48. Davit-Spraul A, Cosson C, Couturier M, et al. Standard treatment of alpha-tocopherol in Alagille patients with severe cholestasis is insufficient. *Pediatr Res*. 2001;49:232–236.
49. Sokol RJ. Fat-soluble vitamins and their importance in patients with cholestatic liver disease. *Gastroenterol Clin North Am*. 1994;23:673–705.
50. Novy MA, Schwartz KB. Nutritional consideration and management of the child with liver disease. *Nutrition*. 1997;13(3):177–184.
51. Squires RH. End-stage liver disease in children. *Curr Treat Options Gastroenterol*. 2001;4(5):409–421.
52. Spinossi NS. Hepatobiliary diseases. In: Hendricks KM, Duggan C, Walker WA, eds. *Manual of Pediatric Nutrition*. 3rd ed. Hamilton, Ontario: Decker; 2000:427–432.
53. Bucuvalas JC, Heubi JE, Specker BL, et al. Calcium absorption in bone disease associated with liver cholestasis during childhood. *Hepatology*. 1990;12:1200–1205.
54. Heubi JE, Hollis BW, Specker B, Tsang RC. Bone diseases in chronic childhood cholestasis. I. vitamin D absorption and metabolism. *Hepatology*. 1989;9:258–264.
55. Bucuvalas JC, Heubi JE, Specker BL, et al. Calcium absorption in bone disease associated with liver cholestasis during childhood. *Hepatology*. 1990;12:1200–1205.
56. Powers SG, Meister L. Urea synthesis and ammonia metabolism. In: Arias M , Jakoby WB, Popper H, Schalter D, Shafritz DA, eds. *The Liver: Biology and Pathology*. New York, NY: Raven Press; 1988:317–330.
57. Hambidge KM, Krebs NF, Lilly JR, Zerbe GO. Plasma and urine zinc in infants and children with extrahepatic biliary atresia. *J Pediatr Gastroenterol Nutr*. 1987;6:872–877.
58. Shepherd RW, Chin SE, Cleghorn GJ, et al. Malnutrition in children with chronic liver disease accepted for liver transplantation: clinical profile and effects on outcome. *J Paediatric Child Health* 1991;27:295–296.
59. Goulet OJ, de Ville de Goyet, Otte JB, Ricour C. Preoperative nutritional evaluation and support of liver transplantation in children. *Transplant Proc*. 1987;19(4):3249–3255.
60. National Institute of Health. National Institute of Health Consensus Development Conference statement: liver transplantation—June 20–23, 1982. *Hepatology*. 1984;4:107S.
61. Whitington PF. Advances in pediatric liver transplantation. In: Barnes LA, ed. *Advances in Pediatrics*. Vol 37. Chicago, Ill: Year Book Publishers; 1990:357–389.
62. Whitington PF, Balistreri WF. Liver transplantation in pediatrics: indications, contraindications, and pretransplant management. *J Pediatr*. 1991;118:169–177.
63. Molleston JP. Acute and chronic liver disease. In: Walker WA, Watkins JB, eds. *Nutrition in Pediatrics*. 2nd ed. Hamilton, Ontario: Decker Inc; 1996:565–571.
64. Santiago, JM. Nutritional therapies in liver disease. *Semin Liver Dis*. 1991;11:278–291.
65. Dunn RL, Stettler N, Mascarenhas MR. Refeeding syndrome in hospitalized pediatric patients. *Nutr Clin Pract*. 2003;18:327–332.
66. Becht MB, Pedersen SH, Ryckman FC, Balistreri WF. Growth and nutrition management of pediatric patients after orthotopic liver transplantation. *Gastroenterol Clin North Am*. 1993;22:367–380.
67. Kelly DA. Nutritional factors affecting growth before and after liver transplantation. *Pediatr Transplant*. 1997;1(1):80–84.
68. Codoner-Franch P, Bernard O, Alvarez F. Long-term follow-up growth in height after successful liver transplantation. *J Pediatr*. 1994;124:368–373.
69. McKiernan PJ, Pearmin GD, Johnson T, Buckels JA, Mayer AD, Kelly DA. Catch up growth in children following orthotopic liver transplantation. *Hepatology*. 1992;16:567.
70. Lee H, Vacanti JP. Liver transplantation and its long term management in children. *Pediatr Clin North Am*. 1996;43:99–124.
71. Ramaccioni V, Soriano HE, Arumugam R, Klish WJ. Nutritional aspects of chronic liver disease and liver transplantation in children. *J Pediatr Gastroenterol Nutr*. 2000;30(4):361–367.
72. Sarna S, Laine J, Sipila I, Koistinen R, Holmberg C. Differences in linear growth and cortisol production between liver and renal transplant recipients on similar immunosuppression. *Transplantation*. 1995;60:656–661.
73. Guthery SL, Pohl JF, Bucuvalas JC, et al. Bone mineral density in long-term survivors following pediatric liver transplantation. *Liver Transpl*. 2003;9:365–370.

74. Argao EA, Balistreri WF, Hollis BW, Ryckman FC, Heubi JE. Effects of orthotopic liver transplantation on bone mineral content and serum vitamin D metabolites in infants and children with chronic cholestasis. *Hepatology.* 1994;20:598–603.

75. Bartosh SM, Alonso EM, Whitington PF. Renal outcome in pediatric liver transplantation. *Clin Transplant.* 1997;11:354–360.

76. Whitington PF, Alonso EM, Piper JB. Pediatric liver transplantation. *Sem Liver Dis.* 1994;14:303–317.

77. Munoz SJ. Hyperlipidemia and other coronary risk factors after orthotopic liver transplantation: pathogenesis, diagnosis, and management. *Liver Transplant Surg.* 1995;1(suppl):29–38.

78. Pirsch J, Simmons W, Sollinger H. *Transplant Drug Manual.* 3rd ed. Austin, Tex: Landes Bioscience; 1999.

79. Lohmann T, List C, Lamesch P, et al. Diabetes mellitus and inlet cell specific autoimmunity as adverse effects of immunosuppression therapy with FK506/tacrolimus. *Exp Clin Endocrinol Diabetes.* 2000;108:347–352.

Chapter 37

Short Bowel

Valeria C. Cohran and Samuel A. Kocoshis

INTRODUCTION

Short gut syndrome is defined as intestinal resection or intestinal failure that results in malabsorption of fluids, electrolytes, and nutrients. Dependence on total parenteral nutrition (PN) is implied by this definition. After surgical resection, a complex process known as intestinal adaptation takes place. This process allows the remaining intestine to compensate for the loss of bowel by increasing its surface area and functional capacity to meet the body's requirements. The time to achieve complete intestinal adaptation depends on the functional state of the remaining bowel and the primary etiology of the short gut syndrome.

The metabolic consequences of short gut syndrome are determined by the region and length of intestine that is resected or affected by an inflammatory or motility disorder (Table 37-1). During good health, the jejunum absorbs 4–5 liters per day of fluid and the ileum absorbs up to 4 liters per day. When the jejunum is absent or not functional, the ileum has the capacity to adapt and so is able to perform both jejunal and ileal functions. The reverse is not true. The terminal ileum and ileocecal valve (ICV) are commonly affected in infants with necrotizing enterocolitis (NEC). Loss of the ICV permits contamination of the distal small intestine by colonic flora resulting in small bowel bacterial overgrowth. Loss of enough ileum (> 60 cm in adults) results in B_{12} deficiency because no other region of the small bowel absorbs B_{12} effectively.[1] Regardless of the primary etiology, management of children with short gut syndrome requires meticulous attention to nutrition and physiology to avoid dehydration, growth failure, and nutritional deficiencies.

In infants, the most common cause of short gut syndrome is NEC (Table 37-2). Although this disorder is primarily seen in premature infants, older, term infants can also develop NEC. Intestinal atresias such as isolated jejunal or jejunal-ileal atresia and gastroschisis with or without midgut volvulus can also result in significant intestinal resections. Older children could develop short gut secondary to intussusception, vascular accidents, hemolytic uremic syndrome, or inflammatory bowel disease such as Crohn's disease. Even in the absence of surgical resection, patients with autoimmune enteropathy, intestinal pseudoobstruction, and microvillus inclusion disorders have a functional short gut syndrome that might require PN for survival.

In 1979, Wilmore reported the outcomes of 50 infants with small bowel resections.[2] In this series, infants who had ileocecal resections and small intestinal lengths < 40 cm died. One infant survived with 15 cm of small bowel, an ileocecal valve, and an intact colon. Sondheimer et al. suggested that if 50% of calories are not received through the enteral route by 3 months adjusted age, there is approximately an 80% chance of permanent intestinal failure defined as persistent PN requirements at 3 years of age.[3] The cohort analyzed by Sondheimer et al. was comprised of

Table 37-1 Metabolic derangements and their consequences.

Derangements	**Consequences**
Early	*Early*
Gastric hypersecretion	Peptic ulceration
Dumping syndrome	Diarrhea, hyperglycemia, reactive hypoglycemia
Rapid intestinal transit	Nutrient malabsorption
High output from enterostomies	Electrolyte disturbances
Late	*Late*
Bile acid and fatty acid malabsorption	Gallstones, steatorrhea
Bowel dilation and stasis	Bacterial overgrowth syndrome, D-lactic acidosis
Anastomotic ulceration	Gastrointestinal bleeding

Table 37-2 The most common causes of short bowel syndrome.

Disorder	*Description*
Necrotizing enterocolitis	The most common condition for which emergency gastrointestinal surgery is required in the neonatal period. Premature infants are at highest risk for this disorder.
Gastroschisis	A disorder in which the intestines fail to be enclosed in the abdominal cavity during development. There might be little or no intestinal resection required. Regardless of the length of bowel, the intestinal motility tends to be poor.
Omphalocele	A disorder in which the intestines are enclosed by peritoneum but fail to rotate back into the abdomen. Other defects, such as cardiac disease, could be associated.
Intestinal atresias	Occurs when part of the intestine fails to develop. Removal of the atretic portion of bowel and anastomosis with the remaining bowel is necessary. Depending on the degree of atresia, these infants might require PN.
Crohn's disease	Inflammatory bowel disease that can affect the entire gastrointestinal tract from the mouth to the anus.

neonates, primarily with NEC, who had undergone surgical resections. The ability to generalize this data to older children and those without NEC might be limited. Quiros et al. reported the outcomes of 78 children who received PN for more than 3 months.[4] Adaptation in this series rarely occurred after 3 years and only 3 of the 17 children who had no more than 15 cm of small bowel achieved intestinal adaptation. Both of these studies support the theory that adaptation occurs more successfully during the neonatal period; it rarely occurs as a late phenomenon.

Until home PN was introduced in the early 1980s, children with short gut syndrome would be hospital bound for years. Now, most major medical centers refer to home health care agencies that provide home programs that assist families of all educational levels to safely deliver PN at home. Despite increasing survival rates, PN is not a benign therapy and can result in devastating complications including hepatic failure, bacteremia, vascular thrombosis, and even death.

Many drugs and trophic hormones have been proposed as enhancers of intestinal adaptation, but to date none have demonstrated universal success. Intestinal lengthening procedures and intestinal transplantation are newer surgical therapies that could allow children to gain intestinal autonomy. The overall survival in children with short gut syndrome is determined by the length and adaptation of the remaining bowel, functional state of pancreas and gallbladder, and lack of associated anomalies.

In this chapter, we review the medical and surgical management of short gut syndrome, including small bowel transplantation. Medical therapy includes enteral nutrition (EN) and management of small bowel bacterial overgrowth. Surgical techniques, including lengthening and tapering procedures such as the Bianchi procedure and the newer serial transverse enteroplasty (STEP) procedure will also be reviewed.

INTESTINAL ADAPTATION

Intestinal adaptation is an intricate process that begins immediately after surgical resection and can potentially lead to intestinal autonomy. By compensating for intestinal loss, the remaining intestine can assume the functions required to sustain life. Adaptation is characterized by an increase in intestinal mass, lengthening of villi to increase surface area, and improved nutritional absorption at the epithelial cell level. Failure of this process leads to permanent intestinal failure and places the patient at risk for the development of PN related complications. The minimal length of bowel capable of attaining autonomy and fully adapting after resection differs for individual patients; however, it is unlikely that the small bowel will adapt if it is less than 20 cm long; early transplantation should be considered for children whose small bowel is this short.[4]

Home PN poses a significant financial burden, estimated at 3 billion dollars a year in 2001 dollars.[5] Therapeutic agents that promote or enhance small bowel adaptation could reduce the financial, medical, and social burden of PN. Several substances, including glutamine, glucagon-like peptide (GLP-2), epidermal growth factor (EGF), and growth hormone are possible mediators of adaptation.

In 1996, Drucker et al. reported that GLP-2 induced small bowel epithelial proliferation in mice with subcutaneous proglucagon-producing tumors, inferring that GLP-2 might play a role in adaptation.[6] Use of GLP-2 as a therapeutic agent in short bowel syndrome was reported by Jeppesen et al.[7] Two balance studies, 5 days each, were conducted in the hospital, 31 days apart. This study included endoscopies with biopsies, intestinal transit studies, and body composition measurements. Subjects were given subcutaneous injections of 400 μg GLP-2 twice daily for 35 days starting on day 5 of the initial balance study. Net intestinal absorption of energy, wet weight, and nitrogen were improved. Body weight and lean body mass increased. The authors concluded that GLP-2 improved nutrient absorption and nutritional status in short gut patients who had no colon. However, only half of the subjects received PN and the average time from their previous intestinal resection was approximately 10 years. Furthermore, 3 of the 8 patients had more than 100 cm of small bowel. Whether results of this study are applicable to typical pediatric short gut patients is not known.

In a cohort of 8 adult patients, high dose growth hormone, glutamine, and a high carbohydrate, low fat diet did not have a positive effect on small bowel morphology, nutrient absorption, or enteral losses.[8] In a 6-week, randomized study of low dose growth hormone in 12 PN dependent patients, Seguy[9] found that patients receiving a hyperphagic Western diet had significant improvement in their intestinal absorption defined in the terms of energy absorption, nutrition, and carbohydrates.

Stern et al. demonstrated a role for EGF in a murine model of adaptation and apoptosis after small bowel resection by enhancing proliferation and inhibiting apoptosis.[10,11] There are no human data testing its efficacy in short gut syndrome.

The mechanism of intestinal adaptation is unknown. Multicenter studies are needed to understand adaptation because patients are sparse at individual centers. As with many clinical trials, the pediatric population is often overlooked as potential participants because of the concern for the "more than minimal risk" label given by institutional review boards. For now, broad use of agents aimed at stimulating adaptation remains a lofty goal.

MEDICAL MANAGEMENT AND THERAPY

Enteral Nutrition

Vanderhoof described a paradigm for the treatment of short bowel syndrome.[12] The cornerstone of this approach is the early introduction and advancement of EN. Stimulation of the intestine by continuous formula is better tolerated and improves the complex process of intestinal adaptation. Without EN, intestinal adaptation is unlikely to be achieved. Casein hydrolysate formulas and elemental amino acid-based formulas such as Pregestamil, Nutramagin, Alimentum, EleCare, and Neocate are commonly used in children with short gut syndrome. As the children age, other formulas such as Peptamen Jr or Neocate Jr can be introduced to supply age-appropriate quantities of nutrients. The propensity for patients with short bowel syndrome to develop enteritis or colitis supports the use of these costly formulas because amino acids or hydrolyzed proteins are less likely to trigger an immune response and might actually enhance intestinal adaptation. Bines reported 4 children who were able to come off PN 15 months after the introduction of Neocate into their diet.[13] In the setting of refractory allergic enteritis or colitis, 5-aminosalicylate products and steroids, systemic or topical, have been used.

Nutrients can be delivered to the small bowel via oral feedings, gastrostomy, gastrojejunostomy, or jejunostomy tubes. Oral feedings have the advantage of being more physiologic and stimulate the secretion of secretin, cholecystokinin, and other gut hormones similar to levels in healthy children. Unfortunately, a large meal can cause dumping syndrome. Furthermore, hypergastrinemia or damaged gastric innervation associated with short gut can lead to delayed gastric emptying, decreasing the likelihood of satisfactory oral alimentation. Hence, continuous gastrostomy tube feedings are preferred by many centers. When vomiting occurs, a gastroduodenal or gastrojejunal tube as short as 20–30 cm can be positioned to deliver nutrients to the intestines. As feedings are tolerated, the infusion rate may be increased by 1 mL/hr or more daily.

In the neonatal period, oral aversion occurs after a critical illness and the prolonged use of nasogastric tubes. Even older children might become averse to eating after a prolonged illness. Oral feedings are often encouraged 2 to 3 times a day, depending on the degree of the aversion. Speech and physical therapists trained in treatment of feeding disorders can be helpful. Despite the most fervent of efforts, feeding disorders sometimes remain refractory for many years.

Advancement of EN is limited by the patient's tolerance of feedings. Symptoms associated with feeding intolerance include severe diarrhea, abdominal distension, perianal rashes, and vomiting. Children with underlying motility disturbances such as those that occur in gastroschisis are particularly susceptible to gastroesophageal reflux and abdominal distension. Unfortunately, after enterostomies are taken down and continuity is restored between small bowel and colon, children with short gut syndrome often develop significant perianal excoriation requiring frequent diaper changes and creams or ointments such as Ilex and Aquaphor. The liberal use of these products can greatly reduce the amount of contact the acidic stool has with the skin. Candidal dermatitis also occurs frequently and requires topical antifungal therapy. Depending on the severity of excoriation, EN can be halted to allow for proper healing of the buttocks.

One way to circumvent feeding intolerance is to concentrate the caloric density of the formulas, often up to 1 kcal/mL (30 kcal/oz). Concentrating formulas provides maximal nutrition with a reduction in volume, especially for children who are fluid sensitive because of abdominal distension or vomiting. As enteral feeds are advanced, additional fluids delivered enterally or parenterally might be required. Daily urine specific gravity and diaper weights are commonly recorded to monitor hydration status. Parents can and should be taught to calculate their children's daily intake and output.

In the hope of improving nutrient absorption, multiple other therapeutic agents can be tried. Antiperistaltic drugs such as loperamide can slow intestinal transit and potentially increase nutrient absorption. Children who have some colon could benefit from the addition of fiber products such as pectin and guar gum to their diets to increase the stool bulk and prevent fluid losses. Animal data suggests that soluble fiber in these agents is fermented to short chain fatty acids (SCFA), butyric and proprionic acid, and they up-regulate the production of the major colonic sodium transporter, increasing cell proliferation in the colon and allowing improved colonic function and fluid absorption.[14] There have been no prospective studies evaluating the impact of these agents in adults or children.

Total Parenteral Nutrition and Related Liver Disease

Inherent in the definition of short gut syndrome is PN dependence. The advent of PN in the late 1960s revolutionized the care of children with short gut. Wilmore first described an infant with intestinal atresia who was exclusively fed using PN for 44 days in 1967.[15] Prior to this, death was a certainty for patients with short gut syndrome. Today, PN is a bridge that supplies fluids and electrolytes until intestinal adaptation is complete. Children can receive up to 5 liters or more of fluid per day depending on their hydration status and diarrheal losses. Vitamins and minerals can be supplemented to prevent deficiencies. The amount and content of the PN depends on the fluid and nutritional requirements of the patient.

Unfortunately, PN is associated with life-threatening complications such as sepsis and cholestasis. Cholestasis is defined as a direct serum bilirubin > 2 mg/dL. Children receiving PN for as short a time as 1 month can develop cholestasis.[16] Although parenteral lipids and/or protein have been implicated in the pathogenesis of PN associated cholestasis, the primary etiology remains unknown.[17]

Younger infants and children with massive intestinal resection are particularly prone to develop cholestasis. In one series of 42 patients dependent on PN because of neonatal short gut syndrome, 17% subsequently developed liver failure.[16] There was no statistical difference in intestinal length between the patients who developed failure and those who did not. Although no correlation was found between cholestasis and duration of PN dependence in this cohort, others have shown an association.[18] In another series of 36 Italian patients, 44% of children with surgical short gut syndrome had liver disease as compared to 25% of children with gastroschisis or other disorders associated with normal intestinal length.[19] Unfortunately, the authors did not describe the ages of the patients, leaving in question whether a patient's age can play a role in the development of cholestasis.

Another associated risk factor for the development of PN cholestasis is the development of sepsis. The large-bore catheters used to infuse PN can become contaminated by unsterile techniques or bacterial translocation from the intestine. In the Sondheimer series, patients who developed hepatic failure experienced the first bacterial infection at a significantly younger age than those who did not (28.5 ± 5 days compared to 48.2 ± 12.2 days).[16] This finding supports the theory that bacteria and various endotoxins might exacerbate or precipitate liver disease.

Children who require chronic administration of PN must be followed closely by subspecialists with an interest in nutrition. Meehan et al. reviewed the pediatric experience at the University of Alabama regarding PN related cholestasis.[20] Over the course of 10 years, 11% of their patients died because of progressive liver failure. Their protocol included the use of taurine, aggressive treatment of bacterial overgrowth, aseptic techniques for catheter care, and limiting intralipid infusions.[17] The UCLA experience also exemplifies the importance of structured care and monitoring which likely contributed to the high survival rate of their cohort.[4] Despite meticulous care and monitoring, PN associated liver disease can progress to end-stage liver disease necessitating liver transplantation or combined liver/small bowel transplantation.

In any center providing care for these children, biochemical tests should be monitored according to a protocol to evaluate the acid-base status and degree of hepatic dysfunction. At a minimum, routine evaluation should include serum electrolytes, aminotransferases, and urinalyses to screen for electrolyte imbalance, hepatic injury, and glycosuria, respectively. Measuring urinary electrolytes is also helpful because reduced urinary sodium in the absence of liver disease indicates inadequate sodium replacement or significant losses in the stool.[21] Analyzing the fecal and urine output can help estimate the salt and bicarbonate requirements for a particular patient. There is a common misconception that a normal serum sodium represents adequate sodium supplementation. Hyponatremia is actually a late finding in sodium deficiency and severe salt depletion can occur prior to the recognition of higher salt requirements. Some children who have fistulas and extreme short gut syndrome require prodigious daily sodium replacement to meet their sodium needs.

Glucose infusion rates (GIR) must be carefully calculated to prevent hyperglycemia. The GIR should be kept below 13 mg/kg/minute to maintain euglycemia without excessive hyperinsulinemia and conversion of glucose to fat.[22] GIR can be maintained by making adjustments in the dextrose concentration or infusion time. Fat can be supplied as intravenously as an emulsion. Water-soluble vitamins are added to the PN in the form of Peds MVI-5 or Peds MVI-12. Most patients who receive vitamins in their PN do not develop vitamin deficiency. Other trace elements such as zinc, selenium, chromium, manganese, and copper are added to the PN. Copper and manganese should be carefully monitored or reduced in cholestatic patients to prevent toxicity.[23,24]

There is no specific drug therapy that can reduce PN cholestasis. However, ursodeoxycholic acid, a synthetic bile acid, is used to improve bile flow in adults with biliary cirrhosis.[25,26] In pediatrics, the data are less supportive. Heubi et al. evaluated 52 infants to determine whether taurourseodeoxycholic acid (TUDCA) could prevent hepatic injury in neonates receiving PN.[27] Twenty-two patients received 30 mg/kg/day of TUDCA and were compared to 30 untreated neonates. There was no difference in serum conjugated bilirubin or serum transaminases between the 2 groups of patients, even when stratified for weight. Despite the lack of prospective evidence to support its use, ursodeoxycholic acid remains a commonly used drug for PN related cholestasis. Another strategy designed to prevent PN related liver disease is to cycle PN over the course of 24 hours such that periods of fasting are interspersed with periods of feeding. This strategy is designed to simulate the daily hormonal expression pattern of the enterally fed individual. Theoretical advantages notwithstanding, there is little experimental evidence that supports this practice.

SMALL BOWEL BACTERIAL OVERGROWTH

The small bowel bacterial overgrowth syndrome is defined as a bacterial load of > 10^5 colonies per mL of luminal fluid. When colony counts exceed this level, the small bowel ecology becomes disturbed, bacteria deconjugate bile salts, fat is malabsorbed, and steatorrhea might ensue. Bacteria can ferment carbohydrates and metabolize proteins, thereby limiting the bioavailability of both macronutrients. Bacteria use iron so it is not available for absorption, and iron deficiency anemia develops. The ICV prevents colonic bacteria from refluxing into the sterile small bowel. Loss of the ICV, particularly in children with NEC, predisposes to small bowel bacterial overgrowth with a variety of anaerobic and aerobic bacteria. Kaufman et al. found that small bowel enteritis correlated with bacterial overgrowth.[28] PN dependence was prolonged in those children with severe enteritis (36 ± 15 months) in comparison to children with mild enteritis and those without small intestinal inflammation (21 ± 14 and 13 ± 11 months, respectively).

Small bowel bacterial overgrowth can cause bacteremia, abdominal distension, worsening diarrhea, and cholestasis.[29] The diagnosis of bacterial overgrowth is usually based on clinical suspicion. Direct culture of duodenal fluid with quantitation of bacterial counts establishes the diagnosis. Indirect tests such as H_2 breath tests have been used, but false negative breath tests occur in the presence of non-H_2 producing bacteria and during antibiotic use. Overall, the diagnostic utility of breath tests is limited in young children who cannot coordinate breathing into the required container for breath collection.

The antibiotic regimen for treatment of bacterial overgrowth should be tailored to the therapeutic goal. If the goal is to improve malabsorption and abdominal distension, an antibiotic directed against anaerobic organisms should be provided. Monthly cycles of metronidazole for 7–14 days may be used to decrease the overall colonization of anaerobes and to minimize the risk of antimicrobial resistance. In the setting of bacterial translocation and recurrent sepsis, selective digestive decontamination, also known as multiple decontamination drugs), is sometimes used. This antibiotic cocktail consists of nonabsorbable drugs such as colistin, tobramycin, and nystatin directed toward reducing the number of aerobic bacteria and yeast while promoting anaerobic flora. There are no prospective trials to establish the efficacy of this treatment in humans, but animal data support its use.[30]

Surgical Therapies

The management of short gut syndrome requires combined medical and surgical approaches. In the setting of bowel dilation and persistent feeding intolerance, surgical lengthening or tapering procedures should be considered. In 1980, Adrian Bianchi described an intestinal loop-lengthening procedure in a series of 7 pigs who had surgical short gut syndrome (Figure 37-1).[31,32] Dilated bowel is lengthened in a longitudinal fashion to double the length of the bowel segment subjected to surgery. Because the bowel diameter is halved, the overall surface area of the bowel remains constant. The hope with this procedure is that motility improves, bacterial overgrowth decreases, and nutrient absorption increases to result in intestinal autonomy.[32]

Short gut syndrome is rare, and so the outcome of a large series of patients managed in a single center is not reported. Bueno et al. reviewed a series of 230 children referred for intestinal transplantation; 27 of these children had intestinal lengthening procedures prior to referral.[33] The authors identified potential risk factors for failure of the Bianchi procedure, including very young age at the time of the procedure, well established cholestasis prior to the procedure, and remnant small intestinal length < 50 cm prior to the procedure. Patients who had more than 50% of their colon had worse survival than patients who had less than 50%. This defies the concept that early establishment of intestinal continuity improves survival in short bowel syndrome.[34] Furthermore, only one third of the group of patients who underwent a lengthening procedure increased their enteral calories by > 50%. Regardless of intestinal length, there was no difference in survival of patients with or without longitudinal intestinal lengthening procedures. By definition, the Bianchi procedure had failed in this cohort referred for transplantation and so the series lacks a denominator of patients with successful Bianchi procedures. Hence, wide generalizations might not be possible.

In 1993, Kimura and Soper showed that the antimesenteric surface of a small bowel

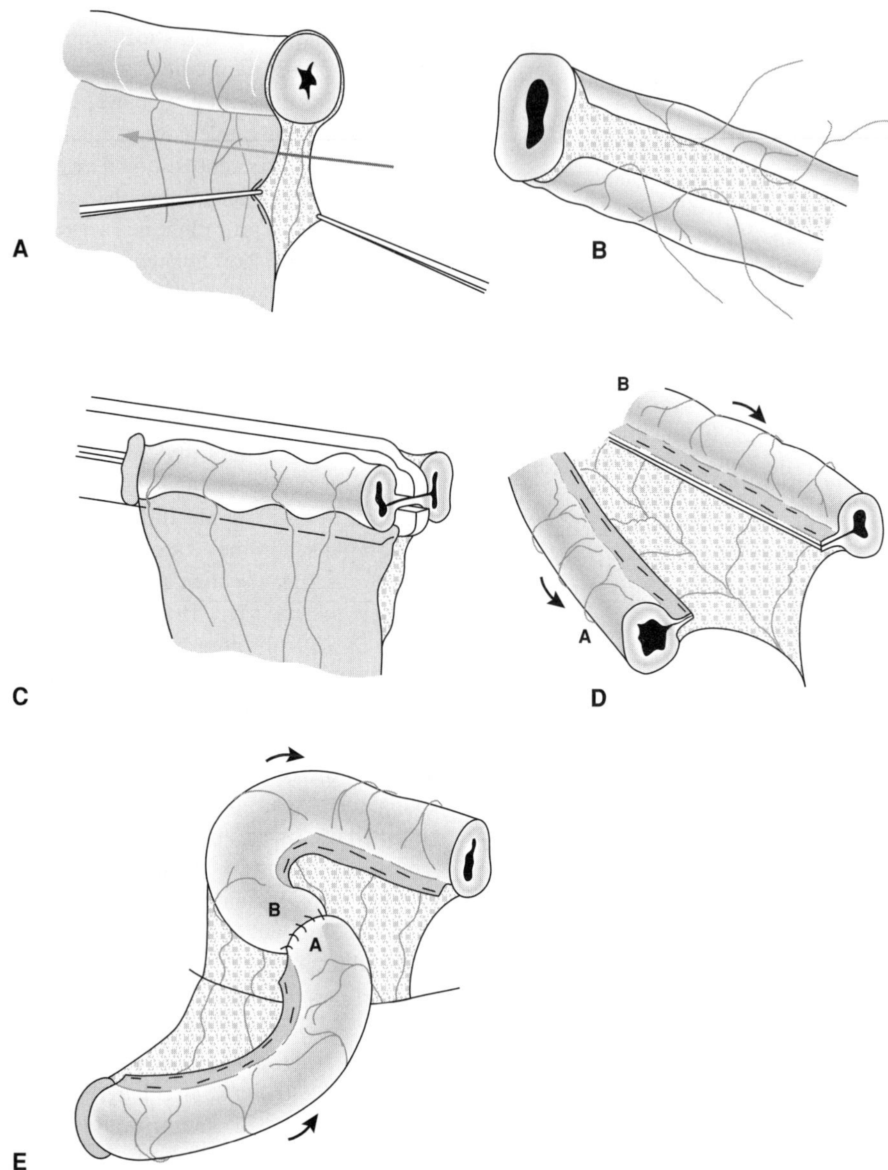

Figure 37-1 The Bianchi procedure. **A.** Dissection between peritoneal leaves of the mesentery. **B.** Intervascular space on mesenteric border of bowel. **C.** Bowel loop between jaws of autostapler prior to division. **D.** Hemiloops resulting from stapling and division of bowel. **E.** Isoperistaltic anastomosis between hemiloops. *Source:* Bianchi A. Intestinal loop lengthening: a technique for increasing small intestinal length. *J Pediatr Surg.* 1980;15(2):145–151. Reprinted with permission from Elsevier.

loop could be arterialized by adhering it to the undersurface of the liver or to the abdominal wall.[35] After the loop had dilated sufficiently, the bowel could be stapled horizontally to yield 2 parallel tubes; each tube was half the diameter of the original bowel. The tubes could be sewn end to end in a fashion analogous to the Bianchi procedure. A patient could then theoretically undergo a Bianchi procedure followed by a Kimura procedure to quadruple the length of a shortened bowel. There are no studies that document the effectiveness of this approach.

The next major advance in autologous bowel reconstruction occurred in 2003, when Kim et al. described a new procedure called a serial transverse enteroplasty (STEP) procedure for intestinal lengthening. This procedure creates a zigzag channel by serial transverse applications of a stapler in opposite directions (Figure 37-2).[36] Initially performing the operation in 6 young pigs, the authors showed that this technique can safely increase intestinal length. The animals gained weight and had no evidence of obstruction by radiologic evaluation. After a failed Bianchi procedure, this same group performed the technique on a 2-year-old male with gastroschisis and a midgut volvulus who did not have PN cholestasis.[37] This child had normal D-xylose absorption and improved texture of his stools after this procedure. Six months after surgery, the child was receiving > 50% of his calories via the enteral route. Further study is required to determine the long term utility of this procedure. Candidates for lengthening procedures should be chosen and evaluated carefully.

In the desire to prevent or decrease PN cholestasis, physicians must weigh the risks of these procedures, including compromised arterial blood supply to the bowel, sepsis, obstruction, worsening liver dysfunction, or persistent intestinal failure against potential benefits. Larger trials, although needed, would be plagued by confounding factors, making it unlikely that these sorts of trials could ever take place.

Small Bowel Transplantation

Despite the best efforts of pediatric gastroenterologists and surgeons, some patients cannot achieve intestinal autonomy and require small intestinal transplantation. Only a handful of small bowel or combined small bowel and liver transplants were performed between 1965 and 1990 when azathioprine, corticosteroid, or cyclosporine were used for immunosuppression. With 1 notable exception, all died within days to months after the transplant.[38] In 1990, tacrolimus, a potent calcineurin inhibitor, allowed small bowel transplantation to become available and made transplantation a viable therapeutic option for children facing certain death. Series reporting adult and pediatric transplantation experience found survival rates of 54% at 5 years and 42% at 10 years.[39,40] These survival rates were considerably better than rates among those who were not transplanted. Bueno et al. described a series of 257 children evaluated for intestinal transplant during 1990–1998 in Pittsburgh.[41] The lowest survival rate among candidates who were not transplanted was among infants with surgical short bowel syndrome and serum bilirubin levels > 3 mg/dL, platelet counts < 100,000/mL, prothrombin time > 15 seconds, or partial thromboplastin time greater than 40 seconds. These findings emphasize the fact that survival after transplantation exceeds survival without transplantation once liver disease develops. Referral for transplantation of infants characterized by the Bueno study[41] should be early before a downhill spiral develops.

There are a number of factors involved in making the decision to list a patient for transplantation. In a position paper on pediatric intestinal transplantation, Kaufman et al. recommended early small bowel transplantation prior to the development of irreversible liver disease manifested by complications of portal hypertension such as bleeding and ascites.[42] Previous work by Sondheimer supported the theory that early infections are associated with worsening liver dysfunction.[16] Hence, recurrent episodes of life-threatening sepsis are an indication for small bowel transplantation.

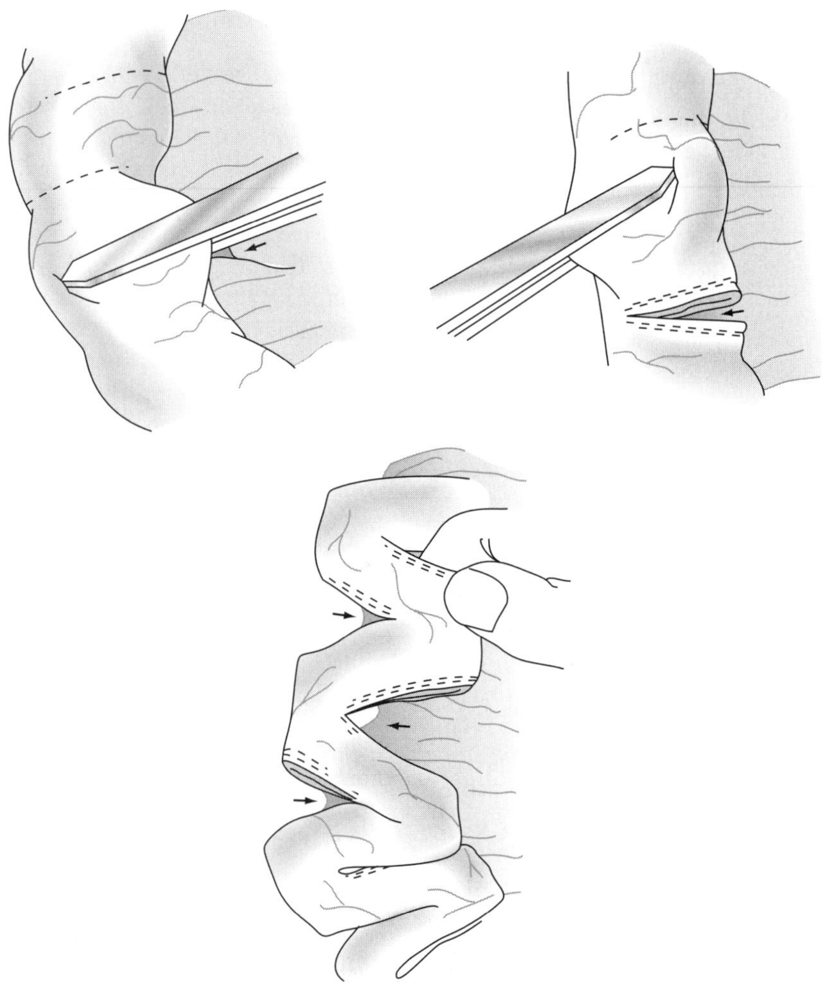

Figure 37-2 Schematic drawing of the serial transverse enteroplasty procedure. The small arrows show the direction of insertion of the ENDO-GIA stapler and the sites of the mesenteric defects. The staplers are placed in the 90° and 270° orientations using the mesentery as the 0° reference point. *Source:* Kim HB, Fauza D, Garza J, Oh JT, Nurko S, Jaksic T. Serial transvere enteroplasty (STEP): a novel bowel lengthening procedure. *J Pediatr Surg.* 2003;38:425–429. Reprinted with permission from Elsevier.

Vascular access is crucial to the delivery of hydration fluids and PN. Pediatric patients have 6 major vessels for insertion of large-bore catheters: the right and left subclavian, the right and left jugular vessels, and the right and left femoral veins. Transplantation must be considered prior to the loss of access sites. In fact, there should be 2 intravenous access sites prior to transplantation because of the persistent need for hydration and PN until the allograft functions. The inability to provide adequate hydration and PN makes transplantation impossible.

In instances of extreme short gut syndrome, the likelihood of intestinal autonomy is minimal. Although Wilmore and Quiros reported children with < 15–20 cm of small bowel who have an

ICV surviving, the overall likelihood of this is minimal at best.[2–4] Kocoshis et al. emphasized the importance of early referral to tertiary care centers that perform transplantation even if transplantation cannot be performed immediately.[43] Specially trained physicians can implement changes in medical or surgical therapies that could allow these patients to be transplanted earlier and maximize their medical care prior to transplantation. Early small bowel transplantation can abort end-stage liver dysfunction.

Despite the fact that living related transplantation[44] and reduced-size grafts[45] are used at some centers, the shortage of intestinal allografts continues to result in disproportionately higher death rates on the waiting list for small bowel transplantation than for many other solid organs.[46] Older and larger children with extreme short gut might be able to receive an isolated small bowel transplant prior to the onset of cholestasis, but cholestasis progresses rapidly among children < 12 months of age on PN. Even if allografts are surgically downsized, few donors are available for infants. Additionally, the donor intestine is less able to withstand hypoxia and hypotension than is the liver. Therefore, if the donor experienced a hypoxic event or required catecholamine support, the small bowel is less likely to be viable than a liver allograft. The difficulty in procuring organs for younger recipients underscores the importance of providing meticulous care in centers experienced in their preoperative management.

Posttransplant Care

The transplant surgery heralds the beginning of another chapter of intense monitoring and care. Posttransplant care of these patients is as intense, if not more so, than pretransplant care. Monitoring requires the expertise of gastroenterologists and surgeons familiar with potential complications including allograft rejection, risk of overwhelming infection, and posttransplant lymphoproliferative disease and high fluid and electrolyte losses. Depending upon the function of the donor allograft, prolonged hydration fluids or PN might remain necessary for weeks to months postoperatively. Gastrointestinal fluid losses could be liters/day and the patients require individualized close monitoring to assure hydration is maintained, as well as to ensure that adequate electrolytes to replenish high ongoing losses are provided.

It is common to require multiple, further surgeries following the initial transplant for peritoneal bleeding—especially in the setting of hepatic insufficiency. Fluid and electrolyte management also remain important until the allograft attains full autonomy. The time children spend in the ICU after a liver or small bowel transplant is variable and depends on their medical condition prior to transplantation and whether complications occur with the transplant itself.

Immunosuppression

One of the most formidable challenges is that the copious lymphoid tissue in the small bowel graft increases the risk of allograft rejection by the recipient. Up to the present time, the cornerstones of immunosuppressive regimens have been corticosteroids and calcineurin inhibitors. Frequently encountered side effects include hypertension, hyperglycemia, and weight gain. Among the many side effects of calcineurin inhibitors, hypertension and nephrotoxicity are common. The requisite higher blood levels of tacrolimus, 15–20 ng/mL, also increase the risk of neurotoxicity.

Recently, the concept of preconditioning the recipient prior to transplantation has gained popularity. Antithymocyte globulin (ATG) is used by some transplant centers to prime the recipient's lymphocytes for the intestinal allograft. The recipient receives 3 mg/kg over 4 to 6 hours just prior to receiving the transplant. On postoperative day 1, another 2 mg/kg are administered to compensate for antibody lost through intraoperative blood loss. By using this antimonoclonal antibody, transplant centers hope to spare prolonged exposure to corticosteroids and reduce the risk of allograft rejection. Employing this type of immune suppression has allowed some transplant centers to stop glucocorticoid administration. Other centers suggest that Campath 1H, a CD52 humanized monoclonal antibody, might reduce the need for glucocortioids.[47,48]

The typical induction regimen for small bowel transplantation also might include a variable course of glucocorticoids, usually beginning with 10 mg/kg of methylprednisolone tapering to a lower corticosteroid dose. On postoperative day 1, tacrolimus is introduced at a dose of 0.2 to 0.3 mg/kg/day delivered every12 hours. The dose is titrated to achieve a blood level of 15–20 ng/mL.

Endoscopic Surveillance

Acute cellular rejection is defined as an immune response to the transplanted organ leading to injury. If severe, the transplanted organ is completely destroyed. Currently, the only reliable method of identifying acute cellular rejection is via endoscopic biopsies with supportive clinical evidence including daily ileostomy output. Early reports suggest that approximately 80% of all patients who undergo intestinal transplantation experienced at least 1 episode of rejection.[49] Despite the more sophisticated preconditioning regimens, vigilant monitoring for rejection is essential. Surveillance endoscopic biopsies are performed twice weekly in the immediate postoperative period. Sigurdsson reported one center's experience where a total of 1,273 endoscopies were performed on 41 children who underwent intestinal or multivisceral transplants between 1990 and 1995.[50] He emphasized that patients remained at risk for rejection even many months postoperatively, and that the histologic changes of rejection are patchy in distribution.

Serum citrulline levels are used as a measure of intestinal function in short bowel syndrome and acute cellular rejection of small bowel allograft. Glutamine is converted to citrulline exclusively in the intestine, and serum citrulline levels reflect the quantity of functional intestinal mass present. Serum citrulline levels of patients experiencing intestinal rejection fall dramatically. Hence some investigators have advocated measuring serum citrulline as a measure of organ rejection.[51,52] Unfortunately, patient-to-patient variability of serum citrulline levels precludes the use of random levels as a marker for intestinal function or for identifying rejection. However, if levels are measured serially, a fall could herald rejection.[51–53] More research is required to better define the role of serum citrulline in rejection. For now, endoscopy remains the gold standard for the diagnosis.

Infections

The intense immunosuppression required for small intestinal transplant renders patients susceptible to infections. In the immediate postoperative period, broad-spectrum antibiotics, such as aminoglycosides, cephalosporins, and penicillins, are used until the invasive catheters and vascular access lines are removed. Fever requires assessment and fast treatment with antibiotics.

Viral infections such as adenovirus and cytomegalovirus (CMV) can be devastating in the perioperative period. Viral status of the recipient determines the type and length of antiviral therapy such as intravenous ganciclovir or cytomegalovirus immune globulin intravenous (human). If symptomatic CMV infections occur, the ganciclovir dose can be increased from a prophylactic to therapeutic dose. Foscarnet is used for ganciclovir-resistant strains.

Adenovirus infections occur frequently early after transplant, and, if disseminated, can portend a poor outcome.[54] Cidofovir is used with varying degrees of success among bone marrow recipients, but it is extremely nephrotoxic and should be used judiciously.[55]

Rotavirus infection, often innocuous in an immunocompetent host, can lead to serious posttransplant setbacks. There is no published experience using oral immunoglobulin for solid organ recipients contracting rotavirus gastroenteritis, but oral immunoglobulin has been used with some success in other immunocompromised hosts.[56]

Candida, a commensal inhabitant of skin and the upper gastrointestinal tract, can pose a significant threat to survival. The threshold for using amphotericin B or fluconazole is low in the setting of suspected sepsis.

Posttransplant Lymphoproliferative Disease

Several months after transplant, Epstein-Barr virus (EBV) infection can cause posttransplant lymphoproliferative disease (PTLD). Any patient undergoing small bowel transplant is at risk for PTLD, but pediatric patients who are EBV naïve and experience a primary infection just before or after transplant are at greatest risk. A primary infection might appear as an incidental serologic finding, infectious mononucleosis, or a frank lymphoma. In the first 6 to 12 months after transplantation, weekly or bimonthly serum EBV-PCR levels may be performed. At the first sign of a primary infection or reactivation of a prior infection, immunosuppression is decreased—the first step in intervention. It is hoped that the patient's immune system will mount an appropriate response. Total body computerized tomography with upper and lower endoscopies are performed to stage the disease. If frank PTLD develops and reduction of immunosuppression is unsuccessful in reducing the tumor burden, a variety of chemotherapeutic regimens is available. A particularly attractive regimen proposed by Gross and others includes low dose cyclophosphamide and corticosteroids.[57,58]

CONCLUSION

Short gut syndrome can be a devastating illness and adversely affect every aspect of a family's life. The presence of invasive catheters and feeding tubes/pumps results in major risks and diminishes the quality of life in patients with short bowel syndrome. Gastroenterologists and surgeons who have specific expertise in the management of short bowel are best suited to manage children experiencing this disorder. Meticulous care by both parents and physicians can allow for intestinal autonomy to be achieved by the majority of children with short gut syndrome. For the small number of patients whose intestine fails to adapt and for whom PN carries excessive risk, small intestinal transplant is a viable therapeutic option.

REFERENCES

1. Hofmann A, Danzinger, RF. Physiologic and clinical significance of ileal resection. *Surgical Annals.* 1972;4:305–325.
2. Wilmore DW. Factors correlating with a successful outcome following extensive intestinal resection in newborn infants. *J Peds.* 1972;80(1):88–95.
3. Sondheimer JM, Cadnapaphornchai M, Sontag M, Zerbe GO. Predicting the duration of dependence on parenteral nutrition after neonatal intestinal resection. *J Pediatr.* 1998;132(1):80–84.
4. Quiros-Tejeira RE, Ament ME, Reyen L, et al. Long-term parenteral nutritional support and intestinal adaptation in children with short bowel syndrome: a 25-year experience. *J Pediatr.* 2004;145(2):157–163.
5. Warner B. GLP-2 as therapy for the short-bowel syndrome. *Gastroenterology.* 2001;120:1041–1043.
6. Drucker DJ, Erlich P, Asa SL, Brubaker PL. Induction of intestinal epithelial proliferation by glucagon-like peptide 2. *Proc Natl Acad Sci U S A.* 1996;93(15):7911–7916.
7. Jeppesen PB, Hartmann B, Thulesen J, et al. Glucagon-like peptide 2 improves nutrient absorption and nutritional status in short-bowel patients with no colon. *Gastroenterology.* 2001;120(4):806–815.
8. Scolapio JS, Camilleri M, Fleming CR, et al. Effect of growth hormone, glutamine, and diet on adaptation in short-bowel syndrome: a randomized, controlled study. *Gastroenterology.* 1997;113(4):1074–1081.
9. Seguy D, Vahedi K, Kapel N, Souberbielle JC, Messing B. Low-dose growth hormone in adult home parenteral nutrition-dependent short bowel syndrome patients: a positive study. *Gastroenterology.* 2003;124(2):293–302.
10. Stern LE, Erwin CR, O'Brien DP, Huang F, Warner BW. Epidermal growth factor is critical for intestinal adaptation following small bowel resection. *Microsc Res Tech.* 2000;51(2):138–148.
11. Stern LE, Falcone RA Jr, Kemp CJ, Braun MC, Erwin CR, Warner BW. Salivary epidermal growth factor and intestinal adaptation in male and female mice. *Am J Physiol Gastrointest Liver Physiol.* 2000;278(6):G871–877.
12. Vanderhoof JA, Langnas AN. Short-bowel syndrome in children and adults. *Gastroenterology.* 1997;113(5):1767–1778.
13. Bines J, Francis D, Hill D. Reducing parenteral requirement in children with short bowel syndrome: impact of

an amino acid-based complete infant formula. *J Pediatr Gastroenterol Nutr.* 1998;26(2):123–128.

14. Musch MW, Bookstein C, Xie Y, Sellin JH, Chang EB. SCFA increase intestinal Na absorption by induction of NHE3 in rat colon and human intestinal C2/bbe cells. *Am J Physiol Gastrointest Liver Physiol.* 2001;280(4): G687–693.
15. Wilmore DW. Growth and development of an infant receiving all nutrients exclusively by vein. *JAMA.* 1968;203(10):140–144.
16. Sondheimer JM, Asturias E, Cadnapaphornchai M. Infection and cholestasis in neonates with intestinal resection and long-term parenteral nutrition. *J Pediatr Gastroenterol Nutr.* 1998;27(2):131–137.
17. Kaufman SS. Prevention of parenteral nutrition-associated liver disease in children. *Pediatr Transplant.* 2002;6(1):37–42.
18. Drongowski RA, Coran AG. An analysis of factors contributing to the development of total parenteral nutrition-induced cholestasis. *JPEN* 1989;13(6):586–589.
19. Diamanti A, Gambarara M, Knafelz D, et al. Prevalence of liver complications in pediatric patients on home parenteral nutrition: indications for intestinal or combined liver-intestinal transplantation. *Transplant Proc.* 2003;35(8):3047–3049.
20. Meehan JJ, Georgeson KE. Prevention of liver failure in parenteral nutrition-dependent children with short bowel syndrome. *J Pediatr Surg.* 1997;32(3):473–475.
21. Schwarz KB, Ternberg JL, Bell MJ, Keating JP. Sodium needs of infants and children with ileostomy. *J Pediatr.* 1983;102(4):509–513.
22. Jones MO, Pierro A, Hammond P, Nunn A, Lloyd DA. Glucose utilization in the surgical newborn infant receiving total parenteral nutrition. *J Pediatr Surg.* 1993;28(9):1121–1125.
23. Sokol RJ, Devereaux MW, O'Brien K, Khandwala RA, Loehr JP. Abnormal hepatic mitochondrial respiration and cytochrome C oxidase activity in rats with long-term copper overload. *Gastroenterology.* 1993;105(1):178–187.
24. Fok TF, Chui KK, Cheung R, Ng PC, Cheung KL, Hjelm M. Manganese intake and cholestatic jaundice in neonates receiving parenteral nutrition: a randomized controlled study. *Acta Paediatr.* 2001;90(9):1009–1015.
25. Poupon RE, Lindor KD, Cauch-Dudek K, Dickson ER, Poupon R, Heathcote EJ. Combined analysis of randomized controlled trials of ursodeoxycholic acid in primary biliary cirrhosis. *Gastroenterology.* 1997;113(3):884–890.
26. Lindor KD, Dickson ER, Baldus WP, et al. Ursodeoxycholic acid in the treatment of primary biliary cirrhosis. *Gastroenterology.* 1994;106(5):1284–1290.
27. Heubi JE, Wiechmann DA, Creutzinger V, et al. Tauroursodeoxycholic acid (TUDCA) in the prevention of total parenteral nutrition-associated liver disease. *J Pediatr.* 2002;141(2):237–242.
28. Kaufman SS, Loseke CA, Lupo JV, et al. Influence of bacterial overgrowth and intestinal inflammation on duration of parenteral nutrition in children with short bowel syndrome. *J Pediatr.* 1997;131(3):356–361.
29. Singh VV, Toskes PP. Small bowel bacterial overgrowth: presentation, diagnosis, and treatment. *Curr Treat Options Gastroenterol.* 2004;7(1):19–28.
30. Lee TK, Heeckt PF, Smith SD, Lee KK, Rowe MI, Schraut WH. Bacterial translocation and the role of postoperative selective bowel decontamination in small intestinal transplantation. *Transplant Proc.* 1994;26(3):1688.
31. Bianchi A. Intestinal loop lengthening—a technique for increasing small intestinal length. *J Pediatr Surg.* 1980;15(2):145–151.
32. Bianchi A. Experience with longitudinal intestinal lengthening and tailoring. *Eur J Pediatr Surg.* 1999;9(4):256–259.
33. Bueno J, Guiterrez J, Mazariegos GV, et al. Analysis of patients with longitudinal intestinal lengthening procedure referred for intestinal transplantation. *J Pediatr Surg.* 2001;36(1):178–183.
34. Gertler JP, Seashore JH, Touloukian RJ. Early ileostomy closure in necrotizing enterocolitis. *J Pediatr Surg.* 1987;22(2):140–143.
35. Kimura K, Soper RT. A new bowel elongation technique for the short-bowel syndrome using the isolated bowel segment Iowa models. *J Pediatr Surg.* 1993;28(6):792–794.
36. Kim HB, Fauza D, Garza J, Oh JT, Nurko S, Jaksic T. Serial transverse enteroplasty (STEP): a novel bowel lengthening procedure. *J Pediatr Surg.* 2003;38(3):425–429.
37. Kim HB, Lee PW, Garza J, Duggan C, Fauza D, Jaksic T. Serial transverse enteroplasty for short bowel syndrome: a case report. *J Pediatr Surg.* 2003;38(6):881–885.
38. Starzl TE, Rowe MI, Todo S, et al. Transplantation of multiple abdominal viscera. *JAMA.* 1989;261(10):1449–1457.
39. Abu-Elmagd KM, Reyes J, Fung JJ, et al. Evolution of clinical intestinal transplantation: improved outcome and cost effectiveness. *Transplant Proc.* 1999;31(1–2):582–584.
40. Abu-Elmagd K, Reyes J, Bond G, et al. Clinical intestinal transplantation: a decade of experience at a single center. *Ann Surg.* 2001;234(3):404–416; discussion 416–407.
41. Bueno J, Ohwada S, Kocoshis S, et al. Factors impacting the survival of children with intestinal failure referred for intestinal transplantation. *J Pediatr Surg.* 1999;34(1):27–32; discussion 32–23.
42. Kaufman SS, Atkinson JB, Bianchi A, et al. Indications for pediatric intestinal transplantation: a position paper

of the American Society of Transplantation. *Pediatr Transplant.* 2001;5(2):80–87.

43. Kocoshis SA, Beath SV, Booth IW, et al. Intestinal failure and small bowel transplantation, including clinical nutrition: Working group report of the second World Congress of Pediatric Gastroenterology, Hepatology, and Nutrition. *J Pediatr Gastroenterol Nutr.* 2004;39(suppl 2):S655–661.
44. Gruessner RW, Sharp HL. Living-related intestinal transplantation: first report of a standardized surgical technique. *Transplantation.* 1997;64(11):1605–1607.
45. de Ville de Goyet J, Mitchell A, Mayer AD, et al. En block combined reduced-liver and small bowel transplants: from large donors to small children. *Transplantation.* 2000;69(4):555–559.
46. Fryer J, Pellar S, Ormond D, Koffron A, Abecassis M. Mortality in candidates waiting for combined liver-intestine transplants exceeds that for other candidates waiting for liver transplants. *Liver Transpl.* 2003;9(7):748–753.
47. Tzakis AG, Kato T, Nishida S, et al. Preliminary experience with campath 1H (C1H) in intestinal and liver transplantation. *Transplantation.* 2003;75(8):1227–1231.
48. Nishida S, Levi D, Kato T, Madariaga J, Nery J, Tzakis A. Induction therapy for adult small bowel transplant with Campath-1H. *Transplant Proc.* 2002;34(5):1889–1891.
49. Fishbein TM, Gondolesi GE, Kaufman SS. Intestinal transplantation for gut failure. *Gastroenterology.* 2003;124(6):1615–1628.
50. Sigurdsson L, Reyes J, Putnam PE, et al. Endoscopies in pediatric small intestinal transplant recipients: five years experience. *Am J Gastroenterol.* 1998;93(2):207–211.
51. Pappas PA, Saudubray JM, Tzakis AG, et al. Serum citrulline as a marker of acute cellular rejection for intestinal transplantation. *Transplant Proc.* 2002;34(3):915–917.
52. Pappas PA, Saudubray JM, Tzakis AG, et al. Serum citrulline and rejection in small bowel transplantation: a preliminary report. *Transplantation.* 2001;72(7):1212–1216.
53. Pappas PA, Tzakis AG, Saudubray JM, et al. Trends in serum citrulline and acute rejection among recipients of small bowel transplants. *Transplant Proc.* 2004;36(2):345–347.
54. Pinchoff RJ, Kaufman SS, Magid MS, et al. Adenovirus infection in pediatric small bowel transplantation recipients. *Transplantation.* 2003;76(1):183–189.
55. Ljungman P, Ribaud P, Eyrich M, et al. Cidofovir for adenovirus infections after allogeneic hematopoietic stem cell transplantation: a survey by the infectious diseases working party of the European Group for Blood and Marrow Transplantation. *Bone Marrow Transplant.* 2003;31(6):481–486.
56. Guarino A, Russo S, Castaldo A, Spagnuolo MI, Tarallo L, Rubino A. Passive immunotherapy for rotavirus-induced diarrhoea in children with HIV infection. *Aids.* 1996;10(10):1176–1178.
57. Orjuela M, Gross TG, Cheung YK, Alobeid B, Morris E, Cairo MS. A pilot study of chemoimmunotherapy (cyclophosphamide, prednisone, and rituximab) in patients with post-transplant lymphoproliferative disorder following solid organ transplantation. *Clin Cancer Res.* 2003;9(10 Pt 2):3945S–3952S.
58. Gross TG. Low-dose chemotherapy for children with post-transplant lymphoproliferative disease. *Recent Results Cancer Res.* 2002;159:96–103.

Appendix A

List of Formulas

Jodi Bettler and Lori Enriquez

Table A-1 Premature Infant Formulas—Nutrients per 100 Calories.

		Human Milk Fortifier (HMF)				
Values listed are for ready to feed formula unless stated as powder	Preterm Human Milk (HM)	Enfamil HMF, 2 Packets (Powder) Mixed with 100 mL Preterm HM	Enfamil HMF, 4 Packets (Powder) Mixed with 100 mL Preterm HM	Similac HMF, 2 packets (Powder) per 100 mL Preterm HM	Similac HMF, 4 packets (Powder) per 100 mL Preterm HM	Similac Natural Care Advance
Manufacture	*	Mead Johnson	Mead Johnson	Ross	Ross	Ross
Volume	149	127	137	127	137	124
Calories	100	100	100	100	100	100
Calories/oz		22	24	22	24	24
% of Total Calories Protein/Fat/Carbohydrate	8/52/40	12/54/35	12/54/35	10/49/41	12/47/42	12/47/41
Protein, g	2.1	2.2	3.09	2.58	2.97	2.71
Source	Preterm HM	Preterm HM, Milk Protein Isolate, Whey Protein Isolate Hydrolysate	Preterm HM, Milk Protein Isolate, Whey Protein Isolate Hydrolysate	Preterm HM, Nonfat Milk & Whey Protein Isolate	Preterm HM, Nonfat Milk & Whey Protein Isolate	Nonfat Milk % Whey Protein Concentrate
Fat, g	5.8	5.93	6.03	5.5	5.24	5.43
Linoleic Acid, mg	550	593	628	498	455	700
Linolenic Acid, mg	55	N/A	N/A	N/A	N/A	101
Arachidonic Acid (ARA), mg	23	N/A	N/A	N/A	N/A	21
Docosahexaenoic Acid (DHA), mg	13	N/A	N/A	N/A	N/A	13
Source	Preterm HM	Preterm HM, MCT (70%) Soy oil	Preterm HM, MCT (70%) Soy oil	Preterm HM, MCT Oil	Preterm HM, MCT Oil	MCT, Soy & Coconut Oils (0.25% DHA, 0.40% ARA)
Carbohydrate, g	9.9	9.2	8.7	10.2	10.4	10.6
Source	Preterm HM	Preterm HM, Corn Syrup Solids, Lactose	Preterm HM, Corn Syrup Solids, Lactose	Preterm HM, Lactose, Corn Syrup Solids	Preterm HM, Lactose, Corn Syrup Solids	Corn Syrup Solids & Lactose
Vitamins						
Vitamin A, IU	581	1167	1652	944	1245	1250
Vitamin D, IU	3	104	187	84	150	150
Vitamin E, IU	1.6	4.6	7	3.6	5.3	4
Vitamin K, mcg	0.3	3	6	6	10	12
Vitamin B_1 (Thiamine), mcg	31	129	211	185	313	250
Vitamin B_2 (Riboflavin), mcg	72	214	331	347	574	620
Vitamin B_6, mcg	22	98	160	162	278	250
Vitamin B_{12}, mcg	0.45	0.18	0.28	0.5	0.85	0.55
Niacin, mcg	224	2227	3884	2611	4587	5000
Folic Acid, mcg	5	21	35	20	32	37
Panthothenic Acid, mcg	269	736	1123	1256	2072	1900
Biotin, mcg	0.6	2.4	3.8	18.1	32.6	37
Vitamin C (Ascorbic Acid), mg	16	23	28	31	44	37
Choline, mg	14	13	12	14	14	10
Inositol, mg	22	20	18	22.5	22.9	5.5
Minerals						
Calcium, mg	38	94	142	112	175	210
Phosphorus, mg	19.5	51	77	62	98	116
Magnesium, mg	4.5	4.8	5	8.9	12.4	12
Iron, mg	0.18	1.1	1.9	0.4	0.6	0.37
Zinc, mg	0.51	0.95	1.31	1.14	1.65	1.5
Manganese, mcg	1	8	13	6	10	12
Copper, mcg	93	117	134	202	289	250
Iodine, mcg	16	14	13	14	13	6
Sodium,mg	37	44	50	44	49	43
Potassium, mg	85	97	106	119	148	129
Chloride, mg	82	83	84	100	115	81
Selenium, mcg	2.2	2.4	2.4	2.3	2.4	1.8
Other						
L-Carnitine, mg	0.35	N/A	N/A	N/A	N/A	N/A
Nucleotides, mg	N/A	N/A	N/A	N/A	N/A	8.9
Osmolality, mOsm/kg water	302	310-340	330-360	290	385	280
Water, g	131	131	108	131	108	109
Potential Renal Solute Load mOsm	18.7	18.7	23	18.7	29.3	26.7

Premature human milk based upon the following references:
Wyeth Nutrition, Internal data. 1992.
American Academy of Pediatrics Committee on Nutrition: Pediatric Nutrition Handbook, 4th Ed. Elk Grove Village: American Academy of Pediatrics, 1998:40, 132-135, 217, 655–658.
The nutrient composition on human milk varies among women.
As products and product composition change frequently, always check with the manufacturer for up-to-date product information.

	Preterm Infant Formulas				Post Discharge Formulas	
Values listed are for ready to feed formula unless stated as powder	Enfamil Premature LIPIL 20 with Iron	Enfamil Premature LIPIL 24 with Iron	Similac Special Care Advance with Iron 20	Similac Special Care Advance with Iron 24	Enfamil Enfacare LIPIL	Similac NeoSure Advance
Manufacture	Mead Johnson	Mead Johnson	Ross	Ross	Mead Johson	Ross
Volume	148	124	148	124	133	134
Calories	100	100	100	100	100	100
Calories/oz	20	24	20	24	22	22
% of Total Calories Protein/Fat/Carbohydrate	12/44/44	12/44/44	11/47/42	11/47/42	11/47/42	11/49/40
Protein, g	3	3	3	3	2.8	2.8
Source	Nonfat Milk, & Whey Protein Concentrate	Nonfat Milk, & Whey Protein Concentrate	Nonfat Milk, & Whey Protein Concentrate	Nonfat Milk, & Whey Protein Concentrate	Nonfat Milk, & Whey Protein Concentrate	Nonfat Milk, & Whey Protein Concentrate
Fat, g	5.1	5.1	5.43	5.43	5.3	5.5
Linoleic Acid, mg	810	810	700	700	950	750
Linolenic Acid, mg	90	90	101	101	95	105
Arachidonic Acid (ARA), mg	34	34	21	21	34	21
Docosahexaenoic Acid (DHA), mg	17	17	13	13	17	8
Source	MCT, Soy, High Oleic Vegetable (Sunflower and Safflower) Oils, DHA & ARA	MCT, Soy, High Oleic Vegetable (Sunflower and Safflower) Oils, DHA & ARA	MCT, Soy & Coconut Oils, DHA & ARA	MCT, Soy & Coconut Oils, DHA & ARA	High Oleic Vegetable (Sunflower and Safflower) Oils, DHA & ARA	Soy, Coconut & MCT Oils, DHA & ARA
Carbohydrate, g	11	11	10.3	10.3	10.4	10.1
Source	Corn Syrup Solids & Lactose	Corn Syrup Solids & Lactose	Corn Syrup Solids & Lactose	Corn Syrup Solids & Lactose	Maltodextrin & Lactose	Corn Syrup Solids & Lactose
Vitamins						
Vitamin A, IU	1250	1250	1250	1250	450	460
Vitamin D, IU	240	240	150	150	80	70
Vitamin E, IU	6.3	6.3	4	4	4	3.6
Vitamin K, mcg	8	8	12	12	8	11
Vitamin B_1 (Thiamine), mcg	200	200	250	250	200	220
Vitamin B_2 (Riboflavin), mcg	300	300	620	620	200	150
Vitamin B_6, mcg	150	150	250	250	100	100
Vitamin B_{12}, mcg	0.25	0.25	0.55	0.55	0.3	0.4
Niacin, mcg	4000	4000	5000	5000	2000	1950
Folic Acid, mcg	40	40	37	37	26	25
Panthothenic Acid, mcg	1200	1200	1900	1900	850	800
Biotin, mcg	4	4	37	37	6	9
Vitamin C (Ascorbic Acid), mg	2	20	37	37	16	15
Choline, mg	20	20	10	10	24	16
Inositol, mg	44	44	40	40	30	35
Minerals						
Calcium, mg	165	165	180	180	120	105
Phosphorus, mg	83	83	100	100	66	62
Magnesium, mg	9	9	12	12	8	9
Iron, mg	1.8 (0.5 without Iron)	1.8 (0.5 without Iron)	1.8 (0.4 without Iron)	1.8 (0.4 without Iron)	1.8	1.8
Zinc, mg	1.5	1.5	1.5	1.5	1.25	1.2
Manganese, mcg	6.3	6.3	12	12	15	10
Copper, mcg	120	120	250	250	120	120
Iodine, mcg	25	25	6	6	21	15
Sodium,mg	58	58	43	43	35	33
Potassium, mg	98	98	129	129	105	142
Chloride, mg	90	90	81	81	78	75
Selenium, mcg	2.8	2.8	1.8	1.8	2.8	2.3
Other						
L-Carnitine, mg	2.4	2.4	N/A	N/A	2	N/A
Nucleotides, mg	4.2	4.2	10.7	8.9	4.2	9.7
Osmolality, mOsm/kg water	260	310	235	280	230	250
Water, g	133	108	133	109	120	120
Potential Renal Solute Load mOsm	27	27	26.2	26.2	24	24

Premature human milk based upon the following references:
Wyeth Nutrition, Internal data. 1992.
American Academy of Pediatrics Committee on Nutrition: Pediatric Nutrition Handbook, 4th Ed. Elk Grove Village: American Academy of Pediatrics, 1998:40, 132-135, 217, 655–658.
The nutrient composition on human milk varies among women.
As products and product composition change frequently, always check with the manufacturer for up-to-date product information.

Table A-2 Term Infant Formulas—Nutrients per 100 Calories.

Values listed are for ready to feed formula unless stated as powder	Term Human Milk (HM)	Enfamil LIPIL	Enfamil with Iron	Enfamil AR LIPIL	Enfamil LactoFree LIPIL
Manufacture	N/A	Mead Johnson	Mead Johnson	Mead Johnson	Mead Johnson
Volume	147	148	148	148	148
Calories	100	100	100	100	100
Calories/oz	20	20	20	20	20
% of Total Calories Protein/Fat/Carbohydrate	6/52/42	8.5/48/43.5	8.5/48/43.5	10/46/44	8.5/48/43.5
Protein, g	1.54	2.1	2.1	2.5	2.1
Source	Term HM	Reduced Minerals Whey, Nonfat Milk	Reduced Minerals Whey, Nonfat Milk	Nonfat Milk	Milk Protein Isolate
Fat, g	5.74	5.3	5.3	5.1	5.3
Linoleic Acid, mg	550	860	860	860	860
Linolenic Acid, mg	63	85	93	85	85
Arachidonic Acid (AA), mg	22	34	none	34	34
Docosahexaenoic Acid (DHA), mg	13	17	none	17	17
Source	Term HM	Palm Olein, Soy, Coconut, High Oleic Sunflower Oils and AA/DHA blend	Palm Olein, Soy, Coconut, High Oleic Sunflower Oils	Palm Olein, Soy, Coconut, High Oleic Sunflower Oils and AA/DHA blend	Palm Olein, Soy, Coconut, High Oleic Sunflower Oils and AA/DHA blend
Carbohydrate, g	10.6	10.9	10.9	11	10.9
Source	Lactose	Lactose	Lactose	Lactose, Rice Starch, Maltodextrin	Corn Syrup Solids
Vitamins					
Vitamin A, IU	331	300	300	300	300
Vitamin D, IU	3	60	60	60	60
Vitamin E, IU	0.6	2	2	2	2
Vitamin K, mcg	0.3	8	8	8	8
Vitamin B_1 (Thiamine), mcg	31	80	80	80	80
Vitamin B_2 (Riboflavin), mcg	51	140	140	140	140
Vitamin B_6, mcg	30	60	60	60	60
Vitamin B_{12}, mcg	0.07	0.3	0.3	0.3	0.3
Niacin, mcg	221	1000	1000	1000	1000
Folic Acid, mcg	7	16	16	16	16
Panthothenic Acid, mcg	265	500	500	500	500
Biotin, mcg	0.6	3	3	3	3
Vitamin C (Ascorbic Acid), mg	6	12	12	12	12
Choline, mg	14	12	12	12	12
Inositol, mg	22	6	6	6	6
Minerals					
Calcium, mg	36	78	78	78	82
Phosphorus, mg	19	53	53	53	55
Magnesium, mg	5.4	8	8	8	8
Iron, mg	0.04	1.8. (0.7 Enfamil LIPIL with Low Iron)	1.8. (0.7 Enfamil Low Iron)	1.8	1.8
Zinc, mg	0.18	1	1	1	1
Manganese, mcg	1	15	15	15	15
Copper, mcg	37	75	75	75	75
Iodine, mcg	16	10	10	10	15
Sodium,mg	26	27	27	40	30
Potassium, mg	78	109	109	108	110
Chloride, mg	62	63	63	75	67
Selenium, mcg	2.2	2.8	2.8	2.8	2.8
Other					
Nucleotides, mg	N/A	4.2	4.2	none added	4.2
Osmolality, mOsm/kg water	286	300	300	240	200
Water, g	132	134	134	134	134
Potential Renal Solute Load mOsm	14.4	19.2	19.2	22	20

Similac Isomil DF has 0.9 g dietary fiber per 100 calories.
*Human milk based upon the following references:
Lawrence, RA. Breastfeeding. A Guide for the Medical Professional, 5th Ed. St. Louis: Mosby Ince, 1999:136, 737.
American Academy of Pediatrics Committee on Nutrition: Pediatric Nutrition Handbook, 4th Ed. Elk Gove Village: American Academy of Pediatrics, 1998:40, 132-135, 217, 655–658.
Wyeth Nutrition, Internal data.
The nutrient composition on human milk varies among women.
As products and product composition change frequently, always check with the manufacturer for up-to-date product information.

Values listed are for ready to feed formula unless stated as powder	Good Start Supreme	Good Start Supreme DHA-ARA	NAN	Good Start Eessentails	Similac Advance
Manufacture	Nestle	Nestle	Nestle	Nestle	Ross
Volume	148	148	148	148	148
Calories	100	100	100	100	100
Calories/oz	20	20	20	20	20
% of Total Calories Protein/Fat/Carbohydrate	9/46/45	9/46/45	9/46/46	9/46/45	8/49/43
Protein, g	2.2	2.2	2.2	2.2	2.07
Source	Partially Hydrolyzed Whey Protein Concentrate	Partially Hydrolyzed Whey Protein Concentrate	Reduced Minerals Whey Protein Concentrate, Nonfat Dry Milk	Reduced Minerals Whey Protein Concentrate, Nonfat Dry Milk	Nonfat Milk & Whey Protein Concentrate
Fat, g	5.1	5.1	5.1	5.1	5.4
Linoleic Acid, mg	900	900	900	900	1000
Linolenic Acid, mg	100	100	78	78	108
Arachidonic Acid (AA), mg	none	32	none	none	21
Docosahexaenoic Acid (DHA), mg	none	16	none	none	8
Source	Palm Olein, Soy, Coconut, High Oleic Safflower Oils	Palm Olein, Soy, Coconut, High Oleic Safflower Oils, DHA, AA	Palm Olein, Soy, Coconut, High Oleic Safflower Oils	Palm Olein, Soy, Coconut, High Oleic Safflower Oils	High Oleic Safflower, Soy & Coconut Oils, DHA, AA
Carbohydrate, g	11.2	11.2	11.2	11.2	10.8
Source	Lactose, Corn Maltodextrin	Lactose, Maltodextrin	Lactose, Corn Syrup	Lactose, Corn Maltodextrin	Lactose
Vitamins					
Vitamin A, IU	300	300	300	300	300
Vitamin D, IU	60	60	60	60	60
Vitamin E, IU	2	2	2	2	1.5
Vitamin K, mcg	8	8	8	8	8
Vitamin B_1 (Thiamine), mcg	60	100	100	80	100
Vitamin B_2 (Riboflavin), mcg	140	140	140	140	150
Vitamin B_6, mcg	75	75	75	65	60
Vitamin B_{12}, mcg	0.33	0.33	0.33	0.25	0.25
Niacin, mcg	1050	1050	1050	1000	1050
Folic Acid, mcg	15	15	15	15	15
Panthothenic Acid, mcg	450	450	450	450	450
Biotin, mcg	4.4	4.4	4.4	3	4.4
Vitamin C (Ascorbic Acid), mg	9	9	9	9	9
Choline, mg	12	12	12	12	16
Inositol, mg	6	6	6	5	4.7
Minerals					
Calcium, mg	64	64	75	75	78
Phosphorus, mg	36	36	42	42	42
Magnesium, mg	7	7	7	7	6
Iron, mg	1.5	1.5	1.5	1.5	1.8
Zinc, mg	0.8	0.8	0.8	0.8	0.75
Manganese, mcg	7	7	7	7	5
Copper, mcg	80	80	80	80	90
Iodine, mcg	12	12	12	10	6
Sodium,mg	27	27	27	24	24
Potassium, mg	108	108	108	105	105
Chloride, mg	65	65	65	63	65
Selenium, mcg	2	2	2	2	1.8
Other					
Nucleotides, mg	4.6	4.6	4.6	4.6	10.7
Osmolality, mOsm/kg water	265	265	300	300	300
Water, g	133	133	133	133	133
Potential Renal Solute Load mOsm	13.5	13.5	13.2	12.6	18.7

Similac Isomil DF has 0.9 g dietary fiber per 100 calories.
*Human milk based upon the following references:
Lawrence, RA. Breastfeeding. A Guide for the Medical Professional, 5th Ed. St. Louis: Mosby Ince, 1999:136, 737.
American Academy of Pediatrics Committee on Nutrition: Pediatric Nutrition Handbook, 4th Ed. Elk Gove Village: American Academy of Pediatrics, 1998:40, 132-135, 217, 655–658.
Wyeth Nutrition, Internal data.
The nutrient composition on human milk varies among women.

Table A-2 Term Infant Formulas—Nutrients per 100 Calories. *(continued)*

Values listed are for ready to feed formula unless stated as powder	Similac with Iron	Similac Lactose Free Advance	Similac PM 60/40 (powder)	Store Brand Milk (powder)	Store Brand Milk with DHA & AA
Manufacture	Ross	Ross	Ross	Wyeth Nutrition	Wyeth Nutrition
Volume	148	148	148	148	148
Calories	100	100	100	100	100
Calories/oz	20	20	20	20	20
% of Total Calories Protein/ Fat/Carbohydrate	8/49/43	9/49/43	9/50/41		
Protein, g	2.07	2.14	2.22	2.2	2.2
Source	Nonfat Milk & Whey Protein Concentrate	Milk Protein Isolate	Whey Protein Concentrate & Sodium Caseinate	Nonfat Milk, Whey Protetin Concentrate	Nonfat Milk, Whey Protetin Concentrate
Fat, g	5.4	5.4	5.59	5.3	5.3
Linoleic Acid, mg	1000	1300	1300	500	500
Linolenic Acid, mg	108	193	71	N/A	N/A
Arachidonic Acid (AA), mg	none	21	none	none	18
Docosahexaenoic Acid (DHA), mg	none	8	none	none	10.7
Source	High Oleic Safflower, Soy & Coconut Oils	Soy & Coconut Oils	Corn, Coconut & Soy Oils	Palm, High Oleic Safflower or Sunflower, Coconut, & Soybean Oils	Palm, High Oleic Safflower or Sunflower, Coconut, & Soybean Oils, DHA, AA
Carbohydrate, g	10.8	10.7	10.2	10.6	10.6
Source	Lactose	Maltodextrin & Sucrose	Lactose	Lactose	Lactose
Vitamins					
Vitamin A, IU	300	300	300	300	300
Vitamin D, IU	60	60	60	60	60
Vitamin E, IU	1.5	3	2.5	1.4	1.4
Vitamin K, mcg	8	8	8	8	8.3
Vitamin B_1 (Thiamine), mcg	100	100	100	100	100
Vitamin B_2 (Riboflavin), mcg	150	150	150	150	150
Vitamin B_6, mcg	60	60	60	62.5	62.5
Vitamin B_{12}, mcg	0.25	0.25	0.25	0.2	0.2
Niacin, mcg	1050	1050	1050	750	750
Folic Acid, mcg	15	15	15	7.5	7.5
Panthothenic Acid, mcg	450	450	450	315	315
Biotin, mcg	4.4	4.4	4.5	2.2	2.2
Vitamin C (Ascorbic Acid), mg	9	9	9	8.5	8.5
Choline, mg	16	16	12	15	15
Inositol, mg	4.7	4.3	24	4.1	4.1
Minerals					
Calcium, mg	78	84	56	63	63
Phosphorus, mg	42	56	28	42	42
Magnesium, mg	6	6	6	7	7
Iron, mg	1.8 (0.7 with Similac Low Iron)	1.8	0.7	1.8	1.2
Zinc, mg	0.75	0.75	0.75	0.8	0.8
Manganese, mcg	5	5	5	15	7.5
Copper, mcg	90	90	90	70	70
Iodine, mcg	6	9	6	9	9
Sodium,mg	24	30	24	22	22
Potassium, mg	105	107	80	83	83
Chloride, mg	65	65	59	56	56
Selenium, mcg	1.8	1.8	1.9	2.1	2.1
Other					
Nucleotides, mg	10.7	10.7	none added	4.5	4.5
Osmolality, mOsm/kg water	300	200	280	280	280
Water, g	133	133	134	135	135
Potential Renal Solute Load mOsm	18.7	19.9	18.3	13.4	13.4

Similac Isomil DF has 0.9 g dietary fiber per 100 calories.
*Human milk based upon the following references:
Lawrence, RA. Breastfeeding. A Guide for the Medical Professional, 5th Ed. St. Louis: Mosby Ince, 1999:136, 737.
American Academy of Pediatrics Committee on Nutrition: Pediatric Nutrition Handbook, 4th Ed. Elk Gove Village: American Academy of Pediatrics, 1998:40, 132-135, 217, 655–658.
Wyeth Nutrition, Internal data.
The nutrient composition on human milk varies among women.
As products and product composition change frequently, always check with the manufacturer for up-to-date product information.

	Soy Based				
Values listed are for ready to feed formula unless stated as powder	Good Start Essentials Soy	Enfamil Prosobee	Enfamil Prosobee LIPIL	RCF	Similac Isomil Advance
Manufacture	Nestle	Mead Johnson	Mead Johnson	Ross	Ross
Volume	148	148	148	148	148
Calories	100	100	100	100	100
Calories/oz	20	20	20	20	20
% of Total Calories Protein/ Fat/Carbohydrate		10/48/42	10/48/42	12/48/40	10/49/41
Protein, g	2.8	2.5	2.5	2.96	2.45
Source	Soy Protein Isolate	Soy Protein Isolate	Soy Protein Isolate	Soy Protein Isolate & L-Methionine	Soy Protein Isolate & L-Methionine
Fat, g	5.1	5.3	5.3	5.33	5.46
Linoleic Acid, mg	920	860	860	1300	1300
Linolenic Acid, mg	90	90	85	N/A	108
Arachidonic Acid (AA), mg	none	none	34	none	21
Docosahexaenoic Acid (DHA), mg	none	none	17	none	8
Source	Palm Olein, Soy, Coconut High Oleic Sunflower Oils	Palm Olein, Soy, Coconut High Oleic Sunflower Oils, DHA & AA	Palm Olein, Soy, Coconut High Oleic Sunflower Oils, DHA & AA	High Oleic Safflower, Soy & Coconut Oils	High Oleic Safflower, Soy & Coconut Oils, DHA, AA
Carbohydrate, g	11.1	10.6	10.6	10.1	10.3
Source	Corn Maltodextrin, & Sucrose	Corn Syrup Solids	Corn Syrup Solids	none in formula - need to add a source	Corn Syrup Solids & Sucrose
Vitamins					
Vitamin A, IU	300	300	300	300	300
Vitamin D, IU	60	60	60	60	60
Vitamin E, IU	3	2	2	1.5	1.5
Vitamin K, mcg	8	8	8	11	11
Vitamin B_1 (Thiamine), mcg	60	80	80	60	60
Vitamin B_2 (Riboflavin), mcg	94	90	90	90	90
Vitamin B_6, mcg	60	60	60	60	60
Vitamin B_{12}, mcg	0.31	0.3	0.3	0.45	0.45
Niacin, mcg	1300	1000	1000	1350	1350
Folic Acid, mcg	16	16	16	15	15
Panthothenic Acid, mcg	470	500	500	750	750
Biotin, mcg	7.8	3	3	4.5	4.5
Vitamin C (Ascorbic Acid), mg	16	12	12	9	9
Choline, mg	12	12	12	12	12
Inositol, mg	18	6	6	5	5
Minerals					
Calcium, mg	105	105	105	105	105
Phosphorus, mg	63	83	83	75	75
Magnesium, mg	11	11	11	7.5	7.5
Iron, mg	1.8	1.8	1.8	1.8	1.8
Zinc, mg	0.9	1.2	1.2	0.75	0.75
Manganese, mcg	34	11	11	25	25
Copper, mcg	120	75	75	75	75
Iodine, mcg	15	15	15	15	15
Sodium,mg	35	38	38	44	44
Potassium, mg	116	120	120	108	108
Chloride, mg	71	80	80	62	62
Selenium, mcg	3	2.8	2.8	1.8	1.8
Other					
Nucleotides, mg	none added	none added	none added	N/A	N/A
Osmolality, mOsm/kg water	200	170	170	168	200
Water, g	133	134	134	133	133
Potential Renal Solute Load mOsm	16.4	24	24	25.8	22.8

Similac Isomil DF has 0.9 g dietary fiber per 100 calories.
*Human milk based upon the following references:
Lawrence, RA. Breastfeeding. A Guide for the Medical Professional, 5th Ed. St. Louis: Mosby Ince, 1999:136, 737.
American Academy of Pediatrics Committee on Nutrition: Pediatric Nutrition Handbook, 4th Ed. Elk Gove Village: American Academy of Pediatrics, 1998:40, 132-135, 217, 655–658.
Wyeth Nutrition, Internal data.
The nutrient composition on human milk varies among women.
As products and product composition change frequently, always check with the manufacturer for up-to-date product information.

Table A-2 Term Infant Formulas—Nutrients per 100 Calories. *(continued)*

	Soy Based			
Values listed are for ready to feed formula unless stated as powder	Similac Isomil	Similac Isomil DF	Store Brand Soy (powder)	Sore Brand Soy with DHA & AA (powder)
Manufacture	Ross	Ross	Wyeth Nutrition	Wyeth Nutrition
Volume	148	148	148	148
Calories	100	100	100	100
Calories/oz	20	20	20	20
% of Total Calories Protein/ Fat/Carbohydrate	10/49/41	11/49/40	11/48/41	11/48/41
Protein, g	2.45	2.66	2.7	2.7
Source	Soy Protein Isolate & L-Methionine	Soy Protein Isolate & L-Methionine	Soy Protein Isolate & L-Methionine	Soy Protein Isolate & L-Methionine
Fat, g	5.46	5.46	5.3	5.4
Linoleic Acid, mg	1300	1300	500	750
Linolenic Acid, mg	105	105	N/A	N/A
Arachidonic Acid (AA), mg	none	none	none	18
Docosahexaenoic Acid (DHA), mg	none	none	none	10.7
Source	High Oleic Safflower, Soy & Coconut Oils	Soy & Coconut Oils	Palm, High Oleic Safflower or Sunflower, Coconut, & Soybean Oils	Palm, High Oleic Safflower or Sunflower, Coconut, & Soybean Oils, AA, DHA
Carbohydrate, g	10.3	10.1	10.2	10.4
Source	Corn Syrup Solids & Sucrose	Corn Syrup Solids & Sucrose	Corn Syrup Solids & Sucrose	Corn Syrup Solids & Sucrose
Vitamins				
Vitamin A, IU	300	300	300	300
Vitamin D, IU	60	60	60	60
Vitamin E, IU	1.5	1.5	1.4	2
Vitamin K, mcg	11	11	8.3	8.3
Vitamin B_1 (Thiamine), mcg	60	60	100	101
Vitamin B_2 (Riboflavin), mcg	90	90	150	150
Vitamin B_6, mcg	60	60	62.5	63
Vitamin B_{12}, mcg	0.45	0.45	0.3	0.3
Niacin, mcg	1350	1350	750	750
Folic Acid, mcg	15	15	7.5	15
Panthothenic Acid, mcg	750	750	450	450
Biotin, mcg	4.5	4.5	5.5	5.3
Vitamin C (Ascorbic Acid), mg	9	9	8.3	9
Choline, mg	12	12	13	13
Inositol, mg	5	5	4.1	4.1
Minerals				
Calcium, mg	105	105	90	90
Phosphorus, mg	75	75	63	63
Magnesium, mg	7.5	7.5	10	10
Iron, mg	1.8	1.8	1.8	1.2
Zinc, mg	0.75	0.75	0.8	0.75
Manganese, mcg	25	25	30	30
Copper, mcg	75	75	70	71
Iodine, mcg	15	15	9	9
Sodium,mg	44	44	30	30
Potassium, mg	108	108	105	105
Chloride, mg	62	62	56	56
Selenium, mcg	1.8	1.8	2.1	2.1
Other				
Nucleotides, mg	N/A	N/A	N/A	N/A
Osmolality, mOsm/kg water	200	240	220	220
Water, g	133	133	135	135
Potential Renal Solute Load mOsm	22.8	24	13.2	13.2

Similac Isomil DF has 0.9 g dietary fiber per 100 calories.
*Human milk based upon the following references:
Lawrence, RA. Breastfeeding. A Guide for the Medical Professional, 5th Ed. St. Louis: Mosby Ince, 1999:136, 737.
American Academy of Pediatrics Committee on Nutrition: Pediatric Nutrition Handbook, 4th Ed. Elk Gove Village: American Academy of Pediatrics, 1998:40, 132-135, 217, 655–658.
Wyeth Nutrition, Internal data.
The nutrient composition on human milk varies among women.
As products and product composition change frequently, always check with the manufacturer for up-to-date product information.

	Protein Hydrolysate				Amino Acid Base	
Values listed are for ready to feed formula unless stated as powder	Nutramigen LIPIL	Pregestimil Liquid	Similac Alimentum Advance	Similac Alimentum	Neocate (powder)	Elecare (powder)
Manufacture	Mead Johnson	Mead Johnson	Ross	Ross	Nutricia. NA	Ross
Volume	148	148	148	148	148	148
Calories	100	100	100	100	100	100
Calories/oz	20	20	20	20	20	20
% of Total Calories Protein/ Fat/Carbohydrate	11/48/41	11/48/41	11/48/41	11/48/41	12/47/41	12/43/43
Protein, g	2.8	2.8	2.75	2.75	3.1	3.01
Source	Casein Hydrolysate & Amino Acids	Casein Hydrolysate & Amino Acids	Casein Hydrolysate, L-Cysteine, L-Tyrosine & L-Trytophan	Casein Hydrolysate, L-Cysteine, L-Tyrosine & L-Trytophan	Free Amino Acids including Taurine & Carnitine	Free L-Amino Acids
Fat, g	5.3	5.6	5.54	5.54	4.5	4.76
Linoleic Acid, mg	860	1120	1900	1900	677	800
Linolenic Acid, mg	85	150	108	95	75	0.1
Arachidonic Acid (AA), mg	34	none	21	none	none	none
Docosahexaenoic Acid (DHA), mg	17	none	8	none	none	none
Source	Palm Olein , Soy, Coconut, High Oleic Sunflower Oils, AA, DHA	Medium Chain Triglyceride, Soy & High Oleic Safflower Oils	Safflower, Medium Chain Trigylceride & Soy Oils, DHA, AA	Safflower, Medium Chain Trigylceride & Soy Oils	High Oleic Safflower Oil, Refined Vegetable Oil (Coconut & Soy)	High Oleic Safflower, Medium Chain Triglyceride & Soy Oils
Carbohydrate, g	10.3	10.2	10.2	10.2	11.7	10.7
Source	Corn Syrup Solids and Modified Corn Starch	Corn Syrup Solids and Modified Corn Starch	Sucrose & Modified Tapoica Starch	Sucrose & Modified Tapoica Starch	Corn Syrup Solids	Corn Syrup Solids
Vitamins						
Vitamin A, IU	300	380	300	300	409	273
Vitamin D, IU	50	50	45	45	87	42
Vitamin E, IU	2	3.8	3	3	1.1	2.1
Vitamin K, mcg	8	18.8	14	14	8.8	6
Vitamin B_1 (Thiamine), mcg	80	80	60	60	92.6	210
Vitamin B_2 (Riboflavin), mcg	90	90	90	90	137.8	105
Vitamin B_6, mcg	60	60	60	60	123.5	101
Vitamin B_{12}, mcg	0.3	0.3	0.45	0.45	0.17	0.42
Niacin, mcg	1000	1000	1350	1350	1540	1680
Folic Acid, mcg	16	16	15	15	10.2	30
Panthothenic Acid, mcg	500	500	750	750	620	421
Biotin, mcg	3	3	4.5	4.5	3.1	4.2
Vitamin C (Ascorbic Acid), mg	12	12	9	9	9.3	9
Choline, mg	12	12	12	12	13.1	8
Inositol, mg	17	17	5	5	23	5.1
Minerals						
Calcium, mg	94	115	105	105	124	108
Phosphorus, mg	63	75	75	75	93.1	81
Magnesium, mg	11	12	7.5	7.5	12.4	8
Iron, mg	1.8	1.88	1.8	1.8	1.85	1.8
Zinc, mg	1	1.1	0.75	0.75	1.66	1.1
Manganese, mcg	23	30	8	8	90	93
Copper, mcg	75	110	75	75	124	126
Iodine, mcg	15	11	15	15	15.4	7
Sodium,mg	47	47	44	44	37.3	45
Potassium, mg	110	110	118	118	155.1	150
Chloride, mg	86	86	80	80	77.2	60
Selenium, mcg	2.8	2.8	1.8	1.8	3.73	2.3
Other						
Nucleotides, mg	none added	none added	N/A	N/A	N/A	none addded
Osmolality, mOsm/kg water	320	280	370	370	375	335
Water, g	133	134	133	133	133	81
Potential Renal Solute Load mOsm	25	26	25.3	25.3	28.3	27.3

Similac Isomil DF has 0.9 g dietary fiber per 100 calories.
*Human milk based upon the following references:
Lawrence, RA. Breastfeeding. A Guide for the Medical Professional, 5th Ed. St. Louis: Mosby Ince, 1999:136, 737.
American Academy of Pediatrics Committee on Nutrition: Pediatric Nutrition Handbook, 4th Ed. Elk Gove Village: American Academy of Pediatrics, 1998:40, 132-135, 217, 655–658.
Wyeth Nutrition, Internal data.
The nutrient composition on human milk varies among women.
As products and product composition change frequently, always check with the manufacturer for up-to-date product information.

Table A-2 Term Infant Formulas—Nutrients per 100 Calories. *(continued)*

	Older Infants and Toddlers				
Values listed are for ready to feed formula unless stated as powder	Good Start 2 Essentials	Good Start 2 Essentials Soy	Enfamil Next Step LIPIL	Enfamil Next Step Prosobee LIPIL	Similac 2 Advance (powder)
Manufacture	Nestle	Nestle	Mead Johnson	Mead Johnson	Ross
Volume	148	148	148	148	148
Calories	100	100	100	100	100
Calories/oz	20	20	20	20	20
% of Total Calories Protein/ Fat/Carbohydrate	10/53/37	12/48/40	10/45/44	13/40/47	8/49/43
Protein, g	2.6	3.1	2.6	3.3	2.07
Source	Nonfat Milk	Soy Protein Isolate	Nonfat Milk	Soy Protein Isolate & L-Methionine	Nonfat Milk & Whey Protein Concentrate
Fat, g	4.1	4.4	5.3	4.4	5.49
Linoleic Acid, mg	680	860	860	720	1000
Linolenic Acid, mg	110	115	N/A	N/A	108
Arachidonic Acid (AA), mg	none	none	34	34	21
Docosahexaenoic Acid (DHA), mg	none	none	17	17	8
Source	Palm Olein, Soy, Coconut, High Oleic Safflower Oils	Palm Olein, Soy, Coconut, High Oleic Safflower Oils	Palm Olein, Soy, Coconut, High Oleic Sunflower Oils	Palm Olein, Soy, Coconut, High Oleic Sunflower Oils	High Oleic Safflower, Coconut & Soy Oils
Carbohydrate, g	13.2	12	10.5	11.8	10.6
Source	Corn Syrup Solids, Lactose, Maltodextrin	Corn Maltodextrin & Sucrose	Corn Syrup Solids & Lactose	Corn Syrup Solids & Sugar	Lactose
Vitamins					
Vitamin A, IU	250	300	300	300	300
Vitamin D, IU	60	60	60	60	60
Vitamin E, IU	2	3	2	2	3
Vitamin K, mcg	8	8	8	8	8
Vitamin B_1 (Thiamine), mcg	80	80	100	80	100
Vitamin B_2 (Riboflavin), mcg	140	94	140	90	150
Vitamin B_6, mcg	65	70	60	60	60
Vitamin B_{12}, mcg	0.25	0.31	0.3	0.3	0.25
Niacin, mcg	900	1300	1000	1000	1050
Folic Acid, mcg	15	16	16	16	15
Panthothenic Acid, mcg	480	470	500	500	450
Biotin, mcg	2.2	7.8	3	3	4.4
Vitamin C (Ascorbic Acid), mg	9	15	12	12	9
Choline, mg	12	12	12	12	16
Inositol, mg	18	12	6	6	4.7
Minerals					
Calcium, mg	120	135	195	195	118
Phosphorus, mg	80	90	130	130	64
Magnesium, mg	8	10	8	11	6
Iron, mg	1.8	1.8	2	2	1.8
Zinc, mg	0.8	0.9	1	1.2	0.75
Manganese, mcg	7	37	15	50	5
Copper, mcg	85	120	75	75	90
Iodine, mcg	10	15	10	15	6
Sodium,mg	39	38	36	36	24
Potassium, mg	135	118	130	120	105
Chloride, mg	90	79	80	80	65
Selenium, mcg	2	2	2.8	2.8	1.8
Other					
Nucleotides, mg	none added	none added	N/A	N/A	N/A
Osmolality, mOsm/kg water	326	200	270	230	300
Water, g	133	133	133	132	133
Potential Renal Solute Load mOsm	12.1	13	26	30	19.5

Similac Isomil DF has 0.9 g dietary fiber per 100 calories.
*Human milk based upon the following references:
Lawrence, RA. Breastfeeding. A Guide for the Medical Professional, 5th Ed. St. Louis: Mosby Ince, 1999:136, 737.
American Academy of Pediatrics Committee on Nutrition: Pediatric Nutrition Handbook, 4th Ed. Elk Gove Village: American Academy of Pediatrics, 1998:40, 132-135, 217, 655–658.
Wyeth Nutrition, Internal data.
The nutrient composition on human milk varies among women.
As products and product composition change frequently, always check with the manufacturer for up-to-date product information.

	Older Infants and Toddlers				
Values listed are for ready to feed formula unless stated as powder	Similac 2 (powder)	Similac Isomil 2 Advance (powder)	Similac Isomil 2 (powder)	Store Brand Formula for Older Infants (Powder)	Store Brand Formula for Older Infants with DHA & AA (powder)
Manufacture	Ross	Ross	Ross	Wyeth	Wyeth
Volume	148	148	148	148	148
Calories	100	100	100	100	100
Calories/oz	20	20	20	20	20
% of Total Calories Protein/ Fat/Carbohydrate	8/49/43	10/49/41	10/49/41	11/49/40	11/49/40
Protein, g	2.07	2.45	2.45	2.6	2.6
Source	Nonfat Milk & Whey Protein Concentrate	Soy Protein Isolate & L-Methionine	Soy Protein Isolate & L-Methionine	Nonfat Milk & Whey Protein Concentrate	Nonfat Milk & Whey Protein Concentrate
Fat, g	5.49	5.46	5.46	5.4	5.4
Linoleic Acid, mg	1000	1000	1000	750	750
Linolenic Acid, mg	108	105	105	N/A	N/A
Arachidonic Acid (AA), mg	none	21	none	none	18
Docosahexaenoic Acid (DHA), mg	none	8	none	none	10.7
Source	High Oleic Safflower, Coconut & Soy Oils	High Oleic Safflower, Coconut & Soy Oils	High Oleic Safflower, Coconut & Soy Oils	Palm, High Oleic Safflower or Sunflower, Coconut, & Soybean Oils	Palm, High Oleic Safflower or Sunflower, Coconut, & Soybean Oils
Carbohydrate, g	10.6	10.2	10.2	10	10
Source	Lactose	Corn Syrup Solids & Sucrose	Corn Syrup Solids & Sucrose	Lactose, & Corn Syrup Solids	Lactose, & Corn Syrup Solids
Vitamins					
Vitamin A, IU	300	300	300	368	370
Vitamin D, IU	60	60	60	65	65
Vitamin E, IU	3	1.5	1.5	2	2
Vitamin K, mcg	8	11	11	9.9	9.8
Vitamin B_1 (Thiamine), mcg	100	60	60	147	150
Vitamin B_2 (Riboflavin), mcg	150	90	90	221	220
Vitamin B_6, mcg	60	60	60	88	90
Vitamin B_{12}, mcg	0.25	0.45	0.45	0.29	0.29
Niacin, mcg	1050	1350	1350	1020	1020
Folic Acid, mcg	15	15	15	15	15
Panthothenic Acid, mcg	450	750	750	440	440
Biotin, mcg	4.4	4.5	4.5	2.9	2.9
Vitamin C (Ascorbic Acid), mg	9	9	9	13	13
Choline, mg	16	12	12	15	15
Inositol, mg	4.7	5	5	4	4
Minerals					
Calcium, mg	118	135	135	120	120
Phosphorus, mg	64	90	90	85	85
Magnesium, mg	6	7.5	7.5	10	10
Iron, mg	1.8	1.8	1.8	1.8	1.8
Zinc, mg	0.75	0.75	0.75	0.88	0.88
Manganese, mcg	5	25	25	5.9	5.9
Copper, mcg	90	75	75	85	85
Iodine, mcg	6	15	15	10	10
Sodium,mg	24	44	44	32	32
Potassium, mg	105	108	108	125	125
Chloride, mg	65	62	62	80	80
Selenium, mcg	1.8	1.8	1.8	2.1	2.1
Other				**N/A**	**N/A**
Nucleotides, mg	N/A	N/A	N/A	N/A	N/A
Osmolality, mOsm/kg water	300	200	200	280	280
Water, g	133	133	133	135	135
Potential Renal Solute Load mOsm	19.5	23.3	23.3	N/A	N/A

Similac Isomil DF has 0.9 g dietary fiber per 100 calories.
*Human milk based upon the following references:
Lawrence, RA. Breastfeeding. A Guide for the Medical Professional, 5th Ed. St. Louis: Mosby Ince, 1999:136, 737.
American Academy of Pediatrics Committee on Nutrition: Pediatric Nutrition Handbook, 4th Ed. Elk Gove Village: American Academy of Pediatrics, 1998:40, 132-135, 217, 655–658.
Wyeth Nutrition, Internal data.
The nutrient composition on human milk varies among women.
As products and product composition change frequently, always check with the manufacturer for up-to-date product information.

Table A-3 Pediatric Formulas—Nutrients per Liter. Standard, no fiber.*

Product name	Enfamil Kindercal TF	Nutren Junior	Pediasure Enteral Formula	Resource Just for Kids
Manufacturer	Mead Johnson	Nestle	Ross	Novartis
Flavor(s)	Vanilla	Vanilla	Vanilla	Vanilla, chocolate, strawberry
Type (powder or liquid)	Liquid	Liquid	Liquid	Liquid
Calories/mL	1.06	1	1	1
Calories	1,060	1,000	1,000	1,000
% protein/% fat/ % carbohydrate	11/37/52	12/44/44	12/36/53	12/44/44
Protein, g/L	30	30	30	30
Protein source	Milk protein concentrate	Milk protein concentrate, whey protein concentrate	Milk protein concentrate	Sodium and calcium caseinates, whey protein concentrate
Fat, g/L	44	49.6	40	50
Fat source	Canola oil, high oleic sunflower oil, MCT, corn oil	Soybean oil, canola oil, MCT, soy lecithin	High oleic safflower oil, soy oil, MCT, soy lecithin, mono- and diglycerides	High oleic sunflower oil, soybean oil, MCT
Carbohydrate, g/L	135	110	132	110
Carbohydrate source	Maltodextrin, sugar	Maltodextrin, sugar	Corn maltodextrin, sucrose, dextrose	Hydrolyzed cornstarch, sucrose, fructose-chocolate only
Fiber, g/L	< 4	0	0	0
Vitamins				
Vitamin A, IU	4,200	4,068	1,600	2,400
Vitamin D, IU	530	560	204	330
Vitamin E, IU	37	28	23	23
Vitamin K, mcg	32	48	60	40
Vitamin B_1 (Thiamine), mg	1.7	2.4	2.7	1.2
Vitamin B_2 (Riboflavin), mg	2.1	2	2.1	1.5
Vitamin B_6, mg	2.1	2.4	2.6	1.6
Vitamin B_{12}, mcg	5.9	6	5.9	2.4
Niacin, mg	21	20	10.1	17
Folic acid, mcg	161	400	300	370
Panthothenic acid, mg	13.1	10	10.1	10
Biotin, mcg	161	300	320	150
Vitamin C (ascorbic acid), mg	250	100	100	100
Choline, mg	270	300	300	400
Inositol, mg	85	80	80	80
Minerals				
Calcium, mg	1,010	1,000	970	1,140
Phosphorus, mg	850	800	840	800
Magnesium, mg	210	200	198	200
Iron, mg	10.6	14	14	14
Zinc, mg	12.7	15.2	5.9	12
Manganese, mg	2.1	1.6	1.5	2
Copper, mg	1.3	1	1	1
Iodine, mcg	127	120	100	120
Sodium, mg	370	460	380	590
Potassium, mg	1,310	1,320	1,310	1,140
Chloride, mg	740	1,080	1,010	510
Selenium, mcg	32	30	32	40
Chromium, mcg	53	30	30	69
Molybdenum, mcg	53	60	36	43
L-carnitine, mg	63	40	17	17
Other				
Osmolality, mOsm/kg water	345	350	335	390 (440 chocolate)
Water, mL	850	852	850	853

* As products and product composition change frequently, always check with the manufacturer for up-to-date product information.

Table A-4 Pediatric Formulas—Nutrients per Liter. Standard, fiber containing.*

Product name	Compleat Pediatric	Enfamil Kindercal TF with Fiber	Nutren Junior with Fiber	Pediasure Enteral Formula with Fiber	Resource Just for Kids with Fiber
Manufacturer	Novartis	Mead Johnson	Nestle	Ross	Novartis
Flavor(s)	Unflavored	Vanilla	Vanilla	Vanilla	Vanilla
Type (powder or liquid)	Liquid	Liquid	Liquid	Liquid	Liquid
Calories/mL	1	1.06	1	1	1
Calories	1,000	1,060	1,000	1,000	1,000
% protein/% fat/ % carbohydrate	15/35/50	11/37/52	12/44/44	12/36/55	12/44/44
Protein, g/L	38	30	30	30	30
Protein source	Beef, sodium, and calcium caseinates	Milk protein concentrate	Milk protein concentrate, whey protein concentrate	Milk protein concentrate	Sodium and calcium caseinates, whey protein concentrate
Fat, g/L	39	44	49.6	40	50
Fat source	High oleic sunflower oil, soybean oil, MCT	Canola oil, high oleic sunflower oil, MCT, corn oil	Soybean oil, canola oil, MCT, soy lecithin	High oleic safflower oil, soy oil, MCT, soy lecithin, mono- and diglycerides	High oleic sunflower oil, soybean oil, MCT
Carbohydrate, g/L	130	138	110	138	110
Carbohydrate source	Hydrolyzed cornstarch, apple juice, vegetables, fruits	Maltodextrin, sugar	Maltodextrin, sugar, pea fiber, inulin	Corn maltodextrin, sucrose, dextrose, FOS, oat fiber, soy fiber	Hydrolyzed cornstarch, sucrose
Fiber, g/L	4.4	6.3	6	8	6
Vitamins					
Vitamin A, IU	3,300	4,200	4,068	1,600	3,500
Vitamin D, IU	480	530	560	204	510
Vitamin E, IU	22	37	28	23	23
Vitamin K, mcg	38	32	48	60	40
Vitamin B_1 (Thiamine), mg	2.6	1.7	2.4	2.7	2.7
Vitamin B_2 (Riboflavin), mg	2	2.1	2	2.1	2.1
Vitamin B_6, mg	2.5	2.1	2.4	2.6	2.6
Vitamin B_{12}, mcg	5.6	5.9	6	5.9	5.9
Niacin, mg	16	21	20	10.1	17
Folic acid, mcg	350	161	400	300	370
Panthothenic acid, mg	9.6	13.1	10	10.1	10
Biotin, mcg	300	161	300	320	320
Vitamin C (ascorbic acid), mg	96	250	100	100	100
Choline, mg	280	270	300	300	400
Inositol, mg	76	85	80	80	80
Minerals					
Calcium, mg	1,000	1,010	1,000	970	1,140
Phosphorus, mg	1,000	850	800	840	800
Magnesium, mg	190	210	200	198	200
Iron, mg	13	10.6	14	14	14
Zinc, mg	12	12.7	15.2	5.9	12
Manganese, mg	2.2	2.1	1.6	1.5	2.5
Copper, mg	1.2	1.3	1	1	1
Iodine, mcg	140	127	120	100	120
Sodium, mg	680	370	460	380	590
Potassium, mg	1,500	1,310	1,320	1,310	1,140
Chloride, mg	720	740	1,080	1,010	510
Selenium, mcg	52	32	30	32	30
Chromium, mcg	88	53	30	30	52
Molybdenum, mcg	56	53	60	36	32
L-carnitine, mg	16	63	40	17	17
Other					
Osmolality, mOsm/kg water	380	345	350	335	390
Water, mL	844	850	848	850	853

* As products and product composition change frequently, always check with the manufacturer for up-to-date product information.

Table A-5 Pediatric Formulas—Nutrients per Liter. Specialized formulas.*

Product name	Elecare†	Neocate Junior Tropical Fruit	Neocate Junior Unflavored	Neocate One*	Pediatric E028	Peptamen Jr.
Manufacturer	Ross	Nutricia, NA	Nutricia, NA	Nutricia, NA	Nutricia, NA	Nestle
Indications	Cow's milk protein intolerance, whole food protein intolerance	Gastrointestinal tract impairment, malabsorption, multiple food protein intolerance, cow's milk protein intolerance	Gastrointestinal tract impairment, malabsorption, multiple food protein intolerance, cow's milk protein intolerance	Cow's milk protein intolerance, multiple food protein intolerance, gastrointestinal reflux	Gastrointestinal tract impairment, malabsorption, gastrointestinal reflux	Gastrointestinal tract impairment, malabsorption, chronic diarrhea, delayed gastric emptying, growth failure, malnutrition
Flavor(s)	Unflavored	Tropical fruit	Unflavored	Unflavored	Orange-pineapple	Unflavored, vanilla
Type (powder or liquid)	Powder	Powder	Powder	Powder	Liquid	Liquid
Calories/mL	1	1	1	1	1	1
Calories	1,000	1,000	1,000	1,000	1,000	1,000
% protein/% fat/ % carbohydrate	14/43/43	12/46/42	13/44/43	10/32/58	10/32/58	12/33/55
Protein, g/L	30	32	30	25	25	30
Protein source	Free amino acids	Free amino acids	Free amino acids	Free amino acids	Free amino acids	Enzymatically hydrolyzed whey protein
Fat, g/L	47.6	49	50	35	35	38.4
Fat source	Safflower oil, MCT, soy oil	Coconut oil, canola oil, safflower oil	Coconut oil, canola oil, safflower oil	Coconut oil, canola oil, safflower oil	Coconut oil, canola oil, safflower oil	Coconut oil, palm kernel oil, soybean oil, canola oil, soy lecithin
Carbohydrate, g/L	107	101	100	146	146	137.6
Carbohydrate source	Corn syrup solids	Corn syrup solids	Corn syrup solids	Corn syrup solids	Maltodextrin, sucrose, corn syrup solids	Maltodextrin, cornstarch, sugar (in flavored)
Fiber, g/L	0	0	0	0	0	0
Vitamins						
Vitamin A, IU	2,730	2,530	2,430	1,170	1,170	4,072
Vitamin D, IU	420	335	322	310	310	560
Vitamin E, IU	21	18	17	8.2	8.2	28
Vitamin K, mcg	60	28	27	15	15	30
Vitamin B_1 (thiamine), mg	2.1	1.04	1	0.55	0.55	2.4
Vitamin B_2 (riboflavin), mg	1.05	1.04	1	0.65	0.65	2
Vitamin B_6, mg	1.01	1.04	1	0.8	0.8	2.4
Vitamin B_{12}, mcg	4.2	2	2	0.7	0.7	6
Niacin, mg	16.8	12	12	9	9	20
Folic Acid, mcg	295	310	300	60	60	400
Panthothenic acid, mg	4.21	4	3.9	2.4	2.4	10
Biotin, mcg	42	21	20	20	20	300
Vitamin C (ascorbic acid), mg	90	96	93	31	31	100
Choline, mg	80	390	376	183	183	300
Inositol, mg	50	229	220	18	18	80
Minerals						
Calcium, mg	1,080	1,180	1,130	620	620	1,000
Phosphorus, mg	810	977	940	620	620	800
Magnesium, mg	80	188	180	90	90	200
Iron, mg	17.7	14	14	7.7	7.7	14
Zinc, mg	11	14	14	7.7	7.7	15.2
Manganese, mg	1.05	2	2	1	1	1.6
Copper, mg	1.26	1.15	1.1	1	1	1
Iodine, mcg	70	100	96	60	60	120
Sodium, mg	450	430	410	200	200	460
Potassium, mg	1,500	1,420	1,370	930	930	1,320
Chloride, mg	600	656	630	350	350	1,080
Selenium, mcg	23.2	31	30	15.4	15.4	30
Chromium, mcg	23.2	39	38	30	30	24.4
Molybdenum, mcg	25.3	47	45	35	35	30
L-carnitine, mg	48	45	43	25	30	40
Other						
Osmolality, mOsm/kg water	551	690	607	610	820	260 unflavored, 360 flavored
Water, mL	833	810	810	850	800	848

* As products and product composition change frequently, always check with the manufacturer for up-to-date product information.
† Also approved for infant use; prepared at 1 kcal/mL.

Product name	Peptamen Jr. with Prebio	Peptamen Jr. Powder	Peptide One*	Portagen	Vivonex Pediatric
Manufacturer	Nestle	Nestle	Nutricia, NA	Mead Johnson	Novartis
Indications	Gastrointestinal tract impairment, malabsorption, chronic diarrhea, delayed gastric emptying, growth failure, malnutrition	Gastrointestinal tract impairment, malabsorption, chronic diarrhea, delayed gastric emptying, growth failure, malnutrition	Gastrointestinal tract impairment, malabsorption, whole protein intolerance	Decreased pancreatic lipase, bile salts, mucosal permeabiliy, or absorptive surface; intestinal lymphatic obstruction (not intended for sole source of nutrition)	Short bowel syndrome, malabsorption, Crohn's disease, trauma, GI disorder, GI enterocutaneous fistula, intractable diarrhea
Flavor(s)	Vanilla	Vanilla	Banana, unflavored	Unflavored	Unflavored
Type (powder or liquid)	Liquid	Powder	Powder	Powder	Powder
Calories/mL	1	1	1	1.01	0.8
Calories	1,000	1,000	1,000	1,010	800
% protein/% fat/ % carbohydrate	12/33/55	12/33/55	12/46/42	14/40/46	12/25/63
Protein, g/L	30	40	31	35	24
Protein source	Enzymatically hydrolyzed whey protein	Enzymatically hydrolyzed whey protein	Free amino acids, hydrolyzed protein (pork, soy)	Sodium caseinates	Free amino acids
Fat, g/L	38.4	38.4	50	48	24
Fat source	Coconut oil, palm kernel oil, soybean oil, canola oil, soy lecithin	Coconut oil, soybean oil, sunflower oil, soy lecithin	Coconut oil, canola oil, safflower oil	MCT, corn oil	MCT, soybean oil
Carbohydrate, g/L	137.6	136	106	115	130
Carbohydrate source	Maltodextrin, sugar, cornstarch, oligofructose, inulin	Maltodextrin, potato starch	Corn syrup solids	Corn syrup solids	Maltodextrin, modified cornstarch
Fiber, g/L	3.6	0	0	0	0
Vitamins					
Vitamin A, IU	4,072	1,500	2,430	7,812	2,500
Vitamin D, IU	560	400	320	780	500
Vitamin E, IU	28	15	16	31.2	30
Vitamin K, mcg	30	40	27	156	40
Vitamin B_1 (thiamine), mg	2.4	0.6	1	1.56	1.5
Vitamin B_2 (riboflavin), mg	2	0.8	1	1.88	1.8
Vitamin B_6, mg	2.4	0.8	1	2.08	2
Vitamin B_{12}, mcg	6	1.52	2	6.25	3
Niacin, mg	20	6	12	20.8	20
Folic Acid, mcg	400	200	300	156.3	200
Panthothenic acid, mg	10	3	4	10.4	5
Biotin, mcg	300	15	20	78.1	100
Vitamin C (ascorbic acid), mg	100	80	93	81.3	100
Choline, mg	300	250	375	130.2	200
Inositol, mg	80	0	220	56.9	60
Minerals					
Calcium, mg	1,000	920	1,130	937.5	970
Phosphorus, mg	800	612	940	708.3	800
Magnesium, mg	200	120	180	208.3	200
Iron, mg	14	10	140	18.75	10
Zinc, mg	15.2	10	14	9.38	12
Manganese, mg	1.6	0.51	2	1.25	2
Copper, mg	1	0.8	1.1	1.56	1.2
Iodine, mcg	1.6	80	96	72.9	120
Sodium, mg	120	660	410	552	400
Potassium, mg	1,320	1,352	1,360	1,250	1,200
Chloride, mg	1,080	812	630	864.6	1,000
Selenium, mcg	30	24	30	0	30
Chromium, mcg	24.4	24	37	0	45
Molybdenum, mcg	30	32	45	0	75
L-carnitine, mg	40	40	21	0	25
Other					
Osmolality, mOsm/kg water	365	305	430 unflavored, 440 flavored	350	360
Water, mL	844	840	872	870	893

* As products and product composition change frequently, always check with the manufacturer for up-to-date product information.

† Also approved for infant use; prepared at 1 kcal/mL.

Table A-6 Adult Formulas—Nutrients per Liter. Standard, no fiber.*

Product name	Ensure	Isocal	Isosource Standard
Manufacturer	Ross	Novartis	Novartis
Indications	For normal protein and calorie needs, recovery from surgery or illness	General tube-feeding needs, inadequate oral intake, malnutrition, barriers to normal ingestion	Normal protein requirements, malnutrition, inadequate oral intake
Flavor(s)	Vanilla, chocolate, butter pecan, strawberry, coffee, eggnog, black walnut, strawberry	Unflavored	Unflavored
Type (powder or liquid)	Liquid	Liquid	Liquid
Calories/mL	1.06	1.06	1.2
Calories	1,060	1,060	1,200
% protein/% fat/ % carbohydrate	14/22/64	13/37/50	14/29/57
Protein, g/L	35	34	43
Protein source	Calcium caseinate, soy protein isolate, whey protein concentrate	Calcium and sodium caseinates, soy protein isolate	Soy isolate
Fat, g/L	26	44	39
Fat source	High oleic safflower oil, canola oil, corn oil, soy lecithin	Soy and MCT oils	Canola, MCT
Carbohydrate, g/L	168	135	170
Carbohydrate source	Sugar, corn syrup, maltodextrin	Maltodextrin	Corn syrup, hydrolyzed cornstarch
Fiber, g/L	0	< 1	0
Vitamins			
Vitamin A, IU	5,263	2,700	4,300
Vitamin D, IU	421	210	340
Vitamin E, IU	32	40	51
Vitamin K, mcg	84	132	80
Vitamin B_1 (thiamine), mg	1.6	2	1.3
Vitamin B_2 (riboflavin), mg	1.8	2.3	1.5
Vitamin B_6, mg	2.1	2.6	2
Vitamin B_{12}, mcg	6.3	7.9	5.1
Niacin, mg	21	26	17
Folic Acid, mcg	421	210	690
Panthothenic acid, mg	11	13.2	8.6
Biotin, mcg	316	159	260
Vitamin C (ascorbic acid), mg	126	159	200
Choline, mg	421	260	340
Minerals			
Calcium, mg	1,263	630	1,200
Phosphorus, mg	1,263	530	1,100
Magnesium, mg	421	210	350
Iron, mg	19	9.5	15
Zinc, mg	16	10.6	19
Manganese, mg	5.5	1.6	1.7
Copper, mg	2.1	1.06	1.7
Iodine, mcg	160	79	150
Sodium, mg	842	530	1,100
Potassium, mg	1,558	1,320	1,900
Chloride, mg	1,305	1,060	1,100
Selenium, mcg	76	53	70
Chromium, mcg	126	64	110
Molybdenum, mcg	160	131	84
L-carnitine, mg	0	0	0
Other			
Osmolality, mOsm/kg water	590	270	490
Water, mL	842	840	819

* As products and product composition change frequently, always check with the manufacturer for up-to-date product information.

Product name	Nutren	Osmolite	Osmolite 1 Cal
Manufacturer	Nestle	Ross	Ross
Indications	For normal protein and calorie needs	For normal protein and calorie needs	For normal calorie needs and elevated protein needs
Flavor(s)	Vanilla, unflavored	Unflavored	Unflavored
Type (powder or liquid)	Liquid	Liquid	Liquid
Calories/mL	1	1.06	1.06
Calories	1,000	1,060	1,060
% protein/% fat/ % carbohydrate	16/33/51	14/29/57	17/29/54
Protein, g/L	40	37	44
Protein source	Calcium-potassium caseinate	Sodium and calcium caseinates, soy protein isolate	Sodium and calcium caseinates, soy protein isolate
Fat, g/L	38	35	35
Fat source	Canola oil, MCT, corn oil, soy lecithin	High oleic safflower oil, canola oil, MCT, soy lecithin	High oleic safflower, canola oil, MCY, soy lecithin
Carbohydrate, g/L	127	151	144
Carbohydrate source	Maltodextrin, corn syrup solids	Maltodextrin	Maltodextrin
Fiber, g/L	0	0	0
Vitamins			
Vitamin A, IU	3,200	2,660	3,790
Vitamin D, IU	267	215	305
Vitamin E, IU	28	24	35
Vitamin K, mcg	50	43	61
Vitamin B_1 (thiamine), mg	2	1.6	1.8
Vitamin B_2 (riboflavin), mg	2.4	1.9	2
Vitamin B_6, mg	4	2.2	2.3
Vitamin B_{12}, mcg	8	6.4	6.9
Niacin, mg	28	22	23
Folic Acid, mcg	540	425	455
Panthothenic acid, mg	14	11	12
Biotin, mcg	400	320	230
Vitamin C (ascorbic acid), mg	140	160	230
Choline, mg	452	320	455
Minerals			
Calcium, mg	668	535	760
Phosphorus, mg	668	535	760
Magnesium, mg	268	215	305
Iron, mg	12	9.6	14
Zinc, mg	14	12	18
Manganese, mg	2.7	2.7	3.8
Copper, mg	1.4	1.1	1.6
Iodine, mcg	100	80	115
Sodium, mg	876	640	930
Potassium, mg	1,248	1,020	1,570
Chloride, mg	1,200	850	1,440
Selenium, mcg	40	38	54
Chromium, mcg	40	64	91
Molybdenum, mcg	120	80	115
L-carnitine, mg	80	80	115
Other			
Osmolality, mOsm/kg water	315 unflavored, 370 vanilla	300	300
Water, mL	848	841	842

* As products and product composition change frequently, always check with the manufacturer for up-to-date product information.

Table A-7 Adult Formulas—Nutrients per Liter. Standard, with fiber.*

Product name	**Compleat**	**Ensure Fiber with FOS**	**Fibersource Standard**
Manufacturer	Novartis	Ross	Novartis
Indications	Semisynthetic blenderized formula for formula related intolerance	For normal protein and calorie needs, recovery from surgery or illness	Normal protein requirements, abnormal bowel function, extended inactivity, neurological impairment, developmentally disabled
Flavor(s)	Unflavored	Vanilla, chocolate	Unflavored
Type (powder or liquid)	Liquid	Liquid	Liquid
Calories/mL	1	1.06	1.2
Calories	1,000	1,060	1,200
% protein/% fat/ % carbohydrate	16/31/53	14/22/64	14/29/57
Protein, g/L	43	37	43
Protein source	Beef, calcium caseinate	Sodium and calcium caseinates, soy protein isolate	Soy concentrate soy isolate
Fat, g/L	37	26	39
Fat source	Canola oil, beef	High oleic safflower oil, canola oil, corn oil	Canola, MCT
Carbohydrate, g/L	140	177	170
Carbohydrate source	Hydrolyzed cornstarch, fruits, vegetables	Maltodextrin, sugar, oat fiber, FOS, soy fiber	Corn syrup, hydrolyzed cornstarch
Fiber, g/L	4.3	12	10
Vitamins			
Vitamin A, IU	3,300	5,263	4,300
Vitamin D, IU	270	421	340
Vitamin E, IU	30	32	51
Vitamin K, mcg	67	84	80
Vitamin B_1 (thiamine), mg	1.5	1.6	1.3
Vitamin B_2 (riboflavin), mg	1.7	1.8	1.5
Vitamin B_6, mg	2	2.1	2
Vitamin B_{12}, mcg	6	6.3	5.1
Niacin, mg	20	21	17
Folic Acid, mcg	270	421	690
Panthothenic acid, mg	6.7	53	8.6
Biotin, mcg	200	316	260
Vitamin C (ascorbic acid), mg	60	126	200
Choline, mg	200	421	340
Minerals			
Calcium, mg	670	1,474	1,000
Phosphorus, mg	730	1,263	940
Magnesium, mg	270	421	350
Iron, mg	12	19	15
Zinc, mg	15	16	19
Manganese, mg	2.7	5.5	1.7
Copper, mg	1.3	2.1	1.9
Iodine, mcg	110	160	150
Sodium, mg	760	842	1,200
Potassium, mg	1,450	1,558	2,000
Chloride, mg	870	1,347	900
Selenium, mcg	67	76	70
Chromium, mcg	100	126	110
Molybdenum, mcg	200	160	130
L-carnitine, mg	43	0	0
Other			
Osmolality, mOsm/kg water	300	500	490
Water, mL	781	821	814

* As products and product composition change frequently, always check with the manufacturer for up-to-date product information.

Product name	Jevity 1 Cal	Nutren Fiber	Ultracal
Manufacturer	Ross	Nestle	Novartis
Indications	General tube feeding needs	For normal protein and calorie needs	General tube-feeding needs, inadequate oral intake, malnutrition, barriers to normal ingestion, need for fiber
Flavor(s)	Unflavored	Vanilla, unflavored	Unflavored
Type (powder or liquid)	Liquid	Liquid	Liquid
Calories/mL	1.06	1	1.06
Calories	1,060	1,000	1,060
% protein/% fat/ % carbohydrate	17/29/54	16/33/51	17/33/50
Protein, g/L	44	40	45
Protein source	Sodium and calcium caseinates, soy protein isolate	Calcium-potassium caseinate	Milk protein concentrate, casein
Fat, g/L	35	38	39
Fat source	High oleic safflower oil, canola oil, MCT, soy lecithin	Canola oil, MCT, corn oil, soy lecithin	Canola oil, MCT, high oleic sunflower oil, corn oil
Carbohydrate, g/L	155	127	142
Carbohydrate source	Maltodextrin, corn syrup solids, soy fiber	Maltodextrin, corn syrup solids, pea fiber	Maltodextrin, microcrystalline cellulose, soy fiber, acacia
Fiber, g/L	14.4	14	14.4
Vitamins			
Vitamin A, IU	3,790	3,200	5,000
Vitamin D, IU	305	267	400
Vitamin E, IU	35	28	90
Vitamin K, mcg	61	50	80
Vitamin B_1 (thiamine), mg	1.7	2	3
Vitamin B_2 (riboflavin), mg	2	2.4	3.4
Vitamin B_6, mg	2.3	4	4
Vitamin B_{12}, mcg	6.9	8	12
Niacin, mg	23	28	40
Folic Acid, mcg	455	540	800
Panthothenic acid, mg	12	14	20
Biotin, mcg	345	400	600
Vitamin C (ascorbic acid), mg	230	140	240
Choline, mg	455	452	550
Minerals			
Calcium, mg	910	668	1,000
Phosphorus, mg	760	668	1,000
Magnesium, mg	305	268	400
Iron, mg	14	12	18
Zinc, mg	18	14	21
Manganese, mg	3.8	2.7	4
Copper, mg	1.6	1.4	2
Iodine, mcg	115	100	150
Sodium, mg	930	876	1,350
Potassium, mg	1,570	1,248	1,850
Chloride, mg	1,310	1,200	1,500
Selenium, mcg	54	40	70
Chromium, mcg	91	40	120
Molybdenum, mcg	115	120	120
L-carnitine, mg	115	80	150
Other			
Osmolality, mOsm/kg water	300	330 unflavored, 410 vanilla	300
Water, mL	829	838	830

* As products and product composition change frequently, always check with the manufacturer for up-to-date product information.

Table A-8 Adult Formulas—Nutrients per Liter. Specialized formulas.*

Product name	Advera†	AlitraQ	Choice DM TF	Comply
Manufacturer	Ross	Ross	Novartis	Novartis
Indications	HIV, AIDS	Metabolic stress, GI impairment, contains glutamine and arginine	Diabetes mellitus, glucose intolerance, stress-induced hyperglycemia	Restricted fluid intake, increased engery needs
Flavor(s)	Vanilla, chocolate	Vanilla	Unflavored	Unflavored
Type (powder or liquid)	Liquid	Powder	Liquid	Liquid
Calories/mL	1.28	1	1.06	1.5
Calories	1,280	1,000	1,060	1,500
%Protein/% Fat/ %Carbohydrate	19/65/16	21/13/66	17/43/40	16/36/48
Protein, g/L	60	52.5	45	60
Protein Source	Soy protein hydrolysate, sodium caseinate	Free amino acids, soy hydrolysate, whey protein concentrate, lactoalbumin hydrolysate	Milk protein concentrate, casein	Calcium and sodium caseinates
Fat, g/L	22.8	15.5	51	61
Fat source	Canola oil, MCT, refined deodorized sardine oil	MCT oil, safflower oil	Canola oil, high oleic sunflower oil, corn and MCT oils	Canola oil, high oleic sunflower oil, corn and MCT oils
Carbohydrate, g/L	216	165	119	180
Carbohydrate source	Maltodextrin, sugar, soy fiber	Maltodextrin, sugar, fructose	Maltodextrin, microcystalline cellulose, soy fiber, acacia	Maltodextrin
Fiber, g/L	8.9	0	14.4	< 1
Vitamins				
Vitamin A, IU	10,788	3,998	5,300	6,000
Vitamin D, IU	338	267	420	480
Vitamin E, IU	38.1	30	127	90
Vitamin K, mcg	101	54	127	144
Vitamin B_1 (thiamine), mg	3.2	2	1.6	1.8
Vitamin B_2 (riboflavin), mg	2.9	2.3	1.8	2
Vitamin B_6, mg	3.4	2.7	2.1	3.4
Vitamin B_{12}, mcg	50.7	8	6.4	18
Niacin, mg	25.4	27	21	24
Folic acid, mcg	507	267	420	600
Panthothenic acid, mg	12.7	14	25	12
Biotin, mcg	381	400	320	360
Vitamin C (ascorbic acid), mg	381	200	250	180
Choline, mg	212	400	530	600
Minerals				
Calcium, mg	1,098	733	1,060	1,200
Phosphorus, mg	1,098	733	1,060	1,200
Magnesium, mg	338	267	420	480
Iron, mg	19.1	15	19	22
Zinc, mg	16	20	21	38
Manganese, mg	5.5	3.4	3.2	3.6
Copper, mg	2.5	1.4	2.1	29
Iodine, mcg	127	100	159	180
Sodium, mg	1,056	1,000	850	1,200
Potassium, mg	2,830	1,200	1,820	1,850
Chloride, mg	1,477	1,300	1,270	1,700
Selenium, mcg	60	50	72	84
Chromium, mcg	71.8	74	210	144
Molybdenum, mcg	228	110	106	120
L-carnitine, mg	127.2	100	159	180
Other				
Osmolality, mOsm/kg water	680	575	300	460
Water, mL	802	846	850	770

* As products and product composition change frequently, always check with the manufacturer for up-to-date product information.

† Vitamin and mineral information for vanilla.

‡ When used as a sole source of nutrition, essential fatty acids, water, and ultratrace minerals should be reviewed.

§ Ready to hang.

Product name	Criticare HN‡	Crucial	Deliver 2.0	Diabetisource AC
Manufacturer	Novartis	Nestle	Novartis	Novartis
Indications	Inflammatory bowel disease, short gut syndrome, nonspecific malabsorptive/maldigestive states, cystic fibrosis	Wound healing, critical illness, increased energy and protein needs	Liver disease, fluid restrictions, volume restriction	Diabetes mellitus, glucose intolerance, stress-induced hyperglycemia, diabetes with wounds
Flavor(s)	Unflavored	Unflavored	Vanilla	Unflavored
Type (powder or liquid)	Liquid	Liquid	Liquid	Liquid
Calories/mL	1.06	1.5	2	1.2
Calories	1,060	1,500	2,000	1,200
%Protein/% Fat/ %Carbohydrate	14/81/5	25/39/36	15/45/40	20/44/36
Protein, g/L	38	94	75	60
Protein Source	Casein hydrolysate, amino acids	Enzymatically hydrolyzed casein, L-arginine	Calcium and sodium caseinates	Soy protein, L-arginine
Fat, g/L	5.3	67.6	101	59
Fat source	Safflower oil, emulsifiers	MCT, fish oil, soy oil, soy lecithin	Soy and MCT oils	Canola oil, MCT
Carbohydrate, g/L	220	135	200	100
Carbohydrate source	Maltodextrin, modified cornstarch	Maltodextrin, cornstarch	Corn syrup	Hydrolyzed cornstarch, vegetables, fruits
Fiber, g/L	none	0	< 1	10
Vitamins				
Vitamin A, IU	2,700	6,000	5,000	4,000
Vitamin D, IU	210	400	400	320
Vitamin E, IU	40	100	75	96
Vitamin K, mcg	131	75	250	64
Vitamin B_1 (thiamine), mg	2	3	3.8	1.5
Vitamin B_2 (riboflavin), mg	2.3	2.4	4.3	1.7
Vitamin B_6, mg	2.7	4	5	2
Vitamin B_{12}, mcg	7.9	8	300	6
Niacin, mg	27	28	50	20
Folic acid, mcg	210	540	400	400
Panthothenic acid, mg	13.1	14	25	10
Biotin, mcg	161	400	300	300
Vitamin C (ascorbic acid), mg	161	1,000	300	240
Choline, mg	270	450	500	200
Minerals				
Calcium, mg	530	1,000	1,010	800
Phosphorus, mg	530	1,000	1,010	800
Magnesium, mg	210	400	400	320
Iron, mg	9.7	18	18.2	14
Zinc, mg	10.6	36	20	15
Manganese, mg	2.7	4	3	1.6
Copper, mg	1.1	3	2	1.6
Iodine, mcg	79	160	148	120
Sodium, mg	630	1,168	800	1,120
Potassium, mg	1,310	1,872	1,690	1,920
Chloride, mg	1,060	1,740	1,180	640
Selenium, mcg	0	100	101	56
Chromium, mcg	0	140	123	140
Molybdenum, mcg	0	220	250	60
L-carnitine, mg	0	150	0	65
Other				
Osmolality, mOsm/kg water	650	490	640	350
Water, mL	850	771	710	818

* As products and product composition change frequently, always check with the manufacturer for up-to-date product information.

† Vitamin and mineral information for vanilla.

‡ When used as a sole source of nutrition, essential fatty acids, water, and ultratrace minerals should be reviewed.

§ Ready to hang.

Table A-8 Adult Formulas—Nutrients per Liter. Specialized formulas.* *(continued)*

Product name	Ensure Plus HN	Ensure Plus HN RTH	EquaLYTE	f.a.a.
Manufacturer	Ross	Ross	Ross	Nestle
Indications	Fluid restrictions, volume limited feedings	Fluid restrictions, volume limited feedings	Fluid and electrolyte replacement	Fat intolerance, severe malabsorption, steatorrhea
Flavor(s)	Vanilla, chocolate	Unflavored	Unflavored	Unflavored
Type (powder or liquid)	Liquid	Liquid	Liquid	Liquid
Calories/mL	1.5	1.5	0.1	1
Calories	1,500	1,500	100	1,000
%Protein/% Fat/ %Carbohydrate	17/30/53	17/30/53	0/0/100	20/10/70
Protein, g/L	62	63	0	50
Protein Source	Sodium and calcium caseinates, soy protein isolate	Sodium and calcium caseinates, soy protein isolate	None	Cystalline L-amino acids
Fat, g/L	50	49	0	11.2
Fat source	Corn oil, soy lecithin	High oleic safflower oil, canola oil, MCT, soy lecithin	None	Soybean oil, MCT, soy lecithin
Carbohydrate, g/L	199	204	30	176
Carbohydrate source	Maltodextrin, sugar	Maltodextrin	Dextrose, FOS	Maltodextrin, cornstarch
Fiber, g/L	0	0	0	0
Vitamins				
Vitamin A, IU	5,263	8,320	0	4,300
Vitamin D, IU	421	400	0	272
Vitamin E, IU	51	45	0	30
Vitamin K, mcg	316	80	0	50
Vitamin B_1 (thiamine), mg	3.2	3	0	2
Vitamin B_2 (riboflavin), mg	3.6	3.4	0	2.4
Vitamin B_6, mg	4.21	4	0	4
Vitamin B_{12}, mcg	12.6	12	0	8
Niacin, mg	42	40	0	28
Folic acid, mcg	842	800	0	540
Panthothenic acid, mg	21	20	0	14
Biotin, mcg	632	600	0	400
Vitamin C (ascorbic acid), mg	316	240	0	340
Choline, mg	632	600	0	448
Minerals				
Calcium, mg	1,053	1,000	0	800
Phosphorus, mg	1,053	1,000	0	700
Magnesium, mg	421	400	0	296
Iron, mg	19	18	0	18
Zinc, mg	24	23	0	24
Manganese, mg	5.5	5	0	2.8
Copper, mg	2.1	2	0	2
Iodine, mcg	160	150	0	150
Sodium, mg	1,179	1,400	1,800	560
Potassium, mg	1,810	1,800	875	1,500
Chloride, mg	1,726	1,700	2,400	1,400
Selenium, mcg	76	70	0	38
Chromium, mcg	126	120	0	34
Molybdenum, mcg	160	150	0	54
L-carnitine, mg	160	150	0	100
Other				
Osmolality, mOsm/kg water	650	525	290	700
Water, mL	728	762	972	824

* As products and product composition change frequently, always check with the manufacturer for up-to-date product information.

† Vitamin and mineral information for vanilla.

‡ When used as a sole source of nutrition, essential fatty acids, water, and ultratrace minerals should be reviewed.

§ Ready to hang.

Product name	Fibersource HN	Glucerna	Glytrol	IMPACT
Manufacturer	Novartis	Ross	Nestle	Novartis
Indications	Elevated protein requirements, abnormal bowel function, extended inactivity, neurological impairment, developmentally disabled	Diabetes mellitus, stress-induced hyperglycemia	Hyperglycemia, diabetes mellitus	Trauma, major surgery, infections or pneumonia, cancer, ventilator dependence, burn injury
Flavor(s)	Unflavored	Vanilla	Unflavored, vanilla	Unflavored
Type (powder or liquid)	Liquid	Liquid	Liquid	Liquid
Calories/mL	1.2	1	1	1
Calories	1,200	1,000	1,000	1,000
%Protein/% Fat/ %Carbohydrate	18/29/53	17/49/34	18/42/40	22/25/53
Protein, g/L	62	42	45	56
Protein Source	Soy isolate, soy concentrate	Sodium and calcium caseinates	Calcium-potassium caseinate	Sodium and calcium caseinates, L-arginine
Fat, g/L	46	54	47.6	28
Fat source	Canola, MCT	High oleic safflower oil, canola oil, soy lecithin	Canola oil, safflower oil, MCT, soy lecithin	Palm kernel oil, sunflower oil, menhaden oil
Carbohydrate, g/L	180	96	100	130
Carbohydrate source	Corn syrup, hydrolyzed cornstarch	Maltodextrin, soy fiber, fructose	Maltodextrin, cornstarch, pea fiber, gum arabic, oligofructose, inulin	Hydrolyzed cornstarch
Fiber, g/L	10	14.1	15	0
Vitamins				
Vitamin A, IU	4,300	6,300	5,080	6,700
Vitamin D, IU	340	285	272	270
Vitamin E, IU	51	32	30	60
Vitamin K, mcg	80	57	50	67
Vitamin B_1 (thiamine), mg	1.5	1.6	2	2
Vitamin B_2 (riboflavin), mg	1.7	1.8	2.4	1.7
Vitamin B_6, mg	2.3	2.2	4	1.5
Vitamin B_{12}, mcg	5.1	6.4	8	8
Niacin, mg	17	22	28	20
Folic acid, mcg	690	425	400	400
Panthothenic acid, mg	8.6	11	14	6.7
Biotin, mcg	260	320	300	200
Vitamin C (ascorbic acid), mg	200	215	140	80
Choline, mg	340	425	400	270
Minerals				
Calcium, mg	1,000	705	720	800
Phosphorus, mg	1,000	705	720	800
Magnesium, mg	350	285	286	270
Iron, mg	17	13	12.8	12
Zinc, mg	19	16	15.2	15
Manganese, mg	1.7	3.6	3	2
Copper, mg	1.9	1.5	1.52	1.7
Iodine, mcg	150	110	120	100
Sodium, mg	1,200	930	740	1,100
Potassium, mg	2,000	1,570	1,400	1,400
Chloride, mg	900	1,440	1,400	1,300
Selenium, mcg	70	50	76	100
Chromium, mcg	110	85	124	100
Molybdenum, mcg	130	110	200	200
L-carnitine, mg	0	145	100	0
Other				
Osmolality, mOsm/kg water	490	355	380 unflavored, 280 vanilla	375
Water, mL	814	853	840	853

* As products and product composition change frequently, always check with the manufacturer for up-to-date product information.

† Vitamin and mineral information for vanilla.

‡ When used as a sole source of nutrition, essential fatty acids, water, and ultratrace minerals should be reviewed.

§ Ready to hang.

Table A-8 Adult Formulas—Nutrients per Liter. Specialized formulas.* *(continued)*

Product name	**IMPACT 1.5**	**IMPACT Glutamine**	**IMPACT with Fiber**	**IntensiCal**
Manufacturer	Novartis	Novartis	Novartis	Novartis
Indications	Fluid restriction, increased energy needs, trauma, major surgery, infections or pneumonia, ventilator dependence, burn injury	Critically ill with GI impairment, trauma, major surgery, infections or pneumonia, cancer, ventilator dependence, burn injury	Trauma, major surgery, infections or pneumonia, cancer, ventilator dependence, burn injury	Multiple trauma, burns, wound healing, sepsis, postsurgical recovery
Flavor(s)	Unflavored	Unflavored	Unflavored	Unflavored
Type (powder or liquid)	Liquid	Liquid	Liquid	Liquid
Calories/mL	1.5	1.3	1.2	1.3
Calories	1,500	1,300	1,200	1,300
%Protein/% Fat/ %Carbohydrate	22/40/38	24/30/46	22/25/53	25/29/46
Protein, g/L	84	78	56	81
Protein Source	Sodium and calcium caseinates, L-arginine	Wheat protein hydrolysate, free amino acids, sodium caseinate	Sodium and calcium caseinates, L-arginine	Casein hydrolysate, L-arginine
Fat, g/L	69	43	28	42
Fat source	MCT, palm kernel oil, sunflower oil, menhaden oil	Palm kernel oil, sunflower oil, menhaden oil	Palm kernel oil, sunflower oil, menhaden oil	Canola oil, MCT and high oleic sunflower oil, corn and menhaden oils
Carbohydrate, g/L	140	150	140	150
Carbohydrate source	Hydrolyzed cornstarch	Maltodextrin	Hydrolyzed cornstarch	Maltodextrin, modified cornstarch
Fiber, g/L	0	10	10	none
Vitamins				
Vitamin A, IU	8,000	8,700	6,700	7,500
Vitamin D, IU	320	400	270	520
Vitamin E, IU	72	78	60	52
Vitamin K, mcg	80	80	67	80
Vitamin B_1 (thiamine), mg	2.4	1.5	2	2.6
Vitamin B_2 (riboflavin), mg	2.1	1.7	1.7	3
Vitamin B_6, mg	1.8	2	1.5	3.5
Vitamin B_{12}, mcg	9.6	6	8	10.5
Niacin, mg	24	20	20	35
Folic acid, mcg	480	400	400	700
Panthothenic acid, mg	8	10	6.7	17.5
Biotin, mcg	240	300	200	530
Vitamin C (ascorbic acid), mg	96	260	80	520
Choline, mg	320	500	80	520
Minerals				
Calcium, mg	960	1,200	800	1,130
Phosphorus, mg	960	1,200	800	1,080
Magnesium, mg	320	400	270	400
Iron, mg	14	18	12	18
Zinc, mg	18	20	15	21
Manganese, mg	2.4	2	2	3.5
Copper, mg	2	2	1.7	2
Iodine, mcg	120	150	100	150
Sodium, mg	1,280	1,200	1,100	1,110
Potassium, mg	1,680	1,800	1,400	1,290
Chloride, mg	1,600	850	1,300	1,470
Selenium, mcg	120	70	100	70
Chromium, mcg	120	120	100	120
Molybdenum, mcg	240	75	200	105
L-carnitine, mg	140	140	0	160
Other				
Osmolality, mOsm/kg water	550	630	375	550
Water, mL	780	807	868	800

* As products and product composition change frequently, always check with the manufacturer for up-to-date product information.
† Vitamin and mineral information for vanilla.
‡ When used as a sole source of nutrition, essential fatty acids, water, and ultratrace minerals should be reviewed.
§ Ready to hang.

Product name	Introlite	Isocal HN	Isocal HN Plus	Isosource 1.5 Cal
Manufacturer	Ross	Novartis	Novartis	Novartis
Indications	For initiation of tube feeding, for adjunct to a full-strength formula	General tube-feeding needs, inadequate oral intake, barriers to normal ingestion	General tube-feeding needs, inadequate oral intake, barriers to normal ingestion	Pulmonary conditions, volume intolerance/fluid restriction, elevated caloric and protein needs, shortened feeding schedules
Flavor(s)	Unflavored	Unflavored	Unflavored	Unflavored
Type (powder or liquid)	Liquid	Liquid	Liquid	Liquid
Calories/mL	0.53	1.06	1.2	1.5
Calories	530	1,060	1,200	1,500
%Protein/% Fat/ %Carbohydrate	17/30/53	17/37/46	18/29/53	18/38/44
Protein, g/L	22	44	54	68
Protein Source	Sodium and calcium caseinates, soy protein isolate	Calcium and sodium caseinates, soy protein isolate	Milk protein concentrate, casein (ready to hang only)	Sodium and calcium caseinates
Fat, g/L	18	45	40	65
Fat source	MCT, corn oil, soy oil, soy lecithin	Soy and MCT oils	Canola oil, MCT and high oleic sunflower oil and corn oil	Canola oil, MCT, soybean oil
Carbohydrate, g/L	71	124	156	170
Carbohydrate source	Maltodextrin	Maltodextrin	Maltodextrin	Hydrolyzed cornstarch, sugar
Fiber, g/L	0	< 1	< 1	8
Vitamins				
Vitamin A, IU	3,790	4,200	5,000	10,700
Vitamin D, IU	305	340	400	430
Vitamin E, IU	35	63	90	64
Vitamin K, mcg	61	106	80	86
Vitamin B_1 (thiamine), mg	1.8	3.2	3	3.2
Vitamin B_2 (riboflavin), mg	2	3.6	3.4	3.6
Vitamin B_6, mg	2.3	4.2	4	4.3
Vitamin B_{12}, mcg	6.9	12.7	12	13
Niacin, mg	23	42	40	43
Folic acid, mcg	455	340	800	640
Panthothenic acid, mg	12	21	20	21
Biotin, mcg	345	250	600	480
Vitamin C (ascorbic acid), mg	230	250	240	320
Choline, mg	455	420	550	540
Minerals				
Calcium, mg	760	850	1,000	1,070
Phosphorus, mg	760	850	1,000	1,070
Magnesium, mg	115	340	400	430
Iron, mg	54	15.2	18	19
Zinc, mg	14	16.9	21	32
Manganese, mg	3.8	2.5	4	2.1
Copper, mg	1.6	1.69	2	2.1
Iodine, mcg	115	127	150	160
Sodium, mg	930	930	1,350	1,290
Potassium, mg	1,570	1,610	1,850	2,250
Chloride, mg	1,440	1,440	1,500	1,610
Selenium, mcg	54	59	70	75
Chromium, mcg	91	101	120	130
Molybdenum, mcg	115	85	120	80
L-carnitine, mg	0	127	150	107
Other				
Osmolality, mOsm/kg water	200	270	390 can, 400 1 liter	650
Water, mL	920	850	810	778

* As products and product composition change frequently, always check with the manufacturer for up-to-date product information.
† Vitamin and mineral information for vanilla.
‡ When used as a sole source of nutrition, essential fatty acids, water, and ultratrace minerals should be reviewed.
§ Ready to hang.

Table A-8 Adult Formulas—Nutrients per Liter. Specialized formulas.* *(continued)*

Product name	Isosource HN	Isosource VHN	Jevity 1.2 Cal	Jevity 1.5 Cal
Manufacturer	Novartis	Novartis	Ross	Ross
Indications	Elevated protein requirements, malnutrition, inadequate oral intake	Increased protein requirements, pressure ulcers, postsurgery/wound healing, calorie restriction	General tube feeding needs	General tube feeding needs with concentrated calories
Flavor(s)	Unflavored	Unflavored	Unflavored	Unflavored
Type (powder or liquid)	Liquid	Liquid	Liquid	Liquid
Calories/mL	1.2	1	1.2	1.5
Calories	1,200	1,000	1,200	1,500
%Protein/% Fat/ %Carbohydrate	18/29/53	25/25/50	19/29/53	17/25/54
Protein, g/L	53	62	56	64
Protein Source	Soy isolate	Sodium and calcium caseinates	Sodium and calcium caseinates, soy protein isolate	Sodium and calcium caseinates, soy protein isolate
Fat, g/L	39	29	39	50
Fat source	Canola, MCT	Canola, MCT	High oleic safflower oil, canola oil, MCT oil, soy lecithin	High oleic safflower oil, canola oil, MCT, soy lecithin
Carbohydrate, g/L	160	130	172	216
Carbohydrate source	Corn syrup, hydrolyzed cornstarch	Hydrolyzed cornstarch	Maltodextrin, corn syrup solids, soy fiber, oat fiber, gum arabic	Corn syrup solids, maltodextrin, FOS, oat fiber, soy fiber
Fiber, g/L	0	10	22	22
Vitamins				
Vitamin A, IU	4,300	8,000	5,000	5,000
Vitamin D, IU	340	320	400	400
Vitamin E, IU	51	48	45	45
Vitamin K, mcg	80	64	80	80
Vitamin B_1 (thiamine), mg	1.3	2.4	2.3	2.3
Vitamin B_2 (riboflavin), mg	1.5	2.7	2.6	2.6
Vitamin B_6, mg	2	3.2	3	3
Vitamin B_{12}, mcg	5.1	9.6	9	9
Niacin, mg	17	32	30	30
Folic acid, mcg	690	480	600	600
Panthothenic acid, mg	8.6	16	15	15
Biotin, mcg	260	360	450	450
Vitamin C (ascorbic acid), mg	200	240	300	300
Choline, mg	340	400	600	600
Minerals				
Calcium, mg	1,200	800	1,200	1,200
Phosphorus, mg	1,200	800	1,200	1,200
Magnesium, mg	350	320	400	1,200
Iron, mg	15	14	18	18
Zinc, mg	19	24	23	23
Manganese, mg	1.7	1.6	5	5
Copper, mg	1.7	1.6	2	2
Iodine, mcg	150	120	150	150
Sodium, mg	1,100	1,380	1,350	1,400
Potassium, mg	1,900	1,800	1,850	1,850
Chloride, mg	1,100	1,360	1,500	1,500
Selenium, mcg	70	56	70	70
Chromium, mcg	110	96	120	120
Molybdenum, mcg	84	60	150	150
L-carnitine, mg	0	80	150	150
Other				
Osmolality, mOsm/kg water	490	300	450	525
Water, mL	818	847	805	760

* As products and product composition change frequently, always check with the manufacturer for up-to-date product information.

† Vitamin and mineral information for vanilla.

‡ When used as a sole source of nutrition, essential fatty acids, water, and ultratrace minerals should be reviewed.

§ Ready to hang.

Product name	Lipisorb	Magnacal Renal	Modulen IBD	Nepro†
Manufacturer	Novartis	Novartis	Nestle	Ross
Indications	HIV infection, inflammatory bowel disease, cystic fibrosis, short bowel syndrome, chronic pancreatitis	Hemodialysis	Crohn's disease	Dialysis for electrolyte and fluid restrictions
Flavor(s)	Vanilla	Vanilla honey graham	Natural	Vanilla, cherry supreme, butter pecan
Type (powder or liquid)	Liquid	Liquid	Powder	Liquid
Calories/mL	1.35	2	1	2
Calories	1,350	2,000	1,000	2,000
%Protein/% Fat/ %Carbohydrate	17/35/48	15/45/40	14/42/44	14/43/43
Protein, g/L	57	75	36	70
Protein Source	Calcium and sodium caseinates	Calcium and sodium caseinates	Casein	Calcium, magnesium, and sodium caseinates, milk protein isolates
Fat, g/L	57	101	46	96
Fat source	MCT and soy oils	Canola oil, high oleic sunflower oil, MCT, and corn oil	Milk, fat, MCT, corn oil, soy lecithin	High oleic safflower oil, canola oil, soy lecithin
Carbohydrate, g/L	161	200	108	223
Carbohydrate source	Maltodextrin, sugar	Maltodextrin, sugar	Corn syrup, sugar	Corn syrup solids, sugar, FOS
Fiber, g/L	< 1	< 4	0	15.6
Vitamins				
Vitamin A, IU	6,300	5,000	2,800	4,215
Vitamin D, IU	510	101	400	85
Vitamin E, IU	38	45	19.6	48
Vitamin K, mcg	101	118	52	85
Vitamin B_1 (thiamine), mg	1.9	3.8	1.16	2.6
Vitamin B_2 (riboflavin), mg	2.2	4.3	1.28	2.9
Vitamin B_6, mg	2.5	10.1	1.64	8.9
Vitamin B_{12}, mcg	7.6	14.8	3.2	11
Niacin, mg	25	50	11.6	34
Folic acid, mcg	510	800	240	1,055
Panthothenic acid, mg	12.7	25	4.8	17
Biotin, mcg	380	300	32	510
Vitamin C (ascorbic acid), mg	76	101	92	105
Choline, mg	210	500	68	635
Minerals				
Calcium, mg	850	1,010	888	1,370
Phosphorus, mg	850	800	600	695
Magnesium, mg	340	200	200	215
Iron, mg	15.2	18.2	10.8	19
Zinc, mg	16.9	20	9.2	24
Manganese, mg	2.5	3	1.95	5.3
Copper, mg	1.7	2	0.96	2.1
Iodine, mcg	127	148	96	160
Sodium, mg	1,350	800	340	845
Potassium, mg	1,690	1,270	1,200	1,055
Chloride, mg	2,200	1,180	728	1,010
Selenium, mcg	59	70	34	105
Chromium, mcg	101	118	48	0
Molybdenum, mcg	85	101	72	0
L-carnitine, mg	194	148	0	261
Other				
Osmolality, mOsm/kg water	630	570	370	665
Water, mL	800	710	875	699

* As products and product composition change frequently, always check with the manufacturer for up-to-date product information.

† Vitamin and mineral information for vanilla.

‡ When used as a sole source of nutrition, essential fatty acids, water, and ultratrace minerals should be reviewed.

§ Ready to hang.

Table A-8 Adult Formulas—Nutrients per Liter. Specialized formulas.* *(continued)*

Product name	NovaSource 2.0	Novasource Pulmonary	Novasource Renal Brik Pak	Nutren 1.5
Manufacturer	Novartis	Novartis	Novarits	Nestle
Indications	Fluid restriction/volume sensitivity, pulmonary conditions, liver disease with ascites, elevated caloric and protein needs, shortened feeding schedules	Ventilator dependency, respiratory disease, pulmonary edema, fluid restriction, COPD, ARDS	Acute renal failure, chronic renal failure, electrolyte restricted, fluid restriction	Increased energy requirements, fluid restricted
Flavor(s)	Vanilla	Unflavored	Vanilla	Unflavored, vanilla
Type (powder or liquid)	Liquid	Liquid	Liquid	Liquid
Calories/mL	2	1.5	2	1.5
Calories	2,000	1,500	2,000	1,500
%Protein/% Fat/ %Carbohydrate	18/39/43	20/40/40	15/45/40	16/39/45
Protein, g/L	85	75	74	60
Protein Source	Calcium and sodium caseinates	Sodium and calcium caseinates	Sodium and calcium caseinates, L-arginine	Calcium-potassium caseinate
Fat, g/L	88	150	100	67.6
Fat source	Canola, MCT	Canola, MCT	High oleic sunflower oil, corn oil, MCT	Canola oil, MCT, corn oil, soy lecithin
Carbohydrate, g/L	220	150	200	169
Carbohydrate source	Corn syrup, sugar, maltodextrin	Corn syrup, sugar	Corn syrup, fructose	Maltodextrin
Fiber, g/L	0	8	0	0
Vitamins				
Vitamin A, IU	5,300	10,700	3,300	4,800
Vitamin D, IU	420	430	80	400
Vitamin E, IU	127	430	45	42
Vitamin K, mcg	84	86	80	75
Vitamin B_1 (thiamine), mg	1.6	3.2	2.5	3
Vitamin B_2 (riboflavin), mg	1.8	3.6	2.9	3.6
Vitamin B_6, mg	2.1	4.3	8	6
Vitamin B_{12}, mcg	6.3	13	10	12
Niacin, mg	21	43	34	42
Folic acid, mcg	420	640	1,000	800
Panthothenic acid, mg	11	21	16	20
Biotin, mcg	320	480	500	600
Vitamin C (ascorbic acid), mg	380	540	80	212
Choline, mg	600	540	330	672
Minerals				
Calcium, mg	1,100	1,070	1,300	1,000
Phosphorus, mg	1,100	1,070	650	1,000
Magnesium, mg	420	430	200	400
Iron, mg	19	19	18	18
Zinc, mg	16	32	25	20
Manganese, mg	2.1	2.1	5	4
Copper, mg	2.1	2.1	2	2
Iodine, mcg	160	160	160	152
Sodium, mg	800	1,390	900	1,168
Potassium, mg	1,520	2,670	810	1,872
Chloride, mg	1,200	1,500	330	1,740
Selenium, mcg	74	75	100	60
Chromium, mcg	130	130	0	60
Molybdenum, mcg	79	80	0	180
L-carnitine, mg	0	110	270	120
Other				
Osmolality, mOsm/kg water	790	650	700	430 Unflavored, 410 vanilla
Water, mL	700	764	709	775

* As products and product composition change frequently, always check with the manufacturer for up-to-date product information.

† Vitamin and mineral information for vanilla.

‡ When used as a sole source of nutrition, essential fatty acids, water, and ultratrace minerals should be reviewed.

§ Ready to hang.

Product name	Nutren 2.0	NutriHep	NutriRenal	NutriVent
Manufacturer	Nestle	Nestle	Nestle	Nestle
Indications	Increased energy requirements, severely fluid restricted	Liver failure, has branched-chain amino acids	Hemodialysis patients	Pulmonary disease
Flavor(s)	Vanilla	Unflavored	Vanilla	Unflavored, vanilla
Type (powder or liquid)	Liquid	Liquid	Liquid	Liquid
Calories/mL	2	1.5	2	1.5
Calories	2,000	1,500	2,000	1,500
%Protein/% Fat/ %Carbohydrate	16/45/39	11/12/77	14/46/44	18/55/27
Protein, g/L	80	40	70	67.5
Protein Source	Calcium-potassium caseinate	Crystalline L-amino acids; whey protein concentrate	Calcium-potassium caseinate	Calcium-potassium caseinate
Fat, g/L	104	21.1	104	94
Fat source	MCT, canola oil, soy lecithin, corn oil	MCT, canola oil, corn oil, soy lecithin	MCT, canola oil, corn oil, soy lecithin	Canola oil, MCT, corn oil, soy lecithin
Carbohydrate, g/L	196	290	204	100
Carbohydrate source	Corn syrup solids, maltodextrin	Maltodextrin, modified cornstarch	Corn syrup solids, maltodextrin	Maltodextrin
Fiber, g/L	0	0	0	0
Vitamins				
Vitamin A, IU	6,400	5,000	1,664	6,000
Vitamin D, IU	532	400	100	420
Vitamin E, IU	56	30	40	42
Vitamin K, mcg	100	120	75	75
Vitamin B_1 (thiamine), mg	4	96	2.24	3
Vitamin B_2 (riboflavin), mg	4.8	1.7	2.56	3.6
Vitamin B_6, mg	8	2	10	6
Vitamin B_{12}, mcg	16	6	12	12
Niacin, mg	56	20	26.7	42
Folic acid, mcg	1,080	400	1,068	812
Panthothenic acid, mg	28	10	15.2	21.2
Biotin, mcg	800	300	400	600
Vitamin C (ascorbic acid), mg	280	96	90	210
Choline, mg	900	400	652	672
Minerals				
Calcium, mg	1,340	956	1,400	1,200
Phosphorus, mg	1,340	1,000	700	1,200
Magnesium, mg	536	376	200	480
Iron, mg	24	18	24	18
Zinc, mg	28	15.2	20	21.2
Manganese, mg	5.2	4	5.28	4
Copper, mg	2.8	2	2.68	2.12
Iodine, mcg	200	152	200	152
Sodium, mg	1,300	160	740	1170
Potassium, mg	1,920	1,320	1,256	1,872
Chloride, mg	1,876	1,144	1,140	1,740
Selenium, mcg	80	0	80	60
Chromium, mcg	80	0	80	60
Molybdenum, mcg	240	0	100	180
L-carnitine, mg	160	120	160	120
Other				
Osmolality, mOsm/kg water	745	790	650	330 unflavored, 450 vanilla
Water, mL	700	760	704	775

* As products and product composition change frequently, always check with the manufacturer for up-to-date product information.

† Vitamin and mineral information for vanilla.

‡ When used as a sole source of nutrition, essential fatty acids, water, and ultratrace minerals should be reviewed.

§ Ready to hang.

Table A-8 Adult Formulas—Nutrients per Liter. Specialized formulas.* *(continued)*

Product name	Optimental	Osmolite 1.2 Cal	Oxepa	Peptamen
Manufacturer	Ross	Ross	Ross	Nestle
Indications	Stress, trauma, Crohn's disease	For increased calorie and protein needs	For modulating inflammation in the mechanically ventilated critically ill	Gastrointestinal tract impairment, malabsorption, chronic diarrhea, delayed gastric emptying, malnutrition
Flavor(s)	Vanilla	Vanilla	Unflavored	Unflavored, vanilla
Type (powder or liquid)	Liquid	Liquid	Liquid	Liquid
Calories/mL	1	1.2	1.5	1
Calories	1,000	1,200	1,500	1,000
%Protein/% Fat/ %Carbohydrate	21/25/55	19/29/53	17/55/28	16/22/51
Protein, g/L	51.3	56	63	40
Protein Source	Soy protein hydrolysate, partially hydrolyzed sodium caseinate, L-arginine	Sodium caseinate and calcium caseinate	Sodium caseinate and calcium caseinate	Enzymatically hydrolyzed whey protein
Fat, g/L	28.4	39	94	39
Fat source	Structured lipid (interesterified sardine oil, MCT), canola oil, soybean oil	High oleic safflower oil, canola oil, MCT, soy lecithin	Canola oil, MCT, refined deodorized sardine oil, borage oil	MCT, soy oil, soy lecithin
Carbohydrate, g/L	139	158	105	127
Carbohydrate source	Maltodextrin, sugar, FOS	Maltodextrin	Sugar, maltodextrin	Maltodextrin, cornstarch
Fiber, g/L	5	0	0	0
Vitamins				
Vitamin A, IU	8,290	5,000	11,910	4,300
Vitamin D, IU	285	400	425	272
Vitamin E, IU	215	45	320	30
Vitamin K, mcg	85	80	85	50
Vitamin B_1 (thiamine), mg	2.2	2.3	3.2	2
Vitamin B_2 (riboflavin), mg	2.4	2.6	3.6	2.4
Vitamin B_6, mg	2.9	3	4.3	4
Vitamin B_{12}, mcg	8.5	9	13	8
Niacin, mg	29	30	43	28
Folic acid, mcg	565	600	850	540
Panthothenic acid, mg	15	15	22	14
Biotin, mcg	425	450	635	400
Vitamin C (ascorbic acid), mg	215	300	850	340
Choline, mg	425	600	635	452
Minerals				
Calcium, mg	1,055	1,200	1,060	800
Phosphorus, mg	1,055	1,200	1,060	700
Magnesium, mg	425	400	425	300
Iron, mg	13	18	20	18
Zinc, mg	16	23	24	24
Manganese, mg	3.6	5	5.3	2.8
Copper, mg	1.5	2	2.2	2
Iodine, mcg	160	150	160	148
Sodium, mg	1,055	1,420	1,310	560
Potassium, mg	1,760	1,940	1,960	1,500
Chloride, mg	1,355	1,540	1,690	1,000
Selenium, mcg	50	70	74	50
Chromium, mcg	85	120	130	40
Molybdenum, mcg	110	150	160	120
L-carnitine, mg	110	150	185	100
Other				
Osmolality, mOsm/kg water	540	360	535	270 unflavored, 380 vanilla
Water, mL	832	820	785	848

* As products and product composition change frequently, always check with the manufacturer for up-to-date product information.
† Vitamin and mineral information for vanilla.
‡ When used as a sole source of nutrition, essential fatty acids, water, and ultratrace minerals should be reviewed.
§ Ready to hang.

Product name	Peptamen 1.5	Peptamen VHP	Peptamen with Prebio	Peptinex Brik Pak
Manufacturer	Nestle	Nestle	Nestle	Novartis
Indications	Gastrointestinal tract impairment, malabsorption, chronic diarrhea, delayed gastric emptying, malnutrition, fluid restriction, elevated protein needs, shortened feeding schedule	Gastrointestinal tract impairment, elevated protein needs, critical illness, protein-losing enteropathy	Gastrointestinal tract impairment, malabsorption, chronic diarrhea, delayed gastric emptying, malnutrition	Bowel resection, malabsorption syndrome, Crohn's disease, GI enterocutaneous fistula, pancreatic disorders, short bowel syndrome, GI disorders related to AIDS
Flavor(s)	Unflavored, vanilla	Unflavored, vanilla	Vanilla	Vanilla
Type (powder or liquid)	Liquid	Liquid	Liquid	Liquid
Calories/mL	1.5	1	1	1
Calories	1,500	1,000	1,000	1,000
%Protein/% Fat/ %Carbohydrate	18/33/49	25/33/42	16/33/51	20/15/65
Protein, g/L	67.6	62.5	40	50
Protein Source	Enzymatically hydrolyzed whey protein	Enzymatically hydrolyzed whey protein	Enzymatically hydrolyzed whey protein	Whey protein hydrolysate
Fat, g/L	56	39	39	17
Fat source	MCT, soy oil, soy lecithin	MCT, soy oil, soy lecithin	MCT, soy oil, soy lecithin	MCT, soybean oil, soy lecithin
Carbohydrate, g/L	188	104.5	127	160
Carbohydrate source	Maltodextrin, cornstarch	Maltodextrin, cornstarch, guar gum	Maltodextrin, cornstarch, inulin, oligofructose	Hydrolyzed cornstarch
Fiber, g/L	0	0	4	0
Vitamins				
Vitamin A, IU	6,460	4,300	4,300	3,330
Vitamin D, IU	408	272	272	270
Vitamin E, IU	45	30	30	26
Vitamin K, mcg	18.8	50	50	53
Vitamin B_1 (thiamine), mg	3	2	2	1.7
Vitamin B_2 (riboflavin), mg	3.6	2.4	2.4	1.9
Vitamin B_6, mg	6	4	4	2.3
Vitamin B_{12}, mcg	12	8	8	6.8
Niacin, mg	42	28	28	23
Folic acid, mcg	812	540	540	450
Panthothenic acid, mg	21	14	14	11
Biotin, mcg	600	400	400	340
Vitamin C (ascorbic acid), mg	512	340	340	170
Choline, mg	676	450	452	230
Minerals				
Calcium, mg	1,000	800	800	670
Phosphorus, mg	1,000	700	700	670
Magnesium, mg	400	300	300	270
Iron, mg	27	18	18	12
Zinc, mg	36	24	24	13
Manganese, mg	4	2.8	2.8	1.7
Copper, mg	3	2	2	1.3
Iodine, mcg	225	150	148	100
Sodium, mg	1,020	560	560	1,010
Potassium, mg	1,860	1,500	1,500	1,490
Chloride, mg	1,740	1,000	1,000	830
Selenium, mcg	76	50	50	61
Chromium, mcg	60	40	40	100
Molybdenum, mcg	180	120	120	65
L-carnitine, mg	150	100	100	100
Other				
Osmolality, mOsm/kg water	550 unflavored, 550 vanilla	270 unflavored, 380 vanilla	300	320
Water, mL	771	844	848	828

* As products and product composition change frequently, always check with the manufacturer for up-to-date product information.

† Vitamin and mineral information for vanilla.

‡ When used as a sole source of nutrition, essential fatty acids, water, and ultratrace minerals should be reviewed.

§ Ready to hang.

Table A-8 Adult Formulas—Nutrients per Liter. Specialized formulas.* *(continued)*

Product name	Peptinex DT	Perative	Probalance	Promote
Manufacturer	Novartis	Ross	Nestle	Ross
Indications	Bowel resection, malabsorption syndrome, Crohn's disease, GI enterocutaneous fistula, pancreatic disorders, short bowel syndrome, GI disorders related to AIDS	Metabolic stress, wounds, burns, surgery	Volume sensitivity, increased energy or protein needs, dietary management of diarrhea and constipation	For risk of protein-energy malnutrition or pressure ulcers, increased protein needs
Flavor(s)	Unflavored	Unflavored	Unflavored, vanilla	Vanilla
Type (powder or liquid)	Liquid	Liquid	Liquid	Liquid
Calories/mL	1	1.3	1.2	1
Calories	1,000	1,300	1,200	1,000
%Protein/% Fat/ %Carbohydrate	20/15/65	21/25/55	18/30/52	25/23/52
Protein, g/L	50	67	54	63
Protein Source	Casein hydrolysate, free amino acids	Partially hydrolyzed sodium caseinate, lactalbumin hydrolysate, L-arginine	Calcium-potassium caseinate	Sodium and calcium caseinates, soy protein isolate
Fat, g/L	17.4	37	40.8	26
Fat source	MCT, soybean oil	Canola oil, MCT, corn oil, soy lecithin	Canola oil, MCT, corn oil, soy lecithin	High oleic safflower oil, MCT, soy lecithin
Carbohydrate, g/L	164	180	156	130
Carbohydrate source	Maltodextrin, food starch modified	Maltodextrin	Maltodextrin, soy polysaccharides, gum arabic	Maltodextrin, sugar
Fiber, g/L	0	6.5	10	0
Vitamins				
Vitamin A, IU	3,300	8,675	10,667	7,250
Vitamin D, IU	270	350	600	400
Vitamin E, IU	20	40	100	45
Vitamin K, mcg	53	70	80	80
Vitamin B_1 (thiamine), mg	1.7	2	2.24	2.3
Vitamin B_2 (riboflavin), mg	1.9	2.3	2.56	2.6
Vitamin B_6, mg	2.2	2.6	4	3
Vitamin B_{12}, mcg	6.7	7.9	12	9
Niacin, mg	22	27	40	30
Folic acid, mcg	440	520	1,200	600
Panthothenic acid, mg	11	14	15	15
Biotin, mcg	330	395	400	450
Vitamin C (ascorbic acid), mg	67	260	240	345
Choline, mg	220	520	452	600
Minerals				
Calcium, mg	670	870	1,250	1,200
Phosphorus, mg	670	870	1,000	1,200
Magnesium, mg	270	350	400	400
Iron, mg	12	16	18	18
Zinc, mg	13	20	24	24
Manganese, mg	1.3	4.4	4	5
Copper, mg	1.3	1.8	2	2
Iodine, mcg	110	135	150	150
Sodium, mg	1,700	1,040	764	1,000
Potassium, mg	800	1,735	1,560	1,980
Chloride, mg	800	1,650	1,296	1,260
Selenium, mcg	47	61	80	70
Chromium, mcg	80	105	100	120
Molybdenum, mcg	50	135	150	150
L-carnitine, mg	67	135	100	150
Other				
Osmolality, mOsm/kg water	460	460	350 unflavored, 450 vanilla	340
Water, mL	830	790	810	837

* As products and product composition change frequently, always check with the manufacturer for up-to-date product information.

† Vitamin and mineral information for vanilla.

‡ When used as a sole source of nutrition, essential fatty acids, water, and ultratrace minerals should be reviewed.

§ Ready to hang.

Product name	Promote with Fiber	Protain XL	Pulmocare†	Renalcal
Manufacturer	Ross	Novartis	Ross	Nestle
Indications	For risk of protein-energy malnutrition or pressure ulcers, increased protein needs	Pressure sores, surgical wounds, burns, tramua	COPD, cystic fibrosis, respiratory failure	Acute renal failure, electrolyte sensitivity
Flavor(s)	Vanilla	Unflavored	Vanilla, strawberry	Unflavored
Type (powder or liquid)	Liquid	Liquid	Liquid	Liquid
Calories/mL	1	1	1.5	2
Calories	1,000	1,000	1,500	2,000
%Protein/% Fat/ %Carbohydrate	25/25/50	22/26/52	17/55/28	7/35/58
Protein, g/L	63	57	63	34.4
Protein Source	Sodium and calcium caseinates	Sodium and calcium caseinates	Sodium and calcium caseinates	Whey protein source, amino acid blend
Fat, g/L	28	30	93	82.4
Fat source	High oleic safflower oil, canola oil, MCT, soy lecithin	Canola oil, high oleic sunflower oil, MCT, and corn oil	Canola oil, MCT, corn oil, high oleic safflower oil, soy lecithin	MCT, canola oil, corn oil, soy lecithin
Carbohydrate, g/L	138	145	106	290.4
Carbohydrate source	Maltodextrin, sugar, oat fiber, soy fiber	Maltodextrin, soy fiber, and microcrystalline cellulose	Sugar, maltodextrin	Maltodextrin, cornstarch
Fiber, g/L	14.4	9.1	0	0
Vitamins				
Vitamin A, IU	7,250	7,000	11,760	0
Vitamin D, IU	400	400	425	0
Vitamin E, IU	45	77	85	0
Vitamin K, mcg	80	120	85	0
Vitamin B_1 (thiamine), mg	2.3	2.4	3.2	1.52
Vitamin B_2 (riboflavin), mg	2.6	2.7	3.6	1.72
Vitamin B_6, mg	3	3.2	4.3	7
Vitamin B_{12}, mcg	9	15	13	6
Niacin, mg	30	32	43	20
Folic acid, mcg	600	480	850	600
Panthothenic acid, mg	15	12	22	10
Biotin, mcg	450	360	635	300
Vitamin C (ascorbic acid), mg	345	240	320	60
Choline, mg	600	500	635	400
Minerals				
Calcium, mg	1,200	800	1,060	0
Phosphorus, mg	1,200	800	1,060	0
Magnesium, mg	400	320	425	0
Iron, mg	18	18	20	0
Zinc, mg	24	30	24	14
Manganese, mg	5	6	5.3	0
Copper, mg	2	2.4	2.2	0
Iodine, mcg	150	150	160	0
Sodium, mg	1,300	920	1,310	0
Potassium, mg	1,980	1,760	1,960	0
Chloride, mg	1,260	1,350	1,690	0
Selenium, mcg	70	100	77	50
Chromium, mcg	120	150	130	0
Molybdenum, mcg	150	150	165	0
L-carnitine, mg	150	150	160	100
Other				
Osmolality, mOsm/kg water	380	340	475	600
Water, mL	830	830	785	700

* As products and product composition change frequently, always check with the manufacturer for up-to-date product information.
† Vitamin and mineral information for vanilla.
‡ When used as a sole source of nutrition, essential fatty acids, water, and ultratrace minerals should be reviewed.
§ Ready to hang.

Table A-8 Adult Formulas—Nutrients per Liter. Specialized formulas.* *(continued)*

Product name	**Replete**	**Replete with Fiber**	**RESOURCE Diabetic§**	**Respalor**
Manufacturer	Nestle	Nestle	Novartis	Novartis
Indications	Wound healing, increased protein needs	Wound healing, increased protein needs	Diabetes mellitus, glucose intolerace, stress-induced hyperglycemia	Limited respiratory function, COPD patients, ventilator-dependent patients
Flavor(s)	Unflavored, vanilla	Unflavored, vanilla	Vanilla, chocolate, strawberry Brik pak	Vanilla
Type (powder or liquid)	Liquid	Liquid	Liquid	Liquid
Calories/mL	1	1	1.06	1.5
Calories	1,000	1,000	1,060	1,500
%Protein/% Fat/ %Carbohydrate	25/30/45	25/30/45	24/40/36	20/40/40
Protein, g/L	62.4	62.4	63	75
Protein Source	Calcium-potassium caseinate	Calcium-potassium caseinate	Sodium and calcium caseinates, soy protein isolate	Sodium and calcium caseinates
Fat, g/L	34	34	47	68
Fat source	Canola oil, MCT, soy lecithin	Canola oil, MCT, soy lecithin	High oleic sunflower oil, Soybean oil	Canola oil, MCT, high oleic sunflower oil, and corn oil
Carbohydrate, g/L	113	113	100	146
Carbohydrate source	Maltodextrin	Maltodextrin, soy polysaccharides	Hydrolyzed cornstarch	Maltodextrin, sugar (in can version)
Fiber, g/L	0	14	12.8	none
Vitamins				
Vitamin A, IU	5,000	5,000	5,100	7,000
Vitamin D, IU	272	272	340	400
Vitamin E, IU	60	60	140	84
Vitamin K, mcg	50	50	68	80
Vitamin B_1 (thiamine), mg	3	3	1.3	3
Vitamin B_2 (riboflavin), mg	2.4	2.4	1.4	3.4
Vitamin B_6, mg	4	4	1.7	4
Vitamin B_{12}, mcg	8	8	5.1	12
Niacin, mg	28	28	17	40
Folic acid, mcg	540	540	340	800
Panthothenic acid, mg	14	14	8.5	20
Biotin, mcg	400	400	250	600
Vitamin C (ascorbic acid), mg	340	340	420	300
Choline, mg	452	452	470	600
Minerals				
Calcium, mg	1,000	1,000	1,100	1,000
Phosphorus, mg	1,000	1,000	1,100	1,000
Magnesium, mg	400	400	340	400
Iron, mg	18	18	15	18
Zinc, mg	24	24	13	24
Manganese, mg	4	4	1.7	4
Copper, mg	2	2	1.7	2
Iodine, mcg	160	160	130	150
Sodium, mg	876	876	1,230	1,270
Potassium, mg	1,500	1,500	1,360	1,480
Chloride, mg	1,300	1,300	930	1,690
Selenium, mcg	100	100	59	84
Chromium, mcg	140	140	100	120
Molybdenum, mcg	220	220	64	120
L-carnitine, mg	100	100	110	180
Other				
Osmolality, mOsm/kg water	300 unflavored, 350 vanilla	310 unflavored, 390 vanilla	300	400
Water, mL	845	835	847	780

* As products and product composition change frequently, always check with the manufacturer for up-to-date product information.

† Vitamin and mineral information for vanilla.

‡ When used as a sole source of nutrition, essential fatty acids, water, and ultratrace minerals should be reviewed.

§ Ready to hang.

Product name	Subdue§	Subdue Plus	Suplena	TOLEREX
Manufacturer	Novartis	Novartis	Ross	Novartis
Indications	Malabsorption/ maldigestion, GI surgery, Crohn's disease, chronic diarrhea, pancreatic disorders, short bowel syndrome, inflammatory bowel disease	Malabsorption/ maldigestion, fluid or volume restrictions, trauma, pancreatic insufficiency, increased caloric needs	Chronic or acute kidney failure without dialysis	Impaired digestion and absorption, specialized nutrient needs
Flavor(s)	Unflavored, chocolate, orange vanilla	Unflavored	Vanilla	Unflavored
Type (powder or liquid)	Liquid	Liquid	Liquid	Powder
Calories/mL	1	1.5	2	1
Calories	1,000	1,500	2,000	1,000
%Protein/% Fat/ %Carbohydrate	20/30/50	20/30/50	6/43/51	8/1/91
Protein, g/L	50	76	30	21
Protein Source	Hydrolyzed whey protein concentrate (cans), casein hydrolysate (1 liter bottle)	Hydrolyzed whey protein concentrate	Sodium caseinate, calcium caseinate	Free amino acids
Fat, g/L	34	51	96	1.5
Fat source	MCT, canola, high oleic sunflower and corn oils, and milk fat (in 1 liter bottles)	MCT, canola, high oleic sunflower and corn oils, and milk fat	High oleic safflower oil, soy oil, soy lecithin	Safflower oil
Carbohydrate, g/L	130	186	255	230
Carbohydrate source	Maltodextrin, modified cornstarch, sugar (in flavor versions)	Maltodextrin, modified cornstarch	Maltodextrin, sugar	Maltodextrin, modified cornstarch
Fiber, g/L	none	none	0	0
Vitamins				
Vitamin A, IU	4,250	5,400	1,060	2,780
Vitamin D, IU	500	630	85	220
Vitamin E, IU	89	127	48	17
Vitamin K, mcg	84	127	85	44
Vitamin B_1 (thiamine), mg	1.28	1.6	2.6	0.83
Vitamin B_2 (riboflavin), mg	1.45	1.8	2.9	0.94
Vitamin B_6, mg	2.5	2.1	8.5	1.1
Vitamin B_{12}, mcg	7.5	6.3	11	3.3
Niacin, mg	17	21	34	11
Folic acid, mcg	500	420	1,060	220
Panthothenic acid, mg	8.5	10.6	17	5
Biotin, mcg	255	320	510	170
Vitamin C (ascorbic acid), mg	150	250	106	33
Choline, mg	350	590	635	41
Minerals				
Calcium, mg	1,100	1,390	1,390	560
Phosphorus, mg	1,050	1,310	730	560
Magnesium, mg	360	440	215	220
Iron, mg	15.3	19	19	10
Zinc, mg	15.8	16.1	24	8.3
Manganese, mg	2.5	440	5.3	1.1
Copper, mg	1.7	2.1	2.1	1.1
Iodine, mcg	128	161	160	89
Sodium, mg	1,100	1,180	790	470
Potassium, mg	1,600	2,000	1,120	1,170
Chloride, mg	1,400	1,820	935	950
Selenium, mcg	70	76	78	39
Chromium, mcg	110	127	0	67
Molybdenum, mcg	110	80	0	42
L-carnitine, mg	80	101	158	0
Other				
Osmolality, mOsm/kg water	330 unflavored can, 525 flavored versions, 440 1 liter bottle	400	600	550
Water, mL	840	760	713	864

* As products and product composition change frequently, always check with the manufacturer for up-to-date product information.
† Vitamin and mineral information for vanilla.
‡ When used as a sole source of nutrition, essential fatty acids, water, and ultratrace minerals should be reviewed.
§ Ready to hang.

Table A-8 Adult Formulas—Nutrients per Liter. Specialized formulas.* *(continued)*

Product name	TraumaCal	TwoCal HN	Ultracal HN Plus	Vital HN
Manufacturer	Novartis	Ross	Novartis	Ross
Indications	Hypermetabolic states, ventilator dependence, cancer	Increased calorie and protein needs, low-volume feedings	General tube-feeding needs, inadequate oral intake, malnutrition, barriers to normal ingestion, need for fiber	Chronically impaired gastrointestinal function, maldigestion, malabsorption
Flavor(s)	Vanilla	Vanilla, butter pecan	Unflavored	Vanilla
Type (powder or liquid)	Liquid	Liquid	Liquid	Powder
Calories/mL	1.5	2	1.2	1
Calories	1,500	2,000	1,200	1,000
%Protein/% Fat/ %Carbohydrate	22/40/38	17/40/43	18/29/53	17/10/74
Protein, g/L	82	84	54	42
Protein Source	Calcium and sodium caseinates	Sodium and calcium caseinates	Milk protein concentrate, casein (in ready to hang only)	Partially hydrolyzed whey, meat, and soy protein, free amino acids
Fat, g/L	68	91	40	11
Fat source	Soy and MCT oils	High oleic safflower oil, MCT, canola oil, soy lecithin	Canola oil, MCT, high oleic sunflower oil, and corn oil	Safflower oil, MCT
Carbohydrate, g/L	144	219	156	185
Carbohydrate source	Corn syrup, sugar	Corn syrup, maltodextrin, sugar, FOS	Maltodextrin, microcrystalline cellulose, soy fiber, and acacia	Maltodextrin, sugar
Fiber, g/L	< 1	0	10	0
Vitamins				
Vitamin A, IU	2,500	5,270	5,000	3,332
Vitamin D, IU	200	425	400	267
Vitamin E, IU	38	51	90	30
Vitamin K, mcg	127	85	80	54
Vitamin B_1 (thiamine), mg	1.9	2.6	3	2
Vitamin B_2 (riboflavin), mg	2.2	2.9	3.4	2.3
Vitamin B_6, mg	2.5	3.4	4	2.7
Vitamin B_{12}, mcg	7.5	10	12	8
Niacin, mg	25	34	40	26.7
Folic acid, mcg	200	675	800	533
Panthothenic acid, mg	12.7	17	20	13.4
Biotin, mcg	148	510	600	400
Vitamin C (ascorbic acid), mg	148	320	240	200
Choline, mg	250	635	550	400
Minerals				
Calcium, mg	750	1,050	1,000	667
Phosphorus, mg	750	1,050	1,000	667
Magnesium, mg	200	425	400	267
Iron, mg	8.9	19	18	12
Zinc, mg	14.8	24	21	15
Manganese, mg	2.5	5.3	4	3.4
Copper, mg	1.5	2.1	2	1.4
Iodine, mcg	75	160	150	100
Sodium, mg	1,180	1,450	1,350	566
Potassium, mg	1,390	2,440	1,850	1,400
Chloride, mg	1,610	1,810	1,500	1,032
Selenium, mcg	0	74	70	47
Chromium, mcg	0	130	120	67
Molybdenum, mcg	0	160	120	100
L-carnitine, mg	0	160	150	0
Other				
Osmolality, mOsm/kg water	560	725	370	500
Water, mL	780	700	810	867

* As products and product composition change frequently, always check with the manufacturer for up-to-date product information.

† Vitamin and mineral information for vanilla.

‡ When used as a sole source of nutrition, essential fatty acids, water, and ultratrace minerals should be reviewed.

§ Ready to hang.

Product name	VIVONEX PLUS	VIVONEX RTF	VIVONEX T.E.N.
Manufacturer	Novartis	Novartis	Novartis
Indications	Bowel resection, irradiated bowel, malabsorption syndrome, trauma, surgery, Crohn's disease, GI enterocutaneous fistula, pancreatic disorders	Bowel resection, irradiated bowel, malabsorption syndrome, trauma, surgery, Crohn's disease, GI enterocutaneous fistula, pancreatic disorders	Bowel resection, irradiated bowel, malabsorption syndrome, trauma, surgery, Crohn's disease, GI enterocutaneous fistula, pancreatic disorders
Flavor(s)	Unflavored	Unflavored	Unfavored
Type (powder or liquid)	Powder	Liquid	Powder
Calories/mL	1	1	1
Calories	1,000	1,000	1,000
%Protein/% Fat/ %Carbohydrate	18/6/76	20/10/70	15/3/82
Protein, g/L	45	50	38
Protein Source	Free amino acids	Free amino acids	Free amino acids
Fat, g/L	6.7	12	2.8
Fat source	Soybean oil	Soybean oil, MCT	Safflower oil
Carbohydrate, g/L	190	175	210
Carbohydrate source	Maltodextrin, modified cornstarch	Maltodextrin, modified cornstarch	Maltodextrin, modified cornstarch
Fiber, g/L	0	0	0
Vitamins			
Vitamin A, IU	2,780	3,300	2,500
Vitamin D, IU	220	270	200
Vitamin E, IU	17	20	15
Vitamin K, mcg	44	53	40
Vitamin B_1 (thiamine), mg	1.7	1.7	1.5
Vitamin B_2 (riboflavin), mg	1.9	1.9	1.7
Vitamin B_6, mg	2.2	2.2	2
Vitamin B_{12}, mcg	6.7	6.7	6
Niacin, mg	22	22	20
Folic acid, mcg	440	440	400
Panthothenic acid, mg	11	11	10
Biotin, mcg	330	330	300
Vitamin C (ascorbic acid), mg	67	67	60
Choline, mg	220	220	200
Minerals			
Calcium, mg	560	670	500
Phosphorus, mg	560	670	500
Magnesium, mg	220	270	200
Iron, mg	10	12	9
Zinc, mg	13	13	11
Manganese, mg	1.1	1.3	1
Copper, mg	1.1	1.3	1
Iodine, mcg	89	110	80
Sodium, mg	610	670	600
Potassium, mg	1,060	800	950
Chloride, mg	940	800	850
Selenium, mcg	39	47	35
Chromium, mcg	67	80	60
Molybdenum, mcg	42	50	38
L-carnitine, mg	67	67	60
Other			
Osmolality, mOsm/kg water	650	630	630
Water, mL	850	848	853

* As products and product composition change frequently, always check with the manufacturer for up-to-date product information.
† Vitamin and mineral information for vanilla.
‡ When used as a sole source of nutrition, essential fatty acids, water, and ultratrace minerals should be reviewed.
§ Ready to hang.

Table A-9 Modulars

	Non-Protein Additives								
Product	Duocal	Product 80056	Microlipid	MCT Oil	Safflower Oil	Moducal	Polycose	Pro-Phree	Benefiber*
Manufacturer	Nutricia, NA	Mead Johnson	Mead Johnson	Mead Johnson		Mead Johnson	Ross	Ross	Novartis
Calories	4.9/gm or 42 kcal/ level Tbsp	5.0/gm	4.5/mL	7.7/mL	9/mL	3.8/gm	3.8/gm Powder 2.0/mL Liquid	5.1/gm	16/Tbsp
Fat Source	Corn, Coconut, MCT Oils	Corn Oil	Safflower Oil	Fractionated Coconut Oil	Safflower	None	None	Palm, Coconut, Soy Oils	None
Carbohydrate Source	Hydrolyzed Cornstarch	Corn Syrup Solids, Modified Tapioca Starch	None	None	None	Maltodextrin	Glucose Polymers	Hydrolyzed Cornstarch	Partially Hydrogenated Guar Gum

*Benefiber contains 3 gm of fiber per Tbsp.

	Protein Additives			
Product	Casec	ProMod	Beneprotein	Complete Amino Acid Module
Manufacturer	Novartis	Ross	Novartis	Nutricia, NA
Calories	17 kcal/ level Tbsp	28 kcal/scoop or 15.5 kcal/Tbsp	25 kcal/scoop or 17/Tbsp	31 kcal/ Tbsp or 3.3 kcal/gm
Protein	4.0 gm/ Tbsp	5.0 gm/scoop or 3.0 gm/ Tbsp	6.0 gm/scoop or 4.0 gm/Tbsp	7.8 gm/Tbsp Protein Equivalents
Source	Calcium Caseinate	Whey Protein Concentrate	Whey Protein Isolate	L-Amino Acids
Fat	Trace	Trace	None	None

It is recommended to use a gram scale with Complete Amino Acid Module instead of household measurements.

As products and product composition change frequently, always check with the manufacturer for up-to-date product information.

Table A-10 Oral Electrolyte Solutions

Oral Electrolyte Solutions						
Solution	Ceralyte-70	Ceralyte-50	Enfalyte	Pedialyte	Rehydralyte	WHO Oral Rehydration Salts
Manufacturer	Cera	Cera	Mead Johnson	Ross	Ross	Jianas
Calories/ oz	4.9	4.9	3.5	3	3	2
Carbohydrate, gm/dL	4	4	3	2.5	2.5	2
Carbohydrate Source	Rice Digest	Rice Digest	Rice Syrup Solids	Dextrose	Dextrose	Dextrose
Na mEq/dL	7	5	5	4.6	2	9
K mEq/dL	2	2	2.5	2	2	2
Osmolality	232	200	170	250	300	330

As products and product composition change frequently, always check with the manufacturer for up-to-date product information.

Table A-11 Concentrating Term Infant Formula

Concentrated formulas have a greater osmolality and renal solute load. Therefore, it is important to monitor fluid and electrolyte status in infants consuming concentrating formulas.

Concentrating Term Infant Formula		
Concentration	**Amount of Formula**	**Amount of Water**
20 kcal/oz or 0.67 kcal/cc	1 scoop powder	2 oz
	1 oz liquid concentrate	1 oz
	1 can (13 oz) liquid concentrate	13 oz
24 kcal/oz or 0.8 kcal/cc	3 scoops powder	5 oz
	3 oz liquid concentrate	2 oz
	1 can (13 oz) liquid concentrate	9 oz
27 kcal/oz or 0.9 kcal/cc	3 scoops powder	4.5 oz
	2 oz liquid concentrate	1 oz
	1 can (13 oz) liquid concentrate	6 oz
30 kcal/oz or 1.0 kcal/cc	3 scoops powder	4 oz
	3 oz liquid concentrate	1 oz
	1 can (13 oz) liquid concentrate	4 oz

*The above table is a guideline to prepare the approximate concentrations. Please contact the specific formula manufacturer for the most accurate guidelines. Note that scoop size may vary from company to company.

As products and product composition change frequently, always check with the manufacturer for up-to-date product information.

Table A-12 Manufacturer Contact Information

Manufacturer	Telephone	Website
Cera Products, LLC.	1-888-237-2598	www.ceraproductsinc.com
Jianas Brothers, Co.	1-866-421-2880	not available
Mead Johnson Nutritionals	1-800-222-9123	www.meadjohnson.com
Nestle, USA, Inc.	1-800-628-2229	www.verybestbaby.com
Novartis Nutrition Corporation	1-800-333-3785	www.novartisnutrition.com
Ross Producers Division, Abbott Laboratories	1-800-227-5767	www.ross.com
Nutricia, NA	1-800-365-7354	www.shsna.com
Wyeth Nutrition	1-800-272-5095	www.storebrandformulas.com www.brightbeginnings.com www.parentschoiceformula.com

Appendix B

Karen Hauff

Table B-1 Recommendations for administration of drugs with possible food-drug interactions.

Drug	*Proposed mechanism*	*Effect of drug*	*Recommendation*
ACE inhibitors (captopril, enalapril, lisinapril)	Possible decreased absorption	No change in hemodynamic effects	Give 1 hour before or 2 hours after a meal or snack; avoid salt substitutes
Ampicillin	Acid labile	Risk of treatment failure at low dose	Give 1 hour before or 2 hours after a meal or snack
Azithromycin (capsule)	Acid labile	Risk of treatment failure	Give 1 hour before or 2 hours after a meal or snack. Note: The tablets and suspension are unaffected by food
Carbamazepine	Absorption favored by bile secretion	Fluctuations in drug effect	Give with consistent relationship to meals
Cephalexin	Acid labile	In young children, might decrease antibacterial activity	Give 1 hour before or 2 hours after a meal or snack; do not give with milk/formula
Ciprofloxacin	Chelation	Risk of treatment failure	Do not give within 2 hours of dairy products or enteral feeds
Cyclosporine	Increased absorption	Drug toxicity	Give at the same time in relation to meals; avoid grapefruit juice
Digoxin	Binds to fiber/ decreased absorption	Change in dietary fiber intake may require dosage adjustment	Give 0.5–1 hour before or 4 hours after bran fiber. Take consistently with or without food.
Erythromycin enteric coated	Acid labile	Risk of treatment failure	Give 1 hour before or 2 hours after a meal or snack
Erythromycin ethyl succinate	Stimulates smooth muscle and gastrointestinal motility leading to the potential for abdomimal pain and cramping	Gastrointestinal irritation	May give without regard to meals unless symptoms occur. Then give with meal or snack since ESS is less susceptible to gastrointestinal acid

Drug	*Proposed mechanism*	*Effect of drug*	*Recommendation*
Erythromycin stearate	Acid labile	Little risk of treatment failure	Give 1 hour before or 2 hours after a meal or snack
Fluoroquinolone	Complexation/ chelation with divalent cations	Risk of treatment failure	Do not give within 2 hours of iron, magnesium, zinc, calcium supplements; dairy products or enteral feedings
Furosemide	Decreased intestinal absorption	Possible reduction in diuretic response	Give 1 hour before or 2 hours after a meal or snack
Gabapentin	Carrier trans-stimulation effect has been proposed	Increased absorption with milk products	May administer without regard to food intake unless inadequate response to therapy
Ganciclovir	Bioavailability may be enhanced	Possible increase in drug effect	Give with food
Griseofulvin	Absorption favored by bile secretion	Treatment failure	Give with food to prevent treatment failure especially in children
Hydralazine	Change in bioavailability	Fluctuations in bioavailability and drug effect	Give with a consistent relationship to meals
Indinavir	Bound by protein to decrease absorption	High risk of treatment failure	Give 1 hour before or 2 hours after a meal or snack
Isoniazid	Delayed or decreased absorption; acid labile	Risk of treatment failure	Give 1 hour before or 2 hours after a meal or snack
Itraconazole capsules	Depends on gastric acid for solubility	Decreased clinical response	Give with a meal
Itraconazole solution. Note: Effect does not occur with capsules	Food increases first-pass metabolism	Maximum and steady state concentrations and AUC may be lowered	Give 1 hour before or 2 hours after a meal or snack
Levothyroxine	Decreased absorption	Decreased clinical response	Give 1 hour before or 2 hours after a meal or snack

Table B-1 Recommendations for administration of drugs with possible food-drug interactions. *(continued)*

Drug	*Proposed mechanism*	*Effect of drug*	*Recommendation*
Monoamine oxidase inhibitors	Blocked deamination of dietary pressor amines	Hypertensive crisis	Give without tyramine-containing food
Melphalan	Competition with dietary amino acids	Risk of treatment failure	Give 1 hour before or 2 hours after a meal or snack
Mercaptopurine	Food causes oxidation into inactive metabolites	Treatment failure	Give 1 hour before or 2 hours after a meal or snack
Methotrexate	Unknown	Risk of treatment failure in children only	Give 1 hour before or 2 hours after a meal or snack
Mycophenolate	Decreased absorption	Treatment failure	Give 1 hour before or 2 hours after a meal or snack
Nifedipine	Decreased absorption rate. Increase in serum concentration caused by inhibition of metabolism	Reduced incidence of adverse effects. Risk of hypotension	Give with a meal or snack Avoid use of grapefruit juice
Nifedipine sustained release	Absorption favored by bile secretion	Food increases hypotensive effect	Give with a consistent relationship to meals
Norfloxacin	Chelation	Risk of treatment failure	Do not administer with milk
NSAIDs	Affects mucosal integrety	Decreased incidence of gastrointestinal side effects	Give with a meal, snack, or milk
Ondansetron	Unknown	None	Give with a meal or snack
Penicillins	Decreased absorption, acid labile	Treatment failure not likely	Give 1 hour before meal or 2 hours after a meal or snack
Phenytoin oral suspension	Chelation/binding to protein components or decreased absorption	High risk of treatment failure	Withhold enteral feeds 2 hours before and after administration
Potassium salts	Food decreases irritation	Risk of gastrointestinal irritation	Give with meal
Potassium-sparing diuretics	Potentiation of increase in serum potassium level	Risk of hyperkalemia	Avoid use of potassium containing salt substitute and excessive potassium intake

Drug	*Proposed mechanism*	*Effect of drug*	*Recommendation*
Pravastatin	Food increase conversion into inactive metabolite	No change in lipid-lowering capacity	None
Rifampin	Food increases first-pass metabolism	Treatment failure is unlikely at higher doses	Give 1 hour before or 2 hours after a meal or snack
Saquinavir	Food increases dissolution	High risk of treatment failure	Give with a meal
Sirolimus	High fat meal increases AUC	Fluctuation of drug levels	Give with consistent relationship to meals
Spironolactone	Pharmacodynamic interaction	Risk of hyperkalemia	Avoid excessive potassium intake
Sucralfate	Binding to protein components of food	Decreased effectiveness	Give 1 hour before or 2 hours after a meal or snack
Tacrolimus	Increased solubility with fat intake	Fluctuations in drug effect	Give with consistent relationship to meals
Theophylline	Decreased hepatic clearance	Monitor serum concentrations	Give with high-carbohydrate/low-protein diet
Theophylline sustained release	Dose dumping with older preparations	Risk of toxicity	Give 1 hour before and 2 hours after a meal or snack, monitor serum concentrations
Warfarin	Antagonism of effect due to vitamin K content of food	Antagonism of the effect of warfarin	Maintain diet balanced in vitamin K content
Zidovudine	Decreased absorption	May decrease peak plasma concentration	May administer without regard to meals unless inadequate response. Then give 1 hour before and 2 hours after a meal or snack.

NAD = Nicotinamide adenine dinucleotide; NSAID = Nonsteroidal anti-inflammatory drug; AUC = area under the curve

Table B-2 Sugar and sorbitol content of selected medications.

Medication	*Sugar content (sucrose, corn syrup, lactulose, fructose, or glucose) gm/5 mL*	*Sorbitol content in gm/5 mL*
Acetaminophen elixir (Tylenol) 160 mg/5 mL; McNeil	1.6	1
Acetaminophen with codeine (Tylenol with codeine) McNeil	3	0
Acetaminophen liquid (Tylenol) 500 mg/mL; McNeil	5.49	1
Acetaminophen suspension (Tylenol) 160 mg/5 mL; McNeil	3.7	1
Acyclovir suspension (Zovirax) 200 mg/5 mL; GlaxoSmithKline	0	0.3
Aluminum hydroxide gel (Alternagel) Johnson & Johnson-Merck	0	0.6
Aluminum with magnesium hydroxide (Gaviscon liquid) Marion Merrell Dow	5.55	0.36
Aluminum with magnesium hydroxide (Maalox) Rorer	0	0.225
Aluminum with magnesium hydroxide (Maalox Extra Strength Plus) Rorer	0	0.5
Aluminum with magnesium hydroxide (Maalox TC) Rorer	0	0.75
Amantadine solution (Symmetrel) 50 mg/5 mL	0	3.6
Aminocaproic acid syrup (Amicar) 250 mg/mL; Xanodyne	0	0.7
Amoxicillin suspension 125 mg/5 mL; Biocraft	2	0
Amoxicillin suspension 250 mg/5 mL; Biocraft	3	0
Amoxicillin suspension 125 mg/5 mL; Lederle	2.08	0
Amoxicillin suspension 250 mg/5 mL; Lederle	1.923	0
Ampicillin suspension 125 mg/5 mL; Lederle	4.021	0

Medication	*Sugar content (sucrose, corn syrup, lactulose, fructose, or glucose) gm/5 mL*	*Sorbitol content in gm/5 mL*
Ampicillin suspension 250 mg/5 mL; Lederle	4.024	0
Azithromycin suspension (Zithromax) 100 mg/5 mL; Pfizer	3.86	0
Azithromycin suspension (Zithromax) 200 mg/5 mL; Pfizer	3.87	0
Calcium carbonate suspension 1250 mg/5 mL; Roxane	0	1.4
Calcium glubionate (NeoCalglucon) 115 mg/5 mL; Sandoz	0	0.45
Carbamazepine suspension (Tegretol) 100 mg/5 mL; Novartis	2	0.6
Cefaclor suspension (Ceclor); Lilly	3	0
Cefuroxime suspension (Ceftin) 125 mg/5 mL; Glaxo	3.214	0
Cephalexin suspension Dista	3	0
Cephalexin suspension 125 mg/5 mL; Lederle	1.4	0
Cephalexin suspension 250 mg/5 mL; Lederle	1.2	0
Cephradine (Velosef) E.R. Squibb	3.3	0
Charcoal, activated (Actidose with Sorbitol) 208 mg/mL; Paddock	0	2
Chloral hydrate syrup 500 mg/5 mL; UDL Laboratories	2.5	1.4
Chlorothiazide suspension (Diuril) Merck	2	0
Cimetidine liquid (Tagamet) 300 mg/5 mL; GlaxoSmithKline	0	2.8
Cisapride suspension (Propulsid) 1 mg/mL; Janssen	0	3.85

Table B-2 Sugar and sorbitol content of selected medications. *(continued)*

Medication	*Sugar content (sucrose, corn syrup, lactulose, fructose, or glucose) gm/5 mL*	*Sorbitol content in gm/5 mL*
Clarithromycin suspension (Biaxin) 125 mg/5 mL; Abbott	3	0
Clarithromycin suspension (Biaxin) 250 mg/5 mL; Abbott	2.28	0
Clindamycin solution (Cleocin) 75 mg/5 mL; Pharmacia & Uphohn	1.825	0
Cyclosporine (Sandimmune) 100 mg/mL; Novartis	0	0
Dexamethasone oral solution Roxane	0	1.2
Diazepam solution Roxane	0	1
Digoxin elixir 50 mcg/mL; Roxane	0	1
Digoxin elixir (Lanoxin) GlaxoSmithKline	1.5	0
Diphenhydramine elixir (Benadryl) 12.5 mg/5 mL; Parke-Davis	0	2.25
EES/sulfisoxazole Lederle	2	0
EES/sulfisoxazole (Pediazole) Ross	2	0
Erythromycin ethyl succinate suspension Abbott	3.5	0
Ethosuximide syrup (Zarontin) 250 mg/5 mL; Park-Davis	3	0
Famotidine suspension (Pepcid) 40 mg/5 mL; Merck	1.186	0
Felbamate suspension (Felbatol) 600 mg/5 mL; Carter-Wallace	0	1.5
Ferrous sulfate drops (Fer-In-Sol) 25 mg Fe/mL; Mead Johnson	1.9	1.55
Ferrous sulfate syrup (Fer-In-Sol) 18 mg/5 mL; Mead Johnson	3	0.325

Medication	*Sugar content (sucrose, corn syrup, lactulose, fructose, or glucose) gm/5 mL*	*Sorbitol content in gm/5 mL*
Fluconazole suspension (Diflucan) 50 mg/5 mL; Pfizer	2.88	0
Fluconazole suspension (Diflucan) 200 mg/5 mL; Pfizer	2.73	0
Furosemide oral solution (Lasix) 10 mg/mL; Hoechst-Roussel	1.75	0
Furosemide solution 10 mg/mL and 40 mg/5 mL; Roxane	0	2.4
Hydrocortisone suspension (Cortef) Upjohn	0.4	0
Hydroxyzine suspension (Vistaril) Pfizer	0	5
Ibuprofen suspension (Advil) 100 mg/5 mL; Whitehall	0	0.5
Ibuprofen suspension (Pedi-Profen) 100 mg/5 mL; McNeil	0	1.55
L-carnitine solution (Carnitor) Sigma Tau	0.2385	0
Lactulose syrup (Cephulac) (Chronolac)	4.67	0
Lactulose Boehringer Ingleheim Roxane	3.3	0
Lorezepam (Intensol)	0	0
Metaproterenol syrup (Alupent) 10 mg/5 mL; Boehringer-Ingelheim	0	1.4
Metaproterenol syrup (Metaprel) 10 mg/5 mL; Sandoz	0	1.4
Metaproterenol syrup 10 mg/5 mL; Biocraft	0	1.7
Methadone oral solution 5 mg/5 mL; Roxane	0	0.7
Metoclopramide syrup 5 mg/5 mL; Biocraft	0	2.1
Metoclopramide syrup 5 mg/5 mL; Roxane	0	1.4

Table B-2 Sugar and sorbitol content of selected medications. *(continued)*

Medication	*Sugar content (sucrose, corn syrup, lactulose, fructose, or glucose) gm/5 mL*	*Sorbitol content in gm/5 mL*
Milk of magnesia Roxane	0.4	1
Midazolam 2 mg/mL Roxane	0	2.35
Morphine sulfate oral solution 10 mg/5 mL; Boehringer Ingelheim Roxane	0	0.7
Multivitamin liquid (Iberet 250) Abbott	0	3.61
Multivitamin liquid (Iberet 500) Abbott	0.62	2.1
Multivitamins (Vi-Daylin liquid) Ross	0.778	0
Multivitamins with minerals (Advanced Formula Centrum) Wyeth	1.67	0
Naproxen suspension (Naprosyn) 125 mg/5 mL; Roche	1.275	0.45
Naproxen Suspension 125 mg/5 ml Boehringer Ingelheim Roxane	1.28	0.4
Nitrofurantoin suspension (Furadantin) 25 mg/5 mL; Procter & Gamble	0	0.7
Nystatin suspension (Nilstat)	3	0
Oxybutynin syrup (Ditropan) 5 mg/5 mL; Marion Merrel Dow	4	1.3
Penicillin VK suspension 125 mg/5 mL; Teva	2.4	0
Phenobarbital elixir 20 mg/5 mL; Lilly	0.65	0
Phenytoin suspension (Dilantin) 125 mg/5 mL; Park Davis	1	0
Potassium chloride 30 mEq/15 mL; Fleming	0	0.54
Prednisolone oral liquid (Pediapred) 5 mg/5 mL; Calltech	0	1.53

Medication	*Sugar content (sucrose, corn syrup, lactulose, fructose, or glucose) gm/5 mL*	*Sorbitol content in gm/5 mL*
Prednisolone oral liquid (Prelone) Muro	1.84	0
Prednisone solution 5 mg/5 mL; Roxane	1.75	0
Prochorperazine syrup (Compazine) Smith Kline Beecham	3.15	0
Propranolol solution 20 mg/5 mL and 40 mg/5 mL; Roxane	0	3.2
Ranitidine syrup (Zantac) 15 mg/mL; Glaxo	0	0.5
Sodium polystyrene sulfonate suspension 15 gm/60 mL; Roxane	0	1.18
Sucralfate suspension (Carafate) 1 gm/10 mL; Axcan	0	0.7
Sulfamethoxazole/trimethoprim suspension Teva	0	0.35
Sulfamethoxazole/trimethoprim suspension (Septra) Monarch	0	2.25
Sulfamethoxazole/trimethoprim suspension (Bactrim) Roche	2.5	0.35
Theophylline liquid (Theoclear) 80 mg/15 mL; Central	0	4
Theophylline liquid (Theolair) 80 mg/15 mL; 3 M	2.5	0.48
Theophylline oral solution 80 mg/15 mL; Roxane	0	2.3
Triprolidine and Pseudoephedrine (Actifed) Liquid, Children's Warner-Lambert	2.6	2.5
Valproic acid syrup (Depakene) 250 mg/5 mL; Abbott	3	0.75
Vitamin E drops (Aquasol E) 15 IU/0.3 mL; Astra	0	1
Zidovudine syrup (Retrovir) 50 mg/5 mL; GlaxoSmithKline	3	0

Table B-3 Summary of drugs that cannot be crushed.

Type	*Description*
Enteric—coated	Designed to pass through the stomach intact. Drug is released in the intestines. Purpose of enteric coating: 1. prevent destruction of drug by stomach acids 2. prevent stomach irritation 3. delay onset of action
Extended-release	Designed to release drug over an extended period of time. Such products include: 1. multiple-layered tablets that release the drug as each layer is dissolved 2. mixed-release pellets that dissolve at different time intervals 3. special (inert) matrixes that contain and slowly release the active drug
Sublingual	Designed to dissolve quickly in oral fluids for rapid absorption by the abundant blood supply of the mouth.
Miscellaneous	Drugs that: 1. irritate the oral mucosa 2. are extremely bitter 3. contain dyes or substances that could stain teeth and mucosal tissue

Table B-4 Osmolality (mOsm/kg) of selected liquid preparations of drugs.

Drug (manufacturer)	*Concentration*	*mOsm/kg*
Acetaminophen elixir (Roxane)	65 mg/mL	5,400
Acetaminophen with codeine elixir (Wyeth)	acetaminophen 120 mg/5 ml codeine phosphate 12 mg/5 ml	4,700
Amantadine HCl solution (Dupont)	10 mg/mL	3,900
Aminophylline liquid (Fisons)	21 mg/mL	450
Amoxicillin suspension (Squibb)	50 mg/mL	2,250
Ampicillin suspension (Squibb)	50 mg/mL	2,250
Ampicillin suspension (Bristol)	100 mg/mL	1,850
Calcium glubionate syrup (Sandoz)	0.36 gm/mL	2,550
Cephalexin suspension (Dista)	50 mg/mL	1,950
Cephalexin suspension (Dista Products Company)	250 mg/5 mL	2,445
Cephalosporin suspension (Eli Lilly and Company)	250 mg/5 mL	2,430
Chloral hyrate syrup (Pharmaceutical Associates)	50 mg/mL	4,400
Cimetidine solution (Smith Kline & French)	60 mg/mL	5,550
Dexamethasone elixir (Organon)	0.1 mg/mL	3,350
Dexamethasone solution (Roxane)	1 mg/mL	3,100
Dicloxacillin suspension (Wyeth Laboratories)	62.5 mg/5 mL	2,980
Digoxin elixir (Burroughs Wellcome)	50 mcg/mL	1,350

Table B-4 Osmolality (mOsm/kg) of selected liquid preparations of drugs. *(continued)*

Drug (manufacturer)	*Concentration*	*mOsm/kg*
Diphenhydramine HCL elixir (Roxane)	2.5 mg/mL	850
Docusate sodium syrup (Pharmaceutical Associates)	3.3 mg/mL	4,700
Docusate sodium syrup (Roxane)	3.3 mg/mL	3,900
EES (Erythromycin) Oral Suspension suspension (Abbott Laboratories)	200 mg/5 mL	1,750
Furosemide oral solution (Hoechst-Roussel Pharmaceuticals, Inc)	10 mg/5 mL	2,050–3,938
Haloperidol concentrate (McNeil)	2 mg/mL	500
Hydroxyzine HCl syrup (Roerig)	2 mg/mL	4,450
Lactulose syrup (Roerig)	0.67 gm/mL	3,600
Lithium citrate syrup (Roxane)	1.6 mEq/mL	6,850
Magnesium citrate solution (Medalist)	1.75 g/30 mL	1,000
Methyldopa suspension (Merck Sharp & Dohme)	50 mg/mL	2,050
Neutra-phos oral solution (Willen)	16.7 mg phosphous/5 mL	250
Nystatin suspension (Squibb)	100,000 units/mL	3,300
Oxacillin oral solution (Bristol Laboratories)	250 mg/5 mL	2,420
Penicillin V suspension (Eli Lilly and Company)	250 mg/5 mL	2,995
Phenytoin suspension (Parke-Davis)	6 mg/mL	2,000
Phenytoin suspension (Parke-Davis)	25 mg/mL	1,500
Potassium chloride injection	2 mEq/mL	3,600

Drug (manufacturer)	*Concentration*	*mOsm/kg*
Potassium chloride liquid 10% (Adria)	20 mEq potassium/15 mL	3,000
Potassium chloride liquid 10% (Roxane)	20 mEq potassium/15 mL	3,300–4,350 (lot dependent)
Potassium phosphate injection	3 mM Phosphorus/mL	5,450
Primidone suspension (Ayerst)	50 mg/mL	450
Prochlorperazine syrup (Smith Kline & French)	1 mg/mL	3,250
Prostaphlin oral solution (Bristol Laboratories)	250 mg/5 mL	2,420
Sodium acetate injection	2 mEq/mL	3,980
Sodium bicarbonate injection	1 mEq/mL	1,730
Sodium chloride injection	4 mEq/mL	7,090
Sodium citrate liquid (Willen)	1 mEq sodium and 1 mEq bicarbonate/mL	2,050
Sodium phosphate injection	3 mM Phosphorus/mL	4,650
Sodium phosphate liquid (Fleet)	0.5 gm/mL	7,250
Spironolactone suspension (Searle & Co.)	25 mg/5 mL	2,245
Theophylline solution (Berlex)	5.33 mg/mL	800
Theophylline solution (Pharmaceutical Associates)	5.33 mg/mL	600
Trimethoprim 40 mg/5 mL Sulfamethoxazole 200 mg/5 mL (Bactrim) (Roche Laboratories)	Trimethoprim 40 mg/5 ml Sulfamethoxazole 200 mg/5 ml	4,560
Trimethoprim 40 mg/5 mL Sulfamethoxazole 200 mg/5 mL (Co-trimoxazole) (Burroughs-Wellcome)	Trimethoprim 40 mg/5 ml Sulfamethoxazole 200 mg/5 ml	2,200

Table B-5 Routes of delivery via feeding tube.

Medications recommended for administration via the gastric route only

Medication	*Comments*
Acetazolamide (Diamox Sequels)	Aspirate the liquid from the gelatin capsule for administration or dissolve the capsule in warm water to administer. Do not administer the undissolved outer gelatin capsule to avoid clogging the feeding tube.
Antacids: • Aluminum hydroxide gel • Aluminum carbonate • Aluminum hydroxide and magnesium trisilicate • Aluminum and magnesium hydroxide • Calcium carbonate • Calcium carbonate and magnesium hydroxide • Magnesium hydroxide • Magaldrate • Magnesium oxide • Sodium bicarbonate • Sodium citrate	Antacids neutralize gastric acidity, resulting in a pH increase of the stomach and duodenal bulb. They also inhibit the proteolytic activity of pepsin and have a local astringent effect. Antacids increase the lower esophageal sphincter tone.
Carbamazepine	Absorption via feeding tubes placed farther down in the GI tract may be unpredictable.
Cephalexin	The primary absorption site is the duodenum. Jejunal administration may be associated with inadequate plasma concentrations.
Cromolyn (Gastrocom)	A microencapsulated form that can be opened and the pellets inside poured down the feeding tube, then flushed with water.
Diltiazem (Cardiazem CD, Cardiazem SR)	A microencapsulated form that can be opened and the pellets inside poured down the feeding tube, then flushed with water.
Ferrous gluconate (Fergon)	A microencapsulated form that can be opened and the pellets inside poured down the feeding tube, then flushed with water.
Fluoxetine (Prozac)	A microencapsulated form that can be opened and the pellets inside poured down the feeding tube, then flushed with water.
Ketoconazole	There is inadequate absorption if administered into a feeding tube placed farther down in the gastrointestinal tract.

Medication	*Comments*
Pancreatic enzymes (Creon, Pancrease, Pancrease MT)	A microencapsulated form that can be opened and the pellets inside poured down the feeding tube, then flushed with water.
Phenytoin	Subtherapeutic levels and decreased response have been associated with jejunal administration immediately before or after feedings are stopped. Tube feedings should be stopped for 2 hours before and after phenytoin administration.
Sucralfate	The drug reacts with gastric acid in the stomach to form a condensed, viscous, adhesive, pastelike substance that buffers acid. It persists in this form as it moves to the alkaline environment of the proximal duodenum, where it adheres to the gastroduodenal mucosa, providing local protection of ulcers.
Valproic acid	Absorption via feeding tube placed farther down in the GI tract may be unpredictable.
Warfarin	Warfarin resistance could occur due to the vitamin K content of enteral formulas or secondary to malabsorption of warfarin. Tube feedings should be stopped for 2 hours before and after warfarin administration.

Table B-5 Routes of delivery via feeding tube. *(continued)*

Medications that may be administered via either the gastric or jejunal route.

Medication	*Comments*
Amoxicillin	Administer via JT only if absolutely necessary since the suspension is hyperosmolar
Ampicillin	Ampicillin is poorly absorbed via the jejunal route. Amoxicillin is more suitable
Calcium salts	Calcium Gluconate Injection is the preparation of choice for administration due to the hyperosmolarity of other liquid oral preparations.
Digoxin	May be associated with a decreased response via the jejunal route necessitating an increase in dosage
Furosemide	There may be decreased absorption via the jejunal route necessitating an increase in dosage
Lansoprazole	It is recommended that the capsules be swallowed. However, when no other option is available lansoprazole, which is acid labile, may be administered via the feeding tube. Open the capsule and mix the contents with 5–10 ml of sodium bicarbonate (1 mEq/ml). The pharmacy department may manufacture a lansoprazole suspension which is stable for 14 days at 24°C and for 30 days in the refrigerator. It may be administered via either route. Flush the tubing
Nifedipine • Adalat, Procardia 10 mg/0.34 ml 20 mg/0.45 ml • Generic Nifedipine UDL: 10 mg/0.34 ml Vangard, Purpac, and Goldline: 10 mg/0.38 ml Novopharm: 10 mg/0.4 ml	Aspirate the liquid from the soft gelatin capsule with a syringe to obtain the appropriate dose. Or, if the whole capsule's contents are to be administered dissolve the capsule in warm water. To avoid causing clogging of the FT do not put the undissoved gelatin down the tube. If administering nifedipine via JT monitor the BP closely. If there is no response attempt administration via GT if available

Medication	*Comments*
Omeprazole	It is recommended that the capsules be swallowed. However, when no other option is available omeparazole, which is acid labile, may be administered via FT. Open the capsule and dissolve the contents in 5–10 ml of sodium bicarbonate (1 mEq/ml). The pharmacy department may compound omeprazole solution that is stable for 14 days at 24°C and for 30 days in the refrigerator that may be administered via FT. Flush the tubing after medication administration
Oxprenolol	Uniform absorption throughout GI tract
Potassium Chloride	Note that some liquid oral products are incompatible with feeding formulations forming a viscous or gelatinous product that may clog a FT. Dilute to < 0.2 mEq/ml prior to administration.

Table B-5 Routes of delivery via feeding tube. *(continued)*

Medications that should not be administered via feeding tube.

Medication	*Comments*
Clarithromycin	Consists of irregularly shaped film-coated macro-granules suspended in a viscous liquid that may cause FT occlusion
Dimetapp Elixir	Causes breakdown of enteral feeding
Feosol Elixir	Gels completely if mixed with enteral feeding
Klorvess Syrup	Forms viscous gelatinous mass with feedings
MCT Oil	Forms adhesive gelatinous mass
NeoCalglucon Syrup	Forms adhesive gelatinous mass immedicately
Nifedipine	Extended release forms
Potassium Chloride effervescent tablets	Solution formed when added to liquid will coagulate when mixed with enteral products
Psyllium or methylcellulose	Administration requires mixing with up to 8 ounces of water per dose. If the resultant mixture is administered via FT it may cause occlusion due to expansion and congealing of the preparation
Renagel	Do not crush, chew, or break into pieces prior to taking, contents expand when mixed with water
Sudafed Syrup	Granular formation

Table B-6 Sodium content of selected injectable medications.

Medication	*mEq sodium/drug amount*
Acetazolamide	0.41 mEq/100 mg
Acyclovir	4.2 mEq/gm
Amikacin	1.3 mEq/gm
Ampicillin	2.9–3.1 mEq/gm
Ampicillin/sulbactam	5 mEq/gm of ampicillin component
Blood products	130–160 mEq/L
Cefazolin	2 mEq/gm
Cefoperazone	1.5 mEq/gm
Cefotaxime	2.2 mEq/gm
Cefotetan	3.5 mEq/gm
Cefoxitin	2.3 mEq/gm
Ceftazidime (Fortaz, Tazicef, Tazidime)	2.3 mEq/gm
Ceftizoxime	2.6 mEq/gm
Ceftriaxone	3.6 mEq/gm
Cefuroxime	2.4 mEq/gm
Chloramphenicol	2.3 mEq/gm
Cyclophosphamide	0.7 mEq/100 mg
Ganciclovir	4 mEq/gm
Hydrocortisone sodium succinate (Solu-Cortef)	2 mEq/gm
Imipenem - Cilastatin Sodium for injection/ suspension for injection	3.2 mEq/gm/2.8 mEq/gm imipenem
Meropenem (Merram)	3.92 mEq/gm
Methylprednisolone sodium succinate (Solu-Medrol)	2.01 mEq/gm
Metronidazole (Flagyl) IV	28 mEq/gm
Midazolam (Versed)	0.14 mEq/mL
Nafcillin	2.9 mEq/gm
Oxazolidinone	1.7 mEq/200 mg bag 3.3 mEq/400 mg bag 5 mEq/600 mg bag

Table B-6 Sodium content of selected injectable medications. *(continued)*

Medication	*mEq sodium/drug amount*
Penicillin G sodium	2 mEq/million units
Penicillin G potassium	0.3 mEq/million units and 1.7 mEq potassium/million units
Piperacillin	1.85 mEq/gm
Piperacillin/tazobactam	2.35 mEq/gm of piperacillin component
Sodium bicarbonate	12 mEq/gm
Ticarcillin	5.2–6.5 mEq/gm
Ticarcillin disodium/clavulanate K	4.75 mEq/gm

Table B-7 Drug-induced electrolyte abnormalities.

Drug	*Electrolyte change*	*Proposed mechanism*
Ace inhibitors (captopril, enalapril, lisinopril)	↑ K	Increase distal renal tubular K secretion due to inhibition of aldosterone biosynthesis.
Acetazolamide	↑ Cl, ↓ Phosphorus, ↓ K	Increased distal renal tubular K secretion.
Albuterol/terbutaline	↓ K	Intracellular shift via stimulation of Na-K ATPase pump; direct beta 2 receptor stimulation of insulin release from pancreas.
Aluminum-containing antacids	↓ Phosphorus	Phosphate binding within the gastrointestinal tract and increased fecal elimination.
Aminoglycosides (amikacin, gentamicin, tobramycin) associated with large doses and prolonged therapy	↓ Mg, ↓ Ca, ↓ K	Defect of Mg conversion by the distal nephron.
Aminophylline, theophylline	↓ K	Increased distal renal tubule secretion.
Amphetamines	↑ K	Cellular shift due to rhabdomyolysis.
Amphotericin B	↓ K, ↓ Mg Note: Liposomal amphotericin B (Ambisome) contains Phosphorusphorus salt and may be associated with ↑ Phosphorus and ↓ Ca	Nephrotoxicity due to azotemia, renal tubular acidosis, and nephrocalcinosis.
Ampicillin (high dose)	↓ K	Increased distal renal tubule secretion.
Arginine	↑ K	Intracellular leak.
Biphosphonates (pamidronate, alendronate, clondronate)	↓ Ca, ↓ Phosphorus	Decrease bone resorption of Ca by inhibiting osteoclast recruitment and activity and shortening the life span of osteoclasts.
Blood products	↓ Ca	Transient complexation with citrated blood.

Table B-7 Drug-induced electrolyte abnormalities. *(continued)*

Drug	*Electrolyte change*	*Proposed mechanism*
Busulfan	↓ K, ↓Ca, ↓ Phosphorus, ↓ Mg	
Calcitonin	↓ Ca, ↓ Phosphorus	Increased renal excretion and increased skeletal uptake.
Calcium salts/antacids	↑ Ca	Excessive intake.
Carbamazepine	↓ Na	SIADH.
Cholestyramine	↑ Na, ↑ Cl, ↓ Ca	Na content; osmotic diuresis.
Cimetidine	↓ Ca	Impairs parathyroid function.
Cisplatin	↓ Mg, ↓ Ca, ↓ K ↓ Na, ↓ Phosphorus	Renal tubular dysfunction with persistent renal Mg leak.
Corticosteroids	↑ Na, ↓ K, ↓ Ca, ↓ Phosphorus	Decreased intestinal absorption of Ca with increased urinary excretion and decreased bone absorption; increased mobilization of K from tissue leading to Na K exchange and K excretion.
Cyclophosphamide	↑ K, ↓ Na	Tumor lysis; SIADH.
Cyclosporine	↑ K, ↓ Mg	Renal tubular excretion.
Digoxin	↑ K associated with toxicity	Inhibition of Na-K ATPase.
Epinephrine	↓ Phosphorus ↓ K	Intracellular K shift.
Fat emulsion	↓ Na	Pseudohyponatremia with lipemic serum sample.
Foscarnet	↓ Ca, ↓ or ↑ Phosphorus, ↓ Mg, ↓ K	Acute tubular necrosis.
Fosphenytoin	↑ Phosphorus, ↓ Ca	Provides exogenous phosphorus.
Glucagon	↓ Ca, ↓ Phosphorus	Increased intestinal Ca absorption; increased bone resorption, and increased renal tubular reabsorption.
Glucose	↓ K, ↓ Phosphorus	Intracellular leak due to increased insulin secretion.

Drug	*Electrolyte change*	*Proposed mechanism*
Heparin	↓ Ca	Pseudohypocalcemia.
Ibuprofen	↓ Na	SIADH.
Ifosfamide	↓ K	Irreversible Fanconi's anemia causing kaliuresis.
Indomethacin	↑ K (only with prolonged treatment)	Anabolic shift of K intracellularly.
Insulin	↓ Mg, ↓ Phosphorus, ↓ K	Intracellular shift.
Iron dextran (high dose)	↓ Ca	Transient. Remains decreased for approximately 4 hours after infusion.
Itraconazole (chronic, high dose)	↓ K	
Lactulose	↑ Na	Fecal water loss in excess of Na resulting in contraction of ECF volume.
Laxatives	↑ Na	Dehydration.
Lithium	↑ Na ↑ Ca ↓ K	Suppression of action of ADH, increased renal water loss; decreased urinary Ca excretion; distal renal tubular acidosis.
Loop diuretics (bumetanide, furosemide, torsemide)	↓ K, ↓ Mg, ↓ Cl, ↑ HCO_3, ↓ Ca	Cl reabsorption is blocked; increased renal excretion; increased distal renal tubular K shift.
Medium chain triglycerides	↑ Ca, ↓ Na, ↓ K	Fecal water, Na, and K excretion in patients with steatorrhea. Might increase Ca absorption.
Mineralocorticoids	↑ K, ↓ Na	K retention; Na wasting due to adrenal insufficiency.
Nafcillin	↓ K	Dose related increase in urinary excretion.
Osmotic diuretics (mannitol, urea)	↓ Ca, ↑ Na or ↓ Na, ↑ K or ↓ K	Osmotic extracellular water shift; increased distal renal tubular K secretion.

Table B-7 Drug-induced electrolyte abnormalities. *(continued)*

Drug	*Electrolyte change*	*Proposed mechanism*
Penicillin G sodium	↑ Na, ↓ K	Increased distal renal tubular secretion.
Phenobarbital	↑K ↓ Ca	Alters vitamin D metabolism due to enzyme induction; abuse may lead to cellular shift due to rhabdomyolysis.
Phenytoin	↓ Ca	Alters vitamin D metabolism due to enzyme induction.
Potassium-sparing diuretics (spironolactone, triamterene, amiloride)	↑ K, ↑ Mg	Aldosterone antagonism; decreased distal renal tubule secretion.
Rifampin	↓ Ca, ↓ Phosphorus	Secondary to decreased 25 and 1,25-vitamin D_3.
Rituximab	↑ K, ↑ Phosphorus	Tumor lysis syndrome.
Saline laxatives (sodium phosphate solution)	↑ Na, ↓ K, ↑ Phosphorus, ↓ Ca,	Due to phosphorus load.
Saquinavir	↑ K	
Sevelamer	↓ Phosphorus, ↑ Ca	Phosphate binder.
Sodium bicarbonate (citrate, acetate, and lactate)	↑ Na ↓ Phosphorus ↓ K	Na content; increased renal excretion and increased cellular uptake; intracellular K distribution due to alkalosis.
Sodium ferric gluconate	↑ K	
Sodium polystyrene sulfonate	↓ K, ↑ Na	Cation exchange resin, increases fecal K elimination.
Succinylcholine	↑ K (transient)	Intracellular shift.
Tacrolimus	↑ K, ↓ Mg	Hyporenin-aldosterone status.
Ticarcillin	↓K	Increased distal renal tubule K secretion.
Trimethoprim	↑ K	Inhibits Na channel in renal distal tubule leading to decreased urinary excretion.

Drug	*Electrolyte change*	*Proposed mechanism*
Thiazide diuretics	↓ Mg, ↓ K, ↓ Phosphorus, ↑ Ca, ↓ Cl	Increased excretion of K, Mg, and phosphorus caused by excess ADH activity; vitamin D hydroxylation is inhibited and Ca excretion is decreased due to direct effect on renal tubule; chloride is decreased due to blocking of reabsorption.
Thyroid replacement	↑ Ca	Increased bone reabsorption.
Vinblastine	↑ K	Tumor lysis syndrome.
Vincristine	↑ K	Tumor lysis syndrome.
Vitamin A	↑ Ca	Only if chronic ingestion of ≥ 50,000 units/day in adults.
Vitamin D (excess)	↑ Ca	Increased renal tubular reabsorption, decreased plasma concentration of 25-OH vitamin D_3 and cholecalciferol, and increased metabolism to inactive metabolite.

SIADH = syndrome of inappropriate antidiuretic hormone; ATP = adenosine triphosphate; ECF = extracellular fluid; ADH = antidiuretic hormone.

Table B-8 Drug-induced acidosis or alkalosis.

Medication	*Mechanism*
Metabolic acidosis	
Acetazolamide	Decreases reabsorption of bicarbonate in the proximal tubule.
Amiloride	Decreases renal H^+ secretion.
Ammonium chloride	Chloride salt.
Amphotericin B	Renal tubular acidosis.
Ampicillin	Diarrheal bicarbonate loss.
Arginine	Hydrochloride salt.
Cholestyramine (prolonged use)	Increased intestinal bicarbonate loss.
Cimetidine	Inhibiton of gastric acid secretion, blunting tendency to metabolic alkalosis.
Clindamycin	Diarrheal bicarbonate loss.
Colchicine	Diarrheal bicarbonate loss.
Cyclosporine	Hyperchloremia secondary decreased bicarbonate.
Famotidine	Inhibition of gastric acid secretion, blunting tendency to metabolic alkalosis.
Foscarnet	Causes hyperchloremia
Ifosphamide	Aminoaciduria.
Propofol	Prolonged use, high doses.
Ranitidine	Inhibition of gastric acid secretion, blunting tendency to metabolic alkalosis.
Saline laxatives	Increased intestinal bicarbonate loss.
Sodium nitroprusside	Lactic acidosis secondary to cyanide toxicity.
Spironolactone	Decreased renal H^+ secretion.
Triamterene	Decreased renal H^+ secretion.

Medication	*Mechanism*
Metabolic alkalosis	
Acetate salts	Metabolized to bicarbonate via extrahepatic metabolism.
Ampicillin	Increase H^+ secretion.
Antacids	Excess pH increase.
Blood products (contain citrate)	Citrate is a bicarbonate precursor.
Bumetanide	Increased renal H^+ secretion.
Calcium gluconate	Gluconate is a bicarbonate precursor.
Chlorothiazide	Increased renal H^+ secretion.
Corticosteroids	Increased H^+ secretion, increased bicarbonate reabsorption.
Furosemide	Increased H^+ secretion.
Hydrochlorthiazide	Increased H^+ secretion.
Ketoralac	Precursor to bicarbonate.
Lactate salts	Metabolized to bicarbonate by the liver.
Sodium bicarbonate	Provides bicarbonate.
Ticarcillin	Increased renal H^+ secretion.
Tromethamine	Bicarbonate precursor.

Table B-9 Medications affecting trace element and vitamin status.

Medication	*Change in level*	*Proposed mechanism*
Aluminum containing phosphate binder	↓ iron	Decreases iron absorption when taken concurrently.
Aminoglycosides	↓ cyanocobalamin	Decreases absorption.
Aminopterin	↓ folic acid	Inhibits conversion of folate to tetrahydrofolate by blocking dihydrofolate reductase.
Antacids	↓ cyanocobalamin ↓ iron ↓ thiamine	Administered concurrently results in instability due to alkaline environment.
Antibiotics (broad spectrum)	↓ vitamin K	Decreases synthesis by altering gut flora.
Ascorbic acid	↑ iron	Increased absorption from gastrointestinal tract.
Aspirin	↓ iron	Chronic intake may lead to intestinal bleeding, antiplatelet effect.
Bicarbonate	↓ iron	Decreases absorption.
Chloramphenicol	↓ cyanocobalamin ↓ iron	Suppresses activity of ferro-chelatase involved in hemoglobin synthesis; antagonizes hematopoietic response.
Cholestyramine/colestipol	↓ iron ↓ vitamin A, ↓ vitamin D, ↓ vitamin K, ↓ folic acid ↓ cyanocobalamin	Binds heme and inorganic iron-blocking absorption; adsorbs bile salts, causing steatorrhea and decreased absorption; prevents formation of cyanocobalamin.
Cimetidine (chronic)	↓ cyanocobalamin	Decreases absorption.

Medication	*Change in level*	*Proposed mechanism*
Cisplatin	↓ copper, ↓ zinc	Induces renal tubular dysfunction.
Colchicine	↓ cyanocobalamin	Decreases absorption by causing histological changes in intestinal mucosa.
Coumadin	↓ iron	May lead to gastrointestinal hemorrhage.
Cyclosporine	↓ vitamin D	Impaired vitamin D activation.
D-penicillamine	↓ copper, ↓ zinc ↓ pyridoxine	Chelates copper and zinc that are then excreted; competes with pyridoxal coenzymes, decreasing activity.
Digoxin	↓ thiamine	
Famotidine (chronic)	↓ cyanocobalamin	Decreases absorption.
5-fluorouracil	↓ niacin	Blocks intracellular synthesis of NAD and NADP.
Furosemide	↓ ascorbic acid	Increased urinary excretion.
Glucorticoids	↓ vitamin D	Interferes with hepatic metabolism of 25-hydroxy cholecalciferol.
Heparin	↓ iron	May lead to GI hemorrhage.
Hydralazine	↓ pyridoxine	Increases excretion.
Iron	↑ ascorbic acid	Increases absorption.
Isoniazid	↓ folic acid ↓ iron ↓ niacin ↓ pyridoxine	Impairs uptake of iron into protoporphyrin; increases excretion due to impaired hormonal metabolism; inhibits conversion of tryptophan to niacin.

Table B-9 Medications affecting trace element and vitamin status. *(continued)*

Medication	*Change in level*	*Proposed mechanism*
Magnesium-containing antacids	↓ riboflavin	Decreases absorption.
6-mercaptopurine	↓ niacin ↓ pantothenic acid	Blocks intracellular synthesis of NAD and NADP; inhibits coenzyme A synthesis.
Methotrexate	↓ folic acid	Inhibits conversion of folate to tetrahydrofolate by blocking dihydrofolate reductase.
Metoclopramide	↓ riboflavin	Decreases absorption by causing peristalsis to increase.
Mineral oil (chronic use)	↓ vitamin A ↓ vitamin D ↓ vitamin E ↓ vitamin K	Impairs micelle formation of bile salts, causing a physical barrier to absorption.
Neomycin	↓ vitamin A ↓ vitamin D	Decreases absorption due to inhibition of pancreatic lipase inactivating bile salts, causing mucosal damage in the small intestine.
Pentamidine	↓ folic acid	Inhibits formation.
Phenobarbital	↓ ascorbic acid ↓ cyanocobalamin ↓ folic acid ↓ vitamin D	Accelerates degradation; increases urinary excretion; interferes with intestinal absorption.
Phenytoin	↓ ascorbic acid ↓ cyanocobalamin ↓ folic acid ↓ vitamin D	Accelerates degradation; increases urinary excretion; interferes with intestinal absorption; inhibits hepatic metabolism.
Potassium	↓ cyanacobalamin	Inhibits absorption by decreasing the pH at the ileal lumen absorption site.

Medication	*Change in level*	*Proposed mechanism*
Primidone	↓ ascorbic acid ↓ cyanocobalamin ↓ folic acid ↓ vitamin D	Accelerates degradation; increases urinary excretion; interferes with intestinal absorption.
Propofol (Diprivan)	↓ zinc	Contains edetate disodium which chelates zinc; loss in pediatrics is approximately 1.5–2 mg/day.
Pyridoxine	Risk for ↓ phenytoin activity	Induces metabolism.
Pyrimethamine	↓ folic acid	Inhibits formation.
Ranitidine	↓ cyanocobalamine	With chronic therapy, decreases absorption.
Triamterene	↓ folic acid	Inhibits formation by blocking dihydrofolate reductase.
Triiodothyronine	↓ vitamin E	Reduction in serum lipid concentration
Trimethoprim	↓ folic acid	Inhibits formation.
Valproic acid	↓ carnitine	Increases urinary excretion.

Table B-10 Induction of hypoglycemia/hyperglycemia.

Drug	***Mechanism***
Hypoglycemia	
α-blockers (prazocin)	Increases insulin secretion.
Ace inhibitors	Usually in diabetic patients secondary increased bradykinin.
Acetaminophen	May cause toxicity to the liver, decreasing hepatic glucose production.
Alcohol	Depletes glycogen stores, inhibits gluconeogenesis, and increases insulin secretion.
β-2 agonists	Increases plasma insulin levels, increases C-peptide levels.
Nonselective β blockers (atenolol, esmolol, labetolol, propranol)	Blocks signs and symptoms of hypoglycemia, may potentiate insulin-induced hypoglycemia, dose dependent.
Octreotide	Decreases glucose absorption.
Pentamidine	Causes toxicity to β-cells, may induce hemorrhagic pancreatitis, may increase plasma insulin levels.
Salicylates overdose	Toxicity causes decreased insulin clearance, decreases hepatic glucose production, inhibits gluconeogenesis.
Theophylline	Augments insulin release.
Hyperglycemia	
Alcohol	Supresses insulin release, increases glycogenolysis, stimulates glucocorticoid release, and inhibits peripheral utilization of glucose.
β-adrenergic agonists (albuterol, terbutaline)	Increases β-cell stimulation, increases glycogenolysis.
Chlorpromazine	Large doses cause inhibition of insulin secretion.
Clonidine	Inhibits secretion of insulin by α-adrenergic stimulation.
Corticosteroids (most effects seen with hydrocortisone, prednisone, and prednisolone)	Stimulates gluconeogenesis, decreases peripheral glucose utilization, may cause insulin resistance, dose related.
Cyclosporine	Dose dependent toxicity to pancreatic β-cells.
L-asparginase	Inhibits insulin synthesis and may destroy pancreatic tissue.

Drug	*Mechanism*
Hyperglycemia	
Loop diuretics	Induce hypokalemia, may increase blood glucose.
Tacrolimus	Dose dependent islet cell damage.
Theophylline	Toxicity is associated with stimulation of catacholamines and decreased serum potassium with resultant hyperglycemia.
Thiazide diuretics	Causes increased insulin secretion secondary to hypokalemia.
Thyroid hormone	Increases glucose production, depletes pancreatic insulin reserves, and decreases secretory capacity of β-cells.

Appendix C

Steven Yannicelli and Kathryn Camp[1]

[1] The views expressed in this chapter are those of the authors and do not reflect the official policy of the Department of the Army, the Department of Defense, or the U.S. Government.

Table C-1. Metabolic medical foods for nutrition therapy of inherited metabolic diseases.

Indications	*Product*	*Company*	*Age Group*	*Description*
Glutaric aciduria Type I	XLys, XTrp Analog	Nutricia North America*	Infants	LYS- and TRP-free protein source, CHO, fat, vitamins and minerals
	Glutarex-1	Ross	Infants and toddlers	LYS- and TRP free protein source, CHO, fat, vitamins and minerals
	XLys, XTrp Maxamaid	Nutricia North America	Children 1–8 yrs	LYS- and TRP-free protein source, CHO, vitamins and minerals; no fat
	Glutarex-2	Ross	Children and adults	LYS- and TRP-free protein source, CHO, fat, vitamins and minerals
	XLys, XTrp, Maxamum	Nutricia North America	Individuals > 8 yrs	LYS- and TRP-free protein source, CHO, vitamins and minerals; no fat
	GA	Mead Johnson	Infants, children, adults	LYS- and TRP-free protein source, CHO, fat, vitamins and minerals
Isovaleric acidemia	XLEU Analog	Nutricia North America	Infants	LEU-free protein source, CHO, fat, vitamins and minerals
	I-Valex-1	Ross	Infants and toddlers	LEU-free protein source, CHO, fat, vitamins and minerals
	XLEU Maxamaid	Nutricia North America	Children 1–8 yrs	LEU-free protein source, CHO, vitamins and minerals; no fat
	I-Valex-2	Ross	Children and adults	LEU-free protein source, CHO, fat, vitamins and minerals
	LMD	Mead Johnson	Children and adults	LEU-free protein source, CHO, fat, vitamins and minerals
	XLEU Maxamum	Nutricia North America	Individuals > 8 yrs	LEU-free protein source, CHO, vitamins and minerals; no fat

Indications	*Product*	*Company*	*Age Group*	*Description*
Propionic and methylmalonic acidemia	OS-1	Milupa	Infants	ILE-, MET-, THR-, and VAL-free concentrated protein source, CHO, vitamins and minerals; no fat
	XMTVI Analog	Nutricia North America	Infants	MET-, THR-, and VAL-free, low ILE protein source, CHO, fat, vitamins and minerals
	OA 1	Mead Johnson	Infants and toddlers	ILE-, MET-, THR-, and VAL-free protein source, CHO, fat, vitamins and minerals
	Propimex-1	Ross	Infants and toddlers	ILE-, MET-, THR-, and VAL-free protein source, CHO, fat, vitamins and minerals
	XMTVI Maxamaid (orange)	Nutricia North America	Children 1–8 yrs	MET-, THR-, and VAL-free, low ILE protein source, CHO, vitamins and minerals; no fat
	OS-2	Milupa	Children	ILE-, MET-, THR-, and VAL-free concentrated protein source, CHO, vitamins and minerals; no fat
	Propimex-2	Ross	Children and adults	ILE-, MET-, THR-, and VAL-free protein source, CHO, fat, vitamins and minerals
	OA 2	Mead Johnson	Children and adults	ILE-, MET-, THR-, and VAL-free protein source, CHO, fat, vitamins and minerals
	XMTVI Maxamum (orange)	Nutricia North America	Individuals > 8 yrs	MET-, THR-, and VAL-free, low ILE protein source, CHO, vitamins and minerals, low fat

Table C-1. Metabolic medical foods for nutrition therapy of inherited metabolic diseases. *(continued)*

Indications	*Product*	*Company*	*Age Group*	*Description*
Hyper-methionemia and homocystinuria	HOM-1	Milupa	Infants	MET-free concentrated protein source, CHO, vitamins and minerals, no fat
	XMET Analog	Nutricia North America	Infants	MET-free protein source, CHO, fat, vitamins and minerals
	Hominex-1	Ross	Infants and toddlers	MET-free protein source, CHO, fat, vitamins and minerals
	HCY 1	Mead Johnson	Infants and toddlers	MET-free protein source, CHO, vitamins and minerals
	HOM-2	Milupa	Children	MET-free concentrated protein source, minimum CHO, vitamins and minerals; no fat
	HCY2 (vanilla)	Mead Johnson	Children and adults	MET-free protein source, CHO, fat, vitamins and minerals
	Hominex-2	Ross	Children and adults	MET-free protein source, CHO, fat, vitamins and minerals
	XMET Maxamaid	Nutricia North America	Children 1–8 yrs	MET-free protein source, CHO, vitamins and minerals; no fat
	HCU Gel	Vitaflo	Children 1–10 yrs	MET-free protein source, CHO, vitamins and minerals; no fat; low volume
	HCU Express	Vitaflo	Individuals > 8 yrs	MET-free protein source, CHO, vitamins and minerals; no fat; low volume
	XMET Maxamum (orange)	Nutricia North America	Individuals > 8 yrs	MET-free protein source, CHO, vitamins and minerals; no fat

Indications	*Product*	*Company*	*Age Group*	*Description*
Phenylketonuria (PKU)	Phenyl-Free 1 (vanilla)	Mead Johnson	Infants and toddlers	PHE-free protein source, CHO, fat, vitamins and minerals
	PKU-1	Milupa	Infants	PHE-free concentrated protein source, minimum CHO, vitamins and minerals; no fat
	XPhe Analog	Nutrica North America	Infants	PHE-free protein source, CHO, fat, vitamins and minerals
	Phenex-1	Ross	Infants and toddlers	PHE-free protein source, CHO, fat, vitamins and minerals
	XPhe Maxamaid (orange or unflavored)	Nutricia North America	Children 1–8 yrs	PHE-free protein source, CHO, vitamins and minerals; no fat
	Phenyl-Free 2 (vanilla)	Mead Johnson	Children and adults	PHE-free protein source, CHO, fat, vitamins and minerals
	Phenyl-Free 2HP (vanilla)	Mead Johnson	Children and adults	PHE-free concentrated protein source, CHO, vitamins and minerals; low fat
	PKU-2	Milupa	Children	PHE-free concentrated protein source, minimum CHO, vitamins and minerals; no fat
	PKU-3	Milupa	Adolescents, adults and pregnant women	PHE-free concentrated protein source, minimum CHO, vitamins and minerals; no fat
	Phenex-2 (vanillla or unflavored)	Ross	Children and adults	PHE-free protein source, CHO, fat, vitamins and minerals

Table C-1. Metabolic medical foods for nutrition therapy of inherited metabolic diseases. *(continued)*

Indications	*Product*	*Company*	*Age Group*	*Description*
Phenylketonuria (PKU)	PhenylAde (strawberry, orange crème, vanilla)	Applied Nutrition	Children and adults	PHE-free protein source, CHO, fat, vitamins and minerals
	PhenylAde40	Applied Nutrition	Children and adults	PHE-free concentrated protein source, CHO, vitamins and minerals; low fat
	XPhe Maxamum powder and Drink (orange, berry or unflavored)	Nutricia North America	Individuals > 8 yrs, pregnant women	PHE-free concentrated protein source, CHO, vitamins and minerals; no fat
	Lophlex	Nutricia North America	Individuals > 9 yrs, pregnant women	PHE-free protein source, vitamins and minerals; no CHO or fat, low volume
	Periflex (orange/ pineapple, chocolate or unflavored)	Nutricia North America	Individuals > 1 yr	PHE-free protein source, CHO, fat, vitamins and minerals
	PhenylAde Amino Acid Blend	Applied Nutrition	Individuals ≥ 1 yr	PHE-free protein source
	PhenylAde MTE Amino Acid Blend	Applied Nutrition	Individuals ≥ 1 yr	PHE-free protein source with minerals
	Phlexy-10 drink mix‡	Nutricia North America	Individuals ≥ 1 yr	PHE-free protein source, CHO, fat
	Phlexy-10 bar	Nutricia North America	Individuals ≥ 1 yr	PHE-free protein source, CHO, fat

Indications	*Product*	*Company*	*Age Group*	*Description*
Phenylketonuria (PKU) *(continued)*	Phlexy-10 capsules	Nutricia North America	Individuals ≥ 1 yr	PHE-free protein source
	Phlexy-10 tablets	Nutricia North America	Individuals ≥ 1 yr	PHE-free protein source
	Phlexy-Vits	Nutricia North America	Individuals > 11 yrs	Powdered supplement of vitamins and minerals for the Phlexy-10 system
	PKU Express powder and Cooler (flavored)	Vitaflo	Children > 8 yrs	PHE-free protein source, CHO, vitamins and minerals; no fat; low volume
	PKU Gel	Vitaflo	Children 1–10 yrs	PHE-free protein source, CHO, vitamins and minerals; no fat; low volume
	PhenylAde amino acid bar (chocolate or white chocolate)	Applied Nutrition	Individuals ≥ 1 yr	PHE-free protein source, CHO, fat
	PhenylAde amino acid bar (crispy chocolate)	Applied Nutrition	Individuals ≥ 1 yr	Low PHE protein source (0.008mg PHE per bar)
Tyrosinemia				
Type I & II	TYR-1	Milupa	Infants	PHE- and TYR-free concentrated protein source, CHO, vitamins and minerals; no fat
Type I	XPTM Analog	Nutricia North America	Infants	PHE-, TYR-, and MET-free protein source, fat, CHO, vitamins and minerals

Table C-1. Metabolic medical foods for nutrition therapy of inherited metabolic diseases. *(continued)*

Indications	*Product*	*Company*	*Age Group*	*Description*
Tyrosinemia *(continued)*				
Type I, II, or III	Tyrex-1	Ross	Infants and toddlers	PHE- and TYR-free protein source, fat, CHO, vitamins and minerals
Type I, II, or III	TYROS 1	Mead Johnson	Infants and toddlers	PHE- and TYR-free protein source, fat, CHO, vitamins and minerals
Type I & II	TYR-2	Milupa	Children	PHE- and TYR-free concentrated protein source, CHO, vitamins and minerals; no fat
Type I & II	XPhe, XTyr Maxamaid (orange)	Nutricia North America	Children 1–8 yrs	PHE- and TYR-free protein source, CHO, vitamins and minerals; no fat
Type I, II, or III	TYROS 2 (vanilla)	Mead Johnson	Children and adults	PHE- and TYR-free protein source, CHO, vitamins and minerals; low fat
Type I, II, or III	Tyrex-2	Ross	Children and adults	PHE- and TYR-free protein source, fat, CHO, vitamins and minerals
Type I, II, or III	TYR gel	Vitaflo	Children 1–10 yrs	TYR- and PHE-free protein source, CHO, vitamins and minerals; no fat; low volume
Type I, II, or III	TYR Express	Vitaflo	Children > 8 yrs	TYR and PHE-free protein source, CHO, vitamins and minerals; no fat; low volume
Maple syrup disease (MSUD)	MSUD 1	Milupa	Infants	VAL-, LEU-, and ILE-free concentrated protein source, CHO, vitamins and minerals; no fat
	MSUD Analog	Nutricia North America	Infants	VAL-, LEU-, and ILE-free protein source, CHO, fat, vitamins and minerals

Indications	*Product*	*Company*	*Age Group*	*Description*
Maple syrup disease (MSUD) *(continued)*	Ketonex-1	Ross	Infants and toddlers	VAL-, LEU-, and ILE-free protein source, CHO, fat, vitamins and minerals
	BCAD1	Mead Johnson	Infants and toddlers	VAL-, LEU-, and ILE-free protein source, CHO, fat, vitamins and minerals
	MSUD 2	Milupa	Children	VAL-, LEU-, and ILE-free concentrated protein source, CHO, vitamins and minerals; no fat
	MSUD Maxamaid (orange)	Nutricia North America	Children 1–8 yrs	VAL-, LEU-, and ILE-free protein source, CHO, vitamins and minerals; no fat
	BCAD 2 (vanilla)	Mead Johnson	Children and adults	VAL-, LEU-, and ILE-free protein source, CHO, fat, vitamins and minerals
	Ketonex-2	Ross	Children and adults	VAL-, LEU-, and ILE-free protein source, CHO, fat, vitamins and minerals
	MSUD gel	Vitaflo	Children 1–10 yrs	VAL-, LEU-, ILE-free protein source, CHO, vitamins and minerals; no fat; low volume
	MSUD Express	Vitaflo	Children > 8 yrs	VAL-, LEU-, ILE-free protein source, CHO, vitamins and minerals; no fat; low volume
	MSUD Maxamum (orange)	Nutricia North America	Individuals > 8 yrs	VAL-, LEU-, and ILE-free protein source, CHO, vitamins and minerals; no fat
	Complex MSUD (vanilla)	Applied Nutrition	Children and adults	VAL-, LEU-, and ILE-free protein source, CHO, fat, vitamins and minerals

Table C-1. Metabolic medical foods for nutrition therapy of inherited metabolic diseases. *(continued)*

Indications	*Product*	*Company*	*Age Group*	*Description*
Maple syrup disease (MSUD) *(continued)*	Acerflex (pineapple)	Nutricia North America	Individuals >1 yrs	VAL-, LEU-, and ILE-free protein source, CHO, fat, vitamins and minerals
	Complex MSUD amino acid bar (chocolate)	Applied Nutrition	Individuals >1 yrs	VAL-, LEU-, and ILE-free protein source, CHO, fat
	Complex MSUD amino acid blend	Applied Nutrition	Children and adults	VAL-, LEU-, and ILE-free protein source
Galactosemia	Isomil	Ross	Infants and children	Milk- and lactose-free powdered soy formula; complete
	Neocate Infant	Nutricia North America	Infants	Galactose- and lactose-free amino acid-based powdered infant formula; complete
	Isomil 2	Ross	Infants 6–18 mos	Milk- and lactose-free powdered soy formula; complete
	Neocate One+	Nutricia North America	Children > 1 yrs	Galactose- and lactose-free amino acid based powdered formula; complete
	EleCare	Ross	Infants, children, and adults	Galactose- and lactose-free amino acid-based powdered formula; complete
	Enfamil Prosobee	Mead Johnson	Infants	Milk- and lactose-free powdered soy formula; complete
	Enfamil Nutramigen	Mead Johnson	Infants	Lactose-free, sucrose-free casein hydrolysate, complete

Indications	*Product*	*Company*	*Age Group*	*Description*
Urea cycle disorders	UCD-1	Milupa	Infants	Nonessential amino acid-free protein source, CHO, vitamin and minerals; no fat
	Cyclinex-1	Ross	Infants and toddlers	Nonessential amino acid-free protein source, CHO, fat, vitamin and minerals
	WND 1	Mead Johnson	Infants and toddlers	Nonessential amino acid-free protein source, CHO, fat, vitamin and minerals
	UCD-2	Milupa	Children	Nonessential amino acid-free protein source, CHO, vitamin and minerals; no fat
	Cyclinex-2	Ross	Children and adults	Nonessential amino acid-free protein source, CHO, fat, vitamin and minerals
	WND-2	Mead Johnson	Children and adults	Nonessential amino acid-free protein source, CHO, fat, vitamin and minerals
	Essential Amino Acid Module	Nutricia North America	Individuals > 1 yr	Essential amino acid powder

LYS = lysine; TRP = tryptophan; CHO = carbohydrate; LEU = leucine; ILE = isoleucine; MET = methionine; THR = threonine; VAL = valine; PHE = phenylalanine

*Name changed from *SHS North America* to *Nutricia North America* as of March, 2006.

MEDICAL FOOD COMPANY REFERENCES

Applied Nutrition Corp.
10 Saddle Road
Cedar Knolls, NJ 07927
1-973-734-0023
1-800-605-0410
http://www.medicalfood.com/

Milupa, North America
22513 Gateway Center Drive
Clarksburg, MD 20871
1-877-2MILUPA (1-877-264-5872)
http://www.milupana.com/

Mead Johnson Nutritionals
2400 West Lloyd Expressway
Evansville, IN 47721
1-812-429-6399
http://www.meadjohnson.com/

Ross Products Division/Abbott Laboratories
PO Box 1317
Columbus, OH 43216
1-800-986-8755
http://www.ross.com/

Nutricia North America (formerly Scientific Hospital Supplies, North America)
PO Box 117
Gaithersburg, MD 20884
1-800-356-7354
http://www.shsna.com/

Vitaflo USA
123 East Neck Road
Huntington, NY 11743
1-888-848-2356
1-631-547-5984
http://www.vitaflousa.com

PRODUCT RESOURCE GUIDE

Amino Acids

Package sizes were obtained from either the company's web site or telephone customer services. Contact the company directly for updated information.

Fisher Scientific
1-800-766-7000
https://www1.fishersci.com
Available in 100-g containers

JoMar Laboratories
583-B Division Street
Campbell, CA 95008
1-408-374-5920
1-800-538-4545
http://www.jomarlabs.com
Available in 150-g and 1-kg containers

Scandinavian Formulas
1-215-453-2507
http://www.scandinavianformulas.com
Available in 1-kg containers

Spectrum Chemicals and Laboratory Products
7400 N. Oracle Road
Tuscon, AZ 85704
1-800-791-3210
http://www.spectrumchemical.com
Available in 25-g, 100-g, and 1-kg containers

Vitaflo USA
123 East Neck Road
Huntington, NY 11734
1-631-547-5984
1-888-848-2356
http://www.vitaflousa.com
Isoleucine and valine available in 50-mg individual packets

Biotin (oral use only)

Mericon Industries, Inc.
8819 North Pioneer Road
Peoria, IL 61615
1-309-693-2150
1-800-242-6464
http://www.mericon-industries.com

Betaine (Cystadane)

Jazz Pharmaceuticals, Inc.
13911 Ridgedale Drive
Minnetonka, MN 55305
1-888-867-7426
http://www.orphan.com

Carnitine

Sigma Tau Pharmaceuticals, Inc.
800 South Frederick Avenue, Suite 300
Gaithersburg, MD 20877
1-301-948-1041
1-800-447-0169
http://www.sigmatau.com

MCT Oil (Fractionated Coconut Oil)

Novartis Medical Nutrition
Consumer & Product Support
445 State Street
Fremont, MI 49412
1-800-333-3785

NTBC (Orfadin)

Rare Diseases Therapeutics, Inc.
1101 Kermit Drive, Suite 608
Nashville, TN 37217
1-615-399-0700
http://www.raretx.com

Parenteral Amino Acid Solutions

Coram Health Care
Clinical Operations Department
1675 Broadway, Suite 900
Denver, CO 80202
1-303-672-8802
1-800-CORAMHC
http://www.coramhc.com

CoEnzyme Q10

Vitaline CoQ10 with vitamin E. Comes in the following doses:
CoQ10, 100 mg with 300 IU vitamin E
CoQ10, 200 mg with 400 IU vitamin E

α-Lipoic Acid (Thioctic acid)

Standard available dosages are 50- and 100-mg capsules. It is available from health food stores and other stores that carry quality vitamins and supplements.

Note: For dietary supplements it is recommended to only use those supplements manufactured as USP (United States Pharmacopoeia) grade. Not all supplements are equal in quality, so it is recommended to use a known brand. For questions, contact the Council for Responsible Nutrition, Washington DC, http://www.crnusa.org/.

SUGGESTED READING AND RESOURCES FOR NUTRITION IN PATIENTS WITH METABOLIC DISEASES

Books

Acosta PB, Yannicelli S. *Nutrition Support Protocols.* 4th ed. Columbus, Ohio: Ross Products Division; 2001.

Clarke JTR. *A Clinical Guide to Inherited Metabolic Diseases.* 2nd ed. Cambridge: University Press; 2002.

Scriver CR, Beaudet AL, Sly WS, Valle D, eds. *The Metabolic and Molecular Bases of Inherited Disease.* 8th ed. New York: McGraw-Hill; 2001.

Zschocke J, Hoffmann GF. *Vademecum Metabolicum Manual of Metabolic Paediatrics.* 2nd ed. Friedrichsdorf, Germany: Milupa Schattauer; 2004.

Journal Articles

Morton DH, Strauss KA, Robinson DL, Puffenberger EG, Kelley RI. Diagnosis and treatment of maple syrup urine disease: a study of 36 patients. *Pediatrics.* 2002;109:900–1008.

Nyhan WL, Rice-Kelts M, Klein J, Barshop BA. Treatment of the acute crisis in maple syrup urine disease. *Arch Pediatr Adolesc Med.* 1998;152:593–598.

Ogier de Baulny H. Management and emergency treatments of neonates with a suspicion of inborn errors of metabolism. *Semin Neonatol.* 2002;7:17–26.

Ogier de Baulny H, Benoist JF, Rigal O, Touati G, Rabier D, Saudubray JM. Methylmalonic and propionic acidaemias: management and outcome. *J Inherit Metab Dis.* 2005;28:415–423.

Prietsch V, Lindner M, Zschocke J, Nyhan WL, Hoffmann GF. Emergency management of inherited metabolic diseases. *J Inherit Metab Dis.* 2002;25:531–546.

Saudubray JM, Nassogne MC, le Lonlay P, Touati G. Clinical approach to inherited metabolic disorders in neonates: an overview. *Semin Neonatol.* 2002;7:3–15.

Summar, M. Current strategies for the management of neonatal urea cycle disorders. *J Pediatrics.* 2001;138(1): S30–S39.

Web Sites

National Newborn Screening and Genetics Resource Center
http://genes-r-us.uthscsa.edu/

New England Consortium of Metabolic Programs
http://web1.tch.harvard.edu/newenglandconsortium/

Index

A

E

G

H

I

N

O

P

Q

R

S

T

U

X

Y

Z